Update on General Medicine

Section 1
2009–2010

(Last major revision 2006–2007)

BASIC AND CLINICAL SCIENCE COURSE

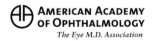

LIFELONG
EDUCATION FOR THE
OPHTHALMOLOGIST

The Basic and Clinical Science Course is one component of the Lifelong Education for the Ophthalmologist (LEO) framework, which assists members in planning their continuing medical education. LEO includes an array of clinical education products that members may select to form individualized, self-directed learning plans for updating their clinical knowledge. Active members or fellows who use LEO components may accumulate sufficient CME credits to earn the LEO Award. Contact the Academy's Clinical Education Division for further information on LEO.

The American Academy of Ophthalmology is accredited by the Accreditation Council for Continuing Medical Education to provide continuing medical education for physicians.

The American Academy of Ophthalmology designates this educational activity for a maximum of 30 *AMA PRA Category 1 Credits*™. Physicians should only claim credit commensurate with the extent of their participation in the activity.

The Academy provides this material for educational purposes only. It is not intended to represent the only or best method or procedure in every case, nor to replace a physician's own judgment or give specific advice for case management. Including all indications, contraindications, side effects, and alternative agents for each drug or treatment is beyond the scope of this material. All information and recommendations should be verified, prior to use, with current information included in the manufacturers' package inserts or other independent sources, and considered in light of the patient's condition and history. Reference to certain drugs, instruments, and other products in this course is made for illustrative purposes only and is not intended to constitute an endorsement of such. Some material may include information on applications that are not considered community standard, that reflect indications not included in approved FDA labeling, or that are approved for use only in restricted research settings. **The FDA has stated that it is the responsibility of the physician to determine the FDA status of each drug or device he or she wishes to use, and to use them with appropriate, informed patient consent in compliance with applicable law.** The Academy specifically disclaims any and all liability for injury or other damages of any kind, from negligence or otherwise, for any and all claims that may arise from the use of any recommendations or other information contained herein.

Copyright © 2009
American Academy of Ophthalmology
All rights reserved
Printed in Singapore

Basic and Clinical Science Course

Gregory L. Skuta, MD, Oklahoma City, Oklahoma, *Senior Secretary for Clinical Education*
Louis B. Cantor, MD, Indianapolis, Indiana, *Secretary for Ophthalmic Knowledge*
Jayne S. Weiss, Detroit, Michigan, *BCSC Course Chair*

Section 1

Faculty Responsible for This Edition

Eric P. Purdy, MD, *Chair*, Fort Wayne, Indiana
James P. Bolling, MD, Jacksonville, Florida
Roger Kaldawy, MD, Franklin, Massachusetts
Rohit Varma, MD, MPH, Los Angeles, California
Jonathan Walker, MD, Fort Wayne, Indiana
Harold E. Shaw, Jr, MD, Greenville, South Carolina
  Practicing Ophthalmologists Advisory Committee for Education
Anne Louise Coleman, MD, PhD, *Consultant*, Los Angeles, California
Gwen Sterns, MD, *Consultant*, Rochester, New York

Dr. Coleman states that she has an affiliation with Allergan, Inc.

The other authors state that they have no significant financial interest or other relationship with the manufacturer of any commercial product discussed in the chapters that they contributed to this course or with the manufacturer of any competing commercial product.

Recent Past Faculty

Emily Y. Chew, MD
Bernard F. Godley, MD, PhD
Patrick S. O'Connor, MD
Michael J. Spedick, MD

Glenn L. Stoller, MD
William G. Tsiaras, MD
Daniel T. Weaver, MD

In addition, the Academy gratefully acknowledges the contributions of numerous past faculty and advisory committee members who have played an important role in the development of previous editions of the Basic and Clinical Science Course.

American Academy of Ophthalmology Staff
    Richard A. Zorab, *Vice President, Ophthalmic Knowledge*
    Hal Straus, *Director, Publications Department*
    Carol L. Dondrea, *Publications Manager*
    Christine Arturo, *Acquisitions Manager*
    D. Jean Ray, *Production Manager*
    Stephanie Tanaka, *Medical Editor*
    Steven Huebner, *Administrative Coordinator*

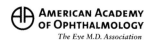

655 Beach Street
Box 7424
San Francisco, CA 94120-7424

Contents

General Introduction xiii
Objectives 1

1 **Infectious Disease** 3
   Recent Developments 3
   General Microbiology 3
   Staphylococcus 5
   Streptococcus 6
   Clostridium difficile 8
   Haemophilus influenzae 10
   Neisseria 12
   Pseudomonas aeruginosa 14
   Treponema pallidum 15
      Stages 16
      Diagnosis 16
      Management 17
   Borrelia burgdorferi 18
      Stages 19
      Diagnosis 19
      Management 20
   Chlamydia trachomatis 21
   Mycoplasma pneumoniae 22
   Mycobacteria 23
      Tuberculosis 23
   Fungal Infections 25
   Toxoplasma 26
   Herpesvirus 27
      Herpes Simplex 27
      Varicella-Zoster 28
      Cytomegalovirus 29
      Epstein-Barr Virus 30
   Influenza 30
   Hepatitis 31
      Hepatitis A 31
      Hepatitis B 31
      Hepatitis C and Other Forms of Hepatitis 31
   Human Papillomavirus 33
   Severe Acute Respiratory Syndrome 33
   Acquired Immunodeficiency Syndrome 36
      Etiology and Pathogenesis 36
      Clinical Syndromes 37
      Seroepidemiology 39

    Modes of Transmission 39
    Prognosis and Treatment. 40
    Opportunistic Infections 45
    Ophthalmologic Considerations. 51
Update on Antibiotics 53
    Antibacterial Agents. 54
    Tetracyclines 72
    Miscellaneous Antibacterial Agents 73
    New Antibiotic Classes. 74
    Antifungal Agents. 75
    Antiviral Agents 76
    Treatment of Hospital-Acquired Infections 77

2 Hypertension 81
Recent Developments 81
Introduction 81
Classification of Blood Pressure and Diagnosis of Hypertension. 82
Etiology and Pathogenesis of Hypertension. 82
Evaluation of Hypertension 84
Treatment of Hypertension. 84
    Lifestyle Modifications. 85
    Pharmacologic Treatment 86
Antihypertensive Drugs 87
    Diuretics. 87
    Beta-Blockers. 92
    Angiotensin-Converting Enzyme Inhibitors 92
    Angiotensin II Receptor Blockers 93
    Calcium Channel Blockers 93
    α_1-Blockers. 93
    Combined α-Adrenergic and β-Adrenergic Antagonists 93
    Centrally Acting Adrenergic Agents 93
    Direct Vasodilators 94
    Parenteral Antihypertensive Drugs 94
Special Considerations 94
    Ischemic Heart Disease 94
    Heart Failure 95
    Diabetes and Hypertension. 95
    Chronic Renal Disease 95
    Cerebrovascular Disease 95
    Obesity and the Metabolic Syndrome 95
    Sleep Disorders 95
    Left Ventricular Hypertrophy 95
    Peripheral Arterial Disease 96
    Orthostatic Hypotension. 96
    Hypertension in Older Patients 96
    Women and Pregnancy 96
    Children and Adolescents 97
    Minority Populations 97

Withdrawal Syndromes 97
Hypertensive Crisis 98
Ophthalmic Considerations 98

3 Cerebrovascular Disease 101
Recent Developments 101
Introduction 101
Cerebral Ischemia 101
Diagnosis and Management 103
Diagnostic Studies 103
Treatment 104
Intracranial Hemorrhage 105
Carotid Artery Disease 107

4 Acquired Heart Disease 111
Recent Developments 111
Ischemic Heart Disease 111
Pathophysiology 112
Risk Factors for Coronary Artery Disease 112
Clinical Syndromes 113
Noninvasive Cardiac Diagnostic Procedures 116
Invasive Cardiac Diagnostic Procedures 119
Management of Ischemic Heart Disease 120
Congestive Heart Failure 125
Symptoms 126
Clinical Signs 126
Diagnostic Evaluation 127
Epidemiology 127
Etiology 128
Pathophysiology and Clinical Course 128
Medical and Nonsurgical Management 129
Invasive or Surgical Management 132
Disorders of Cardiac Rhythm 132
Bradyarrhythmias and Conduction Disturbances 133
Premature Contractions 135
Tachyarrhythmias 136
Ophthalmologic Considerations 141
Amiodarone 141
Beta-Blockers 141
Digoxin 142
Angiotensin-Converting Enzyme Inhibitors 142

5 Hypercholesterolemia 143
Recent Developments 143
Introduction 143
Risk Assessment 144
Management 145

Special Issues. 148
    Use of Statins in Acute Myocardial Syndromes 148
    The Metabolic Syndrome. 148
    Comments on Specific Dyslipidemias 150
Ophthalmologic Considerations 150

6 Pulmonary Diseases 153
Recent Developments 153
Introduction 153
Obstructive Lung Diseases 153
Restrictive Lung Diseases 154
Evaluation 155
Treatment 155
    Nonpharmacologic Approaches 155
    Pharmacologic Therapy 156
Preoperative and Postoperative Considerations 158

7 Hematologic Disorders 159
Recent Developments 159
Ophthalmologic Considerations 159
Blood Composition 159
Erythropoiesis 160
Anemia 160
    Iron Deficiency Anemia 161
    Anemia of Chronic Disease 161
    The Thalassemias 161
    Sideroblastic Anemia 162
    Vitamin B_{12} Deficiency. 162
    Folic Acid Deficiency 162
    Hemolytic Anemias 162
Disorders of Hemostasis 163
    Laboratory Evaluation of Hemostasis and Blood Coagulation 165
    Clinical Manifestations of Hemostatic Abnormalities 166
    Vascular Disorders 166
    Platelet Disorders 166
    Disorders of Blood Coagulation 168
    Primary Hypercoagulable States 170
    Secondary Hypercoagulable States 171

8 Rheumatic Disorders 173
Recent Developments 173
Introduction 173
Rheumatoid Arthritis 173
    Therapy 174
Spondyloarthropathies 175
    Ankylosing Spondylitis 175
    Reactive Arthritis 176
    Other Spondyloarthropathies 177

    Juvenile Idiopathic Arthritis 178
Systemic Lupus Erythematosus 179
    Diagnosis 180
    Ophthalmic Considerations 182
Antiphospholipid Antibody Syndrome. 182
    Diagnosis 183
    Ophthalmic Considerations 184
    Treatment 184
Scleroderma 185
    Ophthalmic Considerations 186
Sjögren Syndrome 186
Polymyositis and Dermatomyositis 186
Relapsing Polychondritis. 187
Vasculitis 188
    Large Vessel Vasculitis 188
    Medium-sized Vessel Vasculitis 191
    Small Vessel Vasculitis 192
Behçet Syndrome 193
    Treatment 193
    Ophthalmic Considerations 194
Medical Therapy for Rheumatic Disorders 194
    Corticosteroids 194
    Nonsteroidal Anti-inflammatory Drugs 196
    Methotrexate 198
    Hydroxychloroquine. 198
    Sulfasalazine 199
    Gold Salts 199
    Anticytokine Therapy and Other Immunosuppressive Agents 199

9 Endocrine Disorders 201
Recent Developments 201
Diabetes Mellitus 201
    Basics of Glucose Metabolism. 202
    Definition 202
    Classification 203
    Clinical Presentation of Diabetes 206
    Diagnosis and Screening 207
    Prevention of Diabetes 207
    Management 207
    The Importance of Glucose Control 214
    Glucose Surveillance. 215
    Acute Complications of Diabetes 216
    Long-Term Complications of Diabetes 216
    Ophthalmologic Considerations. 218
    Surgical Considerations in Diabetes 220
Thyroid Disease 221
    Physiology 221
    Testing for Thyroid Disease. 222

  Hyperthyroidism 223
  Hypothyroidism 225
  Thyroiditis 226
  Thyroid Tumors 227
 The Hypothalamic-Pituitary Axis 227
  Pituitary Adenomas 228
  Pituitary Apoplexy 229
 Multiple Endocrine Neoplasia Syndromes 230

10 Geriatrics 233
 Physiologic Aging and Pathologic Findings of the Aging Eye 235
 Pharmacology 235
 Outpatient Visits 236
 Elder Abuse 236
 Surgical Considerations 237
 Psychology of Aging 238
  Normal Aging Changes 238
  Psychopathology 239
  Treatment 240
  Ophthalmologic Considerations 240
 Osteoporosis 240
  Bone Physiology 241
  Risk Factors 241
  Clinical Features 242
  Diagnostic Evaluation 242
  Who Should Be Tested? 243
  Clinical Evaluation 244
  Treatment 244
  Osteoporosis in Men 246
 Falls 247
 Systemic Diseases 247

11 Cancer 251
 Recent Developments 251
 Incidence 251
 Etiology 252
  Carcinogenic Factors 252
 Therapy 255
  Radiation 255
  Chemotherapy 256
 Ophthalmic Considerations 262

12 Behavioral and Neurologic Disorders 263
 Recent Developments 263
 Introduction 263
 Behavioral Disorders 264
  Mental Disorders Due to a General Medical Condition 264
  Schizophrenia 264

Mood Disorders 265
Somatoform Disorders. 266
Substance Abuse Disorders 267
Pharmacologic Treatment of Psychiatric Disorders 271
Antipsychotic Drugs. 271
Antianxiety and Hypnotic Drugs 273
Ophthalmologic Considerations. 277
Neurologic Disorders 278
Parkinson Disease. 278
Multiple Sclerosis 280
Epilepsy 280
Stroke 284
Pain Syndromes. 284
Alzheimer Disease and Dementia 284

13 Preventive Medicine 291
Recent Developments 291
Screening Procedures 291
Cardiovascular Diseases 292
Cancer. 294
Metabolic Diseases 300
Infectious Diseases 301
Immunization 302
Hepatitis B 303
Influenza. 305
Varicella-Zoster. 306
Measles 306
Mumps 306
Rubella 306
Polio 307
Tetanus and Diphtheria 307
Pneumococcal Pneumonia 308
Haemophilus influenzae 308
Meningococcus. 309
Travel Immunizations 309
New and Future Vaccines. 310

14 Medical Emergencies 313
Recent Developments 313
Introduction 313
Cardiopulmonary Arrest. 313
Shock 317
Classification 317
Assessment. 318
Treatment 318
Anaphylaxis 319
Seizures and Status Epilepticus 320
Toxic Reactions to Local Anesthetics and Other Agents 321
Ocular Side Effects of Systemic Medications 323

15 Perioperative Management in Ocular Surgery ... 327
Preoperative Assessment ... 327
    Adult Patients ... 327
    Pediatric Patients ... 328
    Specific Preoperative Concerns ... 329
    Preoperative Fasting ... 331
    Management of Medications ... 331
    Preoperative Sedation ... 335
Intraoperative Complications ... 335
    Adverse Reactions to Local Anesthesia ... 335
    Malignant Hyperthermia ... 336
Postoperative Care ... 337

16 Using Statistics in Practice and Work ... 339
Obtaining Useful Information From Published Studies ... 339
    Participants and Setting ... 341
    Sample Size Determination ... 342
    Issues Related to Intervention ... 342
    Issues Related to Outcome ... 342
    Validity ... 343
    Clinical Relevance Issues ... 344
Clinical Study Designs ... 345
    Case Reports ... 345
    Case Series ... 346
    Case-Control Studies ... 347
    Cross-sectional Studies ... 349
    Cohort Studies ... 350
    Clinical Trials ... 351
    Systematic Reviews and Meta-analyses of Clinical Trials ... 352
Interpreting Diagnostic or Screening Tests ... 353
    The Straightforward Case ... 353
    Complicating Features ... 355
    Summary ... 360
Discussing Benefits, Risks, Probabilities, and Expected Outcomes
    With Patients ... 360
Applying Statistics to Measure and Improve Clinical Practice ... 362
    Issues in Designing a Measurement System ... 363
    Implementing a Monitoring System ... 364
    Analyzing the Results ... 366
    Methods of Data Presentation to Facilitate Continuous
        Improvement of Practices ... 368
    Other Features of Continuous Quality Improvement ... 370
    Summary ... 370

Basic Texts ... 373
Credit Reporting Form ... 375
Study Questions ... 379
Answers ... 389
Index ... 395

General Introduction

The Basic and Clinical Science Course (BCSC) is designed to meet the needs of residents and practitioners for a comprehensive yet concise curriculum of the field of ophthalmology. The BCSC has developed from its original brief outline format, which relied heavily on outside readings, to a more convenient and educationally useful self-contained text. The Academy updates and revises the course annually, with the goals of integrating the basic science and clinical practice of ophthalmology and of keeping ophthalmologists current with new developments in the various subspecialties.

The BCSC incorporates the effort and expertise of more than 80 ophthalmologists, organized into 13 Section faculties, working with Academy editorial staff. In addition, the course continues to benefit from many lasting contributions made by the faculties of previous editions. Members of the Academy's Practicing Ophthalmologists Advisory Committee for Education serve on each faculty and, as a group, review every volume before and after major revisions.

Organization of the Course

The Basic and Clinical Science Course comprises 13 volumes, incorporating fundamental ophthalmic knowledge, subspecialty areas, and special topics:

1. Update on General Medicine
2. Fundamentals and Principles of Ophthalmology
3. Clinical Optics
4. Ophthalmic Pathology and Intraocular Tumors
5. Neuro-Ophthalmology
6. Pediatric Ophthalmology and Strabismus
7. Orbit, Eyelids, and Lacrimal System
8. External Disease and Cornea
9. Intraocular Inflammation and Uveitis
10. Glaucoma
11. Lens and Cataract
12. Retina and Vitreous
13. Refractive Surgery

In addition, a comprehensive Master Index allows the reader to easily locate subjects throughout the entire series.

References

Readers who wish to explore specific topics in greater detail may consult the references cited within each chapter and listed in the Basic Texts section at the back of the book.

These references are intended to be selective rather than exhaustive, chosen by the BCSC faculty as being important, current, and readily available to residents and practitioners.

Related Academy educational materials are also listed in the appropriate sections. They include books, online and audiovisual materials, self-assessment programs, clinical modules, and interactive programs.

Study Questions and CME Credit

Each volume of the BCSC is designed as an independent study activity for ophthalmology residents and practitioners. The learning objectives for this volume are given on page 1. The text, illustrations, and references provide the information necessary to achieve the objectives; the study questions allow readers to test their understanding of the material and their mastery of the objectives. Physicians who wish to claim CME credit for this educational activity may do so by mail, by fax, or online. The necessary forms and instructions are given at the end of the book.

Conclusion

The Basic and Clinical Science Course has expanded greatly over the years, with the addition of much new text and numerous illustrations. Recent editions have sought to place a greater emphasis on clinical applicability while maintaining a solid foundation in basic science. As with any educational program, it reflects the experience of its authors. As its faculties change and as medicine progresses, new viewpoints are always emerging on controversial subjects and techniques. Not all alternate approaches can be included in this series; as with any educational endeavor, the learner should seek additional sources, including such carefully balanced opinions as the Academy's Preferred Practice Patterns.

The BCSC faculty and staff are continuously striving to improve the educational usefulness of the course; you, the reader, can contribute to this ongoing process. If you have any suggestions or questions about the series, please do not hesitate to contact the faculty or the editors.

The authors, editors, and reviewers hope that your study of the BCSC will be of lasting value and that each Section will serve as a practical resource for quality patient care.

Objectives

Upon completion of BCSC Section 1, the reader should be able to

- describe the ophthalmic manifestations of the major systemic diseases covered in this volume

- summarize the most common human pathogens and their manifestations

- discuss the epidemiology, clinical findings, and treatment of HIV infection

- review the newer antiviral, antifungal, and antibacterial agents and their benefits

- classify levels of hypertension by blood pressure measurements

- list the major classes of antihypertensive medications and some of their characteristics and side effects

- describe the various diagnostic procedures used in the evaluation of patients with coronary artery disease

- review the current treatment options for atrial fibrillation, atrial flutter, and ventricular tachycardia

- discuss the indications for dietary and pharmacologic treatment of hypercholesterolemia

- distinguish between obstructive and restrictive, reversible and irreversible, pulmonary diseases, and give examples of each type

- describe the classification, pathophysiology, presentation, and diagnostic criteria for diabetes mellitus

- review the various therapeutic approaches for diabetes mellitus, including new insulins and oral agents

- list the most prevalent types of cancer for men and for women together with the appropriate screening methods for detecting them

- review current concepts about the etiologies of most malignancies
- describe traditional as well as more novel approaches to the treatment of cancers
- summarize the major behavioral disorders and possible therapeutic modalities for these conditions (including the ocular side effects of psychoactive medications)
- list some of the factors associated with a patient's compliance or noncompliance with medical regimens
- explain the rationale for and value of screening programs for various systemic diseases
- summarize the major disease processes affecting most of the adult population, and briefly explain how preventive measures may reduce the morbidity and mortality they cause
- assess medical literature more critically in regard to appropriate study design and validity of conclusions
- explain the importance of the randomized, controlled clinical study in evaluating the effects of new treatments

---

CHAPTER 1

Infectious Disease

Recent Developments

- Vancomycin-resistant strains of enterococci and staphylococci have emerged in recent years as a cause of life-threatening infection in hospitalized patients.
- DNA probes using polymerase chain reaction (PCR) provide new, more sensitive diagnostic tools for the detection of gonorrhea, syphilis, Lyme disease, and infections caused by *Chlamydia,* mycobacteria, fungi, and many viruses.
- Newer nucleoside analogues and protease inhibitors provide potent drug combinations that are improving survival in HIV-infected patients.
- The incidence of cytomegalovirus (CMV) retinitis in HIV-infected patients has decreased significantly in the era of highly active antiretroviral therapy (HAART).
- Newer antibiotics, such as meropenem, cefepime, linezolid, quinupristin/dalfopristin, evernimicin, telithromycin, daptomycin, grepafloxacin, and teicoplanin, provide expanded antimicrobial coverage and offer treatment options for multidrug-resistant infections.
- Real-time PCR assays for detecting specific mutations for antibiotic resistance offer guidance in selecting more precise antimicrobial therapy.

General Microbiology

Despite formidable immune and mechanical defense systems, the human body harbors an extensive, well-adapted population of microorganisms on the skin and in the gastrointestinal, vaginal, and upper respiratory tracts. The organisms maintain their foothold on these epithelial surfaces chiefly by adherence, and they indirectly benefit the host by excluding pathogenic bacterial colonization and by priming the immune system. If antimicrobial agents alter this host–microbe interplay by eliminating the normal flora, the host's susceptibility to normally excluded pathogenic microorganisms is increased. When the mechanical defenses of the epithelial layers are breached so as to expose normally sterile areas, or if a critical component of the immune system that usually prevents microbial invasion fails, severe infections can result from the normal microbial flora.

However, even when both the mechanical and immune defense systems are intact, pathogenic microbes can cause infections by means of specific virulent characteristics that allow the microbes to invade and multiply. These virulent traits vary among different species.

Following are several mechanisms of virulence:

- *Attachment.* Neisseria gonorrhoeae and Neisseria meningitidis breach epithelial barriers by adhering to host epithelial cell surface receptors by means of a ligand on the bacteria's pili. Presence of the cell surface receptors is genetically determined.
- *Polysaccharide encapsulation.* Streptococcus pneumoniae, N meningitidis, Haemophilus, and Bacteroides evade phagocytosis in the absence of antibody and complement because of their polysaccharide coating.
- *Blocking of lysosomal fusion.* Intracellular existence, as well as protection from humoral immune mechanisms, is a characteristic of Chlamydia, Toxoplasma, Legionella, and Mycobacterium.
- *Antigenic surface variation.* Antigenic shifts in the cell wall of Borrelia recurrentis incapacitate the humoral immune system, which has a lag time in antibody production. Similar antigenic shifts are found in Chlamydia and influenza viruses.
- *IgA protease.* Haemophilus influenzae, N gonorrhoeae, and N meningitidis eliminate the IgA antibody normally found on mucosal surfaces, which would otherwise prevent the microbes' adherence.
- *Endotoxin.* A normal constituent of the gram-negative bacterial cell wall, endotoxin produces dramatic systemic physiologic responses ranging from fever and leukocyte margination to disseminated intravascular coagulation and septic shock.
- *Exotoxin.* Exotoxins are a diverse set of proteins with specific actions on target tissues that can cause severe systemic effects in such diseases as cholera or tetanus.
- *Biofilm formation.* Staphylococci have the ability to develop biofilms on various biomaterials, such as catheters and prosthetic heart valves.
- *Multiple mechanisms.* Some organisms, such as coagulase-positive Staphylococcus aureus, may possess multiple mechanisms of virulence. Also, it appears that nearly any S aureus genotype carried by humans can transform into a life-threatening pathogen, but certain clones are more virulent than others.

The immune system, which makes possible the host's adaptive response to colonization and infection, is classically divided into the humoral and cellular immune systems. The *humoral immune system,* composed of cells derived from the B lymphocyte series, is responsible for antibody-mediated opsonization, complement-mediated bacterial killing, antitoxin, and mediation of intracellular infections. The *cellular immune system,* determined by the T lymphocytes, is responsible for interaction with and stimulation of the humoral immune system, direct cytotoxicity, release of chemical messengers, and control of chronic infections. The successful interplay between the humoral and cellular immune systems mitigates and usually eradicates the infection, allowing for repair and healing. See also Part I, Immunology, in BCSC Section 9, *Intraocular Inflammation and Uveitis.*

Ando E, Monden K, Mitsuhata R, et al. Biofilm formation among methicillin-resistant *Staphylococcus aureus* isolates from patients with urinary tract infection. Acta Med Okayama. 2004;58:207–214.

Melles DC, Gorkink RF, Boelens HA, et al. Natural population dynamics and expansion of pathogenic clones of *Staphylococcus aureus.* J Clin Invest. 2004;114:1732–1740.

Staphylococcus

Staphylococcus aureus colonizes the anterior nares and other skin sites in 15% of community isolates. Of the tertiary-care hospital isolates, 25% are resistant to all β-lactam antibiotics. Transmission of organisms is usually by direct contact. Resistance of organisms to antimicrobials is usually plasmid determined and varies by institution. The increasing prevalence of methicillin-resistant *S aureus* (MRSA) in tertiary referral hospitals appears to be related to the population of high-risk patients at such centers. The natural history of staphylococcal infections indicates that immunity is of short duration and incomplete. Delayed hypersensitivity reactions to staphylococcal products may be responsible for chronic staphylococcal disease.

Conditions caused by staphylococcal infections include stye, furuncle, acne, bullous impetigo, paronychia, osteomyelitis, septic arthritis, deep-tissue abscesses, bacteremia, endocarditis, enterocolitis, pneumonia, wound infections, scalded skin syndrome, toxic shock syndrome, and food poisoning.

Acute serious staphylococcal infections require immediate intravenous antibiotic therapy. A penicillinase-resistant penicillin or first-generation cephalosporin is normally used, pending the results of susceptibility tests. With the emergence of methicillin-resistant staphylococci, vancomycin has become the drug of choice in the treatment of life-threatening infections, pending susceptibility studies. The increasing emergence of vancomycin-resistant enterococci (VRE) has led to concern about cases of vancomycin-resistant *S aureus* (VRSA) infection, mediated through plasmid transfer.

In fact, since 1997, infections due to strains of *S aureus* with reduced susceptibility to vancomycin (glycopeptide-intermediate *S aureus*) have been identified, with increasing frequency, in the United States, Japan, and Europe. Many of the cases occurred after prolonged inpatient treatment with intravenous vancomycin. Some reported cases have been successfully treated with various forms of combination therapy, including rifampin and trimethoprim-sulfamethoxazole; vancomycin, gentamicin, and rifampin; and vancomycin and nafcillin. Other agents with activity against vancomycin-intermediate *S aureus* (VISA) are ampicillin-sulbactam (Unasyn) and some newer antibiotics: trovafloxacin (Trovan), daptomycin (Cubicin), evernimicin (Ziracin), linezolid (Zyvox), and quinupristin/dalfopristin (Synercid). In July 2002, the first case of true VRSA was reported, and many additional cases have been described since then. Exposure to vancomycin-intermediate and vancomycin-resistant isolates of *S aureus* has been shown to increase the organism's resistance to vancomycin and other new agents, such as teicoplanin. Most VISA and nearly all VRSA isolates reported to date have arisen from endemic MRSA and, in the case of VRSA, have acquired genes from VRE. Accordingly, the emergence of VISA and VRSA provides strong motivation for the containment of MRSA and VRE transmission.

Staphylococcus epidermidis is an almost universal inhabitant of the skin, present in up to 90% of skin cultures. It can cause infection when local defenses are compromised. Its characteristic adherence to prosthetic devices makes it the most common cause of prosthetic heart valve infections, and it is a common infectious organism of intravenous catheters and cerebrospinal fluid shunts.

Most isolates are resistant to methicillin and cephalosporin; therefore, the drug of choice is vancomycin, occasionally in combination with rifampin or gentamicin. Unfortunately, there have also been recent reports of vancomycin-resistant infections caused by coagulase-negative staphylococcus. In one recent report, the standard disk diffusion antibiotic sensitivity method was unable to detect these isolates with decreased susceptibility to vancomycin. In addition to antibiotic therapy, management usually involves removal of the infected prosthetic device or vascular catheter.

> Bozdogan B, Ednie L, Credito K, et al. Derivatives of a vancomycin-resistant *Staphylococcus aureus* strain isolated at Hershey Medical Center. *Antimicrob Agents Chemother*. 2004;48(12):4762–4765.
>
> Centers for Disease Control and Prevention (CDC). Vancomycin-resistant *Staphylococcus aureus*—Pennsylvania, 2002. *MMWR Morb Mortal Wkly Rep*. 2002;51:902.
>
> Foster TJ. The *Staphylococcus aureus* "superbug." *J Clin Invest*. 2004;114:1693–1696.
>
> Smith TL, Pearson ML, Wilcox KR, et al. Emergence of vancomycin resistance in *Staphylococcus aureus*. Glycopeptide-Intermediate *Staphylococcus aureus* Working Group. *N Engl J Med*. 1999;340:493–501.
>
> Srinivasan A, Dick JD, Perl TM. Vancomycin resistance in staphylococci. *Clin Microbiol Rev*. 2002;15:430–438.
>
> Tiemersma EW, Bronzwaer SL, Lyytikainen O, et al. Methicillin-resistant *Staphylococcus aureus* in Europe, 1999–2002. *Emerg Infect Dis*. 2004;10:1627–1634.

Streptococcus

Group A β-hemolytic streptococci *(Streptococcus pyogenes)* cause a variety of acute suppurative infections through droplet transmission. The infection is modulated by an opsonizing antibody, which provides a type-specific immunity that lasts for years and is directed against the protein in the cell wall pili. Suppurative streptococcal infections in humans include pharyngitis, impetigo, pneumonia, erysipelas, wound and burn infections, puerperal infections, and scarlet fever. Genetically mediated humoral and cellular responses to certain strains of group A streptococci play a role in the development of the postinfectious syndromes of glomerulonephritis and rheumatic fever, both of which represent delayed, nonsuppurative, noninfectious complications of group A streptococcal infections. Rapid identification with antigen detection tests allows prompt treatment of patients with pharyngitis due to group A β-hemolytic streptococcus and can reduce the risk of spread of infection, enable patients to return to school or work sooner, and possibly reduce the risk of acute morbidity.

Streptococcus pyogenes remains highly susceptible to penicillin G; however, in the presence of allergy, erythromycin or (if no cross-allergy exists) cephalosporin is substituted. In recent years, macrolide-resistant and clindamycin-resistant strains of group A β-hemolytic streptococci have been reported. Antibiotic prophylaxis against recurrent rheumatic fever is administered for procedures that may result in transient bacteremia. However, such prophylaxis may not prevent acute glomerulonephritis.

Streptococcus pneumoniae organisms are lancet-shaped diplococci that cause α-hemolysis on blood agar. Although 10%–30% of the normal population carry 1 or more serologic types of pneumococci in the throat, the incidence and mortality of pneumococcal pneumonia increase sharply after age 50, with a fatality rate approaching 25%. Pneumococcal virulence is determined by its complex polysaccharide capsule, of which there are more than 80 distinct serotypes. The polysaccharide capsule inhibits macrophage engulfment of the organism. Infection is modulated by the development of anticapsular antibodies after 5–7 days; these antibodies allow phagocytosis of the organism by polymorphonuclear leukocytes.

Conditions caused by *S pneumoniae* include pneumonia, sinusitis, meningitis, otitis media, and peritonitis. Pneumococci are usually highly susceptible to penicillin, other β-lactams, erythromycin, or the newer fluoroquinolones. Routine susceptibility testing should be performed on patients with meningitis, bacteremia, or other life-threatening infections. Penicillin-resistant strains of *S pneumoniae* have been reported with increasing frequency in recent years. In several regions of the world, more than 25% of isolates are penicillin resistant; many of these are also resistant to cephalosporins and macrolides. Multidrug resistance was present in 19% of isolates in one recent study. Treatment of highly resistant strains may require vancomycin or meropenem. Prophylaxis is available through use of the 23-valent vaccine (see Chapter 13, Preventive Medicine).

α-Hemolytic streptococci and staphylococci cause the majority of cases of subacute bacterial endocarditis (55% and 30% of cases, respectively). Other pathogens that cause subacute bacterial endocarditis (SBE) include *Enterococcus, Haemophilus,* and fungi. Patients with prosthetic cardiac valves and those with most congenital or acquired cardiac structural or valvular defects should receive prophylaxis for SBE whenever they undergo invasive procedures involving the oral, nasopharyngeal, respiratory, gastrointestinal, or genitourinary regions. Prophylaxis for SBE is usually not considered necessary for routine ocular surgery in an uninfected patient but should be provided for surgery involving the nasolacrimal drainage system or sinuses or for surgical repair of orbital trauma (Tables 1-1 through 1-4).

Blanco-Carrion A. Bacterial endocarditis prophylaxis. *Med Oral Patol Oral Cir Bucal.* 2004;9 suppl:44–51; 37–43.

Cabell CH, Abrutyn E, Karchmer AW. Cardiology patient page. Bacterial endocarditis: the disease, treatment, and prevention. *Circulation.* 2003;107:185–187.

Dajani AS, Taubert KA, Wilson W, et al. Prevention of bacterial endocarditis. Recommendations by the American Heart Association. *JAMA.* 1997;277:1794–1801.

Gerber MA, Shulman ST. Rapid diagnosis of pharyngitis caused by group A streptococci. *Clin Microbiol Rev.* 2004;17:571–580.

Hasenbein ME, Warner JE, Lambert KG, et al. Detection of multiple macrolide- and lincosamide-resistant strains of *Streptococcus pyogenes* from patients in the Boston area. *J Clin Microbiol.* 2004;42(4):1559–1563.

Jacobs MR. *Streptococcus pneumoniae:* epidemiology and patterns of resistance. *Am J Med.* 2004;117 suppl 3A:3S–15S.

Shulman ST. Acute streptococcal pharyngitis in pediatric medicine: current issues in diagnosis and management. *Paediatr Drugs.* 2003;5 suppl 1:13–23.

Tan TQ. Antibiotic resistant infections due to *Streptococcus pneumoniae:* impact on therapeutic options and clinical outcome. *Curr Opin Infect Dis.* 2003;16:271–277.

Taubert KA, Dajani AS. Optimisation of the prevention and treatment of bacterial endocarditis. *Drugs Aging.* 2001;18(6):415–424.

Table 1-1 Cardiac Conditions Associated With Endocarditis

Endocarditis Prophylaxis Recommended

High-risk category
 Prosthetic cardiac valves, including bioprosthetic and homograft valves
 Previous bacterial endocarditis
 Complex cyanotic congenital heart disease (eg, single ventricle states, transposition of the great arteries, tetralogy of Fallot)
 Surgically constructed systemic pulmonary shunts or conduits

Moderate-risk category
 Most other congenital cardiac malformations (other than above and below)
 Acquired valvar dysfunction (eg, rheumatic heart disease)
 Hypertrophic cardiomyopathy
 Mitral valve prolapse with valvar regurgitation and/or thickened leaflets

Endocarditis Prophylaxis Not Recommended

Negligible-risk category (no greater risk than the general population)
 Isolated secundum atrial septal defect
 Surgical repair of atrial septal defect, ventricular septal defect, or patent ductus arteriosus (without residua beyond 6 mo)
 Previous coronary artery bypass graft surgery
 Mitral valve prolapse without valvar regurgitation
 Physiologic, functional, or innocent heart murmurs
 Previous Kawasaki disease without valvar dysfunction
 Previous rheumatic fever without valvar dysfunction
 Cardiac pacemakers (intravascular and epicardial) and implanted defibrillators

Reprinted from Dajani AS, Taubert KA, Wilson W, et al. Prevention of bacterial endocarditis. Recommendations by the American Heart Association. *JAMA*. 1997;277:1795. ©American Medical Association.

Clostridium difficile

Clostridium difficile is an endemic anaerobic gram-positive bacillus that is part of the normal gastrointestinal flora. It has acquired importance because of its role in the development of pseudomembranous enterocolitis following the use of antibiotics. Typically, within 1–14 days of starting antibiotic therapy, patients develop fever and diarrhea. The diarrhea occasionally becomes bloody and typically contains a cytopathic toxin that is elaborated by *C difficile*.

At present, a tissue-culture assay for the toxin is the best diagnostic test. Newer enzyme immunoassay tests allow rapid detection, but these have lower sensitivity than the toxigenic tissue culture has. Also, PCR has been used to detect *C difficile* toxins A and B in fecal samples. The most frequently associated antibiotics include clindamycin, ampicillin, chloramphenicol, tetracycline, erythromycin, and the cephalosporins.

Initial treatment includes discontinuing the causative antibiotic and administering metronidazole or oral metronidazole for 10 days. Vancomycin is also effective, but its use should be limited to decrease the development of vancomycin-resistant organisms such as enterococci and staphylococci. It is also much more expensive than metronidazole. Vancomycin should be limited to those who cannot tolerate or have not responded to metronidazole, or to situations in which metronidazole use is contraindicated, such as during the first trimester of pregnancy. Fusidic acid was shown in 1 study to be as effective

Table 1-2 Surgical Procedures and Endocarditis Prophylaxis

Endocarditis Prophylaxis Recommended

Respiratory tract
- Tonsillectomy and/or adenoidectomy
- Surgical operations that involve respiratory mucosa
- Bronchoscopy with a rigid bronchoscope

Gastrointestinal tract*
- Sclerotherapy for esophageal varices
- Esophageal stricture dilation
- Endoscopic retrograde cholangiography with biliary obstruction
- Biliary tract surgery
- Surgical operations that involve intestinal mucosa

Genitourinary tract
- Prostatic surgery
- Cystoscopy
- Urethral dilation

Endocarditis Prophylaxis Not Recommended

Respiratory tract
- Endotracheal intubation
- Bronchoscopy with a flexible bronchoscope, with or without biopsy†
- Tympanostomy tube insertion

Gastrointestinal tract
- Transesophageal echocardiography†
- Endoscopy with or without gastrointestinal biopsy†

Genitourinary tract
- Vaginal hysterectomy†
- Vaginal delivery†
- Cesarean section
- In uninfected tissue:
  - Urethral catheterization
  - Uterine dilatation and curettage
  - Therapeutic abortion
  - Sterilization procedures
  - Insertion or removal of intrauterine devices

Other
- Cardiac catheterization, including balloon angioplasty
- Implanted cardiac pacemakers, implanted defibrillators, and coronary stents
- Incision or biopsy of surgically scrubbed skin
- Circumcision

*Prophylaxis is recommended for high-risk patients; optional for medium-risk patients.
†Prophylaxis is optional for high-risk patients.

Reprinted from Dajani AS, Taubert KA, Wilson W, et al. Prevention of bacterial endocarditis. Recommendations by the American Heart Association. *JAMA*. 1997;277:1797. ©American Medical Association.

as metronidazole in the treatment of *C difficile* infection. Rifampin, intravenous immunoglobulin, and a new toxin-binding polymer have all been evaluated as potential alternative therapies, and trials are in progress with a new toxoid vaccine. Corticosteroids have been proven to reduce the diarrhea associated with *C difficile* infection.

> Belanger SD, Boissinot M, Clairoux N, et al. Rapid detection of *Clostridium difficile* in feces by real-time PCR. *J Clin Microbiol*. 2003;41:730–734.

Table 1-3 Prophylactic Regimens for Dental, Oral, Respiratory Tract, or Esophageal Procedures

Situation	Agent	Regimen*
Standard general prophylaxis	Amoxicillin	Adults: 2.0 g; children: 50 mg/kg orally 1 h before procedure
Unable to take oral medications	Ampicillin	Adults: 2.0 g intramuscularly (IM) or intravenously (IV); children: 50 mg/kg IM or IV within 30 min before procedure
Allergic to penicillin	Clindamycin *or*	Adults: 600 mg; children: 20 mg/kg orally 1 h before procedure
	Cephalexin† or cefadroxil† *or*	Adults: 2.0 g; children: 50 mg/kg orally 1 h before procedure
	Azithromycin or clarithromycin	Adults: 500 mg; children: 15 mg/kg orally 1 h before procedure
Allergic to penicillin and unable to take oral medications	Clindamycin *or*	Adults: 600 mg; children: 20 mg/kg IV within 30 min before procedure
	Cefazolin†	Adults: 1.0 g; children: 25 mg/kg IM or IV within 30 min before procedure

*Total children's dose should not exceed adult dose.
†Cephalosporins should not be used in individuals with immediate-type hypersensitivity reaction (urticaria, angioedema, or anaphylaxis) to penicillins.

Reprinted from Dajani AS, Taubert KA, Wilson W, et al. Prevention of bacterial endocarditis. Recommendations by the American Heart Association. *JAMA*. 1997;277:1798. ©American Medical Association.

Cavagnaro C, Berezin S, Medow MS. Corticosteroid treatment of severe, non-responsive *Clostridium difficile*–induced colitis. *Arch Dis Child*. 2003;88:342–344.

Nomura K, Matsumoto Y, Yoshida N, et al. Successful treatment with rifampin for fulminant antibiotics-associated colitis in a patient with non-Hodgkin's lymphoma. *World J Gastroenterol*. 2004;10:765–766.

Oldfield EC 3rd. *Clostridium difficile*–associated diarrhea: risk factors, diagnostic methods, and treatment. *Rev Gastroenterol Disord*. 2004;4:186–195.

Stoddart B, Wilcox MH. *Clostridium difficile*. *Curr Opin Infect Dis*. 2002;15:513–518.

Wilcox MH. Descriptive study of intravenous immunoglobulin for the treatment of recurrent *Clostridium difficile* diarrhoea. *J Antimicrob Chemother*. 2004;53:882–884.

Wullt M, Odenholt I. A double-blind randomized controlled trial of fusidic acid and metronidazole for treatment of an initial episode of *Clostridium difficile*–associated diarrhoea. *J Antimicrob Chemother*. 2004;54:211–216.

Haemophilus influenzae

H influenzae is a common inhabitant of the upper respiratory tract in 20%–50% of healthy adults and 80% of children. *H influenzae* is divided into 6 serotypes, based on differing capsular polysaccharide antigens. Both encapsulated and unencapsulated species cause disease, but systemic spread is typical of the encapsulated strain, whose capsule protects it against phagocytosis. The exact mechanism of invasion is unknown, but an acute suppu-

Table 1-4 Prophylactic Regimens for Genitourinary and Gastrointestinal Procedures

Situation	Agents*	Regiment
High-risk patients	Ampicillin plus gentamicin	Adults: ampicillin 2.0 g intramuscularly (IM) or intravenously (IV) plus gentamicin 1.5 mg/kg (not to exceed 120 mg) within 30 min of starting the procedure; 6 h later, ampicillin 1 g IM/IV or amoxicillin 1 g orally Children: ampicillin 50 mg/kg IM or IV (not to exceed 2.0 g) plus gentamicin 1.5 mg/kg within 30 min of starting the procedure; 6 h later, ampicillin 25 mg/kg IM/IV or amoxicillin 25 mg/kg orally
High-risk patients allergic to ampicillin/amoxicillin	Vancomycin plus gentamicin	Adults: vancomycin 1.0 g IV over 1–2 h plus gentamicin 1.5 mg/kg IV/IM (not to exceed 120 mg); complete injection/infusion within 30 min of starting the procedure Children: vancomycin 20 mg/kg IV over 1–2 h plus gentamicin 1.5 mg/kg IV/IM; complete injection/infusion within 30 min of starting the procedure
Moderate-risk patients	Amoxicillin or ampicillin	Adults: amoxicillin 2.0 g orally 1 h before procedure, or ampicillin 2.0 g IM/IV within 30 min of starting the procedure Children: amoxicillin 50 mg/kg orally 1 h before procedure, or ampicillin 50 mg/kg IM/IV within 30 min of starting the procedure
Moderate-risk patients allergic to ampicillin/amoxicillin	Vancomycin	Adults: vancomycin 1.0 g IV over 1–2 h; complete infusion within 30 min of starting the procedure Children: vancomycin 20 mg/kg IV over 1–2 h; complete infusion within 30 min of starting the procedure

*Total children's dose should not exceed adult dose.
†No second dose of vancomycin or gentamicin is recommended.

Reprinted from Dajani AS, Taubert KA, Wilson W, et al. Prevention of bacterial endocarditis. Recommendations by the American Heart Association. *JAMA*. 1997;277:1799. ©American Medical Association.

rative response results, with eventual humoral immunologic modulation of the infection. Long-term immunity follows with the development of bactericidal antibodies to the type B capsule in the presence of complement. Infants are usually protected for a few months by passively acquired maternal antibodies; thereafter, active antibody levels increase with age, being inversely related to the risk of infection. Of the patients with meningitis, roughly 14% develop significant neurological damage. Other infections include epiglottitis, orbital cellulitis, arthritis, otitis media, bronchitis, pericarditis, sinusitis, and pneumonia. Polymerase chain reaction DNA probe assay is available for rapid diagnosis of *H influenzae* type B infections. In the medical literature, *PCR* is also sometimes referred to as *nucleic acid amplification test (NAAT)*.

Treatment of acute infections has been complicated by the emergence of ampicillin-resistant strains, with an incidence approaching 50% in some geographic areas. Current recommendations are to start empirical therapy with amoxicillin-clavulanate (Augmentin), trimethoprim-sulfamethoxazole (Bactrim), a quinolone such as ciprofloxacin, or a third-generation cephalosporin, pending susceptibility testing of the organism. Nearly all isolates of *H influenzae* are now resistant to macrolides. Serious or life-threatening infections should be treated with an intravenous third-generation cephalosporin with known activity against *H influenzae,* such as ceftriaxone or cefotaxime, while results of sensitivity testing are pending. Recent reports note an increase in the number of isolates with reduced sensitivity to cephalosporins, especially in patients with chronic pulmonary disease. A recent case of ofloxacin resistance illustrated the possible emergence of quinolone resistance during prolonged therapy.

Two *H influenzae* type B conjugate vaccines are available for use in infants. Both have demonstrated their effectiveness in protecting infants and older children against meningitis and other invasive diseases caused by *H influenzae* type B. In studies of fully immunized populations, *H influenzae* infection has been nearly eradicated since the *H influenzae* type B vaccines were introduced. Also, the incidence of meningitis, orbital cellulitis, and other infections caused by *H influenzae* has been reduced significantly since *H influenzae* type B conjugate vaccines became available. It is important to remember that immunized patients are still susceptible to infections caused by strains of *H influenzae* other than type B.

> Ambati BK, Ambati J, Azar N, et al. Periorbital and orbital cellulitis before and after the advent of *Haemophilus influenzae* type B vaccination. *Ophthalmology.* 2000;107:1450–1453.
>
> Biedenbach DJ, Jones RN. Five-year analysis of *Haemophilus influenzae* isolates with reduced susceptibility to fluoroquinolones: prevalence results from the SENTRY antimicrobial surveillance program. *Diagn Microbiol Infect Dis.* 2003;46:55–61.
>
> Bozdogan B, Appelbaum PC. Macrolide resistance in Streptococci and *Haemophilus influenzae. Clin Lab Med.* 2004;24:455–475.
>
> Marty A, Greiner O, Day PJ, et al. Detection of *Haemophilus influenzae* type b by real-time PCR. *J Clin Microbiol.* 2004;42:3813–3815.

Neisseria

Most *Neisseria* organisms are normal inhabitants of the upper respiratory and alimentary tracts; however, the commonly recognized pathogenic species are the meningococci and the gonococci.

Meningococci can be cultured in up to 15% of healthy persons in nonepidemic periods. Virulence is determined by the polysaccharide capsule and the potent endotoxic activity of the cell wall, which can cause cardiovascular collapse, shock, and disseminated intravascular coagulation. In 2004, the Centers for Disease Control (CDC) reported that *Neisseria meningitidis* remains the leading cause of fatal sepsis. Resolution of the infection is related to circulating group–specific opsonizing antibodies and complement. Complement-deficient or asplenic persons are at risk for clinical infection. Prolonged immunity is usually acquired through a subclinical or carrier state and becomes more prevalent with increasing age. Diagnostic testing may include Gram stain, blood and cerebrospinal fluid cultures, counterimmunoelectrophoresis, enzyme-linked immunosorbent assay (ELISA), and PCR. A new, automated fluorescent multiplex PCR assay that can simultaneously detect *N meningitidis, H influenzae,* and *S pneumoniae* is now available and can be used for the evaluation of patients with suspected meningitis. This test provides extremely high sensitivity and a specificity of 100% for each organism.

The range of meningococcal infections includes meningitis; mild to severe upper respiratory tract infections; and, less often, endocarditis, arthritis, pericarditis, pneumonia, endophthalmitis, and purpura fulminans. *N meningitidis* serogroup B is the most common cause of bacterial meningitis in children and young adults. A less common infection is chronic meningococcemia, characterized by fever, headache, rash, and arthralgia over a period of days to weeks. This infection occurs sporadically, with the rare development of localized infections. Chronic meningococcemia represents an altered host–organism relationship that is poorly understood. Meningitis with a petechial or puerperal exanthem is the classic presentation, although each may occur in isolation.

Historically, the treatment of choice for meningococcal meningitis has been high-dose penicillin or, in the case of allergy, chloramphenicol or a third-generation cephalosporin. However, in one European study, 39% of asymptomatic carriers and 55.3% of infected patients had isolates with decreased susceptibility to penicillin. Rifampin or minocycline is used as chemoprophylaxis for family members or intimate personal contacts of the infected individual. Polysaccharide vaccines for groups A, C, Y, and W-135 strains are most effective in older children and adults. The routine administration of meningococcal vaccines is not recommended except in patients who have undergone splenectomy, complement-deficient persons, military personnel, travelers to endemic regions, and close contacts of infected patients.

Gonococci are not normal inhabitants of the respiratory or genital flora, and their major reservoir is the asymptomatic patient. Among infected women, 50% are asymptomatic, whereas 95% of infected men have symptoms. Asymptomatic patients are infectious for several months, with a transmissibility rate of 20%–50%. Nonsexual transmission is rare. Following a 13-year decline, the number of reported gonorrhea cases in the United States increased by 9% in 1998. The key to prevention is identification and treatment of asymptomatic carriers and their sexual contacts.

Symptomatic infection is characterized by a purulent response, with systemic manifestations of endotoxemia only in the bacteremic phase of the disease. Immunity to gonococcal infection is poorly understood, and repeated infections are common. *Chlamydia trachomatis* coexists with gonorrhea in 25%–50% of women with endocervical gonorrhea and 20%–33% of men with gonococcal urethritis. Diagnosis of gonococcal infections, as well as infections caused by many other bacteria, mycobacteria, viruses, and mycoplasma, has been enhanced with the development of highly sensitive DNA probes that use DNA amplification through PCR techniques.

The range of gonococcal infections includes cervicitis, urethritis, pelvic inflammatory disease, pharyngitis, conjunctivitis, ophthalmia neonatorum, and disseminated gonococcal disease with fever, polyarthralgias, and rash.

Because penicillin-resistant and tetracycline-resistant gonococcal strains have become common in many areas of the United States, treatment should be tailored to their local prevalence. Most of the original resistant isolates have been traced abroad, where there is a very high incidence of penicillinase-producing strains. Tetracycline is effective for susceptible strains, penicillin-allergic persons, or concurrent chlamydial infections. Ceftriaxone (via intramuscular injection) is the drug of choice for penicillinase-resistant strains; thus far, reduced susceptibility to this antibiotic is extremely rare. Other alternatives include oral cefixime; cefuroxime; azithromycin (a macrolide); and the fluoroquinolones. These drugs were initially so effective against gonococci that single oral-dose therapy became a recommended treatment protocol. The macrolides and fluoroquinolones have the added benefit of excellent activity against concomitant *C trachomatis* infection. Not surprisingly, gonococcal isolates with reduced sensitivity to macrolides and fluoroquinolones have been reported with increasing frequency. In fact, the CDC recently recommended that clinicians no longer use fluoroquinolones as a first-line treatment for gonorrhea in 1 high-risk group, homosexual men.

> Arreaza L, de LaFuente L, Vazquez JA. Antibiotic susceptibility patterns of *Neisseria meningitidis* isolates from patients and asymptomatic carriers. *Antimicrob Agents Chemother.* 2000;44:1705–1707.
>
> Burstein GR, Workowski KA. Sexually transmitted diseases treatment guidelines. *Curr Opin Pediatr.* 2003;15(4):391–397.
>
> Centers for Disease Control and Prevention (CDC). Increases in fluoroquinolone-resistant *Neisseria gonorrhoeae* among men who have sex with men—United States, 2003, and revised recommendations for gonorrhea treatment, 2004. *MMWR Morb Mortal Wkly Rep.* 2004;53:335–338.
>
> Guarner J, Greer PW, Whitney A, et al. Pathogenesis and diagnosis of human meningococcal disease using immunohistochemical and PCR assays. *Am J Clin Pathol.* 2004;122:754–764.
>
> Lyss SB, Kamb ML, Peterman TA, et al. *Chlamydia trachomatis* among patients infected with and treated for *Neisseria gonorrhoeae* in sexually transmitted disease clinics in the United States. *Ann Intern Med.* 2003;139(3):178–185.
>
> Smith K, Diggle MA, Clarke SC. Automation of a fluorescence-based multiplex PCR for the laboratory confirmation of common bacterial pathogens. *J Med Microbiol.* 2004;53:115–117.

Pseudomonas aeruginosa

Pseudomonas aeruginosa is a gram-negative bacillus found free living in moist environments. Together with *Serratia marcescens, P aeruginosa* is 1 of the 2 most consistently antimicrobial-resistant pathogenic bacteria. Infection usually requires either a break in the first-line defenses or altered immunity resulting in a local pyogenic response. The virulence of this organism is related to extracellular toxins, endotoxin, and a polysaccharide protection from phagocytosis. Systemic spread can result in disseminated intravascular coagulation, shock, and death. Humoral immune production of antitoxin is correlated with improved survival in bacteremic patients; however, eradication of infection is probably a multifactorial immune process.

Usual sites of infection include the respiratory system, skin, eye, urinary tract, bone, and wounds. Systemic infections caused by a resistant organism carry a high mortality rate and are usually associated with depressed immunity, often in a hospital setting.

Up to half of *P aeruginosa* isolates are now resistant to aminoglycosides. Therefore, treatment of serious infections relies on combined antimicrobial coverage with either a semisynthetic penicillin or a third-generation cephalosporin with an aminoglycoside. Ceftazidime has been the most effective cephalosporin for treatment of pseudomonal infections. Piperacillin/tazobactam, imipenem, and meropenem remain highly effective against most isolates, but resistance to the carbapenems has been rising gradually. The initial choice of antimicrobials depends on local susceptibility prevalence and should be guided by susceptibility testing. One study revealed that multidrug-resistant *P aeruginosa* arises in a stepwise manner following prolonged exposure to antipseudomonal antibiotics and results in adverse outcomes, with high mortality. Intravenous colistin is an effective treatment option for patients with otherwise untreatable multidrug-resistant *P aeruginosa* infections.

The use of vaccines incorporating multiple *P aeruginosa* serotypes is under investigation for the treatment of patients with severe burns, cystic fibrosis, or immunosuppression. Oral ciprofloxacin and other fluoroquinolones as well as newer macrolides such as azithromycin have been useful as prophylactic agents in patients with cystic fibrosis. Also, inhaled nebulized tobramycin has been shown to be effective as an option for treatment or prophylaxis in cystic fibrosis patients with *P aeruginosa* infection or colonization.

> Bonfiglio G, Marchetti F. In vitro activity of ceftazidime, cefepime and imipenem on 1,005 *Pseudomonas aeruginosa* clinical isolates either susceptible or resistant to beta-lactams. *Chemotherapy*. 2000;46:229–234.
>
> Cheer SM, Waugh J, Noble S. Inhaled tobramycin (TOBI): a review of its use in the management of *Pseudomonas aeruginosa* infections in patients with cystic fibrosis. *Drugs*. 2003;63:2501–2520.
>
> Jones ME, Karlowsky JA, Draghi DC, et al. Rates of antimicrobial resistance among common bacterial pathogens causing respiratory, blood, urine, and skin and soft tissue infections in pediatric patients. *Eur J Clin Microbiol Infect Dis*. 2004;23:445–455.
>
> Klepser ME. Role of nebulized antibiotics for the treatment of respiratory infections. *Curr Opin Infect Dis*. 2004;17(2):109–112.
>
> Linden PK, Kusne S, Coley K, et al. Use of parenteral colistin for the treatment of serious infection due to antimicrobial-resistant *Pseudomonas aeruginosa*. *Clin Infect Dis*. 2003;37:154–160.
>
> Saiman L, Marshall BC, Mayer-Hamblett N, et al. Azithromycin in patients with cystic fibrosis chronically infected with *Pseudomonas aeruginosa*: a randomized controlled trial. *JAMA*. 2003;290:1749–1756.

Treponema pallidum

The spirochete *T pallidum* (syphilis) is exclusively a human pathogen. It dies rapidly on drying and is readily killed by a wide variety of disinfectant agents and soaps. After a low of 6000 cases in 1956, the number of cases reported annually has risen to approximately 25,000 per year in the United States. Infection usually follows direct sexual contact. Less commonly, infection occurs after nongenital contact with an infected lesion or accidental inoculation with infected material. Transplacental transmission from an untreated pregnant woman to her fetus before 16 weeks' gestation results in *congenital syphilis*.

Stages

The course of the disease is divided into 4 stages: primary, secondary, latent, and tertiary (late). Initial inoculation occurs through intact mucous membranes or abraded skin and, within 6 weeks, results in a broad, ulcerated, painless papule called a *chancre*. The chancre is infiltrated with lymphocytes, plasma cells, histiocytes, and spirochetes. The spirochetes readily enter the lymphatic system and bloodstream. The ulcer heals spontaneously, and signs of dissemination appear after a variable quiescent period of several weeks to months.

The secondary stage is heralded by fever, malaise, adenopathy, and patchy loss of hair. Meningitis, uveitis, optic neuritis, and hepatitis are less common. Maculopapular lesions may develop into wartlike condylomata in moist areas, and oral mucosal patches sometimes appear, all of which are highly infectious. The secondary lesions usually resolve in 2–6 weeks, although up to 25% of patients may experience relapse in the first 2–4 years. Without treatment, these persons enter the latent stage of disease.

Latent syphilis, characterized by positive serologic results without clinical signs, is divided into 2 stages. The *early latent stage* is within 1 year of infection. During this time, the disease is potentially transmissible because relapses associated with spirochetemia are possible. The *late latent stage* is associated with immunity to relapse and resistance to infectious lesions.

Tertiary manifestations can occur from 2 to 20 years after infection, and one third of untreated cases of latent disease progress to this stage. The remaining two thirds of cases are either subclinical or they resolve spontaneously. *Tertiary disease* is characterized by destructive granulomatous lesions with a typical endarteritis that can affect the skin, bone, joints, oral and nasal cavities, parenchymal organs, cardiovascular system, eye, meninges, and central nervous system (CNS). Few spirochetes are found in lesions outside the CNS.

Immune mechanisms modulating syphilitic infection can contribute to the manifestations of the later stages of the disease. High titers of treponemal and nontreponemal antibodies are present throughout the secondary stage, conferring immunity to reinfection. The manifestations of the tertiary stage are those of a cellular response; however, the paucity of organisms suggests a delayed hypersensitivity to the spirochete products or an autoimmune-type reaction. Pathologically, obliterative endarteritis with a perivascular infiltrate of lymphocytes, monocytes, and plasma cells is a feature of all active stages of syphilis. Gummas of tertiary syphilis are evidenced by a central area of caseating necrosis with a surrounding granulomatous response.

Diagnosis

Most cases of syphilis are diagnosed serologically. *Nontreponemal tests*, such as the VDRL (Venereal Disease Research Laboratory) test or RPR (rapid plasma reagin) test, depend on the patient's nontreponemal serum antibodies causing immune flocculation of cardiolipin in the presence of lecithin and cholesterol. Nontreponemal test results are usually positive during the early stages of the primary lesion, uniformly positive during the secondary stage, and progressively nonreactive in the later stages. In neurosyphilis, the serum VDRL test result may be negative and the cerebrospinal fluid VDRL result may be positive. These patients require careful evaluation and aggressive treatment with close follow-up. Nontreponemal test results become predictably negative after successful therapy and can be used to assess the efficacy of treatment. Nontreponemal test results can be falsely positive in a variety of autoimmune diseases, especially systemic lupus erythematosus and the antiphospholipid antibody syndrome. In this disorder, the autoantibodies, anticardiolipin, and the lupus anticoagulant may result in vasculopathy and a hypercoagulable state, with arterial and venous thrombosis (including retinal vascular occlusion), preeclampsia, and spontaneous abortions. Less than 50% of patients with the antiphospholipid antibody syndrome have lupus. False-positive VDRL results can also occur in liver disease, diseases with a substantial amount of tissue destruction, pregnancy, or infections caused by other treponemae.

The *fluorescent treponemal antibody absorption test* (FTA-ABS) involves specific detection of antibody to *T pallidum* after the patient's serum is treated with nonpathogenic treponemal antigens to avoid nonspecific reactions. Hemagglutination tests specific for treponemal antibodies also have high sensitivity and specificity for detecting syphilis. These tests include the hemagglutination treponemal test for syphilis (HATTS), the *T pallidum* hemagglutination assay (TPHA), and the microhemagglutination test for *T pallidum* (MHA-TP). Treponemal antibody detection tests are more specific than nontreponemal tests, but the titers do not decrease with successful treatment; thus, such tests should be considered as confirmatory tests, especially in later stages of disease (Table 1-5).

Results of treponemal tests can be falsely positive in 15% of patients with systemic lupus erythematosus, in patients with other treponemal infections or Lyme disease, and, rarely, in patients who have lymphosarcoma or who are pregnant, although the fluorescent staining is typically weak.

Newer, more sensitive diagnostic tests for syphilis are under investigation, including direct antigen, ELISA, Western blot, and DNA PCR techniques. These methods may also improve our ability to diagnose congenital syphilis and neurosyphilis. Laboratory diagnosis of treponemal infection may also involve dark-field microscopy of scrapings from primary and secondary lesions. Scrapings of oral lesions are prone to misinterpretation because spirochetes may be present in normal mouth flora.

Management

Treatment of syphilis is determined by stage and by CNS involvement. *Treponema pallidum* is exquisitely sensitive to penicillin, which remains the antimicrobial of choice (Table 1-6). Erythromycin, azithromycin, chloramphenicol, tetracycline, doxycycline, and the cephalosporins are acceptable alternatives to penicillin. Lumbar puncture should be performed to determine cerebrospinal fluid involvement in a number of circumstances. They are as

Table 1-5 Percent Positive Tests in Untreated Syphilis

	VDRL	FTA-ABS
Primary	70%	80%
Secondary	100%	100%
Tertiary	70%	98%

Table 1-6 Treatment of Syphilis

Syphilis	Drug of Choice and Dosage
Early <1 yr	Penicillin G 2.4 million U IM × 1
Late >1 yr, no CNS	Penicillin G 2.4 million U IM weekly × 3 wks
Neurosyphilis	Penicillin G 2–4 million U IV q 4 hr × 10 days

follows: latent syphilis of more than 1 year's duration; suspected neurosyphilis; treatment failure; HIV coinfection; high RPR titers (>1:32); evidence of other late manifestations (cardiac involvement, gumma). Either penicillin G or a single oral dose of azithromycin has been recommended for treatment of patients recently exposed to a sexual partner with infectious syphilis. There have been some recent reports of syphilis treatment failures with use of azithromycin.

Many reports have described an accelerated clinical course of syphilis in patients infected with HIV; furthermore, such patients may experience an incomplete response to standard therapy. An HIV-infected patient with syphilis often requires a longer and more intensive treatment regimen, ongoing follow-up to assess for recurrence, and complete neurologic workup with an aggressive cerebrospinal fluid investigation for evidence of neurosyphilis. In a recent study, ceftriaxone compared favorably with intravenous penicillin for the treatment of neurosyphilis in HIV-infected patients. Patients with any stage of clinical syphilis should also be tested for HIV status.

> Behbehani R, Sergott RC, Savino PJ. The antiphospholipid antibody syndrome: diagnostic aspects. *Curr Opin Ophthalmol*. 2004;15:483–485.
>
> Centers for Disease Control and Prevention (CDC). Azithromycin treatment failures in syphilis infections—San Francisco, California, 2002–2003. *MMWR Morb Mortal Wkly Rep*. 2004;53:197–198.
>
> Grossman JM. Primary versus secondary antiphospholipid syndrome: is this lupus or not? *Curr Rheumatol Rep*. 2004;6:445–450.
>
> Hook EW III, Stephens J, Ennis DM. Azithromycin compared with penicillin G benzathine for treatment of incubating syphilis. *Ann Intern Med*. 1999;131:434–437.
>
> Marra CM, Boutin P, McArthur JC, et al. A pilot study evaluating ceftriaxone and penicillin G as treatment agents for neurosyphilis in human immunodeficiency virus-infected individuals. *Clin Infect Dis*. 2000;30:540–544.
>
> Palmer HM, Higgins SP, Herring AJ, et al. Use of PCR in the diagnosis of early syphilis in the United Kingdom. *Sex Transm Infect*. 2003;79:479–483.

Borrelia burgdorferi

Borrelia burgdorferi is a large, microaerophilic, plasmid-containing spirochete. When transmitted to humans and domestic animals through the bite of the *Ixodes* genus of ticks, this organism can cause both acute and chronic illness, now known as *Lyme disease*. First recognized in 1975, Lyme disease is the most common vector-borne infection in the United States. Although cases have been reported in 43 states, clusters are apparent in the northeast Atlantic, the upper Midwest, and the Pacific southwest, areas corresponding to the distribution of the *Ixodes* tick population. The range of the disease extends throughout Europe and Asia. In the United States, the number of reported cases has increased 5-fold since 1982, partly because of the rapid growth of the deer population in rural and suburban areas and partly as a result of increased awareness of the disease.

The life cycle of the spirochete depends on its horizontal transmission through a mouse. Early in the summer, an infected *Ixodes* tick nymph (juvenile) bites a mouse, which becomes infected; then, in late summer, the infection is transmitted to an immature uninfected larva after it bites the infected mouse. This immature larva then molts to become a nymph, and the cycle is repeated. Once a nymph matures to an adult, its favorite host is the white-tailed deer, although it can survive with other hosts. Recently, it has been discovered that 2 other tick-borne zoonoses (babesiosis and human granulocytic ehrlichiosis) can be co-transmitted with Lyme disease. *Anaplasma phagocytophilum* is another common tick-borne infection.

Stages

Lyme disease usually occurs in 3 stages following a tick bite: *localized (stage 1), disseminated (stage 2),* and *persistent (stage 3).*

Localized disease (stage 1), present in 86% of infected patients, is characterized by skin involvement, initially as a red macule or papule, which later expands in a circular manner, usually with a bright red border and a central clear indurated area, known as *erythema chronicum migrans.*

Hematogenous dissemination (stage 2) can then occur within days to weeks and is manifested as a flu-like illness with headaches, fatigue, and musculoskeletal aching.

More profound symptoms occur as the infection localizes to the nervous, cardiovascular, and musculoskeletal systems (stage 3). Neurological complications such as meningitis, encephalitis, cranial neuritis (including Bell's palsy), radiculopathy, and neuropathy occur in 15% of patients. Cardiac manifestations include myopericarditis and variable heart block in 5% of patients. Unilateral asymmetrical arthritis occurs in up to 80% of untreated patients.

Late persistent manifestations are usually confined to the nervous system, skin, and joints. Late neurological signs include encephalomyelitis as well as demyelinating and psychiatric syndromes. Joint involvement includes asymmetrical pauciarticular arthritis; skin involvement is characterized by localized scleroderma-type lesions or acrodermatitis chronica atrophicans.

Other systemic manifestations during the initial dissemination or the late persistent state include lymphadenopathy, conjunctivitis, keratitis, neuritis, uveitis, orbital myositis, hematuria, and orchitis. In some studies, serologic testing of patients with chronic fatigue syndrome has shown an increased incidence of positive *B burgdorferi* antibodies.

Diagnosis

During the early stages of infection, the immune response is minimal, with little cellular reactivity to *B burgdorferi* antigens and nonspecific elevation of IgM. The spirochete is most easily seen and cultured from the skin lesions during this early stage. During the disseminated phase, cellular antigenic response is markedly increased and specific IgM is followed by a polyclonal B-cell activation, with development of specific IgG antibody within weeks of the initial infection. The infection is immunologically mediated by both serum-mediated complement lysis and cellular phagocytosis. Histopathology demonstrates lymphocytic tissue infiltration, often in a perivascular distribution. Late manifestations may be either HLA-mediated autoimmune damage or prolonged latency followed by persistent infection.

Laboratory diagnosis of *B burgdorferi* infection depends on serodiagnosis: there is a poor recovery rate from blood, cerebrospinal fluid, and synovial fluid during the early stages of infection. The expensive laboratory media needed and the several weeks required for incubation of the organism diminish the practical value of culture-proven infection. Skin-biopsy specimens with monoclonal antibody staining have demonstrated good sensitivity in identifying the organism. Although serodiagnosis remains the practical solution for establishing the diagnosis, laboratory methodology is not standardized. Variations in antigen preparation, adsorption of cross-reacting antibodies, types of assays employed, and intralaboratory quality control have resulted in significant interlaboratory and intralaboratory discrepancies with the same serum sample.

The most commonly used serologic tests are the *immunofluorescence antibody* assay or the more sensitive *ELISA*. Other immunologic tests available are the *indirect hemagglutination antibody* test and the *immunodot* assay. The ELISA is 50% sensitive during the early stages of the disease, and almost all symptomatic patients are seropositive during the later disseminated and persistent phases of the infection. These tests should be used only to support a clinical diagnosis of Lyme disease, not as the primary basis for making diagnostic or treatment decisions. Serologic testing is not useful early in the course of Lyme disease because of the low sensitivity of tests in early disease. Serologic testing is more helpful in later disease, when the sensitivity and specificity are greater. Early administration of antibiotics can cause antibody titers to remain below the threshold level; however, cellular reactivity to *Borrelia* antigens remains high. False-positive results can occur in patients with syphilis, Rocky Mountain spotted fever, yaws, pinta, *B recurrentis*, and various rheumatologic disorders. Western blot analysis has been advocated in identifying false-positive results; however, up to 10% of infected patients may be asymptomatic. PCR has been used to detect *B burgdorferi* DNA in serum and cerebrospinal fluid, but its sensitivity in neuroborreliosis is no better than that of the ELISA methods. Although the FTA-ABS test result for syphilis may be positive in patients with Lyme disease, the VDRL test result should be nonreactive.

Management

Treatment of *B burgdorferi* infection depends on the stage and the severity of the infection. The organism is highly sensitive in vitro to tetracycline, ampicillin, erythromycin, ceftriaxone, and imipenem; it is less sensitive to penicillin. Early Lyme disease is typically treated with oral doxycycline, amoxicillin, cefuroxime, or erythromycin. Mild disseminated disease is treated with oral doxycycline or amoxicillin. Serious disease (with cardiac or neurological manifestations) is typically treated with ceftriaxone or high-dose penicillin G intravenously for up to 6 weeks. Patients who do not respond to the initial regimen may require alternate or combination therapy. Up to 15% of patients may develop a *Jarisch-Herxheimer reaction,* in which symptoms worsen during the first day of treatment.

A recombinant outer surface protein A vaccine for *B burgdorferi* was developed and studied. It was well tolerated, had an acceptable adverse effect profile, and effectively prevented Lyme disease. This vaccine was recommended only for persons aged 15 to 70 who travel extensively, live, or work outdoors in endemic areas. Unfortunately, it was discontinued because of disappointing vaccine sales. Efforts to decrease the incidence of the disease by pesticide spraying have met with limited success. In endemic areas, adults may be able to reduce their risk by applying insect-repellent sprays containing diethyltoluamide (DEET).

> Carvounis PE, Mehta AP, Geist CE. Orbital myositis associated with *Borrelia burgdorferi* (Lyme disease) infection. *Ophthalmology.* 2004;111:1023–1028.
>
> Chmielewski T, Fiett J, Gniadkowski M, et al. Improvement in the laboratory recognition of lyme borreliosis with the combination of culture and PCR methods. *Mol Diagn.* 2003;7:155–162.
>
> Courtney JW, Kostelnik LM, Zeidner NS, et al. Multiplex real-time PCR for detection of *Anaplasma phagocytophilum* and *Borrelia burgdorferi*. *J Clin Microbiol.* 2004;42:3164–3168.
>
> Hayney MS, Grunske MM, Boh LE. Lyme disease prevention and vaccine prophylaxis. *Ann Pharmacother.* 1999;33:723–729.
>
> Hengge UR, Tannapfel A, Tyring SK, et al. Lyme borreliosis. *Lancet Infect Dis.* 2003;3: 489–500.
>
> Hunfeld KP, Brade V. Zoonotic Babesia: possibly emerging pathogens to be considered for tick-infested humans in Central Europe. *Int J Med Microbiol.* 2004;293 suppl 37:93–103.
>
> Ravishankar J, Lutwick LI. Current and future treatment of Lyme disease. *Expert Opin Pharmacother.* 2001;2:241–251.
>
> Terkeltaub RA. Lyme disease 2000. Emerging zoonoses complicate patient work-up and treatment. *Geriatrics.* 2000;55:34–35, 39–40, 43–44.

Chlamydia trachomatis

Chlamydia is a small, obligate, intracellular parasite that contains DNA and RNA and has a unique biphasic life cycle. This prokaryote uses the host cell's energy-generating capacity for its own reproduction. *C trachomatis* can survive only briefly outside the body. Transmitted by close contact, *C trachomatis* is the most common sexually transmitted infection, with 4 million new cases per year. More than 15% of infected pregnant women and 10% of infected men are asymptomatic.

Infection is initiated by local inoculation and ingestion of the organism by phagocytes, followed by intracellular reproduction and eventual spread to other cells. The mechanism for immunologic eradication of *Chlamydia* is uncertain but appears to involve cell-mediated immunity. Infections in humans include trachoma, inclusion conjunctivitis, nongonococcal urethritis, epididymitis, mucopurulent cervicitis, proctitis, salpingitis, infant pneumonia syndrome, and lymphogranuloma venereum. Genital *C trachomatis* infection can result in pelvic inflammatory disease, tubal infertility, and ectopic pregnancy. In a recent study, 80% of ocular adnexal lymphoma samples carried DNA of a related organism, *Chlamydia psittaci,* suggesting an etiologic role of the organism in some cases of lymphoma.

Diagnostic techniques include culture, direct immunofluorescent antibody testing of exudates, enzyme immunoassay, and newer DNA probes utilizing PCR, such as the Amplicor PCR, the Abbott LCx, and the BD ProbeTec ET. The Gen-Probe APTIMA Combo 2 is a PCR assay for the simultaneous detection of *C trachomatis* and *N gonorrhoeae* from urine and urogenital swab specimens.

Chlamydial infections are readily treated with tetracycline, erythromycin, or 1 of the quinolones or newer macrolides. Although single-dose azithromycin or sparfloxacin therapy for urethritis and cervicitis has been proven effective in some studies, it is usually recommended that patients continue treatment for at least 7 days to ensure complete eradication.

> Boyadzhyan B, Yashina T, Yatabe JH, et al. Comparison of the APTIMA CT and GC assays with the APTIMA combo 2 assay, the Abbott LCx assay, and direct fluorescent-antibody and culture assays for detection of *Chlamydia trachomatis* and *Neisseria gonorrhoeae*. *J Clin Microbiol.* 2004;42:3089–3093.
>
> Ferreri AJ, Guidoboni M, Ponzoni M, et al. Evidence for an association between *Chlamydia psittaci* and ocular adnexal lymphomas. *J Natl Cancer Inst.* 2004;96(8):586–594.
>
> Gaydos CA, Theodore M, Dalesio N, et al. Comparison of three nucleic acid amplification tests for detection of *Chlamydia trachomatis* in urine specimens. *J Clin Microbiol.* 2004;42(7):3041–3045.
>
> Stokes T, Schober P, Baker J, et al. Evidence-based guidelines for the management of genital chlamydial infection in general practice. (Leicestershire Chlamydia Guidelines Group.) *Fam Pract.* 1999;16:269–277.

Mycoplasma pneumoniae

Mycoplasma pneumoniae is a unique bacterium that may cause multiple disorders—including pharyngitis, otitis media, tracheobronchitis, pneumonia, endocarditis, nephritis, encephalopathy, optic neuritis, and facial nerve palsy—and has been implicated in some cases of chronic fatigue and fibromyalgia syndromes. Recent serological studies indicate that *M pneumoniae,* varicella-zoster, and *B burgdorferi* cause a majority of cases of Bell's palsy.

Serious *M pneumoniae* infections requiring hospitalization occur in both adults and children and may involve multiple organ systems. Extrapulmonary complications involving all of the major organ systems can occur in association with *M pneumoniae* infection as a result of direct invasion or autoimmune response. Recent evidence suggests that *M pneumoniae* may play a contributory role in chronic lung disorders such as asthma.

Recently, new PCR assays have been adapted for the direct detection of *M pneumoniae* organisms, but in clinical practice, sensitive serologic tests are usually used initially for the detection of antibodies. Initial treatment of *M pneumoniae* infections usually involves use of a macrolide, tetracycline, or fluoroquinolone.

> Candler PM, Dale RC. Three cases of central nervous system complications associated with *Mycoplasma pneumoniae*. *Pediatr Neurol.* 2004;31(2):133–138.

Daxboeck F, Krause R, Wenisch C. Laboratory diagnosis of *Mycoplasma pneumoniae* infection. *Clin Microbiol Infect.* 2003;9:263–273.

Endresen GK. Mycoplasma blood infection in chronic fatigue and fibromyalgia syndromes. *Rheumatol Int.* 2003;23(5):211–215.

Volter C, Helms J, Weissbrich B, et al. Frequent detection of *Mycoplasma pneumoniae* in Bell's palsy. *Eur Arch Otorhinolaryngol.* 2004;261:400–404.

Waites KB, Talkington DF. *Mycoplasma pneumoniae* and its role as a human pathogen. *Clin Microbiol Rev.* 2004;17:697–728.

Mycobacteria

Mycobacteria include a range of pathogenic and nonpathogenic species distributed widely in the environment. *Mycobacterium tuberculosis* is the most significant human pathogenic species. *M tuberculosis* infects an estimated 1.86 billion persons worldwide (32% global prevalence) and causes approximately 2 million deaths each year. There were 8 million new cases of tuberculosis in 1997 alone, most of these occurring in Africa and Southeast Asia. *Nontuberculous mycobacteria* may be responsible for up to 5% of all clinical mycobacterial infections. Atypical mycobacterial infections are more prevalent in immunosuppressed patients and those with AIDS. Infections caused by nontuberculous mycobacteria include lymphadenitis, pulmonary infections, skin granulomas, prosthetic valve infections, and bacteremia. Despite their low virulence, atypical mycobacterial infections are difficult to treat because of resistance to standard antituberculous regimens.

Tuberculosis

Infection usually occurs through inhalation of infective droplets and rarely by way of the skin or gastrointestinal tract. The organism is able to multiply within macrophages with a minor inflammatory response. Cell-mediated hypersensitivity to tuberculoprotein develops 3–9 weeks after infection, with a typical granulomatous response that slows or contains bacterial multiplication. Most organisms die during the fibrotic phase of the response. Reactivation is usually associated with depressed immunity and aging. Systemic spread occurs with reactivation and results in a granulomatous response to the infected foci. Acquired immunity is cell mediated but incomplete, and the role of delayed hypersensitivity is complex: high degrees of sensitivity to tuberculoprotein can cause caseous necrosis, which leads to spread of the disease. Infections include pulmonary involvement, which can lead to systemic spread with involvement of any organ system.

Laboratory diagnosis involves culture of infective material on Lowenstein-Jensen medium for 6–8 weeks and use of the acid-fast type of Ziehl-Neelsen stain or fluorescent antibody staining of infected material. In addition, ELISA as well as DNA probes using PCR techniques for *M tuberculosis* and other mycobacteria are available. Newer PCR assays can identify resistant strains of tuberculosis by detecting isoniazid and rifampin resistance mutations in organisms from cultures or from smear-positive specimens.

The tuberculin skin test measures delayed hypersensitivity to tuberculoprotein. Purified protein derivative (PPD) produced from a culture filtrate of *M tuberculosis* is standardized and its activity expressed as tuberculin units (TU). Usually, intermediate strength (5 TU) is used; however, if a high degree of sensitivity to tuberculoprotein is suspected, low strength (1 TU) is used to avoid the risk of excessive reaction locally or at the site of an infected focus. A positive high-strength (250 TU) reaction with a doubtful intermediate-strength reaction suggests infection with atypical mycobacteria and resultant cross-sensitization.

A positive PPD reaction is defined as an area of induration 10 mm or greater in the area of intradermal injection of 0.1 mL of PPD read 48–72 hours later. Ninety percent of persons demonstrating 10 mm of induration to 5 TU are infected with *M tuberculosis*. A positive response indicates an infection, although the infection might not be currently active. Induration of 5 mm in persons with HIV infection is sufficient to warrant chemoprophylaxis. For children, the tine test is an easily administered alternative to the PPD.

Among patients in whom skin testing yields positive results, the overall risk of reactivation of the disease is 3%–5%. A positive PPD test result should be considered in light of the individual patient's radiologic and clinical data as well as age to determine the need for prophylactic treatment. Administration of isoniazid daily for 1 year reduces the risk of reactivation by 80%; however, the risk of isoniazid hepatotoxicity increases with age and alcohol use. Patients with a positive tuberculin skin test result who require long-term high-dose steroids or other immunosuppressive agents should be treated prophylactically with isoniazid for the duration of their immunosuppressive therapy in order to prevent reactivation of tuberculosis.

Treatment of active infection involves use of 2 or 3 drugs because of the emergence of resistance and of delay in culture susceptibility studies. Standard regimens employ multiple drugs for 18–24 months, but with the addition of newer agents, treatment for 6–9 months has been found equally effective. Drugs currently used include isoniazid, rifampin, rifabutin, ethambutol, streptomycin, pyrazinamide, aminosalicylic acid, ethionamide, and cycloserine. All of the agents currently used have toxic side effects, especially hepatic and neurologic, which should be carefully monitored during the course of therapy. Isoniazid and ethambutol can cause optic neuritis in a small percentage of patients, and rifampin may cause pink-tinged tears and blepharoconjunctivitis. The BCG (bacille Calmette-Guérin) vaccine causes false-positive reactions to the PPD skin test and thus interferes with the efficacy of the PPD skin test as a diagnostic and epidemiologic tool.

Outbreaks of nosocomial and community-acquired multidrug-resistant tuberculosis (MDRTB) have been reported recently, particularly in the presence of concurrent HIV infection. MDRTB in patients infected with HIV is associated with widely disseminated disease, poor treatment response, and substantial mortality. Infection has also been documented in health care workers exposed to these patients. MDRTB represents a serious public health threat that will require an aggressive governmental and medical response to limit its spread. Newer fluoroquinolones and some of the newer classes of broad-spectrum antibiotics, such as linezolid, are effective against many isolates of MDRTB as well as atypical mycobateria and have been recommended as potential therapeutic alternatives.

Lin SY, Probert W, Lo M, et al. Rapid detection of isoniazid and rifampin resistance mutations in *Mycobacterium tuberculosis* complex from cultures or smear-positive sputa by use of molecular beacons. *J Clin Microbiol.* 2004;42:4204–4208.

Neralla S, Glassroth J. *Mycobacterium tuberculosis:* the treatment of active disease. *Semin Respir Infect.* 2003;18:292–306.

Pottumarthy S, Wells VC, Morris AJ. A comparison of seven tests for serological diagnosis of tuberculosis. *J Clin Microbiol.* 2000;38:2227–2231.

Sperhacke RD, Mello FC, Zaha A, et al. Detection of *Mycobacterium tuberculosis* by a polymerase chain reaction colorimetric dot-blot assay. *Int J Tuberc Lung Dis.* 2004;8:312–317.

Fungal Infections

Candida albicans is a yeast that is normally present in the oral cavity, lower gastrointestinal tract, and female genital tract. Under conditions of disrupted local defenses or depressed immunity, overgrowth and parenchymal invasion occur, with the potential for systemic spread. Increased virulence of *Candida* is related to its mycelial phase, when it is more resistant to the host's cellular immune system, which acts as the primary modulator of infection. DNA PCR techniques have been used to diagnose candidemia. Infections include oral lesions (thrush) and vaginal, skin, esophageal, and urinary tract involvement. Chronic mucocutaneous lesions may occur in persons with specific T-cell defects. Disseminated disease can involve any organ system, most commonly the kidneys, brain, heart, and eye.

Some other important invasive fungal infections are cryptococcosis, histoplasmosis, blastomycosis, aspergillosis, and coccidioidomycosis. Invasive fungal infections have become a major problem in immunocompromised patients. New fungal PCR assays provide more rapid diagnosis of serious fungal infections than do fungal cultures, while offering increased sensitivity.

Treatment of serious systemic infections has traditionally involved the use of intravenous amphotericin B, sometimes in combined therapy with flucytosine or an imidazole. Recently, lipid complex and liposome-encapsulated formulations of amphotericin B (AmBisome, Amphotec) were developed to reduce the drug's nephrotoxicity and myelosuppression. A controlled study revealed that intravenous amphotericin B prophylaxis reduced the incidence of systemic fungal infections in immunocompromised patients with leukemia. Newer imidazoles, such as fluconazole, itraconazole, and voriconazole, are less toxic and better-tolerated alternatives. In fact, itraconazole has replaced ketoconazole as the treatment of choice for nonmeningeal, non–life-threatening cases of histoplasmosis, blastomycosis, and paracoccidioidomycosis. Itraconazole is also effective in treating patients with cryptococcosis and coccidioidomycosis, including those with meningitis. Newer antifungals, such as the echinocandins and the triazoles, are discussed later in this chapter.

Carrillo-Muñoz AJ, Quindos G, Tur C, et al. Comparative in vitro antifungal activity of amphotericin B lipid complex, amphotericin B and fluconazole. *Chemotherapy.* 2000;46:235–244.

de Aguirre L, Hurst SF, Choi JS, et al. Rapid differentiation of *Aspergillus* species from other medically important opportunistic molds and yeasts by PCR-enzyme immunoassay. *J Clin Microbiol.* 2004;42:3495–3504.

Evertsson U, Monstein HJ, Johansson AG. Detection and identification of fungi in blood using broad-range 28S rDNA PCR amplification and species-specific hybridisation. *APMIS.* 2000;108:385–392.

Gallagher JC, MacDougall C, Ashley ES, et al. Recent advances in antifungal pharmacotherapy for invasive fungal infections. *Expert Rev Anti Infect Ther.* 2004;2:253–268.

Imhof A, Schaer C, Schoedon G, et al. Rapid detection of pathogenic fungi from clinical specimens using LightCycler real-time fluorescence PCR. *Eur J Clin Microbiol Infect Dis.* 2003;22:558–560.

Maaroufi Y, Ahariz N, Husson M, et al. Comparison of different methods of isolation of DNA of commonly encountered *Candida* species and its quantitation by using a real-time PCR-based assay. *J Clin Microbiol.* 2004;42(7):3159–3163.

Polak A. Antifungal therapy—state of the art at the beginning of the 21st century. *Prog Drug Res.* 2003; Spec no:59–190.

Subira M, Martino R, Gomez L, et al. Low-dose amphotericin B lipid complex vs. conventional amphotericin B for empirical antifungal therapy of neutropenic fever in patients with hematologic malignancies—a randomized, controlled trial. *Eur J Haematol.* 2004;72(5):342–347.

Toxoplasma

Toxoplasmosis is caused by infection with the protozoan parasite *Toxoplasma gondii*, which infects up to a third of the world's population. Acute infections may be asymptomatic in pregnant women, but they can be transmitted to the fetus and cause severe complications, including mental retardation, blindness, and epilepsy. As many as 4000 new cases of congenital toxoplasmosis occur each year in the United States. Of the nearly 750 US deaths attributed to toxoplasmosis each year, approximately half are believed to be caused by eating contaminated undercooked or raw meat. Toxoplasma can also be transmitted to humans by ingestion of oocysts, an environmentally resistant form of the organism, through exposure to cat feces, water, or soil containing the parasite or from eating unwashed contaminated fruits or vegetables.

Toxoplasma infection can be prevented in large part by cooking meat to a safe temperature, peeling or thoroughly washing fruits and vegetables before eating, and cleaning cooking surfaces and utensils after they have contacted raw meat. Pregnant women should avoid changing cat litter and feeding raw or undercooked meat to cats. Also, they should keep cats indoors, where cats are less likely to eat infected prey and subsequently acquire toxoplasma.

Primary infection is usually subclinical, but in some patients cervical lymphadenopathy or ocular disease can be present. The ocular manifestations include uveitis and chorioretinitis with macular scarring. The clinical picture and histopathology of toxoplasmosis are a reflection of the immune response, which includes an early humoral response, followed by the cellular response, which varies from low-grade mononuclear infiltrate to total tissue destruction. In immunocompromised patients, reactivation of latent disease can cause life-threatening encephalitis.

Diagnosis of toxoplasmosis can be established by direct detection of the parasite or by serological techniques. Real-time PCR is a very sensitive technique for diagnosing infection caused by *T gondii* and for determining the precise genotype of the organism. The most commonly used therapeutic regimen, and probably the most effective, comprises a combination of pyrimethamine with sulfadiazine and folinic acid. Recently, sulfadiazine has been replaced by sulfadoxine, which has a longer half-life and provides a dosing schedule resulting in improved compliance. Newer drugs with potential activity against *T gondii* include azithromycin, atovaquone, and clindamycin, but these require further evaluation in animal models and human studies.

>   Kravetz JD, Federman DG. Toxoplasmosis in pregnancy. *Am J Med.* 2005;118:212–216.
>   Lopez A, Dietz VJ, Wilson M, et al. Preventing congenital toxoplasmosis. *MMWR Recomm Rep.* 2000;49(RR-2):59–68.
>   Montoya JG, Liesenfeld O. Toxoplasmosis. *Lancet.* 2004;363:1965–1976.
>   Rothova A. Ocular manifestations of toxoplasmosis. *Curr Opin Ophthalmol.* 2003;14:384–388.

Herpesvirus

As a class, viruses are strictly intracellular parasites, relying on the host cell for their replication. Herpesviruses, which are large-enveloped, double-stranded DNA viruses, are one of the most common human infectious agents, responsible for a wide spectrum of acute and chronic diseases. The major members of the group are herpes simplex viruses (HSV-1 and HSV-2), varicella-zoster virus, cytomegalovirus (CMV), and Epstein-Barr virus.

Herpes Simplex

HSV has 2 antigenic types, each with numerous antigenic strains. Each type has different epidemiologic patterns of infection. Seroepidemiologic studies demonstrate a high prevalence of HSV-1 antibodies with a lower prevalence of HSV-2 antibodies. Many people with HSV antibodies are asymptomatic. Infection is modulated by a predominantly cellular response. The presence of high titers of neutralizing antibodies to HSV does not seem to retard the cell-to-cell transmission of the virus. The virus can spread within nerves and cause a latent infection of sensory and autonomic ganglia. Latent infection does not result in death of the host cell, and the exact mechanism of viral genome interaction with the host genome is incompletely understood. Reactivation of HSV from the trigeminal ganglia may be associated with asymptomatic excretion or with the development of mucosal herpetic ulceration. Serologic testing, DNA PCR testing, and viral culture can assist in the diagnosis of difficult cases, particularly CNS infections. Real-time PCR testing offers more rapid results than do conventional nested PCR assays for the detection of HSV-1, HSV-2, and varicella-zoster virus in clinical samples.

Herpes simplex type 1 is associated with mucocutaneous superficial infections of the pharynx, skin, oral cavity, vagina, eye, and brain. Ophthalmic infection most often manifests as corneal dendritic or stromal disease, but may present as acute retinal necrosis. (The ocular manifestations of HSV infection are discussed in more detail in BCSC Section 8, *External Disease and Cornea*; and Section 12, *Retina and Vitreous*.) Herpes encephalitis carries a 30% mortality rate. *Herpes simplex type 2* is an important sexually transmitted disease that is associated with genital infections, aseptic meningitis, and congenital infection. *Neonatal herpes infection* involves multiple systems and, if untreated, carries a mortality rate of 80%.

The drug of choice for treating acute systemic infections is acyclovir. Localized disease can be treated with oral acyclovir. Topical treatment of skin or mucocutaneous lesions with acyclovir ointment decreases the healing time. Oral acyclovir can also be used prophylactically for severe and recurrent genital herpes. Long-term suppressive oral acyclovir also reduces the recurrence of herpes simplex epithelial keratitis and stromal keratitis.

Two newer antiviral agents, famciclovir and valacyclovir, are approved for the treatment of herpes zoster and herpes simplex. Compared with acyclovir, these agents have better bioavailability and achieve higher blood levels. HSV is also sensitive to vidarabine. Cidofovir, an antiviral drug used for treating CMV infections, is also very effective against acyclovir-resistant herpes simplex.

Varicella-Zoster

Varicella-zoster virus (VZV), also sometimes referred to as *herpes zoster,* produces infection in a manner similar to herpes simplex. After a primary infection, the virus remains latent in dorsal root ganglia, with host cellular immune interaction inhibiting reactivation. Primary infection usually occurs in childhood in the form of chickenpox (varicella), a generalized vesicular rash accompanied by mild constitutional symptoms. Reactivation may be heralded by pain in a sensory nerve distribution, followed by a unilateral vesicular eruption occurring over 1 to 3 dermatomic areas. New crops of lesions appear in the same area within 7 days. Resolution of the lesions may be followed by postherpetic neuralgia, the mechanism of which is incompletely understood. Other neurological syndromes following herpes zoster involvement include segmental myelitis, Guillain-Barré syndrome, and Ramsay Hunt syndrome. The incidence of herpes zoster is 2 to 3 times higher in patients older than age 60. Postherpetic neuralgia occurs after herpes zoster infection in approximately 50% of patients older than 50 years. The pain of postherpetic neuralgia can be severe and debilitating and may persist for months or even years. Immunosuppressed persons experience recurrent lesions; the incidence of disseminated disease in such patients may be 10 times that of immunocompetent persons.

A recent study revealed no significant differences in the results of treating immunocompetent adults with cutaneous VZV infection with either famciclovir 750 mg once daily, 500 mg 2 times daily, or 250 mg 3 times daily; or acyclovir 800 mg 5 times daily. All treatments were given for 7 days.

Treatment of acute infection in immunocompromised patients or those with visceral involvement may include acyclovir, famciclovir, or valacyclovir. Newer drugs being evaluated for resistant VZV strains or concomitant HIV infection include sorivudine, brivudine, fialuridine, fiacitabine, netivudine, lobucavir, foscarnet, and cidofovir. A live attenuated varicella vaccine (Varivax) is available for prevention of primary disease, and it appears to also reduce the incidence of recurrent VZV infection and neuralgia. This vaccine is recommended for children, patients with chronic diseases or leukemia, and patients receiving immunosuppressive therapy. In some patients, tricyclic antidepressants, carbamazepine, gabapentin, and topical capsaicin cream have reduced the pain of postherpetic neuralgia. For refractory cases, transcutaneous electronic nerve stimulation or nerve blocks are sometimes used.

Johnson RW, Dworkin RH. Treatment of herpes zoster and postherpetic neuralgia. *BMJ.* 2003;326:748–750.

Ormrod D, Scott LJ, Perry CM. Valacyclovir: a review of its long-term utility in the management of genital herpes simplex virus and cytomegalovirus infections. *Drugs.* 2000;59:839–863.

Shafran SD, Tyring SK, Ashton R, et al. Once, twice, or three times daily famciclovir compared with acyclovir for the oral treatment of herpes zoster in immunocompetent adults: a randomized, multicenter, double-blind clinical trial. *J Clin Virol.* 2004;29:248–253.

Weidmann M, Meyer-Konig U, Hufert FT. Rapid detection of herpes simplex virus and varicella-zoster virus infections by real-time PCR. *J Clin Microbiol.* 2003;41(4):1565–1568.

Wu JJ, Brentjens MH, Torres G, et al. Valacyclovir in the treatment of herpes simplex, herpes zoster, and other viral infections. *J Cutan Med Surg.* 2003;7:372–381.

Cytomegalovirus

Cytomegalovirus is a ubiquitous human virus: 50% of adults in developed countries harbor antibodies, which are usually acquired during the first 5 years of life. The virus can be isolated from all body fluids, even in the presence of circulating neutralizing antibody, for up to several years after infection. Cytopathic effects following infection are similar to those of HSV. Serologic and PCR testing are available to assist in the diagnosis of CMV infection.

Clinical syndromes with greatest morbidity include congenital CMV disease, with a 20% incidence of hearing loss or mental retardation and a 0.1% incidence of various other congenital disorders, including jaundice, hepatosplenomegaly, anemia, microcephaly, and chorioretinitis. Infections in adults include heterophile-negative mononucleosis, pneumonia, hepatitis, and Guillain-Barré syndrome. In immunocompromised patients, CMV interstitial pneumonia carries a 90% mortality rate. Disseminated spread to the gastrointestinal tract, CNS, and eye is common in patients with AIDS. Latent infection within leukocytes accounts for transfusion-associated disease. CMV replication itself can further suppress cell-mediated immunity, with resultant depressed lymphocyte response and development of severe opportunistic infections.

CMV retinitis and colitis have been successfully treated with the nucleoside derivative ganciclovir, which is available for intravenous, oral, or intravitreal routes. A slow-release intraocular ganciclovir insert is also available for the treatment of CMV retinitis. It should be noted that the intravitreal and intraocular methods of administration are effective only for CMV retinitis and will not treat colitis or other systemic manifestations. Intravenous foscarnet and cidofovir have also been effective in the treatment of CMV retinitis. One study showed that intravitreal cidofovir given at 6-week intervals was highly effective for treating CMV retinitis. Valganciclovir is a well-tolerated, newer oral agent that is highly effective in the treatment of CMV infection, including retinitis.

Boeckh M, Huang M, Ferrenberg J, et al. Optimization of quantitative detection of cytomegalovirus DNA in plasma by real-time PCR. *J Clin Microbiol.* 2004;42:1142–1148.

Razonable RR, Paya CV. Valganciclovir for the prevention and treatment of cytomegalovirus disease in immunocompromised hosts. *Expert Rev Anti Infect Ther.* 2004;2:27–41.

Schleiss MR, McVoy MA. Overview of congenitally and perinatally acquired cytomegalovirus infections: recent advances in antiviral therapy. *Expert Rev Anti Infect Ther.* 2004; 2:389–403.

Segarra-Newnham M, Salazar MI. Valganciclovir: a new oral alternative for cytomegalovirus retinitis in human immunodeficiency virus-seropositive individuals. *Pharmacotherapy.* 2002;22:1124–1128.

Epstein-Barr Virus

Epstein-Barr virus (EBV) antibodies are found in 90%–95% of all adults. Childhood infections are usually asymptomatic, with symptomatic disease occurring in young adults. Infectious mononucleosis is the usual clinical disease in most symptomatic adults. Transplant recipients on cyclosporine or patients with AIDS may develop lymphoproliferative disorders. EBV is epidemiologically associated with Burkitt lymphoma and nasopharyngeal carcinoma and recently has been reported in EBV-associated hemophagocytic lymphohistiocytosis (EBV-HLH), also known as *EBV-associated hemophagocytic syndrome*, which develops mostly in children and young adults and may be fatal. EBV also has been recently reported as a cause of pediatric acute renal failure. EBV's host range is restricted to B lymphocytes and nasopharyngeal epithelial and uterine epithelial cells; however, latent infection appears to be limited to B cells. The virus does not generally produce cytopathic effects in cells, and the viral DNA remains in a circular nonintegrated form within the cell. Lymphoblastoid cell lines infected with EBV can be cultured indefinitely in vitro. The lymphocytosis of mononucleosis is thought to result from a T-cell reaction to infected B cells. A highly sensitive real-time PCR assay is now available for detection of primary EBV infection and infectious mononucleosis.

Treatment of acute disease is largely supportive, although the EBV DNA polymerase is sensitive to acyclovir and ganciclovir, which decrease viral replication in tissue culture. No vaccine is currently available against EBV, but research is ongoing toward developing a cytotoxic T-cell–based vaccine.

Bharadwaj M, Moss DJ. Epstein-Barr virus vaccine: a cytotoxic T-cell-based approach. *Expert Rev Vaccines.* 2002;1:467–476.

Imashuku S, Kuriyama K, Sakai R, et al. Treatment of Epstein-Barr virus-associated hemophagocytic lymphohistiocytosis (EBV-HLH) in young adults: a report from the HLH study center. *Med Pediatr Oncol.* 2003;41:103–109.

Pitetti RD, Laus S, Wadowsky RM. Clinical evaluation of a quantitative real time polymerase chain reaction assay for diagnosis of primary Epstein-Barr virus infection in children. *Pediatr Infect Dis J.* 2003;22:736–739.

Tsai JD, Lee HC, Lin CC, et al. Epstein-Barr virus-associated acute renal failure: diagnosis, treatment, and follow-up. *Pediatr Nephrol.* 2003;18(7):667–674.

Influenza

See Chapter 13 for a discussion of influenza and immunization.

Hepatitis

Hepatitis A

Hepatitis A is usually transmitted by the oral route and may be acquired from contaminated water supplies and unwashed or poorly cooked foods. Patients at high risk (travelers to endemic areas, military personnel, drug abusers, family contacts of infected patients, and laboratory workers exposed to the virus) should be given the hepatitis A vaccine (Havrix). Many adults in the United States are already immune, so antibody testing can be performed first, followed by vaccination if antibodies are not present.

Hepatitis B

See Chapter 13 for a discussion of hepatitis B and immunization.

Hepatitis C and Other Forms of Hepatitis

Approximately 20%–40% of acute viral hepatitis cases reported in the United States are of the non-A, non-B type; of the group, the majority of cases are caused by the hepatitis C virus (HCV). Worldwide prevalence is approximately 1%. Current estimates suggest that 170,000 new cases of HCV occur annually in the United States; 50%–80% of these patients develop evidence of chronic hepatitis, and 20% of these patients develop cirrhosis. Only 6% of reported cases of hepatitis C are transfusion related. Other recognized risk factors for hepatitis C transmission include parenteral drug use, hemodialysis, and occupational exposure to blood. Although the role of sexual activity in the transmission of HCV remains to be fully elucidated, this mode is clearly not a predominant source of transmission. Of all the hepatitis viruses, HCV causes the most damage in immunocompetent hosts because of direct hepatocyte cytotoxicity and may result in cirrhosis, fulminant hepatitis, and hepatocellular carcinoma. At present, cirrhosis from HCV infection is the most common indication for liver transplantation in the United States.

A new, sensitive enzyme immunoassay has been developed for detecting and quantifying total HCV core antigen in anti-HCV-positive or anti-HCV-negative sera. Also, a 1-step PCR assay is available to detect HCV RNA and provide HCV genotyping.

Treatment of acute hepatitis C infection with interferon-α reduces the rate of acute infections converting to chronic hepatitis C infections. The current treatment of choice for chronic active hepatitis C is combination therapy with peginterferon alfa-2a or peginterferon alfa-2b and the antiviral agent ribavirin. This combination can achieve up to 80% response rates for hepatitis C genotypes 2 and 3 and approximately a 50% response rate for patients with genotype 1, cirrhosis, or nonresponse to previous treatments. Other antiviral agents, such as amantadine, have also shown some success when used in combination therapy. Management of chronic persistent hepatitis C is largely supportive, but some studies advocate prolonged therapy with peginterferon. No vaccine is currently available against HCV, but researchers are hopeful that a vaccine will soon be developed.

Chronic delta hepatitis is a severe form of chronic liver disease caused by hepatitis delta virus (hepatitis D virus) infection superimposed on chronic hepatitis B. Both interferon alfa-2a and lamivudine have been found to be beneficial in the treatment of chronic hepatitis D infection.

Hepatitis E virus is a small, non-enveloped RNA virus that is transmitted enterically and causes sporadic as well as epidemic acute viral hepatitis in many developing countries. As a superinfection in patients with preexisting chronic liver disease, hepatitis E may cause severe liver decompensation, often complicated by hepatic encephalopathy and renal failure. Acute hepatitis E in these patients has a protracted course, with high morbidity and mortality. The virus can be detected in fecal samples, using real-time quantitative PCR.

Hepatitis G virus may cause coinfection with HBV or HCV but usually does not increase their pathogenicity. GB virus-C and the hepatitis G virus (GBV-C/HGV) are variants of the same RNA flavivirus, which was recently found to be a lymphotropic virus that replicates primarily in the spleen and bone marrow.

Transfusion-transmitted virus (TTV) is a virus identified in a small percentage of patients with non-A, G posttransfusion hepatitis. In some patients, the virus causes coinfection with hepatitis C. TTV DNA is common in high-risk populations, such as patients with hemophilia, those on hemodialysis, and intravenous drug abusers. TTV has recently been implicated alone, as well as in coinfection with Epstein-Barr virus, as a potential cause of 30%–50% of cases of lymphoma and Hodgkin disease.

> Delwaide J. Postexposure management of hepatitis A, B or C: treatment, postexposure prophylaxis and recommendations. *Acta Gastroenterol Belg.* 2003;66:250–254.
>
> Farci P, Roskams T, Chessa L, et al. Long-term benefit of interferon alpha therapy of chronic hepatitis D: regression of advanced hepatic fibrosis. *Gastroenterology.* 2004;126:1740–1749.
>
> Fried MW, Hadziyannis SJ. Treatment of chronic hepatitis C infection with peginterferons plus ribavirin. *Semin Liver Dis.* 2004;24 suppl 2:47–54.
>
> Garbuglia AR, Iezzi T, Capobianchi MR, et al. Detection of TT virus in lymph node biopsies of B-cell lymphoma and Hodgkin's disease, and its association with EBV infection. *Int J Immunopathol Pharmacol.* 2003;16:109–118.
>
> Mackiewicz V, Dussaix E, Le Petitcorps MF, et al. Detection of hepatitis A virus RNA in saliva. *J Clin Microbiol.* 2004;42:4329–4331.
>
> Orru G, Masia G, Orru G, et al. Detection and quantitation of hepatitis E virus in human feces by real-time quantitative PCR. *J Virol Methods.* 2004;118:77–82.
>
> Santantonio T. Treatment of acute hepatitis C. *Curr Pharm Des.* 2004;10:2077–2080.
>
> Tang YW, Li H, Roberto A, et al. Detection of hepatitis C virus by a user-developed reverse transcriptase-PCR and use of amplification products for subsequent genotyping. *J Clin Virol.* 2004;31:148–152.
>
> Thomas DL, Astemborski J, Rai RM, et al. The natural history of hepatitis C virus infection: host, viral, and environmental factors. *JAMA.* 2000;284:450–456.
>
> Valcavi P, Medici MC, Casula F, et al. Evaluation of a total hepatitis C virus (HCV) core antigen assay for the detection of antigenaemia in anti-HCV positive individuals. *J Med Virol.* 2004;73:397–403.
>
> Vrolijk JM, de Knegt RJ, Veldt BJ, et al. The treatment of hepatitis C: history, presence and future. *Neth J Med.* 2004;62:76–82.
>
> Wang L, Zhuang H. Hepatitis E: an overview and recent advances in vaccine research. *World J Gastroenterol.* 2004;10:2157–2162.

Human Papillomavirus

Human papillomavirus (HPV) infection is highly prevalent and is closely associated with condylomata (genital warts), cervical intraepithelial neoplasia, cervical cancer (95% of cervical cancers contain HPV DNA), conjunctival intraepithelial neoplasia, and some cases of head and neck squamous cell carcinoma. A recent review suggests that HPV has a possible etiologic role in some cases of lung adenocarcinoma as well. More than 50% of all persons are infected with HPV during their lifetimes, either via intrauterine or sexually transmitted infection. HPV can be detected with PCR assay techniques, and women at high risk for HPV should receive HPV testing at the time of the Papanicolaou test. Vaccines to prevent HPV infection and its sequelae have recently become available. HPV in association with cervical cancer is discussed further in Chapter 13.

>Chen YC, Chen JH, Richard K, et al. Lung adenocarcinoma and human papillomavirus infection. *Cancer.* 2004;101:1428–1436.
>
>Gillison ML. Human papillomavirus-associated head and neck cancer is a distinct epidemiologic, clinical, and molecular entity. *Semin Oncol.* 2004;31:744–754.
>
>Jansen KU, Shaw AR. Human papillomavirus vaccines and prevention of cervical cancer. *Annu Rev Med.* 2004;55:319–331.

Severe Acute Respiratory Syndrome

Severe acute respiratory syndrome (SARS) recently emerged as a rapidly contagious infectious disease with significant morbidity and mortality. A 114-day epidemic in late 2002 and early 2003 swept through 29 countries on 5 continents and affected a reported 8422 people, causing 916 deaths (case fatality rate of 11%). The adverse impact on travel and commerce around the world, particularly in Asia, was enormous.

SARS originated in the Guangdong Province of China in November 2002. Early in the outbreak, the infection was transmitted primarily through household contacts and in health care facilities. Contaminated sewage was found to be responsible for an outbreak in a housing facility in Hong Kong, which affected more than 300 residents. The infection was rapidly spread by air travel to other countries. Mainland China, Hong Kong, and Singapore accounted for 87% of all cases and 84% of all deaths. The mean incubation period was 6.4 days, and the duration between onset of symptoms and hospitalization was 3 to 5 days. The incubation period allowed asymptomatic air travelers to spread the disease globally. The number of individuals infected by each case was estimated to be 2.7. A novel coronavirus (CoV) was identified as the cause of SARS, most likely originating from human contact with wild animals, and the genome of SARS was sequenced within months, after a global report on SARS was issued by the World Health Organization. Aggressive quarantine measures successfully terminated the first emergence of SARS.

The primary clinical features of SARS include persistent fever, chills, myalgia, malaise, dry cough, headache, and dyspnea. Less common symptoms include sputum production, sore throat, nasal congestion, dizziness, nausea, vomiting, and diarrhea. There is a spectrum of severity and rate of progression in SARS, and the stages of viral replication, inflammatory pneumonitis, and residual pulmonary fibrosis are clinically nonspecific. Secondary infections are a common complication in patients with prolonged hospitalization and those on mechanical ventilation.

Older patients may present with malaise, poor appetite, falls, and delirium, often without the typical febrile response. The clinical illness is similar to many acute respiratory infections, although a large proportion of patients experience a rapid deterioration with respiratory distress toward the end of the second week of illness.

The worldwide case fatality rate is 11% (range 7% to 27%) for the most severely affected regions. Several adverse prognostic factors have been identified, including advanced age and the presence of comorbidity. No case fatality has been reported in children, and the outcome in pediatric patients appears to be good.

Common laboratory features include lymphopenia with depletion of CD4 and CD8 lymphocytes; thrombocytopenia; prolonged activated partial thromboplastin time; and elevated levels of alanine transaminase, lactate dehydrogenase, and creatine kinase. The constellation of compatible, nonspecific clinical and laboratory findings, together with characteristic radiological findings, and the lack of clinical response to broad-spectrum antibiotics should suggest the possibility of SARS.

Measurement of serum viral RNA levels by real-time PCR assay detects 80% of SARS cases in the first week of the illness, but the detection rates drop to 75% and 42% on day 7 and day 14, respectively. The sensitivity for urine, nasopharyngeal aspirates, and stool specimens has been reported to be 42%, 68%, and 97%, respectively, on day 14 of the illness. However, positive serology for confirmation of SARS may take up to 28 days to reach a detection rate above 90%.

The pharmacologic treatment of SARS is controversial and mostly anecdotal. Most patients with suspected SARS should initially be treated with broad-spectrum antibiotics before proceeding to SARS antiviral therapy. Although now considered ineffective, ribavirin was used extensively in Hong Kong for the treatment of SARS. Recent retrospective data suggest that the use of Kaletra (ritonavir and lopinavir), a combination of protease inhibitors, could decrease mortality and improve clinical outcomes.

Anecdotal experience supports the use of corticosteroids, at least in treating the subset of "critical SARS" patients, who display persistent clinical instability or deterioration and progressive radiographic deterioration on high-resolution CT scanning. A retrospective study of 72 probable SARS patients revealed that patients receiving pulsed methylprednisolone had reduced oxygen requirement, better radiographic outcome, and less likelihood of requiring rescue pulse steroid therapy. Lower doses of oral corticosteroids, as initial therapy for SARS, have resulted in good clinical outcomes. Other drug treatments, such as convalescence serum and plasmapheresis, have also been tried in critically ill patients with SARS.

Chan KS, Zheng JP, Mok YW, et al. SARS: prognosis, outcome and sequelae. *Respirology.* 2003;8 suppl:S36–40.

Chan-Yeung M, Xu RH. SARS: epidemiology. *Respirology.* 2003;8 suppl:S9–14.

Cheng VC, Tang BS, Wu AK, et al. Medical treatment of viral pneumonia including SARS in immunocompetent adult. *J Infect.* 2004;49:262–273.

Hui DS, Chan MC, Wu AK, et al. Severe acute respiratory syndrome (SARS): epidemiology and clinical features. *Postgrad Med J.* 2004;80:373–381.

Hui DS, Wong PC, Wang C. SARS: clinical features and diagnosis. *Respirology.* 2003;8 suppl: S20–24.

Lam WK, Zhong NS, Tan WC. Overview on SARS in Asia and the world. *Respirology.* 2003;8 suppl:S2–5.

Lau YL. SARS: future research and vaccine. *Paediatr Respir Rev.* 2004;5:300–303.

Leung CW, Chiu WK. Clinical picture, diagnosis, treatment and outcome of severe acute respiratory syndrome (SARS) in children. *Paediatr Respir Rev.* 2004;5:275–288.

Nicholls J, Dong XP, Jiang G, et al. SARS: clinical virology and pathogenesis. *Respirology.* 2003;8 suppl:S6–8.

Stadler K, Masignani V, Eickmann M, et al. SARS—beginning to understand a new virus. *Nat Rev Microbiol.* 2003;1:209–218.

Tsang K, Zhong NS. SARS: pharmacotherapy. *Respirology.* 2003;8 suppl:S25–30.

Vijayanand P, Wilkins E, Woodhead M. Severe acute respiratory syndrome (SARS): a review. *Clin Med.* 2004;4:152–160.

Zhong NS, Wong GW. Epidemiology of severe acute respiratory syndrome (SARS): adults and children. *Paediatr Respir Rev.* 2004;5:270–274.

Other viral infectious diseases have featured prominently in the media as well as the medical literature in recent years, including hantavirus, Ebola virus, and the West Nile virus. The hantavirus is a highly virulent respiratory pathogen transmitted from rodent carriers, particularly deer mice. The resulting hantavirus pulmonary syndrome is manifested by pulmonary edema, respiratory failure, and shock. With no specific treatment available thus far, it is associated with a mortality rate of 40%–50%. An outbreak among American Indians in the southwest United States was reported in 1993, and since then the virus has been isolated in all western states and many eastern states.

Ebola virus is endemic in some regions of Africa and causes Ebola hemorrhagic fever, which often includes respiratory involvement and a very high mortality. Health care workers are at an increased risk of illness when caring for infected patients. After the 1-week incubation period, the infected patient develops fatigue, malaise, headache, backache, vomiting, and diarrhea. Within 1 week later, a hemorrhagic papular rash appears over the entire body. Hemorrhaging generally occurs from the gastrointestinal tract, causing the patient to bleed from both the mouth and the rectum. Mortality is high, nearly 90%, and is usually due to septic shock.

The West Nile virus is a flavivirus, similar to Japanese encephalitis virus, and is transmitted by mosquito vector. It was first discovered in 1937, and since 1999, there has been an increasing incidence of infection in many regions of the United States during summer months. As of July 2004, the infection had spread to 46 states. The illness may vary from a flu-like syndrome to meningitis or encephalitis. Ocular findings may include multifocal choroiditis, vitritis, intraretinal hemorrhages, iritis, optic neuritis, branch retinal artery occlusions, and chorioretinal scarring.

Bakri SJ, Kaiser PK. Ocular manifestations of West Nile virus. *Curr Opin Ophthalmol.* 2004;15:537–540.

Clement JP. Hantavirus. *Antiviral Res.* 2003;57:121–127.

Feldmann H, Jones S, Klenk HD, et al. Ebola virus: from discovery to vaccine. *Nat Rev Immunol.* 2003;3:677–685.

Sampathkumar P. West Nile virus: epidemiology, clinical presentation, diagnosis, and prevention. *Mayo Clin Proc.* 2003;78:1137–1143.

Acquired Immunodeficiency Syndrome

During the 1980s, AIDS emerged as a major public health problem. AIDS was originally described in 1981, when *Pneumocystis carinii* pneumonia (PCP) and Kaposi sarcoma were noted to occur in homosexual men and intravenous drug abusers. Since then, the number of cases has increased exponentially. In 1983, it was discovered that AIDS was caused by the retrovirus HIV (human immunodeficiency virus). Subsequently, it became evident that HIV caused a spectrum of disease, including an asymptomatic carrier state, the AIDS-related complex (ARC), and AIDS itself.

As of the end of 2003, an estimated 929,985 AIDS cases in the United States have been reported to the CDC. The number of adult and adolescent AIDS cases totaled 920,566; of these cases, 749,887 were in males and 170,679 were in females; 9419 cases were estimated in children younger than age 13. The total cumulative number of deaths of persons reported with AIDS was 524,060. It is estimated that between 850,000 and 950,000 Americans are currently infected with HIV, with more than 25% of these persons unaware that they are infected. More than 40,000 new cases of HIV infection occur each year in the United States. Approximately 70% of these new cases are males, and half of them are younger than 25 years. On the positive side, improved antiretroviral therapy in recent years has resulted in a significant decline in the number of AIDS cases in the United States and a 70% reduction in deaths due to AIDS since 1995. Further, AIDS is no longer the leading cause of death in young adults in the United States.

Worldwide, AIDS continues to take a devastating toll, particularly in countries of sub–Saharan Africa and in Asian nations with large, impoverished populations. According to the Joint United Nations Program on HIV/AIDS, as of the end of 2003, 37.8 million people are estimated to be living with HIV/AIDS. Approximately two thirds of those infected live in sub–Saharan Africa and 20% live in Asia and the Pacific. Of these, 2.1 million are children younger than age 15. An estimated 28 million people have died from AIDS since the epidemic began, including 12 million women and 5.5 million children younger than age 15. In 2003 alone, AIDS caused the deaths of an estimated 2.9 million people, including 490,000 children younger than age 15. Women are increasingly affected by HIV: approximately 50%, or 19.2 million, of the estimated 37.8 million adults now living with HIV or AIDS worldwide are women. The overwhelming majority of people with HIV, approximately 95% of the global total, are in developing countries. It is estimated that 16,000 new infections occur worldwide each day. More than 50% of the infections are in young adults between the ages of 15 and 25. Only 10% of the world's HIV-infected people know that they are infected. More than 13 million children have been orphaned because of HIV infection of 1 or both of their parents.

Etiology and Pathogenesis

AIDS is caused by infection with HIV (HIV-1), previously known as the human T-cell lymphotropic virus type III (HTLV-III), lymphadenopathy-associated virus, and AIDS-related virus. Thus far, there are 9 known serotypes of HIV-1 group M, and 1 of HIV-1 groups O and N. In the United States, HIV group M, serotype B is the most common form of HIV. Another human T-cell lymphotropic virus, HIV-2, has been isolated from West Africans and is associated with AIDS as well. HIV-2 is closely related to simian immunodeficiency virus.

HIV belongs to a family of viruses known as *retroviruses.* A retrovirus encodes its genetic information in RNA and uses a unique viral enzyme called *reverse transcriptase* to copy its genome into DNA. Other members of this retrovirus family include the human T-cell lymphotropic retrovirus type I, which can cause adult T-cell leukemia and chronic progressive myelopathy with atrophy of the spinal cord. HTLV-II is associated with hairy cell leukemia.

HIV preferentially infects T cells, especially T-helper (CD4$^+$) lymphocytes. The virus infects mature T cells in vitro, although other cells can serve as targets. CD4 is the phenotypic marker for this subset and is identified by monoclonal antibodies OKT4 and Leu 3.

The hallmark of the immunodeficiency in AIDS is a depletion of the CD4$^+$ helper/inducer T lymphocytes. HIV selectively infects these lymphocytes as well as macrophages; with HIV replication, the helper T cell is killed. Because of the central role of the helper T lymphocyte in the immune response, loss of this subset results in a profound immune deficiency, leading to the life-threatening opportunistic infections indicative of AIDS. This selective depletion of CD4$^+$ helper T cells leads to the characteristic inverted CD4$^+$/ CD8$^+$ ratio (also known as *T4/T8 ratio*). Years may pass between the initial HIV infection and the development of these immune abnormalities.

In addition to the cellular immune deficiency, patients with AIDS have abnormalities of B-cell function. These patients fail to mount an antibody response to novel T cell–dependent B-cell challenges, although they have B-cell hyperfunction with polyclonal B-cell activation, hypergammaglobulinemia, and circulating immune complexes. This B-cell hyperfunction may be a direct consequence of HIV infection: studies have demonstrated that polyclonal activation can be induced in vitro by adding HIV to B cells.

HIV has also been documented to infect the brains of patients with AIDS. It is thought that HIV infection of the brain is responsible for the HIV encephalopathy syndrome. HIV-infected cells in the brain have generally been identified as macrophages.

Clinical Syndromes

The clinical syndrome of AIDS consists of recurrent severe opportunistic infections or unusual neoplasms. In 1982, the CDC published an original case definition of AIDS as the presence of a reliably diagnosed disease at least moderately indicative of an underlying cellular immune deficiency (Kaposi sarcoma in a patient younger than 60 years, PCP, or other opportunistic infection) and the absence of known causes of an underlying immune deficiency or of any other stage of resistance reported to be associated with the disease (immunosuppressive therapy, lymphoreticular malignancy). This original surveillance case definition has been modified by the CDC as new data have become available. HIV-related primary encephalopathy and HIV-associated nephropathy are also frequently encountered in HIV-infected patients. HIV-associated nephropathy, which is a glomerulosclerosis, is the most common cause of chronic renal failure in HIV patients and occurs almost exclusively in blacks. It is now clear that this disorder is caused by a direct infection of renal cells by HIV.

AIDS is now diagnosed when a person presents with 1 or more of the indicator diseases outlined in the following list. These diseases are included in the CDC's current AIDS surveillance case definition and are indicative of an underlying cellular immunodeficiency; presentations with PCP or with Kaposi sarcoma are common.

- candidiasis of bronchi, trachea, or lungs
- candidiasis, esophageal
- cervical cancer, invasive
- coccidioidomycosis, disseminated or extrapulmonary
- cryptococcosis, extrapulmonary
- cryptosporidiosis, chronic intestinal (>1 month's duration)
- cytomegalovirus disease (other than liver, spleen, or nodes)
- herpes simplex: chronic ulcer(s) (>1 month's duration); or bronchitis, pneumonitis, or esophagitis
- histoplasmosis, disseminated or extrapulmonary
- HIV encephalopathy
- isosporiasis, chronic intestinal (>1 month's duration)
- Kaposi sarcoma
- lymphoma, Burkitt (or equivalent term)
- lymphoma, immunoblastic (or equivalent term)
- lymphoma, primary in brain
- *Mycobacterium avium* complex or *M kansasii,* disseminated or extrapulmonary
- *M tuberculosis,* any site (pulmonary or extrapulmonary)
- PCP
- pneumonia, recurrent
- progressive multifocal leukoencephalopathy
- *Salmonella* septicemia, recurrent
- toxoplasmosis of brain
- wasting syndrome due to HIV

AIDS represents the most severe end of the spectrum of HIV infection. Acute infection with HIV often manifests as a transient mononucleosis-like syndrome. This syndrome has been called *primary HIV infection,* or *retroviral syndrome,* the typical symptoms of which are fever, fatigue, weight loss, myalgias, headache, pharyngitis, and nausea. Primary HIV infection is diagnosed when a positive result on the plasma HIV RNA test and a negative result on the Western blot assay are obtained on the same day. To confirm seroconversion, patients should have a repeat HIV antibody test 2–3 weeks after resolution of symptoms.

Patients may then enter a prolonged asymptomatic carrier state (the majority of HIV-infected patients in the United States are in this condition). There is also a syndrome of persistent generalized lymphadenopathy, which is associated with depleted T-helper lymphocytes and HIV infection. Lymphadenopathy with other signs and symptoms has commonly been called the *lymphadenopathy syndrome* or *ARC.* Constitutional symptoms in patients with ARC include fever, weight loss, chronic diarrhea, oral thrush, and lymphadenopathy. Although these patients have immunologic defects similar to those found in patients with AIDS, those with ARC have not developed 1 of the AIDS-defining opportunistic infections or unusual neoplasms. The CDC has classified HIV infection into the 3 groups outlined in Table 1-7. The shaded boxes illustrate clinical conditions now defined as AIDS.

Seroepidemiology

Antibodies to HIV can be detected in HIV-infected persons. Such screening is now performed with commercially available kits, all of which are based on an ELISA using whole disrupted HIV antigens. The ELISA test for HIV antibodies is sensitive (99%) and specific (99%). However, false-negative results can occur, especially in the first weeks after HIV infection. False-positive ELISA results are also possible; thus, the ELISA must yield positive results twice and be confirmed by Western blot analysis or immunofluorescence assay before a patient is said to have antibodies to HIV. Persons with antibodies to HIV should be considered infectious for HIV. Currently, HIV p24 antigen testing or HIV-1 RNA analysis can be performed. These tests yield positive results earlier than anti-HIV antibody tests do.

Seroepidemiologic studies conducted in high-risk populations revealed an increasing prevalence of HIV infection, from almost nil before 1979 to as high as 70% by 1988. The rate of increase of HIV infection slowed during the 1990s in the United States but accelerated in Africa and other developing regions. In the past, 100% of patients with HIV infection ultimately developed AIDS, but this percentage is gradually falling as many patients respond to HAART, resulting in a corresponding decrease in the incidence of opportunistic infections. The median incubation period between acquisition of HIV infection and the development of AIDS is now estimated to be more than 10 years.

Modes of Transmission

Modes of transmission of HIV infection are

- sexual contact
- intravenous drug use
- transfusion
- perinatal transmission from an infected mother to her child

There have been no documented cases of transmission by casual contact. Furthermore, although HIV infection may be transmitted by blood or blood products, the risk of transmission by accidental needle stick appears quite low (<0.5%). Studies of nonsexual household contacts of patients with AIDS have revealed that these people are at minimal or possibly no risk of infection with HIV.

At the beginning of the AIDS epidemic, almost all the cases were confined to gay men in the United States, but that proportion has been steadily decreasing, with corresponding increases in the number of cases in intravenous drug users and in patients infected through heterosexual contact. Furthermore, in Africa the male/female ratio is 1:1, and epidemiologic data have suggested that the disease is transmitted predominantly by

Table 1-7 Revised Classification System for HIV Infection and Expanded AIDS Surveillance Case Definition for Adolescents and Adults*

	Clinical Categories		
	A	B	C
		Symptomatic,	
	Asymptomatic,	not A or C	AIDS-indicator
CD4+ CELL CATEGORIES	or PGL†	conditions	conditions
1. ≥500/mm³	A1	B1	C1
2. 200–499/mm³	A2	B2	C2
3. <200/mm³	A3	B3	C3

*The shaded cells illustrate the expansion of the AIDS surveillance case definition. Persons with AIDS-indicator conditions (category C) are currently reportable to the health department in every state and US territory. In addition to persons with clinical category C conditions (categories C1, C2, and C3), persons with CD4+ lymphocyte counts of less than 200/mm³ (category A3 or B3) are also reportable as AIDS cases in the United States.
†PGL = persistent generalized lymphadenopathy. Clinical category A includes acute (primary) HIV infection.

heterosexual activity, parenteral exposure to blood transfusion and unsterilized needles, and perinatal exposure from infected mothers to their newborns.

Prognosis and Treatment

AIDS is still considered an incurable and eventually fatal disease. Nevertheless, infected patients are living much longer and have had better quality of life than infected patients in previous years, because of significant improvements in antiviral therapy. For that reason, AIDS is now managed more as a chronic illness rather than as a terminal disease. The risk factors that are most closely associated with decreased survival in patients with AIDS are reduced CD4 levels, length of time since diagnosis, low serum albumin levels (<0.30 g/L), previous opportunistic infections, high viral load, and new "clinical progression" events. CD4 counts are good predictors of risk of opportunistic infection. Plasma HIV RNA levels are even better predictors of disease progression and are the best single predictors of response to therapy.

It is now well established that superinfection with a second strain or clade of HIV-1 virus occurs in humans, often following a period of immunologic stability. Detection of an increasing number of viral DNA, which results from infection of a cell by 2 or more HIV clades, suggests that superinfection occurs more frequently than previously thought. The second virus (from a different clade or the same clade as the primary virus) can superinfect cells well after the initial infection, and this is associated with rapid viral rebound and immunologic decline. Primary infection with a specific HIV clade appears to provide inadequate immune protection against superinfection with a different clade or the same clade.

Recommended laboratory studies with a newly diagnosed case of HIV infection often include complete blood count with manual differential, CD4 count, HIV viral load testing (RNA level), electrolytes, renal and liver function tests, urinalysis, PPD (tuberculosis test), anergy panel, and serologic tests for syphilis, hepatitis B virus and HCV, toxoplasma,

CMV, and VZV. Female patients should undergo a Papanicolaou test because of the high risk of invasive cervical cancer in HIV-infected persons. The recommended vaccinations in HIV-positive patients are diphtheria/tetanus (every 5 years), inactivated polio, measles, *Pneumococcus* (every 5 years), hepatitis B virus, hepatitis A virus (especially if the patient is HCV-positive), and influenza virus (yearly). *H influenzae* B vaccine is optional.

In 1986, the drug *zidovudine* (also known as azidothymidine, AZT, or Retrovir), a synthetic analogue of thymidine, became available for the treatment of AIDS. Zidovudine is incorporated into DNA by the DNA polymerase (reverse transcriptase) of HIV and prevents further viral DNA synthesis. In the early AIDS treatment trials, zidovudine decreased mortality among patients with AIDS and ARC and decreased the number of episodes of opportunistic infections. The early zidovudine trials also showed that when symptomatic HIV-infected persons with ARC and asymptomatic HIV-infected persons with CD4 counts less than $500/mm^3$ were treated with zidovudine, progression of the disease to later stages (ie, AIDS) was delayed. Furthermore, the data showed improved short-term survival and improved CD4 counts. The major limiting side effect of this therapy was bone marrow suppression. Currently, zidovudine and other nucleoside analogues are used only in combination therapy, because of the rapid emergence of HIV resistance in patients treated with a nucleoside analogue alone.

Some of the other nucleoside analogue reverse transcriptase inhibitors approved as combined therapy for HIV infection are *didanosine* (ddI, Videx), *zalcitabine* (ddC, Hivid), *lamivudine* (3TC, Epivir), and *stavudine* (d4T, Zerit). These drugs have in vitro activity against HIV similar to that of zidovudine. The primary benefit of these drugs over zidovudine is reduced bone marrow toxicity, which makes them more useful in the setting of concurrent leukopenia or use of other marrow-toxic drugs (eg, ganciclovir). Lamivudine is available as a combination drug with zidovudine (Combivir). *Abacavir* (Ziagen) was the first clinically available guanosine analogue reverse transcriptase inhibitor. Trizivir is a combination drug containing abacavir, lamivudine, and zidovudine. Other newer nucleoside analogues include *adefovir* (Preveon), *emtricitabine* (FTC, Emtriva), and *amdoxovir* (DAPD). They are active against isolates resistant to older nucleoside analogues. *Tenofovir* (PMPA, Viread) is a newer *nucleotide* reverse transcriptase inhibitor (NtRTI) that allows for once-daily dosing and has been well tolerated in clinical trials to date, without evidence of long-term toxicity. Truvada is a combination drug containing emtricitabine and tenofovir.

The major treatment-limiting toxicity of didanosine is acute pancreatitis. This agent's use is therefore contraindicated in the setting of alcoholism or prior pancreatitis. In addition, didanosine should not be used concurrently with pentamidine. Zalcitabine may cause rapidly progressive, severe peripheral neuropathy, which may not be reversible upon discontinuing therapy. Lamivudine has been associated with neutropenia and peripheral neuropathy in a small percentage of patients. Stavudine causes peripheral neuropathy in 15%–20% of patients. Lactic acidosis is a potential adverse effect of several agents in this class.

Several non-nucleoside reverse transcriptase inhibitors (NNRTIs)—*nevirapine* (Viramune), *delavirdine* (Rescriptor), and *atevirdine*—are available, but most of them also share the disadvantage of rapid emergence of viral resistance. Therefore, they are currently used in combination therapy. A newer NNRTI, *efavirenz* (Sustiva), is taken once daily, has excellent activity against HIV, and has fewer side effects than other NNRTIs. This agent has become a cornerstone of antiretroviral therapy, and its efficacy over other antiretrovirals has been established in many clinical trials. Efavirenz is well tolerated in most patients, and the reported adverse effects are dizziness, insomnia, abnormal dreams, and rash. Emivirine (Coactinon), capravirine, calanolide, etravirine, KM-1, and TMC 125 are new investigational NNRTIs. Capravirine has a unique resistance profile. Although single mutations allow resistance to the older NNRTIs, HIV must undergo multiple mutations to achieve resistance to capravirine. Capravirine has potent antiviral activity, even in patients previously treated with other antiviral agents. TMC 125 is now involved in multiple controlled trials, and in 1 study, it possessed such initial antiviral potency as a single agent that it was equivalent to a 5-drug, triple-class antiretroviral regimen.

The protease inhibitors are a class of antiretroviral drugs that prevent the cleavage of precursor proteins into viral elements needed for viral assembly, thereby resulting in the production of nonfunctional, noninfectious virions. These agents are used primarily in multidrug therapy along with 1 or more nucleoside analogues. The protease inhibitors currently approved for the treatment of HIV infection include *saquinavir* (Invirase, Fortovase), *indinavir* (Crixivan), *ritonavir* (Norvir), *nelfinavir* (Viracept), *amprenavir* (Agenerase), *atazanavir* (Reyataz), and a *lopinavir/ritonavir combination* (Kaletra). *Fosamprenavir* (Lexiva, Telzir) is a well-tolerated oral prodrug of amprenavir and is indicated as combination therapy for HIV-infected patients who have not previously received other antiretroviral therapy. *Tiprinavir* (Aptivus) and *brecanavir* are the first of a new subclass of antiretroviral drugs, the nonpeptidic protease inhibitors (NPPIs). They are highly selective for the HIV protease enzyme and demonstrate potent in vitro activity against wild-type strains of HIV-1 and HIV-2. In combination therapy with low-dose ritonavir and efavirenz, tiprinavir is highly effective against HIV isolates resistant to other protease inhibitors. Potential adverse effects of protease inhibitors include hyperlipidemia, pancreatitis, renal failure, lipodystrophy, rhabdomyolysis, and hepatitis.

Fusion inhibitors are a new class of investigational antiviral agents that block fusion of HIV with the human cell by blocking the function of the gp120 envelope glycoprotein. *Enfuvirtide* (T-20, Fuzeon) was approved by the FDA for treatment of HIV infection in 2003. Enfuvirtide provides clinically relevant improvements in CD4 cell counts and reductions in HIV viral load across all subgroups of treatment-experienced patients studied, including those taking few or no other active drugs. *T-1249* and *AMD-3100* are investigational second-generation peptide fusion inhibitors that appear to be very effective in reducing HIV viral load in early studies.

Some other new experimental classes of antiretroviral drugs that are currently under investigation include the entry, coreceptor, integrase, and p7 nucleocapsid zinc finger inhibitors; and the coreceptor CXCR4 and CCR5 antagonists, as well as potential inhibitors of genome transport to the nucleus, HIV interaction with nuclear pores, and virus budding.

In response to the extremely high prices of many AIDS drugs, several states have established AIDS drug assistance programs. Also, many AIDS drug manufacturers now offer patient assistance programs to help patients locate sources for reimbursement or provide drugs free to patients who have no means of obtaining them.

Multidrug therapy, or HAART, is now the standard of care and usually involves drug regimens with 3 or more agents. To prevent early drug resistance, patients should be given all drugs simultaneously rather than sequentially. Most of the recent clinical trials recommend a drug regimen that includes a potent protease inhibitor in combination with 2 nucleoside analogue reverse transcriptase inhibitors or 2 protease inhibitors combined with 1 or 2 nucleoside analogue reverse transcriptase inhibitors. Recently, some alternative treatment regimens have omitted protease inhibitors *(protease-sparing regimen)*. This is a departure from the standard treatment, which has included protease inhibitors since their introduction in the 1990s. Protease inhibitors remain among the most effective and important treatments developed, but some persons experience significant problems while using them, including cross-resistance and intolerance. Protease-sparing regimens such as abacavir/AZT/3TC and drug combinations that include efavirenz appear to be as effective as regimens that contain protease inhibitors.

HAART has been shown to result in dramatic reduction of HIV viral load, increased CD4 cell counts, delay of disease progression, reduction in the number of opportunistic infections, decreased number of hospitalizations, and prolonged survival. Some statistics show up to an 82% decline in the number of opportunistic infections in patients on HAART. These advantages are translating into improved survival and enhanced quality of life for HIV-infected patients. It is interesting to note that the number of AIDS cases in the United States peaked in 1993 and has been gradually decreasing since then. The HIV mortality rate has declined more than 70% since 1995, mostly because of HAART. Just in the 2-year period from 1995 to 1997, the AIDS mortality rate decreased from 29.4 to 8.8 per 100 person-years. Despite the high cost of antiretroviral medications, it is still less expensive to treat HIV-infected patients with HAART and prevent them from developing AIDS than it is to provide the extensive care required once they develop AIDS.

Unfortunately, the benefits of HAART have not reached the 42 million HIV-infected patients in the developing world. The number of AIDS cases and the AIDS-related mortality rate continue to rise relentlessly in these regions, partially because of the socioeconomic barriers to expensive therapy.

At present, the most common treatment end point or goal of HAART is reduction of HIV RNA levels, preferably to undetectable levels (<500 copies/mL). In some studies, HAART reduced HIV RNA to undetectable levels in up to 78% of patients. Baseline levels should be checked before the initiation of or change in antiretroviral therapy, again at 1 month after treatment begins to show efficacy, and then every 3 or 4 months. Available HIV RNA assays include branched DNA (Multiplex) and PCR (Amplicor HIV-1 Monitor). Although both tests provide similar information, concentrations of HIV RNA obtained with the PCR test are approximately 2 times higher than those obtained by the branched DNA method. Thus, for consistency, all HIV RNA testing in a single patient should be obtained via the same assay. New assays are now available for monitoring drug levels of most of the antiretroviral agents. Also, detection of specific mutations for drug resistance helps guide therapy for multidrug-resistant HIV infections.

Discontinuation of HAART after 1 year of successful treatment is usually followed by a rapid rebound of viral load. Viral antigen quickly returns to undetectable levels following reintroduction of HAART. For patients in whom HAART fails because of drug resistance, some recent studies have offered alternative aggressive salvage therapy regimens that use

5 or more agents. HIV drug sensitivity testing is now available for most of the approved antiretroviral agents and should be performed in patients with suspected drug-resistant infections. In some patients, HAART is interrupted because of drug toxicity.

In recent years, drug resistance has emerged as a significant problem in the treatment of HIV infection. HAART does not result in long-term suppression of HIV replication in 20%–50% of treatment-naive patients and in up to 50%–70% of treatment-experienced patients. In the majority of patients with viral rebound, mutations of drug resistance are detected. New HIV infections through transmission of drug-resistant strains to patients who have never been exposed to antiretroviral therapy are increasingly reported. Also, recent reports correlate new infections by drug-resistant HIV with suboptimal treatment response.

The immunomodulators are a diverse group of drugs and immunologic adjuvants that are being evaluated for their efficacy in enhancing the host immune response to HIV and related opportunistic infections. They include agents that enhance or stimulate T-cell and macrophage response: ditiocarb, ampligen, CD4-IgG, human granulocyte colony stimulating factor, sargramostim, lentinan, levamisol, thymosin-α_1, and thymic humoral factor.

Some of these agents induce humoral as well as cellular immune responses, such as interleukin-2 and zinc replacement therapy. Other drugs, like the virostatics, inhibit viral replication and include such diverse drugs as β-interferon, interleukin-10, hydroxyurea, thalidomide, mycophenolic acid, leflunomide and rapamycin (which are currently used for other therapeutic indications), and other new experimental drugs. They employ multiple novel mechanisms of action to suppress HIV replication by targeting host cellular proteins that are not susceptible to mutation. Therefore, drug resistance may be less of a problem with these agents.

These immunomodulators have been primarily used as a supplement to antiretroviral agents in combined therapy study protocols and have been discussed much less in the literature since the availability of HAART. *Hematopoietic agents,* such as erythropoietin and interleukin-3, enhance the proliferation of blood cells and are useful in the treatment of cytopenias. Thalidomide is also beneficial for the treatment of HIV wasting syndrome.

A small percentage of the population appears to be naturally immune to HIV infection. These persons have defective genes for CCR5, a surface receptor that HIV requires to attach to T cells. Also, approximately 50% of long-term survivors of HIV are heterozygous for the CCR5 defect. This has led to some speculation concerning the possibilities for genetic therapy, in which anti-HIV genes could be "injected" into a patient's chromosomes with a harmless viral vector. One drug company is testing a CCR5 receptor antagonist in clinical trials.

Although no highly successful HIV vaccines have been developed, clinical trials of several vaccines are in progress. Viral components, such as gp120 and gp160 envelope glycoproteins, and p17 and p24 viral antigens have been incorporated into vaccines that generate limited immune protection. One study demonstrated improved CD4 levels in patients with AIDS given recombinant envelope glycoprotein gp160 vaccine. Two DNA vaccines are currently being investigated. HIV-1 delta 4 is a vaccine in development that uses a mutated form of the virus. However, there is reluctance to use vaccines made up of whole inactivated virions or live attenuated HIV because of the perceived possible risk of transmitting the infection through the vaccine. Another obstacle for vaccine development is the need to provide protection for the 10 or so known subtypes of HIV now in existence around the world as well as the new mutations that continue to arise.

Many health care providers who have been exposed occupationally to HIV have used zidovudine prophylactically immediately after such exposure. The typical dosage has been 200 mg orally every 4 hours for 6 weeks. Treatment with zidovudine may reduce the risk of HIV infection following percutaneous exposure by as much as 80%. Newer recommendations by the CDC incorporate combination therapy that includes some of the newer antiviral drugs into the prophylactic regimen (Table 1-8). The combination of ritonavir + lamivudine + zidovudine has been recommended as one of the most effective prophylactic drug regimens. To provide protection against HIV transmission to babies of HIV-infected women, nevirapine and zidovudine combined therapy is safe and easy to implement for postexposure prophylaxis.

Opportunistic Infections

Treatment of Pneumocystis carinii *pneumonia*

Pneumocystis carinii pneumonia (PCP) continues to affect a significant percentage of patients with AIDS and is a major cause of mortality in these patients. (The organism was recently renamed *P jiroveci,* but all previous medical literature and textbooks refer to it as *P carinii*.) Therapy and prophylaxis for PCP have continued to improve in recent years. Recent advances in diagnosis and management, appropriately targeting chemoprophylaxis to HIV-infected patients at high clinical risk for *P jiroveci* pneumonia, and the introduction of HAART have contributed to the dramatic reduction in the incidence of PCP. Despite the success of these clinical interventions, PCP remains the most common opportunistic pneumonia and the most common life-threatening infectious complication in HIV-infected patients.

PCP is generally treated with IV trimethoprim-sulfamethoxazole (TMP-SMX—trade names Bactrim, Septra). Inhaled pentamidine prevents the recurrence of PCP (secondary prophylaxis) and appears to be efficacious for primary prophylaxis when used in patients with HIV infection and CD4 counts less than 200/mm^3. The regimen for inhaled pentamidine is generally 300 mg every 4 weeks using a nebulizer. This form of therapy avoids the toxicity of systemically administered pentamidine.

Several studies indicate that oral TMP-SMX prophylaxis is more effective than aerosolized pentamidine for PCP prophylaxis in those patients who can tolerate it. This regimen may also provide systemic prophylaxis against toxoplasmosis infection. However, adverse reactions are frequent in HIV-infected patients. Dapsone, effective for primary and secondary prophylaxis against PCP, is tolerated by most patients who develop rashes with use of TMP-SMX. A combination drug comprising dapsone and trimethoprim is currently in clinical trials for PCP prophylaxis. Primaquine, clindamycin, and atovaquone (Mepron) have been used successfully in treating PCP, but these drugs are reserved for use in patients intolerant of TMP-SMX or pentamidine, or for those with resistant infections. Judicious use of steroids may help reduce morbidity in patients with severe pulmonary inflammation that is caused by PCP. Newer agents such as echinocandins and

Table 1-8 Provisional Public Health Service Recommendations for Chemoprophylaxis After Occupational Exposure to HIV

Type of Exposure	Source Material	Antiretroviral Prophylaxis	Antiviral Regimen*
Percutaneous	**Blood** Highest risk[1]	Recommend	AZT plus 3TC plus IDV
	Increased risk[2]	Recommend	AZT plus 3TC ± IDV
	No increased risk[3]	Offer	AZT plus 3TC
	Fluid containing visible blood, other potentially infectious fluid,[4] or tissue	Offer	AZT plus 3TC
	Other body fluid (urine)	Not offer	
Mucous membrane	**Blood**	Offer	AZT plus 3TC ± IDV
	Fluid containing visible blood, other potentially infectious fluid,[4] or tissue	Offer	AZT ± 3TC
	Other body fluid (urine)	Not offer	
Skin, increased risk	**Blood**	Offer	AZT plus 3TC ± IDV
	Fluid containing visible blood, other potentially infectious fluid,[4] or tissue	Offer	AZT ± 3TC
	Other body fluid (urine)	Not offer	

Dosages for Antiviral Regimens

Drug	Dosage
AZT	200 mg PO TID × 4 weeks
3TC	150 mg PO BID × 4 weeks
IDV	800 mg PO TID × 4 weeks
or	
Saquinavir (substituted for IDV)	600 mg PO TID × 4 weeks

New Basic and Expanded HIV Postexposure Prophylaxis (PEP) Regimens

Basic Regimen
- Zidovudine (RETROVIR; ZDV; AZT) + lamivudine (EPIVIR; 3TC); available as COMBIVIR
  ZDV: 600 mg per day, in 2 or 3 divided doses, and
  3TC: 150 mg twice daily.

Alternate Basic Regimens
- Lamivudine (3TC) + stavudine (ZERIT; d4T)
  3TC: 150 mg twice daily, and
  d4T: 40 mg (if body weight is <60 kg, 30 mg twice daily) twice daily.
- Didanosine (VIDEX, chewable/dispersable buffered tablet; VIDEX EC, delayed-release capsule; ddI) + stavudine (d4T)
  ddI: 400 mg (if body weight is <60 kg, 125 mg twice daily) daily, on an empty stomach.
  d4T: 40 mg (if body weight is <60 kg, 30 mg twice daily) twice daily.

Expanded Regimen
Basic regimen plus 1 of the following:
- Indinavir (CRIXIVAN; IDV)
  800 mg every 8 hours, on an empty stomach.

(Continued)

Table 1-8 *(continued)*

- Nelfinavir (VIRACEPT; NFV)
  750 mg 3 times daily, with meals or snack, or
  1250 mg twice daily, with meals or snack.
- Efavirenz (SUSTIVA; EFV)
  600 mg daily, at bedtime.
  Advantages
    - Does not require phosphorylation before activation and might be active earlier than other antiretroviral agents. (*Note:* this might be only a theoretical advantage of no clinical benefit.)
    - One dose daily might improve adherence.
- Abacavir (ZIAGEN; ABC); available as TRIZIVIR, a combination of ZDV, 3TC, and ABC
  300 mg twice daily.

Antiretroviral Agents for Use as PEP *Only* With Expert Consultation
- Ritonavir (NORVIR; RTV)
- Saquinavir (FORTOVASE, soft-gel formulation; SQV)
- Amprenavir (AGENERASE; AMP)
- Delavirdine (RESCRIPTOR; DLV)
- Lopinavir/ritonavir (KALETRA)

Antiretroviral Agents Generally Not Recommended for Use as PEP
- Nevirapine (VIRAMUNE; NVP)

---

*Abbreviations: IDV = indinavir (Crixivan) or saquinavir (Invirase) substituted for IDV.

1. Highest risk = Both larger volume of blood (eg, deep injury with a large-diameter hollow needle previously in a patient's vein or artery, especially involving an injection of source-patient's blood) and blood containing a high titer of HIV (eg, source with acute retroviral illness or end-stage AIDS; viral load measurement may be considered, but its use in relation to postexposure prophylaxis has not been evaluated).
2. Increased risk = Either exposure to larger volume of blood or blood with a high titer of HIV.
3. No increased risk = Neither exposure to larger volume of blood nor blood with a high titer of HIV (eg, solid suture needle injury from source patient with asymptomatic HIV infection).
4. Includes semen; vaginal secretions; cerebrospinal, synovial, pleural, peritoneal, pericardial, and amniotic fluids.

Reprinted from Gerberding JL. Prophylaxis for occupational exposure to HIV. *Ann Intern Med.* 1996;125: 497–501. Table updated from Recommendations and Reports. APPENDIX C. Basic and Expanded HIV Postexposure Prophylaxis Regimens. *MMWR.* 2001;50(RR-11):47–52. Available at http://www.cdc.gov/mmwr/preview/mmwrhtml%5Crr5011a4.htm.

---

pneumocandins, which inhibit beta-glucan synthesis, or sordarins, which inhibit protein synthesis, may become useful in treating resistant infections.

Treatment of CMV infections

Ganciclovir is still used in the treatment of CMV retinitis and colitis in immunocompromised patients. Studies of ganciclovir suggest a response in 80%–100% of patients treated with ganciclovir for CMV retinitis and remissions in 60%–80% of these patients. Usually recommended for maintenance therapy after intravenous induction, oral ganciclovir is effective and has fewer side effects than the intravenous form.

Ganciclovir's major toxicity is reversible bone marrow suppression. One third of patients using ganciclovir develop significant granulocytopenia, requiring them to discontinue the drug. However, in patients with AIDS, cessation of ganciclovir therapy is universally associated with relapse of CMV retinitis. Because ganciclovir and nucleoside analogue antiretroviral agents have similar toxicities, most patients are not able to tolerate systemic therapeutic doses of these drugs simultaneously. Therapy with intravitreal ganciclovir injections has been effective in the treament of CMV retinitis. Unfortunately, most cases require intravitreal injection of ganciclovir 3 to 4 times a week indefinitely to prevent progression of CMV retinitis. A slow-release ganciclovir implant (Vitrasert) is also approved for the treatment of CMV retinitis. These implants are surgically inserted within the vitreal cavity and attached at the pars plana. Combination therapy with oral ganciclovir and the ganciclovir implant is more effective than the implant alone.

Foscarnet (Foscavir) is also effective for the treatment of CMV infections. Foscarnet inhibits the DNA polymerase of herpesvirus and HIV and demonstrates in vitro activity against CMV, herpes simplex, varicella-zoster, and HIV at concentrations readily achieved with intravenous therapy. Because oral bioavailability is poor, chronic intravenous therapy is required for suppression of CMV retinitis in HIV disease. Foscarnet's primary value is that it is not generally myelosuppressive and therefore may be used without discontinuing zidovudine therapy. Foscarnet's main dose-limiting side effect is nephrotoxicity; aggressive pretreatment hydration may reduce this effect significantly.

Cidofovir (HPMPC, Vistide) is a potent antiviral agent with activity against herpes simplex, herpes zoster, CMV, adenovirus, EBV, and HIV. Cidofovir blocks DNA synthesis by viral DNA polymerase. Cidofovir provides a prolonged antiviral activity that lasts up to several weeks, thereby allowing infrequent dosing. Intravenous (3–5 mg/kg, every other week) and intravitreal cidofovir (20 µg per eye, every 5–6 weeks) have been used successfully in the treatment of CMV retinitis. In a recent study, intravitreal cidofovir led to healing of CMV retinitis in all 53 participating patients. During the follow-up period, only 14% of the patients with previous anti-CMV therapy experienced disease progression; those without previous anti-CMV therapy did not experience disease progression.

Fomivirsen (Vitravene), an antisense drug that targets CMV mRNA, has been shown to be effective in controlling early or advanced CMV retinitis. Valganciclovir is an oral agent that is as effective as IV ganciclovir for the treatment of CMV retinitis.

Recent studies indicate that the incidence and frequency of recurrence of CMV retinitis have decreased since 1995, largely because of enhanced immune system function resulting from HAART.

Treatment of spore-forming intestinal protozoa

Spore-forming intestinal protozoa are a frequent cause of gastrointestinal tract infections in patients with AIDS. This group of infections includes cryptosporidiosis (caused by *Cryptosporidium parvum*), microsporidiosis *(Microsporida)*, isosporiasis *(Isospora belli)*, and cyclosporiasis *(Cyclospora cayetanensis)*.

Cryptosporidiosis can be treated with clarithromycin, azithromycin, rifabutin, albendazole, metronidazole, or a newer, more effective agent, nitazoxanide. In many patients, symptoms can be successfully controlled, but eradication of the organism can be extremely difficult. HIV-infected patients on HAART have a dramatically lower incidence of cryptosporidiosis, attributable to the effects of intestinal immune reconstitution, as well as HAART's beneficial effect on the CD4 cell count. Protease inhibitors have a direct inhibitory effect on cryptosporidium infection, suggesting an additional reason for the reduction in the incidence of cryptosporidiosis.

Isosporiasis and cyclosporiasis have been treated successfully with TMP-SMX. There are no curative drugs for invasive microsporidiosis, but recent studies have revealed that albendazole or fumagillin may control disease symptoms.

It is important to realize that chronic diarrhea in HIV-infected patients also may be caused by many nonprotozoan pathogens, particularly *Salmonella, Shigella, Campylobacter, C difficile, Vibrio parahaemolyticus, Escherichia coli, M avium,* and CMV.

Treatment of tuberculosis and atypical mycobacteria

The incidence of tuberculosis (TB) is currently increasing in HIV-infected patients in Africa and Asia. HIV-induced immunosuppression alters the typical clinical presentation of TB, causing atypical signs and symptoms and more frequent extrapulmonary disease dissemination. Also, the treatment of TB is more difficult to manage in HIV-infected patients, because of drug interactions between protease inhibitors and rifampicin or rifabutin. In addition, increased use of HAART in developed countries may be responsible for a paradoxical worsening of TB clinical manifestations, due to immune restoration and the subsequent inflammatory responses against TB.

Multidrug resistance has become an increasing problem—particularly in Africa and Asia—in patients with AIDS who have TB or atypical mycobacterial *(M avium, M kansasii)* infections. Delay in diagnosis and multidrug resistance are strong risk factors for mortality. These factors, along with poor compliance with patient isolation methods, were thought to be responsible for an urban outbreak of TB in 1994. This infection was caused by strain W, was resistant to 7 antituberculosis drugs, and was documented in 367 patients.

Standard drugs used in treating mycobacterial infections include isoniazid, rifampin, ethambutol, streptomycin, para-aminosalicylic acid, ethionamide, pyrazinamide, cycloserine, kanamycin, and amikacin. Some of the newer drugs found to be effective in treating these refractory infections are clofazimine (also used in treating leprosy), capreomycin, rifabutin, azithromycin, clarithromycin, and the quinolones (ciprofloxacin, ofloxacin, and sparfloxacin). The quinolones are promising because they possess a high level of antimycobacterial activity with few adverse effects. In recent studies, combined therapy with rifampin or rifabutin, ethambutol, clofazimine, and clarithromycin or ciprofloxacin has been successful in treating atypical mycobacterial infections in patients with AIDS. Isoniazid prophylaxis has been recommended in HIV-positive patients at high risk for TB.

Prophylactic therapy with azithromycin, clarithromycin, rifabutin, or combined therapy may help prevent disseminated *M avium* complex (MAC) in patients with AIDS. However, a significant reduction in the incidence of disseminated atypical mycobacterial infections in the HAART era has been documented. Also, the clinical picture of atypical mycobacterial infections in patients treated with HAART has shifted from one of primarily disseminated disease with bacteremia to one of localized infections. Data from several recent controlled trials led to the current practice of discontinuing prophylaxis against disseminated MAC infections when the $CD4^+$ cell counts remain stable at over 100 cells/µL. Furthermore, because of the potential drug interactions and adverse effects of anti-mycobacterial therapy, some authors suggest that routine prophylaxis should not be recommended, even in patients with low CD4+ counts, unless these patients do not respond to HAART.

Treatment of other opportunistic infections
Other opportunistic infections encountered in patients with AIDS include CNS toxoplasmosis, disseminated fungal infections, and coinfection with viral hepatitis, herpes simplex, or herpes zoster infections. Although toxoplasmosis has traditionally been treated with sulfadiazine, pyrimethamine, or clindamycin, more recent data suggest that TMP-SMX may be equally effective, with far fewer side effects. Also, TMP-SMX has been used as prophylactic therapy against PCP as well as toxoplasmosis.

Hepatitis B or C coinfection has been encountered more frequently in HIV-infected patients. Recent guidelines for screening and prevention of opportunistic infections suggest testing all HIV-infected patients for hepatitis B and C. HIV coinfection accelerates HCV-related liver disease, causing more rapid progression to cirrhosis, end-stage liver disease, and hepatocellular carcinoma. Although some antiretroviral agents, such as protease inhibitors, have significant anti-HBV activity, they have little direct impact on HCV infection.

The new antiviral agents valacyclovir and famciclovir, as well as other antiviral agents such as cidofovir, offer alternatives to using acyclovir in the treatment of AIDS in patients with refractory or disseminated herpes simplex or herpes zoster infections.

Treatment of disseminated fungal infections is evolving with the availability of the newer imidazoles, fluconazole and itraconazole. Amphotericin B continues to be important in treating advanced invasive fungal disease. New formulations of amphotericin B in lipid complexes or liposomes reduce systemic toxicity. In addition to the commonly recognized benefits of HAART for opportunistic infections (such as reestablishing immune competency), a recent study has proven that the protease inhibitor indinavir directly inhibits the growth rate of the opportunistic fungal pathogen *Cryptococcus neoformans*.

In the past few years, recommendations have been developed for discontinuing prophylaxis for treatment of opportunistic infections in patients whose CD4+ T lymphocyte counts have increased in response to HAART.

Treatment of AIDS-related malignancies
Kaposi sarcoma is usually a localized disease that can be treated with radiotherapy, but metastatic or disseminated disease may require combined chemotherapy. In addition, immunotherapy with β-interferon has been used in some patients with Kaposi sarcoma. B cell lymphomas in patients with AIDS often involve the lymph nodes, CNS, and lungs and may require treatment with multidrug chemotherapy and sometimes with regional radiotherapy. Since the advent of HAART, the incidence of Kaposi sarcoma in HIV-infected patients has declined dramatically—as much as 87%, according to 1 review.

Hodgkin lymphoma is the most common non–AIDS-defining tumor in HIV-infected patients. Although the introduction of HAART led to a decreased incidence of several malignancies among HIV-infected patients, the incidence of HIV-associated Hodgkin lymphoma has been persistent. This disease's highly aggressive behavior is related to an increased frequency of unfavorable histologic types, higher tumor stages, and extranodal involvement by the time of presentation, as well as poorer therapeutic outcome, when compared with Hodgkin lymphoma in non–HIV-infected patients. Treatment of HIV-associated Hodgkin lymphoma is challenging, because of the underlying immunodeficiency caused by HIV itself, and may increase the risk of opportunistic infections by inducing further immunosuppression. Consequently, less aggressive treatment regimens have been developed to achieve tumor control in HIV-infected patients with Hodgkin lymphoma.

Other malignancies that appear to be associated with HIV infection are cervical carcinoma in situ, anogenital neoplasms, leiomyosarcoma, and conjunctival squamous cell carcinoma.

Immune reconstitution syndromes
Some patients starting HAART develop new or worsening opportunistic infections or malignancies, despite improvements in the clinical markers of HIV infection. These examples of paradoxical clinical worsening, also called *immune reconstitution syndromes (IRS)*, are increased in patients with previous opportunistic infections or low $CD4^+$ T-cell levels. Immune reconstitution syndromes are thought to result from inflammatory response due to reemergence of the immune system's ability to recognize pathogens or tumor antigens that were previously present, but asymptomatic. With the increased availability of HAART, more cases and more new forms of IRS are likely to be recognized.

Ophthalmologic Considerations

The ocular manifestations of AIDS are discussed in BCSC Section 9, *Intraocular Inflammation and Uveitis.*

HIV has been demonstrated in tears, conjunctival epithelial cells, corneal epithelial cells, aqueous, retinal vascular endothelium, and retina. Although transmission of AIDS or HIV infection by ophthalmic examinations or ophthalmic equipment has not been documented, the following precautions are recommended.

Health care professionals performing eye examinations or other procedures involving contact with tears should wash their hands immediately after the procedure and between patients. Hand washing alone should be sufficient, but when practical and convenient, disposable gloves may be worn. The use of gloves is advisable when the hands have cuts, scratches, or dermatologic lesions.

Instruments that come into direct contact with external surfaces of the eyes should be wiped clean and disinfected by a 5- to 10-minute exposure to 1 of the following: (1) a fresh solution of 3% hydrogen peroxide; (2) a fresh solution containing 5000 parts per million (ppm) free available chlorine—a one tenth dilution of common household bleach (sodium hypochlorite); (3) 70% ethanol; or (4) 70% isopropanol. The device should be thoroughly rinsed in tap water and dried before use.

Contact lenses used in trial fitting should be disinfected between fittings with a commercially available hydrogen peroxide contact lens disinfecting system or with the standard heat disinfection regimen (78°–80°C for 10 minutes).

The demonstration of HIV in corneal epithelium has led to the recommendation that all corneal donors be screened for antibodies to HIV and that all potential donor corneas from HIV antibody–positive persons be discarded.

For more specific recommendations, see the AAO Information Statement titled "Updated Recommendations for Ophthalmic Practice in Relation to the Human Immunodeficiency Virus and Other Infectious Agents."

Aaron L, Saadoun D, Calatroni I, et al. Tuberculosis in HIV-infected patients: a comprehensive review. *Clin Microbiol Infect.* 2004;10:388–398.

Blasi E, Colombari B, Orsi CF, et al. The human immunodeficiency virus (HIV) protease inhibitor indinavir directly affects the opportunistic fungal pathogen *Cryptococcus neoformans. FEMS Immunol Med Microbiol.* 2004;42:187–195.

Borroto-Esoda K, Myrick F, Feng J, et al. In vitro combination of amdoxovir and the inosine monophosphate dehydrogenase inhibitors mycophenolic acid and ribavirin demonstrates potent activity against wild-type and drug-resistant variants of human immunodeficiency virus type 1. *Antimicrob Agents Chemother.* 2004;48:4387–4394.

Centers for Disease Control and Prevention. Guidelines for using antiretroviral agents among HIV-infected adults and adolescents: recommendations of the Panel on Clinical Practices for Treatment of HIV. *MMWR.* 2002;51(No. RR-7). Available at http://www.cdc.gov/mmwr/PDF/RR/RR5107.pdf. Accessed December 17, 2003.

Centers for Disease Control and Prevention. *HIV/AIDS Surveillance Report, 2003* (Vol. 15). Atlanta: US Department of Health and Human Services, Centers for Disease Control and Prevention; 2004. Also available at http://www.cdc.gov/hiv/stats/hasrlink.htm.

Chan DJ. HIV-1 superinfection: evidence and impact. *Curr HIV Res.* 2004;2:271–274.

Chapman TM, Plosker GL, Perry CM. Fosamprenavir: a review of its use in the management of antiretroviral therapy–naive patients with HIV infection. *Drugs.* 2004;64:2101–2124.

Clotet B, Raffi F, Cooper D, et al. Clinical management of treatment-experienced, HIV-infected patients with the fusion inhibitor enfuvirtide: consensus recommendations. *AIDS.* 2004;18:1137–1146.

De Clercq E. HIV-chemotherapy and -prophylaxis: new drugs, leads and approaches. *Int J Biochem Cell Biol.* 2004;36:1800–1822.

De Clercq E. New anti-HIV agents and targets. *Med Res Rev.* 2002;22:531–565.

Fortin C, Joly V. Efavirenz for HIV-1 infection in adults: an overview. *Expert Rev Anti Infect Ther.* 2004;2:671–684.

Gallant JE, Pham PA. Tenofovir disoproxil fumarate (Viread) for the treatment of HIV infection. *Expert Rev Anti Infect Ther.* 2003;1:415–422.

Gardner EM, Connick E. Illness of Immune Reconstitution: recognition and management. *Curr Infect Dis Rep.* 2004;6:483–493.

Gewurz BE, Jacobs M, Proper JA, et al. Capravirine, a nonnucleoside reverse-transcriptase inhibitor in patients infected with HIV-1: a phase 1 study. *J Infect Dis.* 2004;190:1957–1961.

Hartmann P, Rehwald U, Salzberger B, et al. Current treatment strategies for patients with Hodgkin's lymphoma and HIV infection. *Expert Rev Anticancer Ther.* 2004;4:401–410.

Herman ES, Klotman PE. HIV-associated nephropathy: epidemiology, pathogenesis, and treatment. *Semin Nephrol.* 2003;23:200–208.

Hu DJ, Vitek CR, Bartholow B, et al. Key issues for a potential human immunodeficiency virus vaccine. *Clin Infect Dis.* 2003;36:638–644.

Kelly LM, Lisziewicz J, Lori F. "Virostatics" as a potential new class of HIV drugs. *Curr Pharm Des.* 2004;10:4103–4120.

Lange CG, Woolley IJ, Brodt RH. Disseminated *Mycobacterium avium-intracellulare* complex (MAC) infection in the era of effective antiretroviral therapy: is prophylaxis still indicated? *Drugs.* 2004;64(7):679–692.

Masur H, Kaplan JE, Holmes KK. Guidelines for preventing opportunistic infections among HIV-infected persons—2002. Recommendations of the US Public Health Service and the Infectious Diseases Society of America. *Ann Intern Med.* 2002;137(5 Pt 2):435–478.

Mathews G, Bhagani S. The epidemiology and natural history of HIV/HBV and HIV/HCV co-infections. *J HIV Ther.* 2003;8:77–84.

Mbulaiteye SM, Parkin DM, Rabkin CS. Epidemiology of AIDS-related malignancies: an international perspective. *Hematol Oncol Clin North Am.* 2003;17:673–696.

Milinkovic A, Martinez E. Nevirapine in the treatment of HIV. *Expert Rev Anti Infect Ther.* 2004;2:367–373.

Patel N, Koziel H. *Pneumocystis jiroveci* pneumonia in adult patients with AIDS: treatment strategies and emerging challenges to antimicrobial therapy. *Treat Respir Med.* 2004;3:381–397.

Sankatsing SU, Weverling GJ, Peeters M, et al. TMC125 exerts similar initial antiviral potency as a five-drug, triple class antiretroviral regimen. *AIDS.* 2003;17:2623–2627.

Smith HV, Corcoran GD. New drugs and treatment for cryptosporidiosis. *Curr Opin Infect Dis.* 2004;17:557–564.

Turpin JA. The next generation of HIV/AIDS drugs: novel and developmental anti-HIV drugs and targets. *Expert Rev Anti Infect Ther.* 2003;1:97–128.

UNAIDS 2004 report on the global AIDS epidemic. Joint United Nations Programme on HIV/AIDS. Available at http://www.unaids.org/bangkok2004/report.html. Accessed March 1, 2005.

Wang LH, Begley J, St Claire RL 3rd, et al. Pharmacokinetic and pharmacodynamic characteristics of emtricitabine support its once daily dosing for the treatment of HIV infection. *AIDS Res Hum Retroviruses.* 2004;20:1173–1182.

Wensing AM, Boucher CA. Worldwide transmission of drug-resistant HIV. *AIDS Rev.* 2003;5:140–155.

Yeni P. Tipranavir: a protease inhibitor from a new class with distinct antiviral activity. *J Acquir Immune Defic Syndr.* 2003;34 suppl 1:S91–94.

Yeni PG, Hammer SM, Carpenter CC, et al. Antiretroviral treatment for adult HIV infection in 2002: updated recommendations of the International AIDS Society—USA Panel. *JAMA.* 2002;288:222–235.

Update on Antibiotics

For half a century, the main trend in infectious disease management has been the evolution and refinement of antibiotic therapy. Factors that have stimulated the development of new antibiotics include a spate of resistant bacteria, economics, and the desire to eliminate undesirable side effects. During the last couple of decades, emphasis gradually shifted from *aminoglycosides* to *β-lactams* and the development of new classes of antibiotics such as *carbapenems* and *monobactams*. In addition, *vancomycin, TMP-SMX, erythromycin,* and *rifampin* have enjoyed a popular resurgence and new applications. Quinolones offer the possibility of treating serious infections on an outpatient basis. Antiviral drugs such as *acyclovir, ganciclovir, zidovudine,* and *ribavirin* are all *nucleoside analogues,* which inhibit viral DNA polymerase (reverse transcriptase) and interrupt the growing viral DNA chain. In addition, several new imidazole compounds have been introduced for treatment of systemic fungal infections.

For the characteristics of selected antibiotics, see Table 1-9. Antiretroviral agents are discussed in detail earlier in this chapter.

Antibacterial Agents

The various antibacterial agents act on bacteria in different ways. For example, unlike humans and other higher animals, most bacteria cannot utilize exogenous folic acid and must, therefore, synthesize their own in order to grow. Sulfonamides and trimethoprim each block a different enzyme in this synthetic pathway. For this reason, bacteria susceptible to both agents are inhibited by lower concentrations of the 2 drugs acting together than are needed with either drug alone. Therefore, these 2 agents often are administered as a fixed-combination drug.

The *quinolones* have a different mechanism of action. To function properly, the double-stranded DNA of the bacterial chromosome must be supercoiled by the enzyme DNA gyrase, and quinolones block this enzyme. A number of newer *fluoroquinolones,* which have very broad spectra of activity against a wide range of gram-negative and gram-positive bacterial species, have become available.

To make proteins, bacteria begin by copying the code for each protein from its gene on the bacterial chromosome onto a newly synthesized strand of the specialized RNA known as *messenger RNA (mRNA).* The antituberculosis drug rifampin selectively blocks the enzyme that synthesizes this mRNA strand. Once synthesized, the strand of mRNA then threads its way through the bacterial ribosomes to direct each ribosome in the sequence of assembling amino acids into a protein. This process is blocked in different ways by the tetracyclines and by chloramphenicol, erythromycin, and clindamycin; however, the process resumes again if the drug is discontinued. Because their effect is reversible, these classes of agents are considered to be *bacteriostatic.* In contrast, the aminoglycosides belong to a class of antibiotics that irreversibly derange ribosomal protein synthesis; the process cannot resume even after the drugs are stopped. These drugs, therefore, are *bactericidal.*

The bacterial proteins themselves or their enzymatic products make up the rest of the bacterial cell, including the membrane that encloses the cell. Polymyxin and colistin damage the cell membrane, making it unable to perform essential barrier functions. Surrounding the bacterium and outside of the cell membrane is the bacterial cell wall. The components of the cell wall are synthesized within the bacterial cell and then transported to the outside through the cell membrane before being assembled on its surface. The drugs that block this transport include bacitracin, a topical polypeptide agent derived from a strain of *Bacillus subtilis,* and vancomycin, a glycopeptide.

The final, crucial step in bacterial growth is formation of the bacterial cell wall. The necessary cross-linking of its components is mediated by special enzymes that are unlike anything in the human cell. The antibiotics that selectively inhibit 1 or more of these enzymes include penicillin and its growing family of related agents. This family includes the semisynthetic penicillins, all of the cephalosporin-like drugs, and β-lactams of novel structure such as imipenem. They are all grouped together under the label of *β-lactam* antibiotics because their structural formulas are marked by a distinctive 4-atom structure known chemically as a *β-lactam ring.* When even a small number of 1 of these β-lactam

Table 1-9 Characteristics of Selected Antibiotics

Antibiotic	Spectrum*	Route	Side Effects/Special Uses
	Antibacterial Agents		
Sulfonamides (bacteriostatic)			
Sulfisoxazole (Gantrisin)	Urinary tract infections, +, −, *Nocardia*, lymphogranuloma venereum, trachoma	PO	Crystalluria, allergic reactions (rashes, photosensitivity, and drug fever), kernicterus in newborns, renal damage, Stevens-Johnson syndrome (more likely with long-acting sulfonamides), blood dyscrasia (agranulocytosis), disseminated vasculitis.
Trimethoprim-sulfamethoxazole, TMP-SMX (Bactrim, Septra)	Urinary tract infections, +, −, shigellosis, *Nocardia*, *Pneumocystis* pneumonia	PO, IV	Same as above, plus nausea and vomiting, diarrhea, rashes, CNS irritability, bone marrow toxicity. Liver damage and Stevens-Johnson syndrome may be fatal.
Penicillin G (bactericidal)			
Aqueous (many brands)	+, *Neisseria*, spirochetes, actinomycosis	IV only	Penicillin allergy,** CNS toxicity with high blood levels, Coombs-positive hemolytic anemia, rare nephritis.
Procaine (many brands)	Same as above	IM only	Same as above, plus -*caine* reactions.
Benzathine (Bicillin)	Spirochetes, *Streptococcus* prophylaxis	IM only	Prolonged penicillin allergy.**
Semisynthetic penicillins (bactericidal)			
Penicillin V (Pen-Vee K)	+, *Neisseria*, spirochetes, actinomycosis	PO	Much better absorption than penicillin G when given orally in the fasting state.
Nafcillin (Unipen)	Penicillinase-producing *Staph*	IV	Penicillin allergy,** phlebitis, interstitial nephritis, diarrhea; rare bone marrow toxicity.
Cloxacillin (Tegopen)	+, especially *Staph*	PO	Penicillin allergy,** GI symptoms. Better absorbed and better tolerated than nafcillin and oxacillin given orally in the fasting state.
Dicloxacillin (Dynapen)	+, especially *Staph*	PO	Same as above.

*Symbols: + = gram-positive; − = gram-negative; *Staph* = penicillinase-producers.
**Penicillin allergy includes spectrum from anaphylaxis to serum sickness.

(Continued)

Table 1-9 Characteristics of Selected Antibiotics (continued)

Antibiotic	Spectrum*	Route	Side Effects/Special Uses
Ampicillin (Polycillin)	+, especially *Enterococcus* (except *Staph*) and some −, especially *Haemophilus influenzae*, *Proteus mirabilis*, *Salmonella* sp, *Escherichia coli*	IV, PO	Penicillin allergy,** GI symptoms (from PO administration). Rash common in viral illnesses (maculopapular eruption that is not necessarily allergy).
Ampicillin-sulbactam (Unasyn)	Same as ampicillin plus beta-lactamase producers and some anaerobes	IV	Penicillin allergy,** diarrhea, elevated liver enzymes.
Amoxicillin (Amoxil)	Same as above, except *Shigella*	PO	Same as above. Better absorbed than oral ampicillin. Should replace *oral* ampicillin for everything except bacillary dysentery.
Amoxicillin–potassium clavulanate (Augmentin)	Same as amoxicillin plus beta-lactamase producers (*Haemophilus influenzae*, *Branhamella* sp, and *Staph* sp)	PO	Same as amoxicillin plus more diarrhea.
Ticarcillin (Ticar)	−, especially *Pseudomonas aeruginosa* and *Proteus* sp, abdominal anaerobes, and some +, except *Staph*	IV	Penicillin allergy,** rare bleeding diathesis, hypokalemia (4.0 mEq Na$^+$/gm), abnormal liver function tests, *Candida* overgrowth.
Ticarcillin-potassium clavulanate (Timentin)	Same as ticarcillin plus beta-lactamase producers (*Klebsiella* sp, *Bacteroides fragilis*, and *Serratia* sp)	IV	Same as ticarcillin plus more diarrhea and nausea. *Candida* overgrowth frequent.
Mezlocillin (Mezlin)	Same as ticarcillin	IV	Same as ticarcillin.
Piperacillin (Pipracil)	−, most active of all semisynthetic penicillins against *Pseudomonas* and many other aerobic gram-negative rods, including *Klebsiella*; abdominal anaerobes	IV	One half as much Na$^+$ as ticarcillin. Similar to ticarcillin, but approximately 25% of patients develop a hypersensitivity reaction and/or diarrhea. Must be used with an aminoglycoside. Rare bleeding diathesis.

*Symbols: + = gram-positive; − = gram-negative; *Staph* = penicillinase-producers.
**Penicillin allergy includes spectrum from anaphylaxis to serum sickness.

Table 1-9 (continued)

Antibiotic	Spectrum*	Route	Side Effects/Special Uses
Piperacillin-tazobactam (Zosyn)	Same as piperacillin with increased coverage of beta-lactamase producers and anaerobes	IV	Same as piperacillin.
Cephalosporins (bactericidal)			
First-generation cephalosporins			
Cefazolin (Kefzol, Ancef)	+ and some –; not a good *Staph* treatment	IM, IV	Thrombophlebitis or pain at injection site, rash, urticaria, eosinophilia, neutropenia.
Cephalexin (Keflex)	+, *Staph*, and some –	PO	Same as above plus GI symptoms.
Cephradine (Anspor, Velosef)	+, *Staph*, and some –	PO	Same as above.
Cefadroxil monohydrate (Duracef)	+, *Staph*, and some –	PO	Rash, urticaria, GI symptoms.
Second-generation (extended-spectrum) cephalosporins			
Cefamandole (Mandol)	+, especially *Staph*, and some –	IV	Less thrombophlebitis than above, rash, drug fever, eosinophilia, hypoprothrombinemia ± bleeding. Extremely effective prophylaxis for *Staph* including MRSE.
Cefoxitin (Mefoxin)	+, –, abdominal anaerobes (the best of all cephalosporins)	IV	Thrombophlebitis, fever, rash, eosinophilia, nausea, vomiting, diarrhea, bone marrow and liver toxicity.
Cefonicid (Monocid)	– and some anaerobes	IV	Often used for prophylaxis with colorectal or gynecologic surgeries; may cause pain at injection site, eosinophilia, GI symptoms, rash.
Cefaclor (Ceclor, Distaclor)	+ and some –, *Haemophilus* sp	PO	Toxicity similar to other cephalosporins. Major uses are treating ENT infections in children and respiratory tract infections in adults with COPD.

*Symbols: + = gram-positive; – = gram-negative; *Staph* = penicillinase-producers.

(Continued)

Table 1-9 Characteristics of Selected Antibiotics (continued)

Antibiotic	Spectrum*	Route	Side Effects/Special Uses
Cefuroxime sodium (IV: Zinacef, Kefurox); cefuroxime axetil (PO: Ceftin)	+ and some −, *Haemophilus* sp	IV, PO	Rash, GI symptoms.
Cefotetan (Cefotan)	−, anaerobes	IM or IV	A long half-life cefoxitin. Hypoprothrombinemia, hemolytic anemia, and disulfiram-like reaction.
Third-generation (ultrabroad-spectrum) cephalosporins			
Cefotaxime (Claforan)	−, including many multidrug-resistant organisms	IV	Cephalosporin hypersensitivity reaction, thrombophlebitis. Good penetration into CSF in meningitis.
Cefoperazone (Cefobid)	−, including *Pseudomonas* sp and many multidrug-resistant organisms, some anaerobes	IM or IV	Cephalosporin hypersensitivity, hypoprothrombinemia, diarrhea. Can be given q 8–12h.
Ceftriaxone (Rocephin)	Like cefotaxime; gonorrhea, *Borrelia burgdorferi*	IM or IV	Very long half-life makes it attractive for outpatient therapy. Treatment of choice for gonorrhea. Effective for all forms of Lyme disease. Good CNS penetration for meningitis.
Ceftazidime (Fortaz, Tazidime, Tazicef)	−, especially *Pseudomonas* sp	IM, IV	Good anti-pseudomonal cephalosporin, long half-life: q 8–12h administration. The best all-purpose third-generation cephalosporin.
Ceftizoxime (Cefizox)	Many − and anaerobes	IV	Rash, GI symptoms, elevated liver enzymes.
Cefixime (Suprax)	+, some − (*Haemophilus influenzae*, *Branhamella catarrhalis*)	PO	Diarrhea, nausea, abdominal pain, flatulence. First oral third-generation cephalosporin.
Cefpodoxime proxetil (Vantin)	+, −, *Enterobacter*, *Pseudomonas*, *Serratia*, *Morganella*, *Enterococcus*, generally resistant infections	PO	Twice daily for ENT, respiratory and urinary tract and soft tissue infections. Single dose for uncomplicated gonorrhea.
Cefprozil (Cefzil)	+, −, including *Haemophilus*	PO	Rash, GI symptoms.

*Symbols: + = gram-positive; − = gram-negative; *Staph* = penicillinase-producers.

Table 1-9 (continued)

Antibiotic	Spectrum*	Route	Side Effects/Special Uses
Ceftibuten (Cedax)	+, −, including *Haemophilus, Moraxella*	PO	No real advantages.
Cefdinir (Omnicef)	+, −, including *Haemophilus*	PO	Rash, GI symptoms.
Cefditoren (Spectracef)	+, −, including *Haemophilus*	PO	Very broad spectrum but not active against *Pseudomonas*.
Fourth-generation (very broad spectrum) cephalosporins			
Cefepime (Maxipime)	+, −, some anaerobes	IV, IM	Expensive; slightly better gram-negative coverage than ceftazidime.
Cefpirome	+, −, some anaerobes	IV, IM	Effective for sepsis.
Carbacephems (bactericidal)			
Loracarbef (Lorabid)	+, −, including *Haemophilus*	PO	Rash, GI symptoms.
Cephamycins (bactericidal)			
Cefmetazole (Zefazone)	Similar to that of second-generation cephalosporins	IV	GI symptoms, rash, seizures in patients with renal insufficiency, more side effects than second-generation cephalosporins.
Monobactams (bactericidal)			
Aztreonam (Azactam)	Most −; no activity for + or anaerobes	IM, IV	First of this class of monocyclic beta-lactams. The spectrum of an aminoglycoside without oto- or nephrotoxicity. No cross-reaction in penicillin-allergic patients.
Carbapenems (bactericidal)			
Imipenem-cilastatin (Primaxin)	+, −, including *Pseudomonas* sp and multidrug-resistant strains, anaerobes	IV	Nausea, diarrhea, phlebitis, elevated serum glutamic-oxaloacetic transaminase (SGOT), elevated serum glutamic-pyruvic transaminase (SGPT), seizures. Prototype of carbapenems. *Candida* superinfection frequent. Extremely broad spectrum.

*Symbols: + = gram-positive; − = gram-negative; *Staph* = penicillinase-producers.

(Continued)

Table 1-9 Characteristics of Selected Antibiotics *(continued)*

Antibiotic	Spectrum*	Route	Side Effects/Special Uses
Meropenem (Merrem)	Similar to imipenem, but less active against +, more active against −	IV	Does not require cilastatin component because more resistant to enzyme degradation; less problem with seizures.
Ertapenem	Similar to meropenem	IM, IV	Similar to meropenem; once-daily dosing.
Faropenem	Similar to meropenem	PO	Similar to meropenem.
Macrolides (bacteriostatic)			
Erythromycin	+, spirochetes, *Mycoplasma*, *Legionella*, *Campylobacter*	PO, IV	GI upset, altered liver function test, hepatic damage, stomatitis, thrombophlebitis (with IV administration). Take with meals or a snack when given orally.
Clindamycin (Cleocin)	+, anaerobes, actinomycosis	PO, IV	GI toxicity can be severe and even lethal.
Azalides			
Clarithromycin (Biaxin)	+, *Mycoplasma*, *Chlamydia*, *Legionella*	PO	Reversible dose-related hearing loss in high doses. Less GI than erythromycin.
Azithromycin (Zithromax)			
Dirithromycin (Dynabac)			
Roxithromycin			
Spiramycin			
Josamycin			
Ketolides			
Telithromycin (Ketek)	+, *Mycoplasma*, *Chlamydia*, *Legionella*. Good for multidrug-resistant +	PO	Similar to above.
Glycopeptides (bactericidal)			
Vancomycin (Vancocin)	+, especially *Staph* and *Enterococcus*, *Clostridia*, and other beta-lactam-resistant +	IV, PO	Thrombophlebitis, leukopenia. Resistant enterococci and reduced-sensitivity *Staph* strains are increasing.

*Symbols: + = gram-positive; − = gram-negative; *Staph* = penicillinase-producers.

Table 1-9 (continued)

Antibiotic	Spectrum*	Route	Side Effects/Special Uses
Teicoplanin (Targocid)	Similar to vancomycin with better activity against *Streptococcus* and *Enterococcus*. Effective for some vancomycin-resistant strains of *Enterococcus*.	IV, IM	Longer half-life (allows daily dosing), lower toxicity, less nephrotoxicity, better tissue penetration than vancomycin.
Tetracyclines† (bacteriostatic) *In order of bacterial activity:*			
Minocycline (Minocin)	+ and −, spirochetes, *Mycoplasma*, lymphogranuloma venereum, psittacosis, *Rickettsia*	PO, IV	Most active. Useful as an alternative to vancomycin for treatment of methicillin-resistant staphylococci, particularly MRSE, and for meningococcal prophylaxis. Vertigo.
Doxycycline (Vibramycin)	Same as above	PO, IV	Hepatic excretion, so may be best in renal failure. Do not use in urinary tract infections. Phototoxic reactions.
Tetracycline	Same as above	PO, IV	Probably best choice for routine use. *Candida* overgrowth.
Aminoglycosides (bactericidal)			
Streptomycin	Tuberculosis, −, *Pasteurella* sp, *Franciscella* sp	IM only	Vestibular damage, drug fever, peripheral neuropathy.
Gentamicin (Garamycin)	Community-acquired −; not effective for + or anaerobes	IM or IV slowly	Vestibular damage, renal damage, curare-like effect.
Tobramycin (Nebcin)	−, especially *Pseudomonas* and *Aeromonas*	IM or IV slowly	Less nephrotoxic than gentamicin. Most active against *Pseudomonas*.
Netilmicin (Netromycin)	−, including some gentamicin/tobramycin-resistant organisms	IM or IV slowly	May be less toxic than gentamicin or tobramycin.

*Symbols: + = gram-positive; − = gram-negative; *Staph* = penicillinase-producers.

†*Side effects of tetracyclines:* GI disturbance; bone lesions; staining and deformity of teeth in children up to 8 years old and in newborns when given to pregnant women after the fourth month; malabsorption; enterocolitis; photosensitivity reaction (most frequent with demethylchlortetracycline). Parenteral doses may cause serious liver damage, especially in pregnant women and patients with renal disease; allergic reactions, blood dyscrasia, interference with protein metabolism, increased intracranial pressure in infants, Fanconi-like syndrome from deteriorated tetracyclines. Take with meals or a snack, but avoid milk and milk products.

(Continued)

Table 1-9 Characteristics of Selected Antibiotics (continued)

Antibiotic	Spectrum*	Route	Side Effects/Special Uses
Amikacin (Amikin)	−, active against many gentamicin/tobramycin-resistant gram-negatives. Ideal for nosocomial gram-negative infection.	IM or IV slowly	Nephrotoxic and ototoxic (more deafness than vestibular effects). Curare-like effect.
Quinolones (bactericidal)	+, most −, including multidrug-resistant isolates, and MRSA and MRSE. Not good for *Enterococcus*.		Expensive, *Candida* overgrowth, photosensitivity reactions, hypoglycemia, hyperglycemia.
Norfloxacin (Noroxin)	Same as above	PO	Very broad treatment for complicated urinary tract infections.
Ciprofloxacin (Cipro)	Same as above	PO, IV	Very broad spectrum makes this a useful oral agent for mixed infections, infectious diarrhea, and multidrug-resistant organisms at any body site except CNS.
New quinolones Ofloxacin (Floxin) Sparfloxacin (Zagam) Enoxacin (Penetrex) Temafloxacin (Omniflox) Lomefloxacin (Maxaquin) Levofloxacin (Levaquin) Trovafloxacin (Trovan) Moxifloxacin (Avelox) Gatifloxacin (Tequin) Gemifloxacin (Factive) Clinafloxacin	Increased activity for + and −	PO	Same as above.
Miscellaneous agents			
Chloramphenicol (Chloromycetin)	+, −, anaerobes, *Rickettsia*; bacteriostatic	PO, IV	"Gray baby" syndrome in newborns, bone marrow toxicity, optic atrophy, and peripheral neuropathy.
Metronidazole (Flagyl, Flagyl IV)	Anaerobes, *Campylobacter*, amoebae, *Trichomonas*, *C difficile*; bacteriostatic	PO, IV	GI upset, vertigo, ataxia, peripheral neuropathy, phlebitis, carcinogenic (?), Antabuse-like reaction.

*Symbols: + = gram-positive; − = gram-negative; *Staph* = penicillinase-producers.

Table 1-9 (continued)

Antibiotic	Spectrum*	Route	Side Effects/Special Uses
Rifampin (Rifadin)	TB, *Staph* (synergy), meningococcal prophylaxis; bactericidal	PO	Hepatotoxicity, flulike syndrome, discoloration of body secretions, drug interactions.
Pentamidine (Pentam 300)	*Pneumocystis* pneumonia	IV, aerosol	Hypotension, hypoglycemia, abnormal liver function tests, azotemia, bone marrow toxicity.
New Antibiotic Classes			
Streptogramins (bactericidal) Quinupristin/dalfopristin (Synercid)	Active against multidrug-resistant + organisms, even those with reduced sensitivity to vancomycin	IV	Bactericidal as a combined drug. No cross-resistance with other antibiotics. GI side effects, rash, myalgias.
Oxazolidinones (bactericidal) Linezolid (Zyvox) Eperezolid (investigational)	Similar to quinupristin/dalfopristin	IV, PO	Has monoamine oxidase (MAO) inhibitor effects, so drug interactions are possible.
Everninomicins (bactericidal) Evernimicin (Ziracin)	Similar to quinupristin/dalfopristin	IV	Effective for methicillin-resistant and vancomycin-intermediate-sensitivity organisms.
Avilamycin	Similar to quinupristin/dalfopristin	IV	Similar to above.
Lipopeptides (bactericidal) Daptomycin (investigational)	Similar to quinupristin/dalfopristin	IV, PO	Most bactericidal of all in a study of new antibiotics for drug-resistant + strain.

*Symbols: + = gram-positive; − = gram-negative; *Staph* = penicillinase-producers.

(Continued)

Table 1-9 Characteristics of Selected Antibiotics *(continued)*

Antibiotic	Spectrum*	Route	Side Effects/Special Uses
Antifungal Agents (Fungistatic)			
Nystatin (Mycostatin)	*Candida*	PO tabs or suspension; topical cream, ointment, powder; GU irrigant, vaginal suppository	Useful for prevention of *Candida* overgrowth or for topical treatment of GI, mucosal, or skin candidiasis.
5-fluorocytosine (Ancobon, Ancotil)	*Candida, Cryptococcus*	PO	GI distress, leukopenia, hepatotoxicity. Particularly toxic in patients with compromised renal function.
Amphotericin B (Fungizone, Amphotec)	Most invasive fungi, oral candidiasis	IV for systemic use; PO only for oral candidiasis	Chills, fever, nausea, vomiting, thrombophlebitis, nephrotoxicity, hypokalemia, bone marrow suppression, shock, cardiotoxicity.
Miconazole (Micatin, Monistat)	*Candida*, dermatophytes	Topical or vaginal cream; IV	Topical treatment of *Candida* and dermatophytes. When used IV thrombophlebitis, thrombocytosis, anemia.
Clotrimazole (Lotrimin, Gyne-Lotrimin, Mycelex)	*Candida*, dermatophytes	Topical solution, vaginal suppository; PO	Same as above.
Ketoconazole (Nizoral)	Many fungi	PO	Rash, pruritus, nausea, gynecomastia, liver toxicity, impaired fertility.
Newer imidazoles			
Fluconazole (Diflucan) Itraconazole (Sporanox) Voriconazole (Vfend) Croconazole	*Candida, Cryptococcus*	PO, IV	Less toxicity than amphotericin and flucytosine. Better tolerated than ketoconazole.
Allylamines			
Terbinafine (Lamisil)	Dermatophytes causing onychomycosis	PO	Headache, GI symptoms, rash.

*Symbols: + = gram-positive; − = gram-negative; *Staph* = penicillinase-producers.

Table 1-9 (continued)

Antibiotic	Spectrum*	Route	Side Effects/Special Uses
Benzylamines			
Butenafine (Mentax)	Dermatophyte skin and nail infections	Topical	Rash.
Antiviral Agents†			
Acyclovir (Zovirax)	HSV, varicella-zoster	IV, PO, topical	Nephrotoxicity, CNS toxicity, nausea, vomiting.
Famciclovir (Famvir)	HSV, varicella-zoster	PO	Less frequent dosing (q 8 hrs) than acyclovir.
Valacyclovir (Valtrex)	HSV, varicella-zoster	PO	Pro-drug for acyclovir. Less frequent dosing (q 8 hrs).
Ganciclovir (Cytovene)	CMV, EBV, HSV	IV, PO, intraocular	Bone-marrow toxicity, phlebitis, headache, disorientation, nausea, anorexia, myalgia, rash.
Foscarnet (Foscavir)	CMV, EBV, HSV	IV	Nephrotoxicity.
Cidofovir (Vistide)	CMV, EBV, HSV	IV, intraocular	Effective for CMV and acyclovir-resistant HSV; prolonged duration of action allows infrequent dosing (every other week for IV).
Valganciclovir (Valcyte)	CMV	PO	Active against CMV strains that are resistant to other agents.
Amantadine (Symmetrel, Symadine)	Influenza A	PO	CNS toxicity, anticholinergic reactions.
Rimantadine (Flumadine)	Influenza A	PO	Fewer side effects than amantadine.
Zanamivir (Relenza)	Influenza A and B	Inhaled	An inhaled neuraminidase inhibitor. Approved for treatment and prophylaxis of contacts.
Oseltamivir (Tamiflu)	Influenza A and B	PO	Oral neuraminidase inhibitor. Fewer side effects and less resistance than with others. Approval for treatment and prophylaxis of contacts.
Ribavirin (Virazole)	Respiratory syncytial virus (RSV), hepatitis C; being studied for use with hantavirus	Inhaled, IV, PO	Synergistic with interferon-α for hepatitis C.

*Symbols: + = gram-positive; − = gram-negative; *Staph* = penicillinase-producers.
†Antiretroviral agents for HIV infection are covered in the AIDS discussion in this chapter.

molecules tag an infecting bacterium, gaps develop in the bacterium's cell wall through which the organism ruptures and is destroyed.

Antibacterial agents can thus be separated into groups according to their specific targets on or within bacteria:

- β-lactams and glycopeptides inhibit cell wall synthesis
- polymyxins distort cytoplasmic membrane function
- quinolones and rifampicins inhibit nucleic acid synthesis
- macrolides, aminoglycosides, and tetracyclines inhibit ribosome function
- trimethoprim and sulfonamides inhibit folate metabolism

All antibiotics facilitate the growth of resistant bacteria consequent to the destruction of susceptible bacteria. Although the wide use of antimicrobial agents for veterinary and agricultural purposes has contributed to the emergence of multiresistant microorganisms, the excessive use of antibiotics, especially in hospitals, has been the most significant catalyst for resistance. Bacteria resist antibiotics by inactivation of the antibiotic, decreased accumulation of the antibiotic within the microorganism, or alteration of the target site on the microbe. For example, resistance to penicillins and cephalosporins is initiated by β-lactamase enzymes that hydrolyze the β-lactam ring, thus destroying the antibiotic's effectiveness. Resistance can be mediated by chromosomal mutations or the presence of extrachromosomal DNA, also known as *plasmid resistance*. Plasmid resistance is more important from an epidemiologic point of view because it is transmissible and usually highly stable; also, it confers resistance to many different classes of antibiotics simultaneously and is often associated with other characteristics that enable a microorganism to colonize and to invade a susceptible host.

Resistance-conferring plasmids have been identified in virtually all bacteria. Moreover, many bacteria contain transposons that can enter plasmids or chromosomes. Plasmids can therefore pick up chromosomal genes for resistance and transfer them to species not currently resistant.

Bacteria that have acquired chromosomal and plasmid-mediated resistance can neutralize or destroy antibiotics in 3 different ways (they can use 1 or more of these mechanisms simultaneously):

- by preventing the antibacterial agent from reaching its receptor site
- by modifying or duplicating the target enzyme so that it is insensitive to the antibacterial agent
- by synthesizing enzymes that destroy the antibacterial agent or modify the agent to alter its entry or receptor binding

Antimicrobial susceptibility testing permits a rational choice of antibiotics, although correlation of in vivo and in vitro susceptibility is not always precise. Disk-diffusion susceptibility testing has provided qualitative data about the inhibitory activity of commonly used antimicrobials against an isolated pathogen, and these data are usually sufficient. In serious infections, such as infective endocarditis, it is useful to quantify the drug concentrations that inhibit and kill the pathogen. The lowest drug concentration that prevents the growth of a defined inoculum of the isolated pathogen is the *minimal inhibitory con-*

centration (MIC); the lowest concentration that kills 99.9% of an inoculum is the *minimal lethal concentration (MLC)*. For bactericidal drugs, the MIC and MLC are usually similar.

The antimicrobial activity of a treated patient's serum can be estimated via measurement of serum bactericidal titers. Clinical experience suggests that intravascular infections usually are controlled when the peak serum bactericidal titer is 1.8 or greater. Bactericidal therapy is preferred for patients with immunologic compromise or life-threatening infection. Other patients may be treated effectively with either bactericidal or bacteriostatic drugs. Although synergistic combinations are useful in certain clinical situations (eg, enterococcal endocarditis, gram-negative septicemia in granulocytopenic patients), combined antimicrobial therapy should be used judiciously so that potential antagonism and toxicity can be minimized.

β-Lactam antibiotics

The β-lactam group includes the penicillins, cephalosporins, and monobactams, all of which possess a β-lactam ring that binds to specific microbial binding sites and interferes with cell wall synthesis. The carbapenems and carbacephems are often grouped with β-lactams but have a slightly different ring structure. As new β-lactam agents emerge, it has become customary to refer to them by generation. The generation not only classifies agents chronologically but also connotes their antimicrobial spectrum. The majority of new agents have been created by side-chain manipulation of the β-lactam ring, which has improved resistance to enzymatic degradation. However, some of the newer antibiotics (such as third-generation cephalosporins) show diminished potency against gram-positive cocci, especially staphylococci.

Penicillins The first *natural penicillins,* types G and V, were degraded by the enzyme penicillinase. The *penicillinase-resistant penicillins,* such as methicillin, nafcillin, oxacillin, and cloxacillin, were developed for treatment of resistant *Staphylococcus* species, and except for a strain of methicillin-resistant S *epidermidis,* they were effective. The next generation of penicillins included the *aminopenicillins,* ampicillin and amoxicillin, created by placement of an amino group on the acyl side chain of the penicillin nucleus. This change broadened their effectiveness to include *H influenzae, E coli,* and *Proteus mirabilis.* The next advance was the *carboxypenicillins,* carbenicillin and ticarcillin, active against aerobic gram-negative rods such as *P aeruginosa, Enterobacter* species, and indole-positive strains of *Proteus.* Therefore, carboxypenicillins are particularly effective for intra-abdominal conditions such as cholangitis, diverticular rupture, and gynecologic infections. The fourth-generation penicillins, known as *acylureidopenicillins,* included azlocillin, mezlocillin, and piperacillin. Currently, their usefulness is for the treatment of Enterobacteriaceae, *P aeruginosa,* and febrile neutropenic patients, as well as for infections secondary to a combination of flora found in skin, soft tissue, intra-abdominal, and pelvic infections. However, because of the possibility of emergence of resistance, the newer penicillins are usually administered with an aminoglycoside. Current data, however, do not indicate that they are superior to the older penicillins in such circumstances.

Allergic reactions are the chief adverse effects encountered with the use of the penicillins. In fact, among antimicrobial agents, the penicillins are the leading cause of allergy.

Allergy to the penicillins may be present in 3%–5% of the general population and in as many as 10% of those who have previously received a penicillin. Furthermore, the reported mortality rate with penicillin-induced anaphylaxis is approximately 10%. Large doses or prolonged administration seems to be associated with a high frequency of untoward reaction. Allergic reactions to penicillin are less frequent when the drug is administered orally. Reactions are somewhat higher in frequency when aqueous crystalline penicillin G is given by injection and distinctly higher when procaine penicillin G is given intramuscularly. Cross-allergenicity among the semisynthetic and natural penicillins apparently reflects their common 6-aminopenicillanic acid nucleus and sensitizing derivatives. Cross-allergenicity to cephalosporins may occur in 3%–5% of patients and should be of particular concern when the allergic reaction to either group of antimicrobial agents has been of the immediate type, such as anaphylaxis, angioneurotic edema, or hives.

Cephalosporins The *first-generation cephalosporins* are active against β-lactamase–producing gram-positive cocci and gram-negative bacilli, which are responsible for most community-acquired infections. *Bacillus fragilis, P aeruginosa,* and *Enterobacter* species are typically resistant, as are methicillin-resistant staphylococci. None of the first-generation cephalosporins cross the meninges in concentrations sufficient for the treatment of meningitis.

The *second-generation extended-spectrum cephalosporins* have expanded coverage against gram-negative bacilli.

Third-generation cephalosporins have greater activity against gram-negative bacilli than the earlier cephalosporins, specifically inhibiting the majority of Enterobacteriaceae. Unfortunately, none of the third-generation cephalosporins is effective against enterococci. In general, third-generation cephalosporins are less active than their predecessors against gram-positive organisms, especially *S aureus*. Activity against *B fragilis* varies. Third-generation cephalosporins penetrate the cerebrospinal fluid and have been used successfully to treat meningitis caused by susceptible microorganisms. It is advisable to limit these expensive antibiotics to situations in which they offer a clear advantage, such as in gram-negative bacillary infections or in place of more toxic agents. With the possible exception of ceftazidime, none of these agents is effective enough to be used by itself against *P aeruginosa* or in a febrile neutropenic patient. Likewise, these agents are not to be used for surgical prophylaxis because of their limited activity against gram-positive organisms. Although several oral third-generation cephalosporins are now available, their antimicrobial spectrum is not as broad as that of the parenteral third-generation cephalosporins.

The *fourth-generation cephalosporins,* cefepime and cefpirome, have a very broad spectrum of activity and are active against most gram-positive bacteria, as well as *Pseudomonas* and other gram-negative organisms that are resistant to other β-lactam antibiotics. The fourth-generation cephalosporins also provide good coverage for most anaerobic infections. A new investigational cephalosporin, cefozopran, has similar activity and antibacterial spectrum. Two others, S-3578 and BAL9141, have activity against methicillin-resistant staphylococci and penicillin-resistant *S pneumoniae*.

In recent years, the benefits of continuous intravenous infusion of β-lactam antibiotics, such as nafcillin and ceftazidime, have been demonstrated. This method of dosing provides continuous and stable therapeutic blood and tissue levels of an antibiotic.

Parenteral cephalosporins have a direct effect on prothrombin production and on suppression of vitamin K–producing intestinal flora. The risk of hemorrhagic complications is increased in patients who are taking parenteral cephalosporins in conjunction with heparin, possibly the result of an additive or synergistic pharmacologic effect. The hypoprothrombinemic effects of oral anticoagulants may be increased by such cephalosporins as cefoxitin, leading to a coagulopathy. Acute intolerance to alcohol may occur in persons receiving cephalosporins that possess an N-methylthiotetrazole side chain, such as cefamandole or cefoperazone. Patients should avoid alcohol during therapy and for 2–3 days after completion.

Carbapenems Carbapenems are a class of antibiotics with a basic ring structure similar to that of penicillins, except that a carbon atom replaces sulfur at the number 1 position. The antibacterial spectrum of the carbapenems is broader than that of any other existing antibiotic and includes *S aureus, Enterobacter* species, and *P aeruginosa*. However, carbapenem-resistant strains of *Staphylococcus, Pseudomonas, Klebsiella, Acinetobacter,* and *Bacteroides* have been reported recently. Carbapenems also have excellent activity against anaerobic bacteria, including *Bacteroides fragilis*. Cross-resistance between the carbapenems and between carbapenems and piperacillin/tazobactam has been reported recently in *Pseudomonas* isolates. Carbapenems produce a postantibiotic killing effect against some organisms, with a delay in regrowth of damaged organisms similar to that seen with aminoglycosides but not with cephalosporins or acylureidopenicillins. This quality can be particularly important for settings in which host defenses are compromised, such as granulocytopenia or sequestered foci of infection.

Imipenem-cilastatin (Primaxin) combines imipenem, a carbapenem, with cilastatin, an inhibitor of renal dehydropeptidase. Cilastatin has no antimicrobial activity and is present solely to prevent degradation of imipenem by dehydropeptidase. As monotherapy for mixed infections, imipenem-cilastatin is an appropriate compound. Up to 50% of penicillin-allergic patients are also allergic to imipenem.

Meropenem (Merrem), *biapenem, panipenem, ertapenem, faropenem,* and *ritipenem* are newer penems that have increased stability against degradation by dehydropeptidases. *Doripenem* is a new agent that appears to be the most effective for the treatment of carbapenem-resistant gram-negative bacilli and penicillin-resistant streptococci.

Loracarbef (Lorabid) is an oral *carbacephem,* a class of antibiotic that is structurally similar to cephalosporins but that possesses a broader spectrum due to higher stability against both plasmid and chromosomally mediated β-lactamases. Loracarbef provides good coverage for most gram-positive and gram-negative aerobic bacteria. Newer parenteral carbacephems are currently being evaluated.

Clavulanic acid, sulbactam, and *tazobactam* are β-lactam molecules that possess little intrinsic antibacterial activity, but they are potent inhibitors of many plasmid-mediated class A β-lactamases. Currently, 4 combinations of β-lactam antibiotics plus β-lactamase inhibitors are available in the United States: *Augmentin* (oral amoxicillin and clavulanic acid), *Timentin* (intravenous ticarcillin and clavulanic acid), *Unasyn* (intravenous ampicillin and sulbactam), and *Zosyn* (intravenous piperacillin and tazobactam). These drugs have excellent activity against β-lactamase–producing gram-positive and gram-negative bacteria as well as many anaerobes. Recent research has illuminated new broad spectrum inhibitors that are capable of simultaneously inactivating several classes of β-lactamases (including classes A, C, and D) and has explored potential new cephalosporin-derived β-lactamase inactivators.

Monobactams are a monocyclic class of antibiotics utilizing only the β-lactam ring as their core structure. This group possesses excellent activity against aerobic gram-negative bacilli but is ineffective against both gram-positive cocci and anaerobes. The monobactams are similar in antimicrobial spectrum to the aminoglycosides and are generally better tolerated. However, the use of monobactams is limited by their narrow spectrum: many nosocomial infections are polymicrobial, involving gram-positive bacteria or anaerobes in addition to gram-negative aerobic bacilli. Despite the presence of a β-lactam ring, cross-allergenicity with penicillins and cephalosporins appears to be minimal. *Aztreonam,* the first approved monobactam antibiotic, has an excellent safety profile and good success rate in the treatment of infections caused by aerobic gram-negative bacilli. Aztreonam is usually combined with a semisynthetic antistaphylococcal penicillin or clindamycin in presumptive therapy of known mixed infections. Other new monobactams are currently under evaluation in microbiologic and clinical trials.

Aminoglycosides

The aminoglycoside antibiotics inhibit protein synthesis by binding to bacterial ribosomes. Gentamicin, tobramycin, amikacin, kanamycin, streptomycin, and netilmicin can be considered as a group because of their similar activity, pharmacology, and toxicity. Because of poor gastrointestinal absorption, parenteral administration is necessary to produce therapeutic levels.

Aminoglycosides are used for treatment of serious infections caused by gram-negative bacilli, including bacteremia in immunocompromised hosts, hospital-acquired pneumonia, and peritonitis. They may be combined with penicillin for the treatment of enterococcal endocarditis. Aminoglycosides are not effective against meningitis because they do not cross the blood–brain barrier. Aminoglycosides are not used for most gram-positive infections because the β-lactams are less toxic.

The major adverse effects of the aminoglycosides are nephrotoxicity and ototoxicity. Baseline blood urea nitrogen and creatinine levels should be measured, and serial studies should be performed twice a week. Aminoglycoside peak and trough serum levels should be obtained in patients with known renal disease. Combined administration of a loop diuretic such as furosemide with aminoglycosides has a synergistic ototoxic effect, potentially leading to permanent loss of cochlear function.

Penicillins may decrease the antimicrobial effectiveness of parenteral aminoglycosides, particularly in patients with impaired renal function. Aminoglycosides may exacerbate the neuromuscular blocking effects of nondepolarizing muscle relaxants such as tubocurarine. Their combined use during surgery can cause a prolonged respiratory depression accompanied by extended apnea. Oral aminoglycosides are used for bowel sterilization before gastrointestinal surgery; however, they may cause malabsorption of vitamin K, amplifying the effects of oral anticoagulants.

Once-daily aminoglycoside dosing regimens have been employed in recent years to decrease systemic toxicity, reduce variability in the timing of drug administration, and lower the costs associated with nursing care for intravenous antibiotic administration and drug level monitoring.

Macrolides

The macrolide *erythromycin* is often employed for the initial treatment of community-acquired pneumonia. This agent is effective against infections caused by pneumococci, group A streptococci, *Mycoplasma pneumoniae,* and *Chlamydia*. It is also effective against *Legionella* species, which have been recognized as a significant cause of community-acquired pneumonia. Erythromycin is used to treat upper-respiratory tract infections and sexually transmitted diseases in penicillin-allergic patients.

Clarithromycin (Biaxin), *azithromycin* (Zithromax), and *dirithromycin* (Dynabac) are newer macrolide antibiotics chemically related to erythromycin. All are well-tolerated alternatives to erythromycin and may offer particular advantages in the treatment of gonococcal and *Chlamydia* infections and in the treatment of *M avium* and other recalcitrant infections associated with AIDS. Azithromycin is subclassified as an *azalide,* and it possesses far fewer drug interactions than erythromycin. Increasing cross-resistance among the macrolides has been demonstrated. Additional new macrolide antibiotics, such as roxithromycin, spiramycin, and josamycin, are being evaluated and have similar antimicrobial spectra. Telithromycin, a new ketolide antibiotic that belongs to a new class of semisynthetic 14-membered-ring macrolides, is discussed later in this chapter.

Clindamycin has a gram-positive spectrum similar to that of erythromycin and is also active against most anaerobes, including *B fragilis*. Except for treatment of anaerobic infection, clindamycin is rarely the drug of choice. It is well absorbed orally, and parenteral formulations are available. Its major adverse effect is diarrhea, which may progress to pseudomembranous enterocolitis in some patients.

Glycopeptides

Vancomycin regained popularity because of the emergence of methicillin-resistant staphylococci and the recognition that *C difficile* is a cause of pseudomembranous colitis. Vancomycin has excellent activity against *Clostridium* and against most gram-positive bacteria, including methicillin-resistant staphylococci, *Corynebacterium* species, and other diphtheroids. Vancomycin has been used alone to treat serious infections caused by methicillin-resistant staphylococci. In cases of prosthetic-valve endocarditis caused by methicillin-resistant *S epidermidis,* a combination of vancomycin, rifampin, and gentamicin has been shown to be effective.

In recent years, several cases of vancomycin-resistant enterococcal infection have been reported. In 1 study of hospitalized patients, approximately 1% carried vancomycin-resistant enterococci in their gastrointestinal tract. These infections are very difficult or impossible to treat because of multidrug resistance. In vitro studies have shown that plasmid-mediated vancomycin resistance can be easily transferred to staphylococci; indeed, since July 2002, there have been reports of *S aureus* and *S epidermidis* infections resistant to vancomycin.

The CDC has issued recommendations regarding appropriate use of vancomycin to help counteract the emergence of bacterial drug resistance. These guidelines include discouraging the use of vancomycin for routine surgical prophylaxis, avoiding its empirical use in febrile neutropenic patients unless there is strong evidence for a β-lactam–resistant gram-positive infection, and avoiding prophylactic therapy for patients with intravascular catheters or vascular grafts. The rationale for these recommendations is that inappropriate use of this drug will only hasten the emergence of new resistant bacterial strains. Similarly, many authors think that prophylactic use of vancomycin in routine ophthalmic surgery is not advisable from an infectious disease and public health standpoint.

Teicoplanin (Targocid), a newer glycopeptide, has several advantages over vancomycin, including longer half-life, lower nephrotoxicity, and no requirement for monitoring drug levels. Teicoplanin is effective for treatment of staphylococcal infections, including endocarditis, bacteremia, osteomyelitis, and septic arthritis. The once-daily or alternate-day dosage allows home administration of treatment of serious infections caused by MRSA and enterococci, with significant savings in hospital costs and enhanced quality of life. Teicoplanin may be preferable to vancomycin for surgical prophylaxis because of its excellent tissue penetration, lower toxicity, and long half-life, allowing single-dose administration in several surgical procedures. The antibacterial activity of teicoplanin is similar to that of vancomycin but with increased potency, particularly against *Streptococcus* and *Enterococcus*. Teicoplanin is active against vancomycin-resistant organisms such as VanB-resistant and VanC-resistant strains. Teicoplanin is an investigational drug and is available from the manufacturer for compassionate use. The new investigational glycopeptides oritavancin, telavancin, and dalbavancin and the glycolipodepsipeptide ramoplanin are highly active against vancomycin-resistant infections.

Tetracyclines

The tetracyclines are bacteriostatic agents that reversibly inhibit ribosomal protein synthesis. Although they have a broad spectrum of activity (including *Rickettsia, Chlamydia, Nocardia,* and *Actinomyces*), resistance is widespread, especially among *S aureus* and gram-negative bacilli. The principal clinical uses of tetracyclines are in treatment of nongonococcal urethritis, Rocky Mountain spotted fever, chronic bronchitis, and sebaceous disorders such as acne rosacea. In addition, tetracyclines are an alternative for the penicillin-allergic patient with syphilis. Tetracyclines are well absorbed when taken on an empty stomach; however, their absorption is decreased when taken with milk, antacids, calcium, or iron. Tetracyclines are distributed throughout the extracellular fluid, but cerebrospinal fluid penetration is unreliable. Adverse effects include oral or vaginal candidiasis with prolonged use, gastrointestinal upset, photosensitivity, elevation of the blood urea nitrogen level, and pseudotumor cerebri. Tetracyclines should not be administered to pregnant women or to children younger than age 10 because of effects on developing bone and teeth. Lymecycline is a newer tetracycline agent available in Europe.

Quinolones

In 1962, *nalidixic acid* was discovered as an accidental by-product of research on quinolones as antimalarial agents. Nalidixic acid has relatively good activity against aerobic gram-negative bacteria but only limited activity against gram-positive species. Nalidixic acid can provide adequate therapy for urinary tract infections, but if taken orally, it does not produce tissue concentrations sufficient to treat systemic infections. When administered intravenously, it produces CNS and cardiac toxicity. Consequently, the quinolones were not considered an important class of drugs, particularly in the United States.

Recently, however, the introduction of a fluorine into the basic quinolone nucleus has produced compounds known as *fluoroquinolones,* which have excellent gram-positive activity. The subsequent addition of piperazine produced compounds such as *norfloxacin* (Noroxin) and *ciprofloxacin* (Cipro) that have a broad spectrum of activity, encompassing staphylococci and most of the significant gram-negative bacilli, including *Pseudomonas.* Ciprofloxacin is available in both oral and parenteral forms and can be used to treat urinary tract infections, gonorrhea, and diarrheal diseases, as well as respiratory, skin, and, particularly, bone infections. Fluoroquinolones introduced more recently into the US market include ofloxacin (Floxin), temafloxacin (Omniflox), lomefloxacin (Maxaquin), enoxacin (Penetrex), sparfloxacin (Zagam), levofloxacin (Levaquin), moxifloxacin (Avelox), gatifloxacin (Tequin), trovafloxacin (Trovan), and gemifloxacin (Factive). So far, more than 10,000 fluoroquinolone agents have been synthesized and tested since the discovery of nalidixic acid in 1962. Newer drugs awaiting FDA approval include clinafloxacin, sitafloxacin, garenoxacin, pazufloxacin, nadifloxacin, prulifloxacin, and ABT-492. The new fluoroquinolones possess even greater activity against gram-positive and gram-negative bacteria. Either moxifloxacin or levofloxacin appears to be a good treatment choice for pneumococcal infections that are resistant to penicillin and the macrolides. Oral quinolones are an alternative form of therapy to β-lactams and aminoglycosides and have permitted physicians to treat more patients outside the hospital setting.

Miscellaneous Antibacterial Agents

Rifampin was originally developed as an antituberculosis agent, but it is also used to treat a host of intractable bacterial infections. Rifampin is usually employed adjunctively because bacteria develop resistance to the drug when it is used as a single agent. Rifampin often demonstrates higher effectiveness in vivo than in vitro, perhaps because it penetrates directly into leukocytes and kills phagocytosed bacteria. It also penetrates well into bone and abscess cavities. Rifampin in combination with other agents is used successfully in the treatment of *S aureus* and prosthetic valve endocarditis caused by *S epidermidis.* Rifampin is effective in eradicating the carrier state of nasal *S aureus.* This drug is also effective prophylactically against *N meningitidis* and may be useful for treating oropharyngeal carriers of *H influenzae* type B.

Another oral antibiotic with potential for the treatment of deep-seated infections is TMP-SMX. After a single oral dose, the mean serum levels of trimethoprim and sulfamethoxazole are approximately 75% of the concentration that would be achieved through the intravenous route. In addition to its excellent pharmacokinetics, TMP-SMX has an extremely broad spectrum of activity (against Enterobacteriaceae, it is usually comparable to that of a third-generation cephalosporin or even an aminoglycoside). A number of unusual microorganisms that are resistant to cephalosporins are susceptible to TMP-SMX. One misconception is that TMP-SMX has limited activity against gram-positive bacteria; however, most streptococci, staphylococci, and *Listeria monocytogenes* are susceptible to this drug. Beyond the broad-spectrum effect of TMP-SMX, the concomitant use of *metronidazole* creates an antibiotic combination with activity against microorganisms surpassing that of a third-generation cephalosporin. TMP-SMX has seen increasing use in the treatment and prophylaxis of *Pneumocystis* infection and toxoplasmosis in recent years.

Chloramphenicol is a bacteriostatic agent that reversibly inhibits ribosomal protein synthesis. This drug is active against a wide variety of gram-negative and gram-positive organisms, including anaerobes. The major concern with this agent is hematopoietic toxicity, including reversible bone marrow suppression and irreversible aplasia. Aplastic anemia is an idiosyncratic late reaction to the drug and is usually fatal. Reversible leukopenia, thrombocytopenia, and suppression of erythropoiesis are dose related and can usually be avoided when peak serum levels are maintained at less than 25 µg/mL. Other adverse effects include hemolysis, allergy, and peripheral neuritis.

New Antibiotic Classes

Pharmacologic research is providing entirely new classes of antibiotics that offer additional treatment options for emerging resistant bacterial strains. Most of the new drugs that have been recently developed are targeted against resistant strains of gram-positive bacteria.

The first approved *streptogramin* antibiotic is *quinupristin/dalfopristin* (Synercid). Streptogramins, also called *synergistins,* represent a unique class of antibiotics notable for their outstanding antibacterial activity and their unique mechanism of action. These antibiotics, which are produced naturally by *Streptomyces* species, bind bacterial ribosomes and inhibit protein synthesis. Oral streptogramins have been available in Europe for years, but quinupristin/dalfopristin (Q/D) is the first parenteral drug in this class.

Synercid is composed of 2 semisynthetic pristinamycin derivatives, quinupristin and dalfopristin. Individually, each component drug has bacteriostatic activity; together, they exhibit synergy, resulting in bactericidal activity and up to 16 times more potency than either drug alone. Streptogramins have excellent activity against multidrug-resistant gram-positive organisms in vitro and in vivo. This class is noted for rapid bacterial killing and lacks cross-resistance with other antimicrobials. In a recent study, Q/D displayed excellent activity against all staphylococcal species tested regardless of the resistance pattern to other drug classes, including methicillin and macrolide-resistant strains. Q/D was 2 to 4 times more active than vancomycin. Q/D also has activity against mycoplasma, *N gonorrhoeae, H influenzae, Legionella,* and *Moraxella catarrhalis.* Despite a short half-life, an extended postantibiotic effect allows the drug to be administered every 8–12 hours. Adverse effects include rash, itching, diarrhea, vomiting, arthralgia, myalgias, and reversible elevation of serum alkaline phosphatase levels. Also, Q/D appears to be safe and effective in critically ill immunocompromised children with renal or hepatic impairment.

Linezolid (Zyvox) is the first approved *oxazolidinone* antibiotic and is highly active against multidrug-resistant strains of gram-positive bacteria. Linezolid is as effective as vancomycin for treatment of methicillin-resistant staphylococcal infections and active against vancomycin-resistant enterococci, penicillin-resistant and multidrug-resistant pneumococci, and macrolide-resistant streptococci. In 1 study, linezolid was the most potent new antibiotic tested against gram-positive cocci, including multiresistant strains.

Because it has monoamine oxidase inhibitor effects, drug interaction precautions are necessary. *Furazolidone* (Furoxone) and newer experimental agents eperezolid, ranbezolid, and AZD2563 are other similar oxazolidinones.

Evernimicin (Ziracin) is a new *oligosaccharide* antibiotic of the everninomicin class. This drug offers outstanding activity against drug-resistant gram-positive strains. In a recent multicenter, multinational, in vitro study, evernimicin outperformed vancomycin and Q/D against methicillin-resistant *Staphylococcus* and all other gram-positive organisms tested. *Avilamycin* is another, newer member of this antibiotic family.

Telithromycin (Ketek) is a new *ketolide* that belongs to a new class of semisynthetic 14-membered-ring macrolides, which also have expanded activity against multidrug-resistant gram-positive bacteria. In some studies, these drugs are 8 to 10 times more potent than other macrolides. Telithromycin was specifically designed for the treatment of community-acquired respiratory tract infections and offers a wide spectrum of activity against common respiratory pathogens, such as *S pneumoniae, H influenzae, S pyogenes, M catarrhalis, Chlamydia pneumoniae, Legionella pneumophila,* and *M pneumoniae*. Telithromycin is active against β-lactam–resistant and macrolide-resistant bacteria and does not appear to induce cross-resistance to other antimicrobials. In 1 study, it was more effective than oral cephalosporins, macrolides, and quinolones. Orally administered telithromycin achieves good plasma levels and is highly concentrated in pulmonary tissues and leukocytes. In clinical trials, telithromycin given once daily for 5–10 days was effective for the treatment of community-acquired pneumonia, acute exacerbations of chronic bronchitis, acute sinusitis, and streptococcal pharyngitis. Cethromycin (ABT-773) and rokitamycin are new investigational macrolides that appear to possess antimicrobial activity similar to that of telithromycin.

Daptomycin, a new cyclic *lipopeptide* antibiotic, is also highly active against multidrug-resistant gram-positive bacteria. In one comparative study, daptomycin demonstrated greater bactericidal activity against MRSA and *S epidermidis*, vancomycin-resistant enterococci, and vancomycin-intermediate *S aureus* than did vancomycin, linezolid, and Q/D. An added benefit of this drug is that it has been shown to reduce the nephrotoxicity of aminoglycosides, but the mechanism of this protection is unknown.

Other new antibiotics for the treatment of multidrug-resistant infections include the glycylcycline antibiotic tigecycline (Tigacyl), which is related to the tetracyclines; the bacteriocins, nicin and sakacin; the temporins, temporin A and temporin L; the DNA nanobinders; the peptide deformylase inhibitors; a folic acid antagonist, iclaprim; nucleoside analogues; bacteriophage endolysins, which are derived from viral phage-infected bacterial cells; and antimicrobial proteins (AMPs), natural endogenous proteins able to kill bacteria, fungi, and viruses at nanomolar concentrations.

Antifungal Agents

Fluconazole (Diflucan) and *itraconazole* (Sporanox) are newer antifungal *imidazoles* for the treatment of cryptococcal meningitis, candidiasis, and other invasive fungal infections. These drugs are more effective and better tolerated than ketoconazole in the treatment of candidiasis and invasive fungal disease. Imidazoles function by inhibiting fungal cytochrome P-450–dependent enzymes, thereby blocking synthesis of the fungal cell membrane. The newer imidazoles offer a less toxic alternative to amphotericin B in the treatment of cryptococcal meningitis and may play a role in chronic suppression of *Cryptococcus* after remission of acute infection in severely immunocompromised patients. *Voriconazole* (Vfend), the first approved second-generation triazole, is available in both intravenous and oral formulations. It offers a better treatment option for invasive aspergillosis and other serious fungal infections. In a recent randomized trial, voriconazole demonstrated superior efficacy compared with parenteral amphotericin B, which is followed by other antifungal agents. Additional new investigational imidazoles include *flutrimazole, croconazole, ravuconazole, posaconazole, sertaconazole, albaconazole, lanoconazole, bifonazole, eberconazole,* and *luliconazole.*

Treatment of serious deep-seated systemic fungal infections may require the use of intravenous amphotericin B, sometimes in combined therapy with either flucytosine or an imidazole. Lipid complex and liposome-encapsulated formulations of amphotericin B (AmBisome, Amphotec) are available to reduce the drug's toxicity. Nystatin is classified as a topical antifungal agent and is structurally similar to amphotericin B. However, a new intravenous liposomal formulation of nystatin is currently in clinical trials for treatment of systemic fungal infections.

Terbinafine (Lamisil) is an *allylamine* oral antifungal agent that is effective in controlling onychomycosis due to chronic dermatophyte infections. Treatment must be continued for 6–12 weeks to eradicate the nail infection. *Butenafine* (Mentax) is a benzylamine that effectively treats skin and nail infections caused by dermatophytes.

Several novel antifungal agents include echinocandins, pneumocandins, and improved imidazoles. *Caspofungin* (Cancidas), *micafungin* (Mycamine), and *anidulafungin* (Eraxis) are echinocandins that have recently been approved for treatment of invasive *Candida* and *Aspergillus* infections. Other promising new drugs in preclinical development include inhibitors of fungal protein, fatty acid, lipid, and cell wall synthesis.

Antiviral Agents

Acyclovir (Zovirax) is a nucleoside analogue that is effective against herpes simplex and varicella-zoster infections. It inhibits viral DNA replication. One phosphorylation step of acyclovir is catalyzed by the enzyme thymidine kinase. The viral-induced thymidine kinase is far more active than the host cell thymidine kinase. Therefore, acyclovir is very active against viruses within infected host cells and yet is generally well tolerated.

Acyclovir has proven effective in the treatment of a variety of herpetic infections. A topical 5% ointment may be used in treating localized primary episodes of genital herpes. Oral acyclovir 200 mg 5 times daily is effective in treatment of acute severe genital herpes. Also, long-term suppressive therapy with oral acyclovir has demonstrated efficacy in immunocompetent patients with frequently recurring genital herpes. Intravenous acyclovir 30 mg/kg every 8 hours is the treatment of choice for herpes simplex encephalitis. Acyclovir 500 mg/M^2 every 8 hours has been used successfully for the treatment of herpes zoster infections in immunocompromised patients. This dosage is also used in patients with acute retinal necrosis syndrome.

Oral acyclovir may be used to treat herpes zoster ophthalmicus: 800 mg 5 times daily is usually effective in reducing the incidence of ocular complications of herpes zoster ophthalmicus. However, postherpetic neuralgia is not affected by this therapy. A randomized controlled study of acyclovir and oral corticosteroids demonstrated that the steroids did not help to reduce the incidence of postherpetic neuralgia when added to oral acyclovir.

Famciclovir (Famvir) and *valacyclovir* (Valtrex) are currently approved for the treatment of herpes zoster infections and have also been shown to be effective against herpes simplex in numerous studies. Both of these newer drugs allow less frequent dosing intervals (every 8–12 hours, depending on the indication). *Valganciclovir* (Valcyte) is used for the prevention and treatment of CMV infections in organ transplant patients and AIDS patients. In a few studies, it has also been found to be effective for the treatment of acute retinal necrosis caused by varicella-zoster virus.

Adefovir (Preveon) is a nucleoside analogue and is a potent inhibitor of many viruses, such as HIV, HSV, hepatitis B, HPV, and EBV. The nucleoside analogue *brivudine* appears to have a stronger antiviral effect against the varicella-zoster virus compared with acyclovir or penciclovir. The efficacy of brivudine has been documented in several clinical trials in patients with herpes simplex and herpesvirus-related infections, particularly in patients with herpes zoster.

Ganciclovir (Cytovene), foscarnet (Foscavir), and cidofovir (Vistide) are antiviral agents used for the treatment of CMV infections, including retinitis. These drugs and the antiretroviral agents are discussed in more detail under the earlier heading Acquired Immunodeficiency Syndrome.

Amantadine and rimantadine are M2 protein inhibitors effective for the treatment of influenza A and for the prophylactic treatment of contacts of infected patients. Rapid onset of drug resistance, ineffectiveness against influenza B, and CNS side effects have limited wide acceptance of these agents. Oseltamivir is an oral neuraminidase inhibitor with excellent efficacy against influenza in humans. Oseltamivir provides approximately 90% protection for household contacts of patients with influenza. Recent studies have shown a very low incidence of viral resistance to this agent. It is approved for the treatment and prophylaxis of influenza. Another neuraminidase inhibitor, zanamivir, appears to be effective for influenza, but resistance has recently been reported.

Treatment of Hospital-Acquired Infections

Decisions concerning antibiotic administration in the treatment of serious hospital-acquired infections present important considerations for the prescribing physician. Three distinct stages of therapy tend to occur in such infections. (*Note:* Especially in the latter 2 stages, cost containment is enhanced by close monitoring of mode, level, and frequency of antibiotic dosing.)

The *first stage* of therapy typically lasts about 3 days, during which time uncertainty exists about the causative organism. Therapy is given empirically, often with the combination of an aminoglycoside and a β-lactam antibiotic.

The *second stage* begins about the fourth day, at which time definitive microbiological and clinical data are available that should allow for streamlining of antibiotic therapy, usually from combination therapy to less expensive monotherapy. It is at this stage in the patient's hospital stay that routine assessment of antibiotic management offers the first opportunity to reduce hospital antibiotic costs without compromising the clinical outcome.

The *third stage* of therapy typically begins around the seventh day, when the patient is usually clinically stable and afebrile. At this point, often the only reason the patient is kept hospitalized is to continue treatment with parenteral antibiotics. In many patients, however, therapy can be switched to daily intravenous dosing or oral antibiotics, facilitating outpatient therapy. Streamlining antibiotic therapy by changing modes and frequency of administration is a major step toward effective, responsible cost containment.

Abbanat D, Macielag M, Bush K. Novel antibacterial agents for the treatment of serious Gram-positive infections. *Expert Opin Investig Drugs.* 2003;12:379–399.

Bhavnani SM, Owen JS, Loutit JS, et al. Pharmacokinetics, safety, and tolerability of ascending single intravenous doses of oritavancin administered to healthy human subjects. *Diagn Microbiol Infect Dis.* 2004;50:95–102.

Boucher HW, Groll AH, Chiou CC, et al. Newer systemic antifungal agents: pharmacokinetics, safety and efficacy. *Drugs.* 2004;64:1997–2020.

Bozdogan B, Esel D, Whitener C, et al. Antibacterial susceptibility of a vancomycin-resistant *Staphylococcus aureus* strain isolated at the Hershey Medical Center. *J Antimicrob Chemother.* 2003;52:864–868.

Bronson JJ, Barrett JF. Quinolone, everninomycin, glycylcycline, carbapenem, lipopeptide and cephem antibacterials in clinical development. *Curr Med Chem.* 2001;8:1775–1793.

Brumfitt W, Salton MR, Hamilton-Miller JM. Nisin, alone and combined with peptidoglycan-modulating antibiotics: activity against methicillin-resistant *Staphylococcus aureus* and vancomycin-resistant enterococci. *J Antimicrob Chemother.* 2002;50:731–734.

Buynak JD. The discovery and development of modified penicillin- and cephalosporin-derived beta-lactamase inhibitors. *Curr Med Chem.* 2004;11:1951–1964.

Carpenter CF, Chambers HF. Daptomycin: another novel agent for treating infections due to drug-resistant gram-positive pathogens. *Clin Infect Dis.* 2004;38:994–1000.

Centers for Disease Control and Prevention (CDC). Vancomycin-resistant *Staphylococcus aureus*—New York, 2004. *MMWR Morb Mortal Wkly Rep.* 2004 Apr 23;53(15):322–323.

Cui L, Ma X, Sato K, et al. Cell wall thickening is a common feature of vancomycin resistance in *Staphylococcus aureus*. *J Clin Microbiol.* 2003;41:5–14.

Dalhoff A, Thomson CJ. The art of fusion: from penams and cephems to penems. *Chemotherapy.* 2003;49:105–120.

Decousser JW, Pina P, Picot F, et al. Comparative in vitro activity of faropenem and 11 other antimicrobial agents against 250 invasive *Streptococcus pneumoniae* isolates from France. *Eur J Clin Microbiol Infect Dis.* 2003;22:561–565.

Delgado G Jr, Neuhauser MM, Bearden DT, et al. Quinupristin-dalfopristin: an overview. *Pharmacotherapy.* 2000;20:1469–1485.

Deshpande L, Rhomberg PR, Fritsche TR, et al. Bactericidal activity of BAL9141, a novel parenteral cephalosporin against contemporary Gram-positive and Gram-negative isolates. *Diagn Microbiol Infect Dis.* 2004;50:73–75.

Gallagher JC, MacDougall C, Ashley ES, et al. Recent advances in antifungal pharmacotherapy for invasive fungal infections. *Expert Rev Anti Infect Ther.* 2004;2:253–268.

Graninger W, Zeitlinger M. Clinical applications of levofloxacin for severe infections. *Chemotherapy.* 2004;50 suppl 1:16–21.

Hoellman DB, Lin G, Ednie LM, et al. Antipneumococcal and antistaphylococcal activities of ranbezolid (RBX 7644), a new oxazolidinone, compared to those of other agents. *Antimicrob Agents Chemother.* 2003;47:1148–1150.

Johnson MD, Perfect JR. Caspofungin: first approved agent in a new class of antifungals. *Expert Opin Pharmacother*. 2003;4:807–823.

Jones RN, Hare RS, Sabatelli FJ, et al. In vitro gram-positive antimicrobial activity of evernimicin (SCH 27899), a novel oligosaccharide, compared with other antimicrobials: a multicentre international trial. *J Antimicrob Chemother*. 2001;47:15–25.

Jones RN, Huynh HK, Biedenbach DJ. Activities of doripenem (S-4661) against drug-resistant clinical pathogens. *Antimicrob Agents Chemother*. 2004;48:3136–3140.

Klein JO. Amoxicillin/clavulanate for infections in infants and children: past, present and future. *Pediatr Infect Dis J*. 2003;22(8 suppl):S139–148.

Mercier RC, Kennedy C, Meadows C. Antimicrobial activity of tigecycline (GAR-936) against *Enterococcus faecium* and *Staphylococcus aureus* used alone and in combination. *Pharmacotherapy*. 2002;22:1517–1523.

Montecalvo MA. Ramoplanin: a novel antimicrobial agent with the potential to prevent vancomycin-resistant enterococcal infection in high-risk patients. *J Antimicrob Chemother*. 2003;51(suppl 3):31–35.

Peck R, Gimple SK, Gregory DW, et al. Progressive outer retinal necrosis in a 73-year-old man: treatment with valganciclovir. *AIDS*. 2003;17(7):1110–1111.

Rybak MJ, Hershberger E, Moldovan T, et al. In vitro activities of daptomycin, vancomycin, linezolid, and quinupristin-dalfopristin against Staphylococci and Enterococci, including vancomycin-intermediate and -resistant strains. *Antimicrob Agents Chemother*. 2000;44:1062–1066.

Savant V, Saeed T, Denniston A, et al. Oral valganciclovir treatment of varicella zoster virus acute retinal necrosis. *Eye*. 2004;18(5):544–545.

Spiers KM, Zervos MJ. Telithromycin. *Expert Rev Anti Infect Ther*. 2004;2:685–693.

Stevens DL, Dotter B, Madaras-Kelly K. A review of linezolid: the first oxazolidinone antibiotic. *Expert Rev Anti Infect Ther*. 2004;2:51–59.

Welliver R, Monto AS, Carewicz O, et al. Effectiveness of oseltamivir in preventing influenza in household contacts. A randomized controlled trial. *JAMA*. 2001;285:748–754.

CHAPTER 2

Hypertension

Recent Developments

- Normal blood pressure is less than 120/80 mm Hg, according to guidelines published in 2003 by the Joint National Committee on Prevention, Detection, Evaluation, and Treatment of High Blood Pressure (The JNC 7 Report).
- Individuals with systolic blood pressure of 120–139 mm Hg or diastolic blood pressure of 80–89 mm Hg are considered to have prehypertension and should adopt healthy lifestyle measures to decrease blood pressure and prevent progression to hypertension.
- The risk of cardiovascular disease, beginning at 115/75 mm Hg, doubles with each 20/10 mm Hg rise in blood pressure.
- In persons older than age 50, systolic blood pressure higher than 140 mm Hg is a more important cardiovascular risk factor than diastolic blood pressure.
- A thiazide diuretic, either alone or in combination with other classes of antihypertensive drugs, can be used to treat most patients with uncomplicated hypertension.
- Antihypertensive drug classes other than diuretics (angiotensin-converting enzyme inhibitors, angiotensin II receptor blockers, beta-blockers, calcium channel blockers) are indicated in high risk conditions such as heart disease, kidney disease, and diabetes.
- Most patients with hypertension require 2 or more antihypertensive drugs to achieve blood pressure control (less than 140/90 mm Hg, or less than 130/80 mm Hg for patients with diabetes or kidney disease).
- Hypertension in children and adolescents is more common than previously recognized and has substantial long-term health implications.

Introduction

Hypertension affects an estimated 65 million people in the United States and approximately 1 billion people worldwide. Those with hypertension are at greater risk for stroke, myocardial infarction (MI), heart failure, peripheral vascular disease, kidney disease, and retinal vascular complications. The prevalence of hypertension increases with age and tends to be familial. Hypertension is more common in blacks than in whites, and the incidence of devastating complications is higher in lower socioeconomic groups because of greater prevalence, delayed detection, and poor control rates. Antihypertensive therapy

Classification of Blood Pressure and Diagnosis of Hypertension

A new classification of blood pressure for adults 18 years or older was published in 2003 by the Joint National Committee on Prevention, Detection, Evaluation, and Treatment of High Blood Pressure. Under the guidelines outlined in Table 2-1, normal blood pressure is less than 120/80 mm Hg. *Hypertension* is defined as systolic blood pressure of 140 mm Hg or higher or diastolic blood pressure of 90 mm Hg or higher. A new category, designated *prehypertension,* is systolic blood pressure of 120–139 mm Hg or diastolic blood pressure of 80–89 mm Hg. Stage 1 hypertension is systolic blood pressure of 140–159 mm Hg or diastolic blood pressure of 90–99 mm Hg. Stage 2 hypertension is systolic blood pressure of 160 mm Hg or higher or diastolic blood pressure of 100 mm Hg or higher. The classification is based on the average of 2 or more properly measured seated blood pressure readings on each of 2 or more office visits.

Patients in whom blood pressure is increased only in a physician's office are said to have "white coat" hypertension. Ambulatory blood pressure monitoring is warranted in these individuals and also may be helpful in assessing patients who have labile hypertension, resistant hypertension, hypotensive episodes, or postural hypotension. Ambulatory blood pressure readings are usually lower than measurements in the office and correlate better with target-organ injury than do office measurements. Blood pressure in most individuals decreases by 10% to 20% during the night (dipping pattern); those without such a decrease (nondipping pattern) are at greater risk for cardiovascular events. Individuals with a mean self-measured blood pressure of greater than 135/85 mm Hg at home are generally considered to be hypertensive.

Etiology and Pathogenesis of Hypertension

Approximately 90% of cases of hypertension are *primary (essential),* in which the etiology is unknown, and 10% are secondary to identifiable causes. Primary hypertension most likely results from diverse pathophysiologic mechanisms that increase peripheral

Table 2-1 Classification of Blood Pressure for Adults Aged 18 Years or Older

Blood Pressure Classification	Systolic, mm Hg		Diastolic, mm Hg
Normal	<120	and	<80
Prehypertension	120–139	or	80–89
Stage 1 hypertension	140–159	or	90–99
Stage 2 hypertension	≥160	or	≥100

Adapted from Chobanian AV, Bakris GL, Black HR, et al. The Seventh Report of the Joint National Committee on Prevention, Detection, Evaluation, and Treatment of High Blood Pressure: the JNC 7 report. *JAMA.* 2003;289:2561. ©2003 American Medical Association.

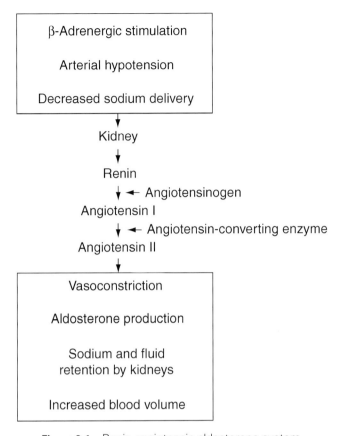

Figure 2-1 Renin-angiotensin-aldosterone system.

vascular resistance and cardiac output. Abnormal sodium transport, increased sympathetic nervous system activity, abnormal vasodilation, excess transforming growth factor β (TGF-β), and renin-angiotensin-aldosterone system (Fig 2-1) derangements all have been implicated as possible pathogenic factors for hypertension.

Causes of *secondary hypertension* are outlined in Table 2-2. Among the signs associated with secondary hypertension are

- *polycystic kidney disease:* flank mass
- *renovascular disease:* unilateral abdominal bruit in a young female with marked hypertension; new-onset hypertension with severe end-organ disease
- *pheochromocytoma:* markedly labile blood pressure with tachycardia and headache
- *hyperaldosteronism:* persistent hypokalemia in the absence of diuretic therapy
- *coarctation of aorta:* delayed or absent femoral pulses in a young patient
- *Cushing syndrome:* truncal obesity and abdominal striae

Secondary causes of hypertension should be suspected in persons who have accelerating hypertension, hypertension unresponsive to medication, or a sudden change in previously well-controlled blood pressure. Causes of resistant hypertension are listed in Table 2-3.

Table 2-2 Causes of Secondary Hypertension

> Renal parenchymal disease
> Renovascular disease
> Hyperaldosteronism
> Pheochromocytoma
> Chronic steroid therapy and Cushing syndrome
> Coarctation of the aorta
> Thyroid or parathyroid disease
> Sleep apnea
> Drugs (see Table 2-3)

Adapted from Chobanian AV, Bakris GL, Black HR, et al. The Seventh Report of the Joint National Committee on Prevention, Detection, Evaluation, and Treatment of High Blood Pressure: the JNC 7 report. *JAMA.* 2003;289:2563. ©2003 American Medical Association.

Evaluation of Hypertension

The evaluation of patients with hypertension should include an assessment of lifestyle and identification of other cardiovascular risk factors (Table 2-4), a search for causes of secondary hypertension, and determination of the presence or absence of target-organ damage and cardiovascular disease.

The physical examination should include measurement of blood pressure in both arms; ophthalmoscopic examination; calculation of body mass index (measurement of waist circumference also may be useful); auscultation for carotid, abdominal, and femoral bruits; examination of the thyroid gland; examination of the heart and lungs; examination of the abdomen for masses and aortic pulsation; examination of the lower extremities for edema and pulses; and neurological assessment.

Laboratory tests recommended before starting treatment include an electrocardiogram; urinalysis; blood glucose; hematocrit; serum potassium, creatinine (or the corresponding estimated glomerular filtration rate), calcium, and uric acid; and a lipid profile that includes high-density-lipoprotein cholesterol (HDL-C), low-density-lipoprotein cholesterol (LDL-C), and triglycerides. More extensive testing for identifiable causes of hypertension usually is not indicated unless blood pressure control is not achieved or there are other clinical findings.

Treatment of Hypertension

The primary objective of antihypertensive therapy is to reduce cardiovascular and renal morbidity and mortality. Controlling systolic blood pressure is the major concern because, in patients older than 50 years, systolic blood pressure greater than 140 mm Hg is a more important cardiovascular risk factor than diastolic blood pressure. Diastolic blood pressure usually is controlled when the systolic goal is reached. Maintaining blood pressure at less than 140/90 mm Hg decreases cardiovascular complications. In hypertensive patients with diabetes or renal disease, the blood pressure goal is less than 130/80 mm Hg. Effective blood pressure control can be attained in most patients with hypertension, but the majority require 2 or more medications. It is important for patients to understand that

Table 2-3 Causes of Resistant Hypertension

Improper blood pressure measurement
Volume overload and pseudotolerance
   Excess sodium intake
   Volume retention from kidney disease
   Inadequate diuretic therapy
Drug-induced or other causes
   Nonadherence
   Inadequate doses
   Inappropriate combinations
   Nonsteroidal anti-inflammatory drugs; cyclooxygenase-2 inhibitors
   Cocaine, amphetamines, other illicit drugs
   Sympathomimetics (decongestants, anorectics)
   Oral contraceptives
   Adrenal steroids
   Cyclosporine and tacrolimus
   Erythropoietin
   Licorice (including some chewing tobacco)
   Selected over-the-counter dietary supplements and medicines (eg, ephedra, ma huang, bitter orange)
Associated conditions
   Obesity
   Excess alcohol intake
Identifiable causes of hypertension (see Table 2-2)

Adapted from Chobanian AV, Bakris GL, Black HR, et al. The Seventh Report of the Joint National Committee on Prevention, Detection, Evaluation, and Treatment of High Blood Pressure: the JNC 7 report. *JAMA*. 2003;289:2569. ©2003 American Medical Association.

lifelong treatment is usually necessary and that symptoms are not a reliable indicator of the severity of hypertension.

In considering the appropriate therapy for an individual patient, the physician should weigh multiple factors: stage of hypertension, target-organ disease, cardiovascular risk factors, cost, compliance, side effects, and comorbid conditions. In general, the higher the blood pressure, the greater the damage to target organs; and the greater the risk factors for cardiovascular disease, the sooner treatment should be initiated. For example, patients with severe hypertension and encephalopathy require emergent treatment, whereas those with mild hypertension may attempt lifestyle modifications before drug therapy is initiated.

Lifestyle Modifications

Obesity, sedentary lifestyle, excessive sodium intake, high daily alcohol consumption, and inadequate intake of vitamins and minerals such as potassium, calcium, magnesium, and folate can contribute to the development of hypertension. Smoking is also important as a major contributor to cardiovascular disease in patients with hypertension. Lifestyle modifications, including weight reduction, the Dietary Approaches to Stop Hypertension (DASH) eating plan, dietary sodium reduction, physical activity, and moderation of alcohol consumption can decrease blood pressure, enhance antihypertensive drug efficacy,

Table 2-4 Cardiovascular Risk Factors

Major Risk Factors*
   Hypertension†
   Cigarette smoking
   Obesity (BMI ≥30)†
   Physical inactivity
   Dyslipidemia†
   Diabetes mellitus†
   Microalbuminuria or estimated GFR <60 mL/min
   Age (>55 years for men, >65 years for women)
   Family history of premature cardiovascular disease (men <55 years of age or women <65 years of age)

Target-Organ Damage
   Heart
      Left ventricular hypertrophy
      Angina or prior myocardial infarction
      Prior coronary revascularization
      Heart failure
   Brain
      Stroke or transient ischemic attack
   Chronic kidney disease
   Peripheral arterial disease
   Retinopathy

*BMI indicates body mass index calculated as weight in kilograms divided by the square of height in meters; GFR, glomerular filtration rate.
†Components of the metabolic syndrome.

Adapted from Chobanian AV, Bakris GL, Black HR, et al. The Seventh Report of the Joint National Committee on Prevention, Detection, Evaluation, and Treatment of High Blood Pressure: the JNC 7 report. *JAMA.* 2003;289:2563. ©2003 American Medical Association.

and reduce cardiovascular disease risk (Table 2-5). Such healthy lifestyle habits are essential for the prevention and control of hypertension.

Pharmacologic Treatment

Several classes of drugs effectively lower blood pressure and reduce the complications of hypertension. The most commonly prescribed antihypertensive drugs include diuretics, beta-blockers, angiotensin-converting enzyme (ACE) inhibitors, angiotensin II receptor blockers (ARB), and calcium channel blockers (CCB). Tables 2-6 and 2-7 list these and other types of oral antihypertensive drugs.

    Numerous studies have confirmed the efficacy of diuretics in preventing the cardiovascular complications of hypertension. A thiazide-type diuretic is the preferred choice for initial therapy in most patients with hypertension, used either alone or in combination with other classes of antihypertensive medications. The use of other antihypertensive drugs as initial therapy is indicated in high-risk conditions such as heart failure, post-MI, high coronary disease risk, diabetes mellitus, and chronic kidney disease, and for recurrent stroke prevention (Table 2-8). In some cases, when blood pressure is more than 20/10 mm Hg above goal, cautiously initiating treatment with 2 drugs may be appropriate. Figure 2-2 provides an algorithm for the treatment of hypertension.

Table 2-5 Lifestyle Modifications to Manage Hypertension*

Modification	Recommendation	Approximate Systolic BP Reduction, Range
Weight reduction	Maintain normal body weight (BMI, 18.5–24.9)	5–20 mm Hg/10 kg weight loss
Adoption of DASH eating plan	Consume a diet rich in fruits, vegetables, and low-fat dairy products with a reduced content of saturated and total fat	8–14 mm Hg
Dietary sodium reduction	Reduce dietary sodium intake to no more than 100 mEq/L (2.4 g sodium or 6 g sodium chloride)	2–8 mm Hg
Physical activity	Engage in regular aerobic physical activity such as brisk walking (at least 30 minutes per day, most days of the week)	4–9 mm Hg
Moderation of alcohol consumption	Limit consumption to no more than 2 drinks per day (1 oz or 30 mL ethanol [eg, 24 oz beer, 10 oz wine, or 3 oz 80-proof whiskey]) in most men and no more than 1 drink per day in women and lighter-weight persons	2–4 mm Hg

Abbreviations: BMI, body mass index calculated as weight in kilograms divided by the square of the height in meters; BP, blood pressure; DASH, Dietary Approaches to Stop Hypertension.

*For overall cardiovascular risk reduction, stop smoking. The effects of implementing these modifications are dose- and time-dependent and could be higher for some individuals.

Adapted from Chobanian AV, Bakris GL, Black HR, et al. The Seventh Report of the Joint National Committee on Prevention, Detection, Evaluation, and Treatment of High Blood Pressure: the JNC 7 report. *JAMA.* 2003;289:2564. ©2003 American Medical Association.

Antihypertensive Drugs

Diuretics

Diuretics are categorized by their site of action in the kidney and are divided into thiazide, loop, and potassium-sparing types.

Thiazide diuretics increase the sodium load on the kidney's distal tubules and initially decrease plasma volume and cardiac output through natriuresis. As the renin-angiotensin-aldosterone system compensates for plasma volume, cardiac output returns to normal and peripheral vascular resistance is lowered.

Loop diuretics act on the ascending loop of Henle and block sodium reabsorption, causing an initial decrease in plasma volume. As with thiazide diuretics, blood pressure is eventually reduced because of decreased peripheral vascular resistance. Loop diuretics are used primarily in treating patients with renal insufficiency. They are not as helpful for long-term use in patients with good renal function.

Potassium-sparing diuretics may competitively block the actions of aldosterone to prevent potassium loss from the distal tubule, or they may act directly on the distal tubule to inhibit aldosterone-induced sodium reabsorption in exchange for potassium. They are often used as adjuncts to the thiazides or loop diuretics to counteract potassium depletion.

Table 2-6 Oral Antihypertensive Drugs*

Class	Drug (Trade Name)	Usual Dose, Range, mg/d	Daily Frequency
Thiazide diuretics	Chlorothiazide (Diuril)	125–500	1
	Chlorthalidone (generic)	12.5–25	1
	Hydrochlorothiazide (Microzide, HydroDIURIL)	12.5–50	1
	Indapamide (Lozol)	1.25–2.5	1
	Metolazone (Mykrox)	0.5–1.0	1
	Metolazone (Zaroxolyn)	2.5–5	1
	Polythiazide (Renese)	2–4	1
Loop diuretics	Bumetanide (Bumex)	0.5–2	2
	Furosemide (Lasix)	20–80	2
	Torsemide (Demadex)	2.5–10	1
Potassium-sparing diuretics	Amiloride (Midamor)	5–10	1–2
	Triamterene (Dyrenium)	50–100	1–2
Aldosterone-receptor blockers	Eplerenone (Inspra)	50–100	1–2
	Spironolactone (Aldactone)	25–50	1–2
β-Blockers	Atenolol (Tenormin)	25–100	1
	Betaxolol (Kerlone)	5–20	1
	Bisoprolol (Zebeta)	2.5–10	1
	Metoprolol (Lopressor)	50–100	1–2
	Metoprolol extended release (Toprol-XL)	50–100	1
	Nadolol (Corgard)	40–120	1
	Propranolol (Inderal)	40–160	2
	Propranolol long-acting (Inderal LA)	60–180	1
	Timolol (Blocadren)	20–40	2
	Nebivolol (Bystolic)†	2.5–40	1
β-Blockers with intrinsic sympathomimetic activity	Acebutolol (Sectral)	200–800	2
	Penbutolol (Levatol)	10–40	1
	Pindolol (generic)	10–40	2
ACE inhibitors	Benazepril (Lotensin)	10–40	1–2
	Captopril (Capoten)	25–100	2
	Enalapril (Vasotec)	2.5–40	1–2
	Fosinopril (Monopril)	10–40	1
	Lisinopril (Prinivil, Zestril)	10–40	1
	Moexipril (Univasc)	7.5–30	1
	Perindopril (Aceon)	4–8	1–2
	Quinapril (Accupril)	10–40	1
	Ramipril (Altace)	2.5–20	1
	Trandolapril (Mavik)	1–4	1
Angiotensin II antagonists	Candesartan (Atacand)	8–32	1
	Eprosartan (Teveten)	400–800	1–2
	Irbesartan (Avapro)	150–300	1
	Losartan (Cozaar)	25–100	1–2
	Olmesartan (Benicar)	20–40	1
	Telmisartan (Micardis)	20–80	1
	Valsartan (Diovan)	80–320	1

(Continued)

Table 2-6 *(continued)*

Class	Drug (Trade Name)	Usual Dose, Range, mg/d	Daily Frequency
Calcium channel blockers: non-dihydropyridines	Diltiazem extended release (Cardizem CD, Dilacor XR, Tiazac)	180–420	1
	Diltiazem extended release (Cardizem LA)	120–540	1
	Verapamil immediate release (Calan, Isoptin)	80–320	2
	Verapamil long-acting (Calan SR, Isoptin SR)	120–360	1–2
	Verapamil (Covera-HS Verelan PM)	120–360	1
Calcium channel blockers: dihydropyridines	Amlodipine (Norvasc)	2.5–10	1
	Felodipine (Plendil)	2.5–20	1
	Isradipine (DynaCirc CR)	2.5–10	2
	Nicardipine sustained release (Cardene SR)	60–120	2
	Nifedipine long-acting (Adalat CC, Procardia XL)	30–60	1
	Nisoldipine (Sular)	10–40	1
α_1-Blockers	Doxazosin (Cardura)	1–16	1
	Prazosin (Minipress)	2–20	2–3
	Terazosin (Hytrin)	1–20	1–2
Combined α- and β-blockers	Carvedilol (Coreg)	12.5–50	2
	Labetalol (Normodyne, Trandate)	200–800	2
Central α_2-agonists and other centrally acting drugs	Clonidine (Catapres)	0.1–0.8	2
	Clonidine patch (Catapres-TTS)	0.1–0.3	1 weekly
	Guanfacine (generic)	0.5–2	1
	Methyldopa (Aldomet)	250–1000	2
	Reserpine (generic)	0.05–0.25	1‡
Direct vasodilators	Hydralazine (Apresoline)	25–100	2
	Minoxidil (Loniten)	2.5–80	1–2
Direct renin inhibitor	Aliskiren (Tekturna)§	150–300	1

ACE = angiotensin-converting enzyme.

*Dosages may vary from those listed in the *Physicians' Desk Reference,* which may be consulted for additional information. Many of the drugs in this table are available in generic formulations.

†Nebivolol is a novel β-blocker that combines β_1 selectivity with endothelium-dependent vasodilation.

‡0.1-mg dose may be given every other day to achieve this dosage.

§Aliskiren, an oral renin inhibitor, is the first new class of antihypertensive drug approved by the FDA in more than a decade.

Adapted from Chobanian AV, Bakris GL, Black HR, et al. The Seventh Report of the Joint National Committee on Prevention, Detection, Evaluation, and Treatment of High Blood Pressure: the JNC 7 report. *JAMA.* 2003;289:2565–2566. ©2003 American Medical Association.

Adverse effects of diuretics vary according to class. Thiazide diuretics can cause weakness, muscle cramps, impotence, hypokalemia, hyperglycemia, hyperlipidemia, hyperuricemia, hypercalcemia, hypomagnesemia, hyponatremia, azotemia, and pancreatitis. On a positive note, they may also slow demineralization that occurs with osteoporosis. Loop diuretics can cause ototoxicity as well as electrolyte abnormalities such as hypokalemia,

Table 2-7 Combination Drugs for Hypertension

Combination Type	Fixed-Dose Combination, mg*	Trade Name
ACE inhibitor and CCB	Amlodipine/benazepril hydrochloride (2.5/10, 5/10, 5/20, 10/20)	Lotrel
	Enalapril maleate/felodipine (5/5)	Lexxel
	Trandolapril/verapamil (2/180, 1/240, 2/240, 4/240)	Tarka
ACE inhibitor and diuretic	Benazepril/hydrochlorothiazide (5/6.25, 10/12.5, 20/12.5, 20/25)	Lotensin HCT
	Captopril/hydrochlorothiazide (25/15, 25/25, 50/15, 50/25)	Capozide
	Enalapril maleate/hydrochlorothiazide (5/12.5, 10/25)	Vaseretic
	Lisinopril/hydrochlorothiazide (10/12.5, 20/12.5, 20/25)	Prinzide
	Moexipril HCl/hydrochlorothiazide (7.5/12.5, 15/25)	Uniretic
	Quinapril HCl/hydrochlorothiazide (10/12.5, 20/12.5, 20/25)	Accuretic
ARB and diuretic	Candesartan cilexetil/hydrochlorothiazide (16/12.5, 32/12.5)	Atacand HCT
	Eprosartan mesylate/hydrochlorothiazide (600/12.5, 600/25)	Teveten HCT
	Irbesartan/hydrochlorothiazide (75/12.5, 150/12.5, 300/12.5)	Avalide
	Losartan potassium/hydrochlorothiazide (50/12.5, 100/25)	Hyzaar
	Telmisartan/hydrochlorothiazide (40/12.5, 80/12.5)	Micardis HCT
	Valsartan/hydrochlorothiazide (80/12.5, 160/12.5)	Diovan HCT
Beta-blocker and diuretic	Atenolol/chlorthalidone (50/25, 100/25)	Tenoretic
	Bisoprolol fumarate/hydrochlorothiazide (2.5/6.25, 5/6.25, 10/6.25)	Ziac
	Metoprolol tartrate/hydrochlorothiazide (50/25, 100/25)	Lopressor HCT
	Nadolol/bendroflumethiazide (40/5, 80/5)	Corzide
	Propranolol LA/hydrochlorothiazide (40/25, 80/25)	Inderide
	Timolol maleate/hydrochlorothiazide (10/25)	Timolide
Centrally acting drug and diuretic	Methyldopa/hydrochlorothiazide (250/15, 250/25, 500/30, 500/50)	Aldoril
	Reserpine/chlorothiazide (0.125/250, 0.25/500)	Diupres
	Reserpine/hydrochlorothiazide (0.125/25, 0.125/50)	Hydropres
Diuretic and diuretic	Amiloride HCl/hydrochlorothiazide (5/50)	Moduretic
	Spironolactone/hydrochlorothiazide (25/25, 50/50)	Aldactone
	Triamterene/hydrochlorothiazide (37.5/25, 50/25, 75/50)	Dyazide, Maxzide

Abbreviations: ACE, angiotensin-converting enzyme; ARB, angiotensin II receptor blocker; CCB, calcium channel blocker; HCl, hydrochloride; HCT, hydrochlorothiazide; LA, long-acting.

*Some drug combinations are available in multiple fixed doses. Each drug dose is reported in milligrams.

Adapted from Chobanian AV, Bakris GL, Black HR, et al. The Seventh Report of the Joint National Committee on Prevention, Detection, Evaluation, and Treatment of High Blood Pressure: the JNC 7 report. *JAMA*. 2003;289:2567. ©2003 American Medical Association.

Table 2-8 Compelling Indications for Individual Drug Classes

High-Risk Condition	Diuretic	β-Blocker	ACE Inhibitor	ARB	CCB	Aldosterone Antagonist
Heart failure	•	•	•	•		•
Post–myocardial infarction		•	•			•
High coronary disease risk	•	•	•		•	
Diabetes	•	•	•	•	•	
Chronic kidney disease			•	•		
Recurrent stroke prevention	•		•			

ACE = angiotensin-converting enzyme; ARB = angiotensin II receptor blocker; CCB = calcium channel blocker.

Adapted from Chobanian AV, Bakris GL, Black HR, et al. The Seventh Report of the Joint National Committee on Prevention, Detection, Evaluation, and Treatment of High Blood Pressure: the JNC 7 report. *JAMA.* 2003;289:2568. ©2003 American Medical Association.

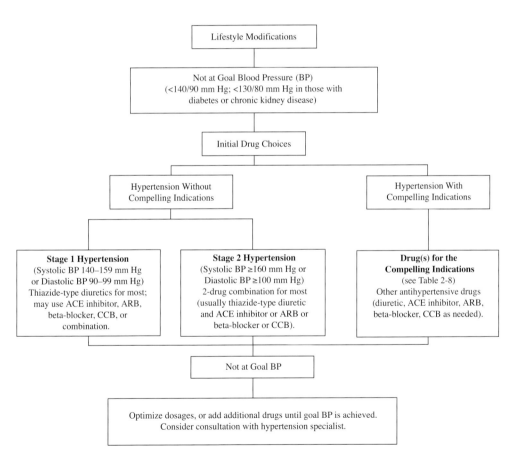

Figure 2-2 Algorithm for treatment of hypertension. *(Adapted with permission from Chobanian AV, Bakris GL, Black HR, et al. The Seventh Report of the Joint National Committee on Prevention, Detection, Evaluation, and Treatment of High Blood Pressure: the JNC 7 report. JAMA. 2003;289:2564. ©2003 American Medical Association.)*

hypocalcemia, and hypomagnesemia. Potassium-sparing diuretics can cause hyperkalemia, renal calculi, renal tubular damage, and gynecomastia.

Beta-Blockers

There are 2 types of β-adrenergic receptor sites: $β_1$ is present in vascular and cardiac tissue, and $β_2$ is found in the bronchial system. Circulating or locally released catecholamines stimulate β sites, resulting in vasoconstriction, bronchodilation, tachycardia, and increased myocardial contractility. Beta-blockers inhibit these effects. They also decrease plasma renin, reset baroreceptors to facilitate lower blood pressure, induce release of vasodilatory prostaglandins, decrease plasma volume, and may have a central nervous system–mediated antihypertensive effect.

Beta-blockers are divided into those that are nonselective ($β_1$ and $β_2$), those that are cardioselective (primarily $β_1$), and those that have intrinsic sympathomimetic activity (ISA). The cardioselective agents may be prescribed with caution in patients with pulmonary disease, diabetes, or peripheral vascular disease, but at higher doses they lose their $β_1$ selectivity and can cause adverse effects in these patients. Beta-blockers with ISA minimize the bradycardia caused by other beta-blockers.

Adverse effects of beta-blockers include bronchospasm, bradycardia, heart failure, masking of insulin-induced hypoglycemia, insomnia, fatigue, depression, impotence, impaired peripheral circulation, impaired exercise tolerance, nasal congestion, and hypertriglyceridemia (except beta-blockers with ISA). Angina pectoris and increased blood pressure can be precipitated by abrupt cessation of beta-blocker therapy. Beta-blockers generally should be avoided in patients with asthma, reactive airways disease, or second-degree or third-degree heart block. Beta-blockers are beneficial in the treatment of atrial fibrillation and tachyarrhythmias, migraine, thyrotoxicosis, and essential tremor.

Angiotensin-Converting Enzyme Inhibitors

Angiotensin-converting enzyme catalyzes the conversion of angiotensin I to angiotensin II. Angiotensin II, a potent vasoconstrictor, is the primary vasoactive hormone of the renin-angiotensin-aldosterone system, and it plays a major role in the pathophysiology of hypertension. ACE inhibitors block the conversion of angiotensin I to angiotensin II, resulting in vasodilation with decreased peripheral vascular resistance and natriuresis. They also decrease aldosterone production and increase levels of vasodilating bradykinins. Some ACE inhibitors stimulate production of vasodilatory prostaglandins. The efficacy of ACE inhibitors is enhanced when they are used together with diuretics, and they can reduce hypokalemia, hypercholesterolemia, hyperglycemia, and hyperuricemia caused by diuretic therapy. ACE inhibitors are beneficial in patients with left ventricular dysfunction and with kidney disease.

Adverse effects of ACE inhibitors include a dry cough (5%–20% of patients), angioneurotic edema, hypotension, hyperkalemia, abnormal taste, leukopenia, proteinuria, and renal failure in patients with preexisting renal insufficiency. ACE inhibitors should be avoided in patients with a history of angioedema; they are contraindicated in pregnancy.

Angiotensin II Receptor Blockers

Angiotensin II receptor blockers inhibit the vasoconstrictor and aldosterone-secreting effects of angiotensin II by selectively blocking angiotensin II receptors that are found in such tissues as vascular smooth muscle and the adrenal gland, resulting in decreased peripheral vascular resistance. ARBs are effective in the management of hypertension in a variety of situations, including patients with heart failure who are unable to tolerate ACE inhibitors.

Side effects of ARBs are similar to those occurring with ACE inhibitors, although less common. The cough caused by ACE inhibitors generally does not occur with ARBs, and angioedema is rare. Like ACE inhibitors, ARBs are contraindicated in pregnancy.

Calcium Channel Blockers

Calcium channel blockers block the entry of calcium into vascular smooth muscle cells, resulting in reduced myocardial contractility and decreased systemic vascular resistance. CCBs are divided into dihydropyridine and non-dihydropyridine types.

Adverse effects of CCBs vary according to the agent but include constipation, headache, fatigue, dizziness, nausea, palpitations, flushing, edema, gingival hyperplasia, arrhythmias, and cardiac ischemia. Because of their negative inotropic effects, CCBs generally should be avoided in patients with cardiac conduction abnormalities or heart failure associated with left ventricular dysfunction and in the setting of acute MI. CCBs may be helpful in Raynaud syndrome and in some arrhythmias.

α_1-Blockers

α_1-Adrenergic antagonists block postsynaptic α-receptors, resulting in arterial and venous vasodilation. Selective α_1-blockers have replaced older nonselective agents in the treatment of hypertension. These agents are not as effective as diuretics, CCBs, and ACE inhibitors, but they may be prescribed as adjunct therapy in selected cases.

Adverse effects include "first-dose effect," in which blood pressure is decreased more with the initial dose than with subsequent doses; orthostatic hypotension; headache; dizziness; and drowsiness.

Combined α-Adrenergic and β-Adrenergic Antagonists

These dual-property agents block the action of catecholamines at both α-adrenergic and β-adrenergic receptor sites. Side effects are similar to those of other α-adrenergic and β-adrenergic antagonists.

Centrally Acting Adrenergic Agents

Centrally acting adrenergic drugs are potent antihypertensive agents that stimulate presynaptic α_2-adrenergic receptors in the central nervous system, causing decreased sympathetic tone, cardiac output, and peripheral vascular resistance.

Adverse effects include fluid retention, dry mouth, drowsiness, dizziness, orthostatic hypotension, rash, impotence, positive direct antibody (Coombs') test, positive ANA test, hepatitis, heart failure in patients with decreased left ventricular dysfunction, and severe rebound hypertension when the drug is abruptly discontinued.

Older centrally acting sympatholytic agents (eg, reserpine) have significant side effects and are now seldom used.

Direct Vasodilators

These potent antihypertensive agents decrease peripheral vascular resistance by direct arterial vasodilation. They are generally reserved for special situations, such as pregnancy or intractable hypertension. They should be avoided or used with caution in patients with ischemic heart disease.

Adverse effects include headache, tachycardia, edema, nausea, vomiting, a lupus-like syndrome, and hypertrichosis. Because of the sympathetic hyperactivity and the sodium and fluid retention caused by direct vasodilators, they are often used in conjunction with diuretics or beta-blockers to mitigate unwanted effects.

Parenteral Antihypertensive Drugs

Parenteral antihypertensive therapy is indicated for immediate reduction of blood pressure in hypertensive emergencies.

Sodium nitroprusside (Nitropress), a direct arterial and venous vasodilator, is the drug of choice for most hypertensive emergencies. Nitroglycerin (generic) may be preferable in patients with severe coronary insufficiency or advanced kidney or liver disease. Labetalol (Normodyne, Trandate) is also effective and is the drug of choice in hypertensive emergencies that occur in pregnancy. Esmolol (Brevibloc) is a cardioselective β-adrenergic antagonist that can be used in hypertensive emergencies when beta-blocker intolerance is a concern; also, it is useful in the treatment of aortic dissection. Phentolamine (generic) is effective in the management of hypertension with acute drug intoxication or withdrawal. Nicardipine (Cardene) is an IV calcium antagonist that is used for postoperative hypertension. Enalaprilat (Vasotec IV) is an IV ACE inhibitor that can be effective, although unpredictable results have been reported with its use. Diazoxide (Hyperstat) and hydralazine (generic) are used infrequently now, but hydralazine does have a long-established safety profile and may be useful in pregnancy-related hypertensive emergencies.

Special Considerations

Ischemic Heart Disease

For patients with hypertension and stable angina pectoris, a beta-blocker is generally the initial drug of choice; alternatively, CCBs can be used. ACE inhibitors and beta-blockers are recommended as first-line drugs in hypertensive patients with acute coronary syndromes (unstable angina or MI). In patients with post-MI, beta-blockers, ACE inhibitors, and potassium-sparing diuretics (aldosterone antagonists) are beneficial.

Heart Failure

In asymptomatic patients with ventricular dysfunction, ACE inhibitors and beta-blockers are recommended. In patients with symptomatic ventricular dysfunction or end-stage heart failure, ACE inhibitors, beta-blockers, ARBs, aldosterone antagonists, and loop diuretics are useful.

Diabetes and Hypertension

To achieve a blood pressure goal of less than 130/80 mm Hg, patients usually need 2 or more antihypertensive drugs. Thiazide diuretics, beta-blockers, ACE inhibitors, ARBs, and CCBs reduce cardiovascular complications in patients with diabetes. ACE inhibitors and ARBs are beneficial for those with diabetic nephropathy.

Chronic Renal Disease

Aggressive treatment, often with 3 or more drugs, is needed to achieve a blood pressure goal of less than 130/80 and to prevent deterioration of renal function and cardiovascular complications in patients with chronic renal disease. ACE inhibitors and ARBs favorably alter the progression of diabetic and nondiabetic nephropathy. For cases of advanced renal disease, loop diuretics may be useful in combination with other drug classes.

Cerebrovascular Disease

The combination of an ACE inhibitor and a thiazide diuretic lowers the risk of recurrent stroke. The optimal blood pressure level during an acute stroke remains undetermined, but consensus favors intermediate control in the range of 160/100 mm Hg until patient stabilization is achieved.

Obesity and the Metabolic Syndrome

Obesity (body mass index ≥30) is a risk factor for the development of hypertension and has become a major concern in the United States, where an estimated 122 million adults are overweight or obese. Closely related to obesity is the *metabolic syndrome,* defined as the presence of 3 or more of the following conditions: abdominal obesity, glucose intolerance, blood pressure of 130/85 mm Hg or higher, hypertriglyceridemia, or low HDL-C level. Patients with these conditions should adopt healthy lifestyle habits and use drug therapy if necessary.

Sleep Disorders

Obstructive sleep apnea frequently coexists with obesity and appears to be an independent risk factor for hypertension and other cardiovascular diseases.

Left Ventricular Hypertrophy

Left ventricular hypertrophy is a risk factor for cardiovascular disease, but it can undergo regression with treatment of hypertension. All antihypertensive drug classes, except the direct vasodilators, are effective for treatment of left ventricular hypertrophy.

Peripheral Arterial Disease

The risk of peripheral arterial disease parallels that of ischemic heart disease in patients with hypertension. All classes of antihypertensive agents are useful in treating hypertensive patients with peripheral arterial disease.

Orthostatic Hypotension

Orthostatic hypotension is a postural drop in systolic blood pressure of more than 10 mm Hg associated with dizziness or fainting. It occurs more frequently in elderly patients with systolic hypertension, in patients with diabetes, and in those taking diuretics, vasodilators, and certain psychotropic drugs. Blood pressure in these individuals should be monitored in the upright position, medication dosages should be carefully titrated, and volume depletion should be avoided.

Hypertension in Older Patients

Hypertension is present in the majority of individuals older than age 65. Treatment recommendations for this group are generally the same as for others with hypertension. In older patients with isolated systolic hypertension, a diuretic with or without a beta-blocker, or a dihydropyridine CCB alone, is the preferred treatment.

Antihypertensive drug therapy in elderly patients can produce side effects such as dizziness and hypotension that increase the risk of falls. Appropriate precautions should be taken to reduce risks and enhance patient safety.

Dementia occurs more commonly with hypertension. In some patients, antihypertensive therapy may slow the progression of cognitive impairment.

Women and Pregnancy

Women taking oral contraceptives should have regular blood pressure checks, as use of oral contraceptives increases the risk of hypertension. Hypertension in women who are pregnant potentially increases maternal and fetal morbidity and mortality. Also, the possibility of adverse effects of antihypertensive drugs on fetal development must be considered. Hypertension in women who are pregnant may be classified as follows:

- Preeclampsia or eclampsia. *Preeclampsia* is defined as pregnancy, hypertension, proteinuria, generalized edema, and possibly coagulation and liver function abnormalities after 20 weeks' gestation. *Eclampsia* includes those abnormalities plus generalized seizures.
- Chronic hypertension. This is defined as blood pressure of more than 140/90 mm Hg before 20 weeks' gestation.
- Chronic hypertension with superimposed preeclampsia or eclampsia.
- Transient hypertension. This condition is characterized by hypertension without proteinuria or central nervous system manifestations during pregnancy and by the return of normal blood pressure within 10 days of delivery.

Methyldopa, beta-blockers, and vasodilators are the recommended agents for treatment of hypertension in pregnancy. ACE inhibitors and ARBs are contraindicated in pregnancy because of teratogenic effects, and they should also be avoided in women who are likely to become pregnant.

Children and Adolescents

Considerable advances have been made in the detection, evaluation, and management of hypertension in children and adolescents. Current evidence indicates that primary hypertension in the young occurs more commonly than previously recognized and has substantial long-term health implications. Hypertension in this group is defined as average systolic blood pressure and/or diastolic blood pressure that is in the 95th percentile or higher for gender, age, and height on 3 or more occasions. Blood pressure between the 90th percentile and the 95th percentile in childhood is now designated as *prehypertension* and is an indication for lifestyle modifications. It is recommended that children older than 3 years who are seen in a medical setting should have their blood pressure measured.

Hypertensive children and adolescents are frequently overweight, and some have sleep disorders. Secondary hypertension occurs more commonly in children than in adults.

Indications for antihypertensive drug therapy in children include uncontrolled hypertension despite nonpharmacologic measures, symptomatic hypertension, secondary hypertension, hypertensive target-organ damage, and hypertension with diabetes. Acceptable drug choices for treatment of hypertension in children include diuretics, beta-blockers, ACE inhibitors, ARBs, and CCBs.

Minority Populations

Significant racial and ethnic disparities in awareness, treatment, and control of hypertension exist in the United States. Blood pressure control rates are lowest in Mexican Americans and Native Americans. The prevalence and severity of hypertension are increased in blacks, in whom beta-blockers, ACE inhibitors, and ARBs are less effective than diuretics and CCBs in lowering blood pressure. In general, treatment of hypertension is similar in all demographic groups; unfortunately, in many minority patients, socioeconomic and lifestyle factors continue to be barriers to treatment.

Withdrawal Syndromes

Hypertension can be associated with withdrawal from drugs such as alcohol, cocaine, amphetamines, and opioid analgesics. Withdrawal syndromes can occur with acute drug intoxication or as the result of abrupt discontinuation of a drug after chronic use. Phentolamine, sodium nitroprusside, and nitroglycerin are all effective in the acute management of these situations. Beta-blockers should not be used in this setting, as unopposed α-adrenergic stimulation can exacerbate the hypertension.

Monoamine oxidase inhibitors taken with certain drugs or with tyramine-containing foods can cause accelerated hypertension by increasing catecholamines. Phentolamine, sodium nitroprusside, and labetalol are effective for treating this type of hypertension.

Abrupt discontinuation of antihypertensive therapy can cause severe rebound hypertension. This occurs most commonly with centrally acting adrenergic agents (particularly clonidine) and with beta-blockers but can occur with other drug classes as well, including diuretics. When an acute withdrawal syndrome occurs and parenteral antihypertensive treatment is needed, sodium nitroprusside is the drug of choice.

Hypertensive Crisis

Patients with severe blood pressure elevation and acute target-organ damage (eg, encephalopathy, MI, unstable angina, pulmonary edema, stroke, head trauma, eclampsia, or aortic dissection) should be hospitalized for emergency parenteral antihypertensive therapy. Patients with marked blood pressure elevation but without target-organ damage may not require hospitalization, but they should be treated urgently with combination oral antihypertensive agents. Identifiable causes of hypertension should be sought, and these patients should be carefully monitored for target-organ damage.

Ophthalmic Considerations

Retinal vascular complications (hypertensive retinopathy, retinal vein occlusions, retinal arterial occlusions), glaucoma, ischemic optic neuropathy, microvascular cranial nerve palsies, and stroke-related disorders of the afferent and efferent visual system are commonly associated with hypertension. Moreover, ophthalmic surgical patients with poorly controlled hypertension may be more susceptible to operative and perioperative complications.

There is strong evidence that certain signs of hypertensive retinopathy, independent of other risk factors, are associated with increased cardiovascular risk. Based on these reported associations, a simplified classification of hypertensive retinopathy recently has been proposed (Table 2-9).

The JNC 7 report emphasizes that control of hypertension is possible only if patients are motivated to take their prescribed medications and to maintain healthy lifestyle habits. Motivation improves when individuals develop empathy with and trust in their physi-

Table 2-9 Classification of Hypertensive Retinopathy With Systemic Associations

Grade of Retinopathy	Retinal Signs	Systemic Associations
None	No detectable signs	None
Mild	Generalized and/or focal arteriolar narrowing, arteriovenous nicking, opacity ("copper wiring") of arteriolar wall, or a combination of these signs	Modest association with risk of stroke, coronary artery disease, and death
Moderate	Hemorrhage (blot, dot, or flame-shaped), microaneurysm, cotton-wool spot, hard exudates, or a combination of these signs	Strong association with stroke, cognitive decline, and death from cardiovascular causes
Malignant	Signs of moderate retinopathy plus swelling of the optic disc	Strong association with death

Adapted from Wong TY, Mitchell P. Hypertensive retinopathy. *N Engl J Med.* 2004;351:2314. ©2004 Massachusetts Medical Society.

cians. As members of the health care team, ophthalmologists have an important role in the detection, monitoring, and shared management of patients with hypertension.

Beers MH, Porter RS, Jones TV, eds. *The Merck Manual of Diagnosis and Therapy*. 18th ed. Rahway, NJ: Merck Research Laboratories; 2006.

Centers for Disease Control and Prevention. Racial/ethnic disparities in prevalence, treatment, and control of hypertension—United States, 1999–2002. *MMWR Morb Mortal Wkly Rep*. 2005 Jan 14;54:7–9.

Chobanian AV, Bakris GL, Black HR, et al. The seventh report of the Joint National Committee on Prevention, Detection, Evaluation, and Treatment of High Blood Pressure: the JNC 7 report. *JAMA*. 2003;289:2560–2572.

Cooper DH, Krainik AJ, Lubner SJ, Reno H, eds. *The Washington Manual of Medical Therapeutics*. 32nd ed. Philadelphia: Lippincott Williams & Wilkins; 2007.

Initial therapy of hypertension. *Med Lett Drugs Ther*. 2004 Jul 5;46(1186):53–55.

National High Blood Pressure Education Program Working Group on High Blood Pressure in Children and Adolescents. The fourth report on the diagnosis, evaluation, and treatment of high blood pressure in children and adolescents. *Pediatrics*. 2004;114:555–576.

Physicians' Desk Reference. 62nd ed. Montvale, NJ: Thomson PDR; 2008.

US Department of Health and Human Services, National Heart, Lung, and Blood Institute. National High Blood Pressure Education Program Web site. Available at http://www.nhlbi.nih.gov/about/nhbpep/index.htm. Accessed August 7, 2008.

Wong TY, Mitchell P. Hypertensive retinopathy. *N Engl J Med*. 2004;351:2310–2317.

CHAPTER 3

Cerebrovascular Disease

Recent Developments

- Intravenous recombinant tissue plasminogen activator (TPA) is strongly recommended for carefully selected patients who can be treated within 3 hours of onset of ischemic stroke, as it improves neurological outcomes.
- Carotid endarterectomy (CEA) is beneficial for symptomatic patients with recent nondisabling carotid artery ischemic events and ipsilateral 70%–99% carotid artery stenosis. Carotid endarterectomy is not beneficial for symptomatic patients with 0%–29% or 100% stenosis. The potential benefit of CEA for symptomatic patients with 30%–69% stenosis is uncertain.
- Patients with acute ischemic stroke presenting within 48 hours of symptom onset should be given aspirin (160–325 mg/day) to prevent recurrent stroke, reduce stroke mortality, and decrease morbidity, provided contraindications such as allergy and gastrointestinal bleeding are absent and recombinant tissue-type plasminogen activator was not or will not be used as treatment.
- Subcutaneous unfractionated heparin may be considered for deep venous thrombosis (DVT) prophylaxis in at-risk patients with acute ischemic stroke.
- Statin use reduces the risk of stroke and other coronary events in patients with coronary artery disease and in those who have had an ischemic stroke of atherosclerotic origin.

Introduction

Vascular stroke is the third leading cause of death in developed countries, ranking behind heart disease and cancer. In the United States, approximately 750,000 strokes occur annually, with a mortality rate exceeding 20%. Stroke is the leading cause of long-term disability in America today.

Vascular stroke results from 2 major causes: cerebral ischemia and intracranial hemorrhage. For extensive discussion of the ophthalmic manifestations of cerebrovascular disease, see BCSC Section 5, *Neuro-Ophthalmology*.

Cerebral Ischemia

Cerebral ischemia results from interference with the circulation to the brain. Usually, cerebral circulation is maintained by a very efficient collateral arterial system that includes the 2 carotid and the 2 vertebral arteries, anastomoses in the circle of Willis, and collateral circulation in the cerebral hemispheres. However, atheromas and congenital arteriovenous (AV) malformations can lead to a reduction in cerebral blood flow. This reduction may be generalized or localized. If the cerebral blood flow is compromised for less than 1 hour, no residual neurological effects are present. However, longer interruptions in cerebral blood flow can result in permanent neurological deficits, depending on the extent and duration of the cerebral ischemia.

There are varying degrees of ischemia, which may be classified by severity and duration. A *transient ischemic attack (TIA)* is a focal loss of neurological function of sudden onset, persisting for less than 24 hours and clearing without residual signs. Most TIAs last only a few minutes, and the symptoms are primarily associated with insufficiency of the internal carotid, middle cerebral, or vertebrobasilar arteries. An *evolving stroke* is a progressively enlarging cerebral infarct that produces neurological deficits which worsen over 24 to 48 hours. A *completed stroke* is an ischemic event that produces a stable permanent neurological disability. Most ischemic strokes consist of small regions of complete ischemia in conjunction with a large area of incomplete ischemia. This ischemic but not infarcted area has been termed the *penumbra*. Recent studies have demonstrated that the penumbra is dynamic, resulting in changes to the once passive approach to treating patients with acute cerebral ischemia.

Emboli or thrombi caused by atherosclerosis, hypertension, or diabetes mellitus and located in medium and small arteries account for the majority of strokes. Strokes caused by emboli of cardiac origin account for 20% of the total. Mural thrombi forming on the endocardium in conjunction with myocardial infarction (MI) account for 8%–10%. Atrial fibrillation, mitral stenosis, mitral valve prolapse, and atrial myxoma are other cardiac conditions associated with intracranial embolism.

Nonarteriosclerotic causes of thrombotic occlusion leading to TIA and stroke include aortic dissection and inflammatory arteritis (eg, collagen vascular disease, giant cell arteritis, meningovascular syphilis, acute and chronic meningitis, and moyamoya disease).

Ischemia must be distinguished from hypoxemia (decreased oxygenation or oxygen-carrying capacity), which can be caused by carbon monoxide poisoning, chronic obstructive pulmonary disease, profound anemia, or pulmonary emboli. Ischemia can also be caused by increased viscosity of the blood due to pregnancy and the postpartum period, use of oral contraceptives, postoperative and posttraumatic states, hyperviscosity syndromes, polycythemia, and sickle cell disease.

Although cerebral ischemia can occur as a result of embolus or thrombus in any artery, the most common sites include the middle cerebral artery and its branches, the tortuous portion of the internal carotid artery extending from the carotid canal to its bifurcation in the anterior and middle cerebral arteries (carotid siphon), and the basilar artery.

Clinical manifestations of cerebral ischemia reflect the functions associated with the area of ischemia and include paresis, paresthesia, amaurosis fugax, and facial paresthesias. Vertebrobasilar symptoms include vertigo, diplopia, binocular visual loss, ataxia, paresis, paresthesia, dysarthria, headache, nausea, and vomiting.

Diagnosis and Management

The diagnosis of TIAs should be differentiated from the diagnosis of diabetic and convulsive seizures, migraine, vertigo, and neoplasms. While the presentation of stroke is usually characteristic, the diagnosis should be differentiated from that of other conditions that may mimic strokes, such as multiple sclerosis, subdural hematoma, cranial nerve palsy, encephalitis, hypoglycemia, seizures, brain tumor, hypertensive encephalopathy, syncope, migraine, and functional disorder.

A detailed history including the time and duration of onset is important. Also, an assessment of risk factors is critical for the treatment of the patient. Nonmodifiable risk factors include age older than 60 years, male gender, and family history or prior history of stroke or TIAs. Modifiable risk factors include diabetes mellitus, hypertension, hyperlipidemia, cardiac arrhythmias, smoking, alcoholism, illicit drug use, migraine, and hypercoagulable states.

The clinical severity of a stroke can be determined using the National Institutes of Health Stroke Scale, which assesses gaze palsy, visual field loss, facial palsy, motor function of the arms and legs, ataxia, sensation, language, dysarthria, and inattention. The assessment is on a 0–2 or 0–3 scale, with *0* being the lowest score and *42* being the highest. The higher the score, the more severe the neurological deficit.

Diagnostic Studies

Laboratory studies should include testing to determine the presence of the various causes of stroke listed previously. However, specific imaging studies need to be performed to differentiate the various causes of ischemia, such as hemorrhage, hematoma, and tumor.

Investigation of the systemic arteries and the heart is essential in determining the cause of cerebral ischemia. Differences between upper limb pulse rates and blood pressure may indicate serious subclavian disease. Multiple bruits may suggest widespread arterial disease but may be present without significant occlusion. Evidence for a cardiac embolic source should be pursued aggressively, especially in younger normotensive persons with cerebral ischemia. *Electrocardiography* should be routine to exclude cardiac dysrhythmia and occult myocardial infarction.

Echocardiography is often helpful in excluding intracardiac emboli. *Transesophageal Doppler echocardiography* is most sensitive in this regard. *Lumbar puncture* is required in rare cases of stroke or TIA, particularly if meningovascular syphilis or meningitis is a serious consideration. *Duplex ultrasonography* is a noninvasive technique to detect obstructive or stenotic carotid artery disease; *transcranial Doppler* continues arterial examination to the intracranial branches of the internal carotid artery.

Ideally, all suspected cases of stroke and threatened stroke should prompt *computed tomography (CT)* of the brain. Computed tomography is very sensitive to the presence of intracranial hemorrhage. *Magnetic resonance imaging (MRI)* is often more sensitive than CT in detecting an evolving stroke within hours of its onset and an early cerebral infarction, whereas CT results may be negative for up to several days after an acute cerebral infarct. These techniques can distinguish among cerebral hemorrhage, old and recent infarction, and hemorrhagic infarction; they can also exclude unsuspected space-occupying lesions. *Magnetic resonance cerebral angiography* may be needed if the neurological event cannot be differentiated by clinical criteria from an arteriovenous malformation, cerebrovascular malformation, or giant aneurysm. *Diffusion-weighted* and *perfusion-weighted MRI* are useful in the evaluation of early cerebral ischemia and regional blood flow. By helping to detect these conditions early in their course, these techniques may provide an opportunity for early treatment, which is beneficial in salvaging tissue at risk. *Cerebral arteriography* is required only if the cause is unclear or if intra-arterial thrombolysis or surgical intervention is being strongly considered.

Treatment

Treatment of threatened stroke includes reduction of risk factors when possible. Hypertension should be controlled, although blood pressure reduction during acute ischemic stroke may cause harmful decreases in local perfusion. Control of both hyperlipidemia and diabetes is indicated. Cigarette smoking and excessive alcohol consumption should be eliminated. The use of anticoagulant drugs, such as heparin and warfarin sodium, is widely accepted in threatened stroke from emboli arising in mural thrombi following myocardial infarction and in nonvalvular atrial fibrillation.

Controlled studies have *not* demonstrated the effectiveness of anticoagulants in the treatment of TIAs in the carotid and vertebrobasilar territory. Heparin is not helpful in patients with completed stroke but can be useful in ischemic stroke to prevent deep venous thrombosis. Because of the associated risk of hemorrhage in the ischemic area, there is no consensus on the best time to start anticoagulant therapy.

Antiplatelet therapy with aspirin is beneficial in patients with cardiac cerebral emboli who cannot tolerate long-term use of anticoagulant drugs. Recent clinical trials indicate that aspirin offers a moderate benefit in the prevention of recurrent stroke. Low doses of aspirin (160–300 mg daily) cause less gastrointestinal discomfort than higher doses, and they reduce the incidence of stroke in patients with unstable angina or acute myocardial infarction. Ticlopidine (Ticlid) is a platelet-inhibiting drug proven beneficial in clinical trials. It alters platelet membrane fibrinogen interaction but does not affect the cyclooxygenase pathway. Adverse effects include bone marrow suppression, rash, and commonly (22% of cases) diarrhea. Clopidogrel (Plavix) prevents clot formation similar to the way that ticlopidine does and initially appears to have a more promising side effect profile. Clopidogrel is more likely to cause rash and diarrhea than aspirin is.

Recent studies have further investigated the role of thrombolytic agents for treatment of acute ischemic stroke. The National Institute of Neurologic Disorders and Stroke Recombinant Tissue Plasminogen Activator Stroke study supports the use of recombinant TPA for the treatment of acute ischemic stroke in patients who meet certain eligibility requirements, if treatment is initiated within 3 hours after the onset of symptoms. Tissue plasminogen activator is administered intravenously. However, use of this agent incurred a 6.4% risk of symptomatic intracerebral hemorrhage. The risk of intracerebral hemorrhage was unacceptably high in trials utilizing another thrombolytic agent, intravenous streptokinase. An additional thrombolytic agent in the treatment of acute ischemic stroke is urokinase, which has been used intra-arterially up to 6 hours after symptom onset. Urokinase may play a role in treating patients with occlusion of the middle cerebral artery and possibly those with basilar artery occlusion. Ancrod, a fibrinogenolytic enzyme derived from snake venom, has also been shown to improve functional outcomes after stroke.

Intracranial Hemorrhage

Intracranial hemorrhage constitutes approximately 15% of acute cerebrovascular disorders. Bleeding from aneurysms of arteries composing the circle of Willis, bleeding from arterioles damaged by hypertension or arteriosclerosis, and trauma are the most common causes of intracranial hemorrhage. Although there are many causes of intracranial hemorrhage, the anatomic location of the bleeding greatly influences the clinical picture. By location, hemorrhages can be grouped into the following general categories:

- subarachnoid hemorrhage
- intracerebral hemorrhage
- surface bleeding that extends into the brain
- intraventricular hemorrhage

Aneurysms that rupture entirely into the subarachnoid space present with features of meningeal irritation or a transient increase in intracranial pressure. The most common symptom of subarachnoid hemorrhage is the sudden development of a violent, usually localized, headache. This headache is at first frontal or temporal, later becoming occipital and then spreading to involve the entire head and neck. In an adult not prone to headaches, a moderately intense headache (with or without associated neck stiffness) that disappears in 2–3 days may be a sign of a warning leak. Brief loss of consciousness or a seizure preceded by an awareness of dizziness or vertigo and by vomiting is common at the onset. Common physical signs include neck rigidity, fundus or preretinal hemorrhages, and cranial nerve palsies.

Vascular malformations within and on the surface of the brain parenchyma commonly present with seizures and headaches, less often with hemorrhage. Arteriovenous malformations produce symptoms more commonly than other types of cerebrovascular malformations.

Hypertensive-arteriosclerotic intracerebral hemorrhages are often catastrophic events. Headache is a predominant feature at the onset in at least one half of hemorrhages and, by contrast, in less than one fourth of thromboembolisms. Vomiting is prominent as an early symptom. Restlessness and vomiting are more common with hemorrhage than with infarction. Generalized seizures are common with intracerebral hemorrhage, are less frequent with subarachnoid hemorrhage, and are uncommon (less than 10% of cases) with cerebral infarction.

Arterial "berry" aneurysms are round or saccular dilatations characteristically found at arteriole bifurcations on the circle of Willis and its major branches or connections. Intracranial aneurysms occur in all age groups but most commonly rupture in the fifth, sixth, and seventh decades of life. Approximately 85% of congenital berry aneurysms develop in the anterior part of the circle of Willis derived from the internal carotid artery in its major branches. The most common site is at the origin of the posterior communicating artery from the internal carotid artery. Such an aneurysm typically presents with headache and third nerve palsy involving the pupil. Vascular malformations within and on the surface of the brain parenchyma constitute approximately 7% of cases with subarachnoid hemorrhage. Four varieties are recognized:

- capillary telangiectasia
- cavernous angioma
- venous angioma
- arteriovenous malformation (AVM)

Capillary telangiectasias are most commonly discovered as incidental postmortem findings in the brain stem. Venous angiomas are cerebrovascular abnormalities often associated with the Sturge-Weber syndrome. These lesions are best identified by MRI.

The most important clues in the diagnosis of hypertensive intracranial hemorrhage are explosive onset, history of high blood pressure, early decline of the level of consciousness, and detection of meningeal irritation and blood in the spinal fluid (preferably by CT) with evidence of a focal lesion. Little other than the past history clinically distinguishes the symptoms of subarachnoid hemorrhage resulting from the rupture of an AVM from those caused by a ruptured aneurysm. Focal neurological signs and evidence of the sudden development of a mass lesion frequently accompany a rupture.

Findings that suggest an AVM as the cause of subarachnoid hemorrhage include a history of previous focal seizures, slow stepwise progression of focal neurological signs, and, occasionally, recurrent unilateral throbbing headache resembling migraine. In addition to meningeal irritation and focal neurological signs reflecting bleeding, a bruit is present over the orbit or skull in approximately 40% of patients.

Immediate CT examination demonstrates blood in the subarachnoid space in approximately 95% of the cases of ruptured aneurysm or AVM. Computed tomography scans identify the size and location of intracerebral hemorrhages, as well as the degree of surrounding edema and the amount and location of any distortion of the brain. Computed tomography scans can identify blood in the subarachnoid space or brain and ventricles in 95% of patients with subarachnoid hemorrhage.

If subarachnoid hemorrhage is suspected and CT results are negative, lumbar puncture is indicated. Computed tomography should always be carried out first to rule out a mass lesion. Arteriography remains the definitive procedure to identify an aneurysm or AVM. Angiography is essential to identify areas of local or general vasospasm and should be performed when cases of subarachnoid hemorrhage are considered reasonable operative risks or when the diagnosis is in doubt.

Initial restoration of normal blood pressure and its maintenance at normal levels are mandatory in the treatment of ruptured aneurysms. Surgical intervention is best accomplished by placing a small clip or ligature across the neck of the sac. If the aneurysm cannot be directly obliterated, surgical ligation of a proximal vessel may be necessary. Symptomatic AVMs can sometimes be dissected and removed, depending on their location. Proton-beam irradiation remains controversial. Ligation of the feeding vessels, coupled with balloon catheter embolization, may be carried out. Results of treatment of intracerebral hemorrhage are mostly unsatisfactory.

Carotid Artery Disease

Asymptomatic carotid bruits occur in 4% of the population over age 40. The annual stroke rate in patients with an asymptomatic bruit is 1.5%. This same population has an annual mortality rate of 4%, primarily from complications of heart disease. Bruit is more a marker for the presence of arteriosclerotic disease than a predictor of stroke. Patients with asymptomatic carotid bruits should be screened for risk factors related to atherosclerosis: hypertension, smoking, and hypercholesterolemia. The degree and severity of stenosis should be determined by noninvasive studies. Patients with asymptomatic carotid stenosis have a 2% annual risk of ipsilateral stroke.

In the Asymptomatic Carotid Atherosclerosis Study, patients with asymptomatic stenosis of greater than 60% were randomized to either CEA or medical treatment. Although the estimated 5-year risk of stroke was 53% lower (5.1% vs. 11.0%) for the CEA group, the only significant difference was in the frequency of TIA or minor stroke ipsilateral to the CEA. No significant differences were discerned between the medical and surgical groups with regard to major ipsilateral stroke or death, and the benefits disappear with operative risk of greater than 3%. Therefore, patients with asymptomatic carotid stenosis of greater than 60% may be considered for elective CEA; patients with less than 60% stenosis should be retested at intervals of 6–12 months and followed up for disease progression. Aspirin (325 mg daily) and risk factor reduction are also employed in this patient group.

Ocular and cerebral conditions associated with carotid stenosis include amaurosis fugax, ocular ischemic syndromes, TIAs, and stroke. The ophthalmologist is often the first physician to see a patient with amaurosis fugax or ocular ischemia. Amaurosis is usually embolic, having either a carotid or a cardiac source. The annual stroke rate among patients with isolated amaurosis fugax, retinal infarcts, or TIAs is approximately 2%, 3%, and 8%, respectively. Untreated patients with amaurosis fugax, retinal infarcts, or TIAs have a 30% risk of myocardial infarction and an 18% risk of death over a 5-year period. A cardiac source of embolization should be excluded for all patients presenting with isolated amaurosis fugax or transient visual loss. The best procedure for this is transesophageal cardiac ultrasonography.

If evidence suggests that a carotid lesion is the cause of the amaurosis fugax, or if venous stasis retinopathy is present, duplex scanning should be performed to determine the presence of vessel wall disease or carotid stenosis.

No hard data are currently available from which to make a clear recommendation about an appropriate course of therapy. It appears that a trial of aspirin (325 mg/day) should be the initial approach for all patients. Ticlopidine or clopidogrel therapy may be considered for patients unable to take aspirin. Carotid endarterectomy with electroencephalographic monitoring should be considered only if the surgeon has a perioperative morbidity rate of less than 3% and if any of the following conditions exist:

- Antiplatelet therapy proves to be ineffective.
- Stenosis appears to be progressive.
- The patient has no operative risk factors.

Patients with TIA or previous stroke in the territory of carotid stenosis are judged to be symptomatic. The risk of stroke within a year of onset of symptoms is 8% in patients with TIA; the risk thereafter is approximately 6% per year, with a 5-year risk of 35%–50%.

In the North American Symptomatic Carotid Endarterectomy Trial, carotid endarterectomy was evaluated in patients with a recent (within 120 days) hemispheric or retinal TIA or a recent nondisabling stroke, who had high-grade (70%–99%) stenosis in the ipsilateral carotid artery. All of the patients received optimal medical care, including antiplatelet therapy with aspirin, as well as treatment of hypertension, hyperlipidemia, or diabetes, when appropriate. The surgical group experienced lower rates of ipsilateral stroke (9.0% vs. 26.0%), any stroke (12.6% vs. 27.6%), major or fatal stroke (3.7% vs. 13.1%), and death from all causes (4.6% vs. 6.3%). The perioperative mortality rate was only 0.6%, and the perioperative rate of major stroke or death was 2.1%. The benefit of surgery for reducing the risk of ipsilateral stroke increased with higher degrees of stenosis: 12% risk reduction for 70%–79% stenosis; 18% risk reduction for 80%–89% stenosis; and 26% risk reduction for 90%–99% stenosis. The European Carotid Surgery Trial also demonstrated a statistically significant benefit for CEA in selected patients with greater than 70% stenosis. However, there is still uncertainty regarding CEA for symptomatic stenosis in the range of 30%–69%.

The risks of major morbidity and mortality with CEA are proportional to the severity of neurological illness and comorbid factors such as ischemic heart disease. The risks for patients with symptomatic unilateral high-grade stenosis and favorable comorbidity are 1%–3% in the hands of capable surgeons. The long-term restenosis rate following CEA is approximately 10% at 5 years.

It is feasible to reopen the internal carotid artery after acute (less than 8 hours) occlusion. The risks are high with emergency CEA, however, and the success rate is less than 50%. Patients with carotid occlusion are usually placed on warfarin therapy for several months in the hope of decreasing distal thrombus progression and subsequent embolic stroke.

In summary, patients with symptomatic carotid stenosis exceeding 70% should be considered for CEA unless there is acute stroke, maximal neurological defect, or other medical contraindication to surgery. The major perioperative morbidity and mortality rates for the surgical team should not exceed 5% for patients with TIA, 7% for patients with minor stroke, or 10% for patients with recurrent stenosis.

The following approach to a patient presenting with a cerebral or retinal TIA should be considered:

- The patient should be evaluated for the presence of risk factors that are associated with atherogenesis: hypertension, diabetes mellitus, obesity, hyperlipidemia, and smoking.
- Appropriate medical therapy should be instituted.
- The presence of coronary artery disease and a cardiac source of emboli should be excluded by appropriate testing.
- The patency of the extracranial carotid artery system should be determined using duplex ultrasonography.

If ipsilateral carotid stenosis exceeds 70%, if bilateral carotid stenosis greater than 50% is present, or if long-term evidence indicates progressive disease, CEA should be considered—but only if the surgeon's perioperative stroke and death rate is less than 3%. Otherwise, antiplatelet therapy with aspirin (325 mg/day), clopidogrel, or ticlopidine should be initiated. A patient presenting with TIA symptoms who has previously undergone CEA should be evaluated and treated similarly. Special attention should be paid to the evaluation of early restenosis and thrombosis.

As an additional note, elevated plasma homocysteine levels have been linked to extracranial carotid stenosis and, directly, to an increased risk of stroke and occlusive vascular disease. Treatment with folic acid reduces this risk by lowering plasma homocysteine levels. Folates naturally occur in green vegetables and are supplemented in bread and in breakfast cereals in the United States. Therefore, increasing dietary folic acid intake can be recommended to all patients with carotid stenosis and generalized cardiovascular disease. Dietary antioxidants (ie, vitamin C and vitamin E) may also play a role in the pathophysiology of stroke. Because of the low cost and low risk of these supplements, physicians may choose to recommend them for patients at risk. See also BCSC Section 5, *Neuro-Ophthalmology*.

> Adams H, Adams R, Del Zoppo G, et al. Guidelines for the early management of patients with ischemic stroke: 2005 guidelines update a scientific statement from the Stroke Council of the American Heart Association/American Stroke Association. *Stroke*. 2005;36:916–923.
>
> Barnett HJ, Eliasziw M, Meldrum HE. Drugs and surgery in the prevention of ischemic stroke. *N Engl J Med*. 1995;332:238–248.
>
> Beauchamp NJ, Bryan RN. Acute cerebral ischemic infarction: a pathophysiologic review and radiologic perspective. *AJR Am J Roentgenol*. 1998;171:73–84.
>
> Brott T, Bogousslavsky J. Treatment of acute ischemic stroke. *N Engl J Med*. 2000;343:710–722.
>
> Moore WS, Barnett HJ, Beebe HG, et al. Guidelines for carotid endarterectomy: a multidisciplinary consensus statement from the ad hoc Committee, American Heart Association. *Stroke*. 1995;26:188–201.
>
> Selhub J, Jacques PF, Bostrom AG, et al. Association between plasma homocysteine concentrations and extracranial carotid-artery stenosis. *N Engl J Med*. 1995;332:286–291.

CHAPTER 4

Acquired Heart Disease

Recent Developments

- Atherosclerotic coronary artery disease remains by far the number one killer in the United States and around the world.
- It is clear that markers of inflammation like C-reactive protein (CRP) are strong risk factors for coronary artery disease (CAD). Their additive value in patients with known cardiometabolic risk is unclear.
- Primary prevention of CAD at a public health level requires lifestyle changes, including reduced intake of saturated fat and cholesterol, increased physical activity, and weight control.
- Smoking remains the number one preventable risk factor for cardiovascular disease worldwide.
- Many times, a patient presenting for an ophthalmologic examination has been using a statin. Recent trials suggest that, regardless of cholesterol level, any patient at significant risk for vascular events should be given a statin.
- Heart failure is increasing in prevalence as the aging population increases.
- Primary percutaneous coronary intervention (PCI) is superior to thrombolysis for the treatment of acute myocardial infarction (MI), if it is performed by experienced operators.
- Stenting is now widely used in patients with acute MI and requires some postoperative dual antiplatelet therapy.
- Prophylactic implantable cardioverter-defibrillators (ICDs) are indicated for patients who have survived a cardiac arrest or an episode of hemodynamically unstable ventricular tachycardia. ICDs are also indicated for severe left ventricular dysfunction after MI. ICDs are not indicated for patients who do not have a reasonable expectation of survival with an acceptable functional status of at least 1 year.
- Pharmacologic adjuncts for the management of acute coronary syndromes (ACS) include low-molecular-weight heparin and glycoprotein IIb/IIIa inhibitors.

Ischemic Heart Disease

Atherosclerotic CAD is by far the number one killer not only in the United States, but also in the world. It is estimated that every minute, 1 person dies in the United States because of CAD. The number of women who die from cardiovascular disease is 10 times that of breast cancer.

Pathophysiology

Abnormal cholesterol intake and metabolism are central factors in ischemic heart disease (IHD). The "fatty streak" is an accumulation of lipids and lipid-laden macrophages under the endothelium of the coronaries. These macrophages are then called "foam" cells, and they organize in a plaque. As the plaque becomes calcified, the lumen of the vessel narrows. The plaque can also become unstable and rupture. This rupture leads to turbulence and activation of the coagulation cascade, causing intravascular thrombosis. The result is partial or complete vessel occlusion, which causes the symptoms of unstable angina or MI.

Ischemia is defined as a local, temporary oxygen deprivation associated with inadequate removal of metabolites caused by reduced tissue perfusion. *Ischemic heart disease* is typically caused by decreased perfusion of the myocardium secondary to stenotic or obstructed coronary arteries. The balance between arterial supply and myocardial demand for oxygen determines whether ischemia occurs. Significant coronary stenosis, thrombosis, occlusion, reduced arterial pressure, hypoxemia, or severe anemia can impede the supply of oxygen to the myocardium. On the demand side, an increase in heart rate, ventricular contractility, or wall tension (which is determined by systolic arterial pressure, ventricular volume, and ventricular wall thickness) may each cause increased utilization of oxygen. When the demand for oxygen exceeds the supply, ischemia occurs. If this ischemia becomes prolonged, infarction and myocardial necrosis result. The necrotic process begins in the subendocardium, usually after approximately 20 minutes of coronary obstruction, and progresses to transmural and complete infarction in 4–6 hours.

Risk Factors for Coronary Artery Disease

The majority of patients with CAD have some identifiable risk factors. These risk factors are evident when epidemiological studies are performed and include a positive family history, male gender, lipid abnormalities, diabetes mellitus, hypertension, physical inactivity, obesity, and smoking. Many of these risk factors are preventable, such as smoking. Although the number of people who smoke is decreasing in the United States, it is estimated that 25% of men and 21% of women smoke. The risk of CAD can be decreased by 50% in just 1 year after an individual stops smoking. Also included among preventable risk factors are lipid abnormalities. Higher low-density-lipoprotein (LDL) and lower high-density-lipoprotein (HDL) levels increase the risk of CAD. The *metabolic syndrome* is defined as a constellation of 3 or more of the following: abdominal obesity; hypertriglyceridemia; low HDL-C level; fasting glucose level of 110 mg/dL or more; and hypertension (see Chapter 5, Table 5-8, for a more detailed definition). This syndrome is increasing in prevalence in the United States and is a major contributor to heart disease. In addition, obesity is being reported more often in the United States (20% of the population). A diet low in saturated fat is widely accepted and promoted as a way of reducing weight in obese men and women. Eating fish rich in omega-3 fatty acids may help protect against vascular disease. Recently, it became clear that markers of inflammation are strong risk factors for CAD. High sensitivity C-reactive protein is the best marker and is now available for clinical use. C-reactive protein levels less than 1, between 1 and 3, and greater than 3 µg/mL identify patients at low, medium, and high risk, respectively, for future cardiovascular events.

Clinical Syndromes

Clinical presentations of IHD include

- angina pectoris: stable angina, variant (Prinzmetal) angina
- acute coronary syndromes: unstable angina, non–Q wave MI, Q wave MI
- congestive heart failure
- sudden cardiac death
- asymptomatic IHD

Angina pectoris

The cardinal symptom in patients with IHD is *angina pectoris,* usually manifested as precordial chest pain or tightness that is often triggered by physical exertion, emotional distress, or eating. Angina pectoris is usually due to atherosclerotic heart disease. Coronary vasospasm may occur at the site of a lesion or even in otherwise normal coronaries. Angina typically lasts 5–10 minutes and is usually relieved by rest, nitroglycerin, or both. Patients may present with pain radiating into other areas, including the jaw, arm, neck, shoulder, back, chest wall, or abdomen. Occasionally, angina may be misinterpreted as indigestion or musculoskeletal pain. The level of physical activity that results in angina pectoris is clinically significant, and it is useful in determining the severity of CAD, treatment, and prognosis. Myocardial ischemia may be painless in diabetic patients, often delaying the diagnosis until the disease is more advanced. The pain associated with MI is similar to that of angina, but classically it is usually more severe and more prolonged.

Stable angina pectoris   Angina is considered stable if it responds to rest or nitroglycerin and if the patterns of frequency, ease of onset, duration, and response to medication have not changed substantially over 3 months.

Variant (Prinzmetal) angina   Variant angina occurs at rest and is not related to physical exertion. The ST segment is elevated on electrocardiography during the anginal episodes, which are caused by coronary artery spasm. Underlying atherosclerosis is present in 60%–80% of cases, and thrombosis and occlusion may result during the episodes of coronary spasm.

Acute coronary syndrome

Acute coronary syndrome (ACS) comprises the spectrum of unstable cardiac ischemia, from unstable angina to acute MI. Plaque rupture is considered to be the common underlying event.

Acute myocardial infarction   If a coronary thrombus is occlusive and if it persists, MI can result. The location and extent of the infarction depend on the anatomic distribution of the occluded vessel, the presence of additional stenotic lesions, and the adequacy of collateral circulation. If the patient has chest pain at rest, unstable angina is the diagnosis. If the ischemia is severe enough to cause myocardial necrosis, infarction results.

In non–Q wave MI, the electrocardiogram (ECG) typically demonstrates ST-segment depression, T wave inversion, or both. If it is established that no biochemical marker of myocardial necrosis has been released, the patient may be considered to have experienced *unstable angina*. When clinical evidence of necrosis is detected by cardiac enzyme testing and no pathologic Q waves evolve on the ECG, the diagnosis is *non–Q wave MI*, a condition midway between unstable angina and Q wave infarction. Plaque rupture in unstable angina and non–Q wave MI is typically accompanied by a less obstructive thrombus or lesser amounts of fibrin formation compared with what occurs in Q wave MI.

Q wave MI usually occurs when plaque rupture results in a completely occlusive thrombus. Typically, ST-segment elevation is apparent on the ECG. Necrosis involving the full or nearly full thickness of the ventricular wall in the distribution of the affected artery ultimately occurs, leading to Q waves on the ECG.

Myocardial infarction may occur suddenly, without warning, in a previously asymptomatic patient or in a patient with stable or variant angina; MI may also follow a period of unstable angina. Patients commonly experience chest pain, nausea, vomiting, diaphoresis, weakness, anxiety, dyspnea, lightheadedness, and palpitations. Nearly 25% of myocardial infarcts are painless; painless MI is more common in persons with diabetes and with increasing age. These patients may present with congestive heart failure or syncope. Symptoms may begin during or after exertion or at rest.

The clinical findings in IHD vary and depend on the location and severity of myocardial ischemia or injury. Approximately half of all infarctions involve the inferior myocardial wall, and most of the remaining half involve the anterior regions. Examination may reveal pallor, coolness of the extremities, low-grade fever, signs of pulmonary congestion and increased central venous pressure (if left ventricular dysfunction is present), an S_3 or S_4 gallop, an apical systolic murmur (caused by papillary muscle dysfunction), hypertension, or hypotension. The ECG may demonstrate a variety of ST-segment and T wave changes and arrhythmias.

Subendocardial (non–Q wave, nontransmural) infarcts usually result in a smaller region of myocardial injury and cause less ventricular dysfunction and heart failure. However, the patient with a non–Q wave infarction may be considered to have an incomplete infarction, with potential for reocclusion of the affected artery. Not surprisingly, these patients experience a greater incidence of post-MI angina and reinfarction during the initial hospitalization and during the first 6 months following the infarction. Approximately 20% experience an acute Q wave infarction within 3 months. Although the in-hospital prognosis for patients with non–Q wave infarction is better than that for patients with Q wave infarction, the prognosis at 6–12 months tends to equalize. As such, patients with non–Q wave infarction constitute a specific subgroup requiring aggressive diagnostic evaluation and treatment. Detection and dilation or bypass of a high-grade coronary stenosis may prevent subsequent reinfarction.

Approximately 60% of patients who die of cardiac disease expire suddenly before reaching the hospital. The prognosis for those hospitalized with MI, on the other hand, has become remarkably good. In some studies using thrombolytic therapy, the mortality rate has been in the range of 5%–8%. Mortality is affected by a wide variety of factors, such as the degree of heart failure, myocardial damage, severity of the underlying atherosclerotic process, heart size, and previous ischemia.

Immediate coronary angiography and primary PCI (including stenting) of the infarct-related artery have been shown to be superior to thrombolysis when done by experienced operators in high-volume centers with rapid time from first medical contact to intervention ("door-to-balloon"). If this time is kept under 90 minutes, outcome is improved, more so if there is a contraindication to thrombolysis to start with. Such a contraindication would limit the therapeutic options to stenting. This intervention, in conjunction with the platelet glycoprotein IIb/IIIa antagonist abciximab, is now widely used in patients with acute MI.

The complications of MI depend on its severity. Regional and global ventricular contractile dysfunction may result in CHF or pulmonary edema. Mild to moderate heart failure occurs in nearly 50% of patients following MI, and severe heart failure in approximately 15%. Cardiogenic shock, which results in a dramatic fall in systemic blood pressure, is observed in 10% of patients with MI and carries a mortality rate of more than 75%. Rupture of the ventricular septum or a papillary muscle is uncommon, with each occurring in about 5% of patients. Rupture of the left ventricular wall, which may occur at any time within 2 weeks of MI, has been found to be the cause of sudden death in about 9% of autopsies after acute MI. Some patients experience post-MI pericarditis, characterized by a pericardial friction rub 2–3 days after infarction. When this rub is accompanied by fever, arthralgia, and pleuropericardial pain, the diagnosis is most likely *post-MI,* or *Dressler, syndrome.* This condition is treated with aspirin, nonsteroidal anti-inflammatory agents, or corticosteroids. Injury along the conduction pathways of the atria or ventricles may result in bradycardia, heart block, supraventricular tachycardias, or ventricular arrhythmias. Arrhythmias often exacerbate ischemic injury by reducing the perfusion pressure in the coronary arteries. Most acute deaths from MI result from arrhythmia.

An important aim of a good cardiac program is to enable patients to return to their usual jobs after discharge from the hospital. Approximately 80%–90% of patients with uncomplicated MI can return to work within 2–3 months. Patients are advised to modify or eliminate their risk factors for atherosclerosis. Dietary programs, reduction of physiologic and psychological stress, and a cardiac rehabilitation program benefit many patients.

Congestive heart failure secondary to IHD
Congestive heart failure is discussed later in this chapter.

Sudden cardiac death
Sudden cardiac death (SCD) is defined as unexpected nontraumatic death occurring within 1 hour after onset of symptoms in clinically stable patients. A disproportionate number of sudden deaths occur in the early morning hours. Sudden cardiac death is usually caused by a severe arrhythmia, such as ventricular tachycardia, ventricular fibrillation, profound bradycardia, or asystole. Sudden cardiac death may result from MI, occur during an episode of angina, or occur without warning in a patient with frequent arrhythmias secondary to underlying IHD or ventricular dysfunction. Other causes of SCD

are Wolff-Parkinson-White syndrome, long QT syndrome, torsades de pointes, atrioventricular block, aortic stenosis, myocarditis, cardiomyopathy, ruptured or dissecting aortic aneurysm, and pulmonary embolism. There is evidence that prophylactic ICDs are the preferred first-line therapy for patients who have survived a cardiac arrest or an episode of hemodynamically unstable ventricular tachycardia. ICDs are also the preferred first-line therapy for severe left ventricular dysfunction after MI, although results from the Multicenter Automatic Defibrillator Implantation Trial II (MADIT II) indicate that the cost of this treatment, if applied to all affected patients, is too high.

Asymptomatic IHD

Asymptomatic patients with IHD are at particular risk for unexpected MI, life-threatening arrhythmias, and SCD. These patients may develop advanced CAD and experience multiple infarcts before the correct diagnosis is made and appropriate treatment is initiated. Elderly persons and individuals with diabetes are more likely to have painless ischemia. Approximately 25% of MIs may be asymptomatic and detected on a subsequent ECG. A patient who has unexplained dyspnea, weakness, arrhythmias, or poor exercise tolerance requires cardiac testing to evaluate for the presence of undiagnosed IHD.

Noninvasive Cardiac Diagnostic Procedures

Noninvasive diagnostic testing in IHD includes electrocardiography, serum enzyme measurements, echocardiography, various types of stress testing, and imaging studies such as positron emission tomography (PET) and magnetic resonance cardiac imaging.

Electrocardiography

The ECG may appear normal between episodes of ischemia in patients with angina. During angina, the ST segments often become elevated or depressed by up to 5 mm. T waves may be inverted; they may become tall and peaked; or inverted T waves may normalize. These ECG findings, when associated with characteristic anginal pain, are virtually diagnostic of IHD. However, absence of ECG changes does not exclude, with certainty, myocardial ischemia.

During MI, QT interval prolongation and peaked T waves may appear. The ST segments may be depressed or elevated. ST-segment elevation may persist for several days to weeks, then return to normal. T wave inversion appears in the leads corresponding to the site of the infarct. Q waves or a reduction in the QRS amplitude appear with the onset of myocardial necrosis. Q waves are typically absent in a subendocardial (nontransmural) infarction. ST-segment elevation, T wave inversion, and Q waves (if present) usually occur in the ECG leads related to the site of the infarct and may be accompanied by reciprocal ST depression in the opposite leads. Tachycardia and ventricular arrhythmias are most common within the first few hours after the onset of infarction. Bradyarrhythmias such as heart block are more common with inferior infarction; ventricular tachycardia and fibrillation are more common with anteroseptal infarction.

Serum enzyme testing

Cardiac enzymes are released into the bloodstream when myocardial necrosis occurs and are therefore valuable in differentiating MI from unstable angina and noncardiac causes of chest pain. With the advent of assays for cardiac-specific troponins, serum enzyme testing has also proven useful in identifying those patients with ACS at greatest risk for adverse outcomes.

Cardiac-specific troponins are gaining acceptance as the primary biochemical cardiac marker in ACS. Cardiac isoforms of troponins (troponins T and I) are important regulatory elements in myocardial cells and, unlike creatine kinase MB (CK-MB), are not normally present in the serum of healthy persons. Troponins T and I have been shown to be more cardiac specific and sensitive than CK-MB, allowing for more accurate diagnosis of cardiac injury. Moreover, unlike CK-MB, levels of troponins T and I are not elevated in patients with skeletal muscle injury. Troponin levels remain elevated from 3 hours to 14 days after MI (long after CK-MB levels have normalized). Therefore, for patients who delay seeking medical attention for MI, troponin assays are the test of choice. However, troponin T is a less sensitive marker than CK-MB in the early stages of infarction (6–12 hours). The greater sensitivity of cardiac troponin assay allows for the detection of lesser amounts of myocardial damage. In fact, mildly elevated troponin levels may be observed in patients with unstable angina as a result of "microinfarctions."

Apart from their diagnostic value, troponin levels also confer prognostic information. It has been demonstrated that patients with an ACS who present with normal CK-MB and elevated troponin T levels have an increased risk of death, recurrent nonfatal infarction, and need for revascularization with *percutaneous transluminal coronary angioplasty (PTCA)* or *coronary artery bypass graft (CABG)*. Similarly, studies have shown that patients with elevated troponin levels at the time of hospital admission are at increased risk for death, cardiogenic shock, or CHF. Finally, a quantitative relationship between the amount of troponin I measured and the risk of death in patients who present with ACS has been demonstrated (Fig 4-1). Therefore, patients who are at greatest risk for adverse outcomes can be identified in the emergency room setting, allowing for more appropriate medical decisions and therapeutic triage.

Until recently, CK-MB isoenzyme has been the principal serum cardiac marker used in the evaluation of ACS. Although not quite as sensitive or specific as the troponins, CK-MB by mass assay remains a useful marker for the detection of more than minor myocardial damage. Serial plasma samples should be drawn for CK and CK isoenzymes after the onset of chest pain. CK levels begin to rise approximately 4 hours after MI, peaking between 12 and 24 hours after the event. However, CK is nonspecific, and levels can also be elevated following injury to skeletal muscles or the brain (perioperative or traumatic).

Three isoenzymes of CK can be identified. The *MB* isoenzyme is relatively specific for myocardium, although it constitutes only about 15% of the total CK released after infarction, the remainder being *MM*, or skeletal muscle isoenzyme. The third isoenzyme is *BB*, which is found primarily in the brain and kidneys. An abnormally elevated CK-MB isoenzyme level is the hallmark for diagnosis of MI. The CK-MB level returns to normal within 36–48 hours after an initial MI. Therefore, in patients who arrive at the hospital more than 36 hours after the onset of chest pain, elevated CK-MB levels will be missed unless a reinfarction occurs.

Serum *myoglobin* is the first marker to rise following myocardial damage, and levels can be elevated between 1 and 20 hours after infarction. Although myoglobin might appear

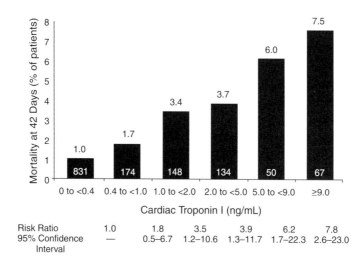

Figure 4-1 Relationship between cardiac troponin levels and risk of death in patients with ACS. *(From Antman EM, Tanasijevic MJ, Thompson B, et al. Cardiac-specific troponin I levels to predict the risk of mortality in patients with acute coronary syndromes. N Engl J Med. 1996;335:1342–1349.)*

to be ideal for early detection of MI, its performance is not consistent and its specificity for cardiac events is poor. Therefore, for the identification of patients with MI, myoglobin should not be the *only* diagnostic marker that is used, but myoglobin's early appearance with myocardial injury makes its absence useful in ruling out myocardial necrosis.

Routine *lactate dehydrogenase* analysis is no longer advocated.

Echocardiography

Echocardiography employs 1- and 2-dimensional ultrasound and color flow Doppler techniques to image the ventricles and atria, the heart valves, left ventricular contraction and wall-motion abnormalities, left ventricular ejection fraction, and the pericardium. Patients with IHD, particularly following infarction, commonly have regional wall-motion abnormalities that correspond to the areas of myocardial injury. Other less frequent complications of infarction, such as mitral regurgitation from papillary muscle injury, ventricular septal defect, ventricular aneurysm, ventricular thrombus, and pericardial effusion, can also be detected with echocardiography. Color flow Doppler provides information on the flow of blood across abnormal valves, pressure differences within the chambers, intracardiac shunts, and cardiac output.

Exercise echocardiography (stress echocardiography) is useful for imaging cardiac valve and wall-motion abnormalities and ventricular dysfunction induced by ischemia during exercise. Predischarge exercise stress echocardiography provides useful prognostic information following acute MI.

Exercise stress testing

Patients with angina may have normal findings on clinical examination, ECG, and echocardiography between episodes of ischemia. Standardized exercise tests have been developed to induce myocardial ischemia under controlled conditions. The ECG, heart rate, blood pressure, and general physical status of the patient are monitored during the procedure. The end point in angina patients is a symptom or sign of cardiac ischemia, such as chest pain, dyspnea, ST-segment depression, arrhythmia, or hypotension. The level of exercise required to induce ischemia is inversely correlated with the likelihood of significant CAD. False-positive and false-negative results occur, and the sensitivity increases with the number of coronary arteries involved. A modified exercise stress test is also performed in patients with a recent MI to help determine functional status and prognosis.

Radionuclide scintigraphy and scans

The sensitivity of exercise testing can be increased via radionuclide techniques. A relatively new agent, *technetium Tc99m Sestamibi (Cardiolite)*, has higher energy than prior substances and thus may provide better image resolution and less soft tissue attenuation. Other techniques include *thallium-201 myocardial* and *technetium-99 pyrophosphate (Tc-99) scintigraphy,* or *blood-pool isotope scans.*

Thallium accumulates in normal myocardium and reveals a perfusion defect in areas of myocardial ischemia. Thallium scans have a high sensitivity and specificity for CAD. Reversible thallium/technetium 99m sestamibi defects consist of a defect that is present during exercise but resolves during rest. This correlates with myocardial ischemia. In contrast, a fixed thallium/Cardiolite defect is present during both exercise and rest and represents a region of prior infarction/nonviable tissue. For those patients unable to exercise vigorously enough to reach the required heart rates, a thallium scan or echocardiogram in conjunction with a pharmacologic stress test using intravenous adenosine, dipyridamole, or dobutamine may provide information similar to that of an actual exercise examination. *Tomographic imaging* of myocardial perfusion is possible with thallium 201 via a technique called *single-photon emission computed tomography (SPECT)*. This technique provides better imaging of infarcts and improved detection of multivessel disease.

Technetium-99 pyrophosphate is an infarct-avid imaging agent. Tc 99 accumulates in necrotic myocardial cells rather than normal myocardium, creating a "hot spot" on imaging. A new infarct is visualized best between 24 and 48 hours after onset with Tc-99 scintigraphy. Other imaging tests that are being evaluated for the detection and management of IHD are *positron emission tomography, ultrafast computed tomography, cardiac magnetic resonance imaging,* and *magnetic resonance fluoroscopy.*

Invasive Cardiac Diagnostic Procedures

Intravascular ultrasound imaging is an evolving invasive modality for studying the intraluminal coronary anatomy. Technologic limitations and uncertainty about long-term safety are a concern. However, as the technology matures, this technique might assume an expanding role in interventional cardiology.

Coronary arteriography and *ventriculography* provide valuable information about the presence and severity of CAD and about ventricular function. These techniques can indicate the specific areas of coronary artery stenosis or occlusion, the number of involved vessels, the ventricular systolic and diastolic volumes, the ejection fraction, and regional wall-motion abnormalities. Multiple gated acquisition (MUGA) can also be obtained for these purposes. This information assists the cardiologist and cardiac surgeon in planning appropriate treatment of the patient.

Coronary artery stenosis is hemodynamically significant when the arterial lumen diameter is narrowed by more than 50% or the cross-sectional area is reduced by more than 75%. Common indications for coronary arteriography are

- ACS
- post-MI angina
- stable angina unresponsive to medical therapy
- a markedly positive exercise stress test result
- recent MI in a patient younger than 40 years
- valvular heart disease
- ventricular septal defect or papillary muscle dysfunction
- cardiomyopathy of unknown cause
- unexplained ventricular arrhythmias

Management of Ischemic Heart Disease

The goals of management for the patient with CAD are to reduce the frequency of or eliminate angina, prevent myocardial damage, and prolong life. The first line of attack should include eliminating or reducing risk factors for atherosclerosis. Recent studies have reported actual regression of atherosclerotic lesions following intensive lipid-lowering therapy. Antiplatelet therapy with daily aspirin has also been advocated for all patients with CAD because of the significant reduction in risk of MI.

Treatment of stable angina pectoris

Medical management of angina pectoris is designed to deliver as much oxygen as possible to the potentially ischemic myocardium, to reduce the oxygen demand to a level where symptoms are eliminated or reduced to a comfortable level, or both. Oxygen delivery through the coronary arteries may be maximized via coronary vasodilators. *Nitroglycerin* or other *nitrates* may be given sublingually for acute episodes of angina and are the drugs of choice. Long-acting orally administered nitrates or topically applied nitroglycerin ointments or transdermal patches may be administered for prevention and long-term control of angina. The systemic effects of nitrates include venous dilation and a decline in arterial pressure; these physiologic effects contribute to the therapeutic effects. Oxygen demands can be reduced by decreasing the heart rate and contractility.

The best agents for reducing heart rate and contractility are the *β-adrenergic blockers*. Their favorable properties have made them the first line and mainstay of treatment for these patients. Beta-blockers are useful in the management of stable and unstable angina. The *slow-channel calcium-blocking agents* (such as *diltiazem, nifedipine, verapamil, nicardipine,* and *amlodipine*) are effective in the treatment of chronic angina and may be useful in preventing episodes of coronary spasm. However, β-adrenergic blockers and calcium channel blockers (particularly verapamil) must be used with caution when left ventricular dysfunction is present. Myocardial oxygen requirements can also be reduced by decreasing ventricular wall tension through controlling systemic hypertension and by reducing the ventricular volume with venous dilators such as nitrates. In addition, routine administration of aspirin reduces the likelihood of thrombus formation. Improving the oxygen-carrying capacity of the blood by treating anemia or coexisting pulmonary disease provides some additional benefit. Patients in whom medical therapy is unsuccessful may be candidates for revascularization with either PTCA or CABG.

Revascularization provides the opportunity to improve coronary blood flow, control of angina, and exercise tolerance. In high-risk patients (Table 4-1), risk of infarction is reduced and long-term survival is enhanced.

PTCA was developed as an alternative to surgical revascularization. Angioplasty involves passing a balloon catheter into a stenosed vessel and inflating the balloon at the site of the narrowing to widen the lumen. A high-grade proximal stenosis (70%) that is smooth, concentric, less than 0.5 cm in length, and noncalcified is considered the lesion most amenable to PTCA. The immediate success rate for PTCA for patients with favorable lesions exceeds 85%. However, the risk of restenosis is considerable, approximately 25%–40% at 6 months. The insertion of a wire-mesh *stent* with PTCA improves patency and reduces the risk of restenosis by nearly 50%. Because stent placement can trigger *acute thrombosis* (heralded by angina) or *subacute thrombosis* (manifested by acute infarction or death), the procedure is followed immediately by 2–4 weeks of potent antiplatelet therapy.

Primary PCI is superior to thrombolysis for the treatment of acute MI if performed by experienced operators. Stenting, in conjunction with abciximab, is now widely used in patients with acute MI.

When angioplasty is inappropriate or ineffective and medical therapy has failed to control symptoms in severe multivessel disease, CABG may be considered. CABG is the treatment of choice in persons with *high-risk disease* (ie, those with significant *left-main, proximal left-anterior descending,* or *3-vessel disease,* especially if accompanied by left ventricular dysfunction) because CABG is superior to medical therapy for prevention of infarction and prolongation of survival. The bypass graft provides a shunt from the aorta

Table 4-1 Risk Stratification for Patients With Stable Angina

Low risk	No angina currently or minimal angina
	Normal left ventricular function (normal ejection fraction)
	Small amount of myocardium at risk (probable single-vessel disease)
Moderate risk	Moderate angina
	Normal left ventricular function (normal ejection fraction)
	Moderate amount of myocardium at risk (probable 2-vessel or proximal left anterior descending artery disease)
High risk	Severe angina
	Impaired left ventricular function (ejection fraction <0.40)
	Extensive amount of myocardium at risk (probable 3-vessel, left main, or "left main equivalent" disease)

Adapted from Goroll AH, Mulley AG, eds. *Primary Care Medicine: Office Evaluation and Management of the Adult Patient.* Philadelphia: Lippincott Williams & Wilkins; 2000.

to the diseased coronary artery beyond the area of obstruction in order to increase blood flow, thereby eliminating angina and often reducing the risk of infarction and cardiac death or preventing these altogether. Coronary artery bypass grafting has also been shown to increase left ventricular function, improve quality of life, and increase life expectancy compared with medical treatment for patients with significant high-risk disease. Saphenous veins are most commonly used as the bypass material, but use of the internal mammary artery has become the standard for the left anterior descending artery because of its improved long-term patency rate. Some patients now receive "off the pump bypass surgery," in which the grafts are sewn onto a beating heart. This technique avoids the adverse effects of cardiopulmonary bypass, which include memory, cognitive, and other neurological deficits.

Alternative methods of revascularization under investigation include atherectomy devices employing *excimer* and *argon lasers, atheroma-cutting blades,* and *high-speed rotary devices and water-jets.* Thus far, outcomes remain disappointing because of unacceptably high complication rates due to debris and endothelial damage associated with these procedures.

Treatment of acute coronary syndromes

Patients with a definite ACS are admitted to the hospital for monitoring and treatment. They are initially treated aggressively with anti-ischemic pharmacotherapy. Once these initial measures are instituted, further management and triage of patients with an ACS is based on the presence or absence of ST-segment elevation. Patients with ST-segment elevation ACS are given reperfusion therapy with either thrombolysis or catheter-based interventions; patients with a non-ST-segment elevation ACS may be appropriately followed up with either medical treatment alone or a more aggressive interventional approach.

Management of non-ST-segment elevation ACS In general, myocardial oxygen demands are managed with medications and supplemental oxygen. Patients are given 160–325 mg of aspirin, which has been demonstrated to be effective in reducing the mortality of MI. The first dose of aspirin should be chewed rather than swallowed to achieve rapid blood levels. As long as the patient is not hypotensive or bradycardic, nitroglycerin is given. Nitroglycerin may be administered sublingually or intravenously. Intravenous administration of nitrates permits careful titration, allowing control of anginal symptoms without causing excessive hypotension. When nitroglycerin does not provide pain relief, morphine sulfate may be administered. Beta-blocker therapy reduces myocardial oxygen demands and should be considered for all patients with evolving MI if no contraindication exists.

For patients who do not receive reperfusion therapy, beta-blocker therapy provides a survival benefit, particularly for the high-risk subset of patients, which includes elderly patients and patients with previous MI and mild pulmonary venous congestion. When beta-blockers cannot be used, heart rate–slowing calcium antagonists (eg, verapamil or diltiazem) offer an alternative; however, rapid-release, short-acting dihydropyridine-type calcium channel blockers (eg, nifedipine) should be avoided in the absence of adequate concurrent beta blockade in ACS, because controlled trials suggest that, in this setting, there is an increased risk of MI and cardiac death. Moreover, the risk of cardiac death is significantly increased when calcium channel blockers are used in the setting of left ventricular failure.

Angiotensin-converting enzyme (ACE) inhibitors such as captopril (Capoten), lisinopril (Prinivil), and ramipril (Altace), given orally during the acute phase of MI, can potentially decrease the risk of immediate mortality when initiated within the first 24 hours of acute MI. ACE inhibitors confer benefit with or without concomitant reperfusion therapy. Patients receiving the greatest benefit are those in high-risk groups, including those with anterior infarctions, evidence of left ventricular systolic dysfunction, mild CHF, and previous MI. ACE inhibitors are contraindicated in patients with hypotension and should be used with caution in patients with renal insufficiency. If CHF or pulmonary edema is present, management should include vasodilators, diuretics, digoxin, or other inotropic agents. Patients with an ACS are also commonly given an antithrombin agent. A glycoprotein IIb/IIIa inhibitor should also be considered.

Largely because of clinical experience, clinicians usually use unfractionated heparin as the antithrombin. However, there is evidence that the newer antithrombin class, the low-molecular-weight heparins (LMWHs—eg, *enoxaparin* [Lovenox]), is superior. Antithrombin therapy with unfractionated heparin has several important disadvantages, such as a variable anticoagulant effect, an inability to inhibit clot-bound thrombin, and the potential to cause thrombocytopenia. LMWHs have increased anti-factor Xa activity and improved bioavailability, and they can be administered by subcutaneous injection. The ESSENCE and TIMI 11B trials have demonstrated that for patients with unstable angina/non–Q wave MI, LMWHs are superior to traditional unfractionated heparin.

The glycoprotein IIb/IIIa receptor is present on the surface of platelets. When platelets are activated, this receptor increases its affinity for fibrinogen and other ligands, resulting in platelet aggregation. This mechanism constitutes the final and obligatory pathway for platelet aggregation. The platelet GP IIb/IIIa receptor antagonists *tirofiban* (Aggrastat), *abciximab* (ReoPro), and *eptifibatide* (Integrilin) act by preventing fibrinogen binding and thereby preventing platelet aggregation. Platelets are involved in the development of both ACS and complications after PCI. Glycoprotein IIb/IIIa inhibitors have been shown to reduce the risk of death and MI in patients with non-ST-segment elevation ACS, as well as after coronary angioplasty and stenting. In addition to percutaneous interventions, the glycoprotein IIb/IIIa inhibitors are also indicated in the treatment of non-ST-segment elevation ACS. However, the benefit in these patients is less than that observed with percutaneous interventions. Patients with a non-ST-segment elevation ACS and an elevated troponin level may constitute a subset of patients who are particularly likely to receive a treatment benefit from platelet GP IIb/IIIa inhibitors and LMWH. Glycoprotein IIb/IIIa inhibitors are also being used in ST-segment elevation MI.

Once unstable angina and non-ST-segment elevation MI have been managed as described above, patients may be evaluated with either a conservative noninvasive approach or an early invasive (angiographic) strategy, depending on their level of risk for adverse outcome. In the early conservative strategy, coronary angiography is reserved for patients with evidence of recurrent ischemia (angina or ST-segment changes at rest or with minimal activity) or a strongly positive stress test result despite vigorous medical therapy. In the early invasive strategy, patients without clinically obvious contraindications to coronary revascularization are routinely recommended for coronary angiography and angiographically directed revascularization, if possible. The decision to proceed from diagnostic angiography to revascularization is influenced not only by the coronary anatomy but by a number of additional factors, including anticipated life expectancy, ventricular function, comorbidity, functional capacity, severity of symptoms, and quantity of viable myocardium at risk.

Management of ST-segment elevation ACS Modern therapy for evolving Q wave MI involves rapid and effective reperfusion because necrosis is a time-dependent process. Not surprisingly, optimal myocardial salvage requires that nearly complete reperfusion be achieved as soon as possible. Benefit is maximized if reperfusion therapy can be instituted within 1 hour of symptom onset; a significant benefit is retained if reperfusion therapy is instituted within 6 hours of symptom onset, and some benefit is still obtained if reperfusion therapy is instituted 6–12 hours after symptom onset. The benefit of reperfusion therapy after 12 hours of symptom onset has not been established.

Methods of reperfusion include thrombolysis and catheter-based percutaneous interventions (balloon angioplasty with or without stent placement). Adjuncts to therapy may include LMWH and glycoprotein IIb/IIIa inhibitors.

Percutaneous interventions require the availability of a cardiac catheterization laboratory and an experienced interventional cardiologist. Such facilities are available in fewer than 20% of hospitals worldwide. Even when these resources are available, a considerable delay (>90 minutes) may be encountered in transferring patients to the cardiac catheterization laboratory. Given the limited worldwide ability to perform timely catheterization, most patients with evolving ST-segment elevation MI are considered for intravenous thrombolytic therapy as soon as the diagnosis is made.

Thrombolysis Indications for thrombolysis include patients with ischemic chest pain lasting 30 minutes to 12 hours with ST-segment elevation of greater than 1 mm in 2 contiguous leads. Currently, several intravenous thrombolytic agents are available, which effectively lyse coronary thrombi and restore coronary blood flow in most patients. The most frequently used agents are *streptokinase* (1.5 million units administered over 30–60 minutes), the recombinant tissue plasminogen activator (TPA) *reteplase* (Retavase), the TPA *alteplase* (Activase), and *anisoylated plasminogen streptokinase activator complex* (30 units given as a bolus). The "front-loaded" alteplase regimen, used most frequently in the United States, consists of a 15-mg bolus followed by 0.75 mg/kg every 30 minutes (maximum, 50 mg) and then 0.50 mg/kg every 60 minutes (maximum, 35 mg). The efficacy of reteplase is similar to that of alteplase, but reteplase's administration (2 bolus injections of 10 IU at 30-minute intervals) is easier. When either is used, intravenous heparin should be administered concurrently.

The disadvantage of streptokinase therapy is that the rate of recanalization of the infarct-related artery is significantly lower than when TPA is used. With front-loaded TPA and heparin therapy, approximately 50% of infarct-related arteries recanalize, providing normal flow to the ischemic myocardium. The major disadvantage of TPA is a slightly greater risk of intracranial hemorrhage compared with streptokinase. Also, TPA therapy is more expensive than streptokinase therapy. Although most studies have restricted the use of these drugs to patients aged 75 or younger, older patients experience distinctly more infarction mortality and therefore may benefit from thrombolytic therapy. Contraindications include known sites of potential bleeding, a history of prior cerebrovascular accident, recent surgery, or prolonged cardiopulmonary resuscitation efforts.

Catheter-based reperfusion Another way of recanalizing the infarct-related artery is via mechanical means using balloon angioplasty (PTCA) with or without a stent. Mechanical reperfusion of a thrombotic coronary occlusion with normal arterial flow can be achieved in at least 90% of patients with ST-segment elevation and acute MI, a significantly greater percentage than is achieved with thrombolysis. Compared with thrombolysis, primary angioplasty has a greater potential to reduce the risk of 30-day mortality for patients with acute MI. Better survival is observed, particularly in high-risk patients with anterior MI, patients with previous MI, and patients with evidence of left ventricular dysfunction. A delay in the institution of reperfusion therapy significantly reduces the magnitude of the treatment's benefits, which apart from decreasing the risk of mortality include preserving left ventricular function and decreasing the risk of CHF.

Therefore, if a considerable delay (>90 minutes) is anticipated before primary angioplasty can be performed, thrombolysis is preferable. Primary PTCA is the preferred reperfusion strategy for patients with contraindications to thrombolytic therapy and for those in cardiogenic shock. Primary PTCA may also be preferable for patients with increased risk of intracranial hemorrhage and in patients who have undergone previous CABG. PTCA is also indicated for patients in whom thrombolytic reperfusion has apparently failed (ie, those with persistent chest pain and ST-segment elevation). Although recent trials suggest that primary angioplasty may be at least as beneficial as thrombolytic therapy for treatment of acute MI, additional questions surrounding the respective roles of these 2 treatments remain. Randomized trials comparing primary angioplasty and thrombolytic therapy are still relatively small, and no trial to date has compared immediate angioplasty with accelerated reteplase plus IV heparin or with newer thrombolytic regimens. The cost-effectiveness of primary angioplasty has not been fully evaluated.

> American Heart Association. *Heart Disease and Stroke Statistics—2003 Update*. Dallas, Tex: American Heart Association, 2002.
>
> Boersma E, Harrington RA, Moliterno DJ, et al. Platelet glycoprotein IIb/IIIa inhibitors in acute coronary syndromes: a meta-analysis of all major randomized clinical trials. *Lancet*. 2002;359:189–198.
>
> Gibbons RJ, Balady GJ, Bricker JT, et al. ACC/AHA 2002 guideline update for the management of patients with unstable angina and non-ST-segment elevation myocardial infarction—summary article. *J Am Coll Cardiol*. 2002;40:1366–1374.

Congestive Heart Failure

The epidemiologic magnitude of CHF is staggering. It is estimated that $60 billion are spent on heart failure every year in the United States alone. Many of the patients consulting an ophthalmologist belong to the elderly population, a group especially prone to this condition. If the heart cannot meet the metabolic demands of the metabolizing tissues, heart failure is the diagnosis. The cardiac pump may be in failure, or it may be near normal but unable to keep up with demand. The direct result of heart failure is circulatory failure.

Symptoms and signs of CHF may occur when the heart is not able to pump a sufficient amount of blood for a prolonged period to meet the body's requirements. *Compensated CHF* refers to patients whose clinical manifestations of CHF have been controlled by treatment. *Decompensated CHF* represents heart failure with symptoms that are not under control. *Refractory CHF* exists when previous therapeutic measures have failed to control the clinical manifestations of the syndrome. Pulmonary edema usually results from severe left ventricular failure with increased pulmonary capillary pressure, causing parenchymal and intra-alveolar fluid accumulation in the lung. Table 4-2 shows the New York Heart Association classification for heart failure symptoms.

Symptoms

Heart failure causes a variety of symptoms, depending on the severity of ventricular dysfunction. Symptoms may result from inadequate tissue perfusion caused by pump failure or from the failing heart's inability to empty adequately, leading to edema and fluid accumulation in the lungs, extremities, and other sites. The most frequent symptoms of left ventricular failure are dyspnea with exertion or at rest, orthopnea, paroxysmal nocturnal dyspnea, diaphoresis, generalized weakness, fatigue, anxiety, and lightheadedness. With more severe CHF, the patient may also experience a productive cough; copious pink, frothy sputum; and mental confusion. Angina may also occur if the CHF results from IHD. Right-sided heart failure may occur separately from or secondary to chronic left-sided heart failure. Patients with right-sided heart failure typically develop peripheral edema.

Clinical Signs

Examination findings in acute left ventricular failure may include respiratory distress, use of the respiratory accessory muscles, pinkish sputum or frank hemoptysis, coarse rales on pulmonary auscultation, expiratory wheezes, a rapid heart rate, an S gallop, diaphoresis, and deterioration in mental status. Blood pressure is often markedly elevated but may be reduced during MI. Long-standing cases of CHF show signs of right ventricular failure, especially elevated central venous pressure, pedal edema, hepatomegaly, and cyanosis. In some patients, pleural effusion or ascites may be detected.

Table 4-2 New York Heart Association Classification for Heart Failure Symptoms

Symptom Class	Symptom
I	No symptoms
II	Comfortable at rest; symptoms with ordinary activity
III	Comfortable at rest; symptoms with less than ordinary activity
IV	Symptoms at rest

Diagnostic Evaluation

The history and clinical examination are the most important components in the diagnostic assessment of CHF. Helpful diagnostic studies in the evaluation of CHF and its underlying causes include chest radiograph, ECG, blood gases, hemoglobin level, serum electrolytes, and urinalysis. If the primary mechanism of heart failure is unclear, additional tests may prove useful in selected patients. Such tests may include echocardiography, exercise stress testing, cardiac nuclear imaging studies, coronary arteriography, right-sided and left-sided heart catheterization, Holter monitoring, pulmonary function tests, and thyroid function tests.

The ECG may reveal acute ischemic changes, acute or old MI, ventricular hypertrophy, chamber enlargement, and atrial fibrillation or other arrhythmias. Typical chest radiographic findings are prominent pulmonary vessels, interstitial or alveolar pulmonary edema, cardiomegaly, and pleural effusions. Patients with severe pump failure may have abnormal serum electrolytes owing to poor renal perfusion. Abnormalities in the blood or urine may help detect severe anemia or renal failure as a precipitating factor in CHF. Abnormal liver enzymes are common if venous congestion is present as a result of right ventricular failure. Echocardiography and other cardiac studies can help differentiate the many cardiac causes of CHF, including IHD, valvular heart disease, cardiomyopathies, and cardiac arrhythmias.

Ejection fraction (EF) is the calculated percentage of blood ejected by the ventricle during a single or average contraction. In patients without CHF, the EF is more than 0.50. An EF of 0.40–0.50 indicates mild impairment; 0.25–0.40, moderate impairment; and less than 0.25, severe impairment. Ejection fraction can be measured using echocardiography, radionuclide ventriculography, and contrast ventriculography. Echocardiography is the most useful and least invasive method of determining and sequentially following EF and the systolic state of the ventricles.

Epidemiology

In a large percentage of patients with CHF, the epidemiology parallels that of IHD because IHD is currently the primary cause of heart failure. Accordingly, the same risk factors for atherosclerosis apply to ischemic CHF. Patients with CHF are more sensitive to a high intake of sodium and should therefore receive dietary instructions to achieve a low-sodium diet. When CHF is not the result of IHD, other causes must be investigated. A history of rheumatic fever, atrial fibrillation, pernicious anemia, hyperthyroidism, or other disorders may suggest one of the less common causes of CHF. Although CHF is most common in adults, it can also occur in children with congenital heart or valve defects, cardiomyopathy, myocarditis, or, in rare instances, following infarction from Kawasaki disease.

The prognosis for patients with CHF depends directly on the degree of ventricular impairment. The New York Heart Association classification system of CHF by symptoms (see Table 4-2) correlates well with survival. In a study from Duke University, patients with class IV CHF had 1-year and 3-year mortality rates of 55% and 82%, respectively. In the Framingham study, the overall 5-year mortality rate was 62% in men with CHF and 42% in women.

Etiology

As was noted previously, IHD is the most common cause of CHF. Cumulative injury to the ventricular myocardium from ischemia and infarction can lead to impaired ventricular systolic and diastolic function, and, ultimately, pump failure. Additional causes of systolic dysfunction are

- valvular heart disease (primarily aortic stenosis and aortic or mitral regurgitation)
- cardiomyopathies (which may be idiopathic or which may have metabolic, infectious, toxic, or connective tissue causes)
- myocarditis (from viral or inflammatory diseases)

Diseases that impair the relaxation and filling properties of the left ventricle can result in diastolic dysfunction. Such disorders include infiltrative diseases (eg, amyloidosis, sarcoidosis, and metastatic disease) and left ventricular hypertrophy (which can be caused by arterial hypertension, idiopathic hypertrophic subaortic stenosis, and coarctation of the aorta).

Actually, systolic dysfunction and diastolic dysfunction often occur simultaneously in the common causes of CHF—namely, IHD, valvular disease, and the congestive cardiomyopathies. Some of the causes of high-cardiac output heart failure are

- severe anemia
- hyperthyroidism
- arteriovenous fistulas
- beriberi
- Paget disease

In high-output failure, the demand for oxygen is so great that the heart eventually fails because it cannot maintain the excessive cardiac output indefinitely. Some patients may have more than 1 mechanism for heart failure, such as a patient with IHD who develops CHF after becoming severely anemic. Pure right ventricular failure may result from chronic pulmonary disease, pulmonary hypertension, tricuspid or pulmonary valve disease, right ventricular infarction, or constrictive pericarditis.

Pathophysiology and Clinical Course

The left and right ventricles function as pumping chambers, and their action can be subdivided into a *systolic,* or contraction, phase and a *diastolic,* or relaxation, phase. During *systole,* the ventricular muscle actively contracts, developing pressure and ejecting blood into the aorta or pulmonary artery for forward perfusion. During *diastole,* the ventricular muscle actively and passively relaxes and allows a refilling of the ventricle from the corresponding atrium. Either or both of these phases may become impaired, leading to dysfunction of systole, diastole, or both. Some of the symptoms and clinical signs of CHF can be distinguished as being attributable to systolic or diastolic impairment. Treatment varies, depending on which type of dysfunction predominates.

Systolic dysfunction

The ability of the heart to contract and eject blood is determined by preload, afterload, and contractility. *Preload* refers to the amount of stretch to which muscle fibers are subjected at the end of diastole, or refilling. Preload is determined by blood volume and venous return. Excessive preload is often called *volume overload*. Up to a point, as the preload increases, the force of contraction also increases, allowing adequate emptying of the ventricle.

Afterload is the amount of tension or force in the ventricular muscle mass just after onset of contraction, as the ventricle begins emptying. Clinically, afterload represents the pressure that the ventricle must withstand during contraction. Thus, the aortic pressure determines afterload for the left ventricle, whereas the pulmonary artery pressure determines afterload for the right. Even a normal ventricle may fail with extremely high preload or afterload.

Contractility refers to the intrinsic ability of the myocardial fibers to contract, independent of the preload or afterload conditions. Contractility can be adversely affected by metabolic, ischemic, or other structural derangement of the myocardial cells. Abnormal intracellular modulation of calcium ions is a key component in heart failure. Clinical disorders that affect preload, afterload, or contractility result in systolic dysfunction. Likewise, therapy directed toward improvements in these parameters can be used to treat systolic dysfunction.

Diastolic dysfunction

Several of the disorders that impair the diastolic, or relaxation, properties of the ventricle were listed previously among the causes of CHF. Diastolic dysfunction causes elevated filling pressures in the ventricles and atria. In the left ventricle, diastolic dysfunction causes pulmonary venous hypertension and its clinical manifestations, such as dyspnea on exertion, orthopnea, and paroxysmal nocturnal dyspnea. Clinical signs of diastolic dysfunction are pulmonary edema with rales, lung congestion visible on chest radiograph, and hypoxemia.

The clinical course of CHF may follow a downward spiral of left ventricular systolic and diastolic dysfunction, ventricular dilation, and a decline in the EF, followed by right-sided heart failure. A continuous reduction in cardiac output and tissue perfusion may be accompanied by increasing pulmonary and systemic venous congestion. Appropriate treatment may slow or even halt progression in some patients. B-type natriuretic peptide (BNP), which is synthesized in the cardiac ventricles and whose release is directly proportional to ventricular volume expansion and pressure overload, may indicate the course of CHF. Levels of BNP correlate with left ventricular pressure, the amount of dyspnea, and the state of neurohumoral modulation. In addition, BNP levels correlate well with the New York Heart Association classification system of CHF.

Medical and Nonsurgical Management

In the management of heart failure, treatment strategies can be directed at systolic or diastolic ventricular dysfunction. Specific treatment for some causes of right-sided heart failure is also available.

Systolic dysfunction

If the preload is reduced, systolic function can occasionally be improved by carefully increasing preload by volume infusion. This increase in preload dilates the ventricle and is 1 of the mechanisms by which the heart intrinsically attempts to compensate for poor systolic function. However, this mechanism fails and systolic function is impaired when the ventricle becomes overly dilated.

Reducing afterload is the most effective way to manage systolic dysfunction in most clinical situations. Reducing vascular resistance and lowering arterial blood pressure decrease the burden on the left ventricle and enhance contraction and ejection. Regardless of the baseline values, lowering blood pressure (while maintaining adequate tissue perfusion) is the mainstay of treatment of systolic dysfunction. The most effective drugs for reducing afterload in current clinical practice are the *ACE inhibitors,* which include *captopril* (Acenorm, Capoten), *enalapril* (Vasotec), *lisinopril* (Zestril), and *ramipril* (Altace). These drugs effectively decrease the clinical manifestations of CHF and have been demonstrated in clinical trials to lower both mortality and morbidity rates among patients with CHF, *morbidity* being defined as hospitalization (or therapy) for worsening heart failure. These beneficial effects can be seen in patients with idiopathic dilated cardiomyopathy as well as in those with diminished left ventricular function after an MI. *Angiotensin-receptor antagonists* have been developed as therapy for CHF, and many physicians have used them as alternative therapy for the management of the ACE-intolerant patient. However, the potential benefits of angiotensin-receptor antagonists have not been assessed in large multicenter randomized studies, and use of these drugs cannot be recommended at present.

Other drugs that reduce afterload by lowering blood pressure and peripheral vascular resistance are *hydralazine, clonidine,* and *calcium channel blockers.* However, calcium channel blockers have generally been found to be of little benefit in patients with CHF. In fact, diltiazem (Cardizem) was associated with increased mortality when used in patients with CHF. Amlodipine (Norvasc) is the only calcium channel blocker that has been shown to be safe in patients with CHF and is therefore the calcium channel blocker of choice in patients with CHF and ongoing IHD not controlled by other means. The *α-adrenergic blockers* such as *prazosin* or *doxazosin* can also be considered for patients who cannot tolerate ACE inhibitors because of renal dysfunction or other relative contraindications. Hospitalized patients with more severe CHF, particularly pulmonary edema, may require more aggressive afterload reduction with intravenous agents such as *nitroprusside, nitroglycerin,* or *enalapril.*

For patients with systolic dysfunction, the contractility of the left ventricle can be enhanced with inotropic agents. *Digitalis,* the time-honored drug for increasing contractility, is a mainstay of treatment, especially for long-term outpatient maintenance therapy. With the exception of digoxin, oral inotropic agents have not proved safe or effective in patients with chronic CHF. However, intravenous inotropic agents play a key role in the treatment of patients hospitalized for worsening heart failure. Three intravenous inotropic agents are FDA-approved as therapy for acute exacerbations of CHF: the adrenergic agonist *dobutamine* (Dobutrex), the phosphodiesterase inhibitor *milrinone* (Primacor), and the dopaminergic/adrenergic agonist *dopamine* (Intropin). For patients with disease refractory to either dobutamine or milrinone, both drugs can be used together to take advantage of synergistic actions. Patients on these potent drugs require close monitoring of blood pressure, heart rate, cardiac output, and urine production.

Patients with CHF have an increased adrenergic drive that is associated with a worsened prognosis. High levels of norepinephrine are both arrhythmogenic and cardiotoxic. The use of beta-blockers such as carvedilol (Coreg), bisoprolol (Zebeta), and metoprolol (Lopressor) has clearly been shown to improve heart failure symptoms and to reduce all-cause mortality and the risk of hospitalization in patients with CHF. These benefits are most obvious in patients with moderate to severe symptoms; however, several important caveats should be noted. First, beta-blocker therapy has not been assessed in patients with bradycardia, hypotension, or class IV symptoms. Similarly, the effects of beta-blockers have not been assessed in patients with left ventricular dilatation but compensated function and the absence of symptoms. In addition, as many as 6% of patients may not tolerate even small amounts of a beta-blocker. Therefore, the initial doses of beta-blocker must be very low, with gradual and careful upward titration over 3–6 months.

Diastolic dysfunction

Diastolic function can be improved by reducing preload, which in turn lowers filling pressures in the ventricle. Preload can be reduced by reducing circulating blood volume, by increasing the capacitance of the venous bed, and by improving systolic function to more effectively empty the ventricle. Diuretics are the most effective agents for reducing blood volume. *Oral thiazide* or *loop diuretics* are effective for long-term diuresis, but *intravenous loop diuretics* such as *furosemide* or *bumetanide* are more potent for severe CHF or pulmonary edema. Venous capacitance can be increased by administering venous dilators, particularly the nitrates. Intravenous *furosemide* and *morphine* also have some venodilation effects, partially explaining their effectiveness in treating pulmonary edema. Any of the measures previously discussed that improve systolic function also indirectly enhance diastolic function by reducing the residual blood volume in the ventricle following contraction.

Other approaches to CHF

Other strategies for managing CHF include seeking the underlying causes or contributing factors responsible for the failure and correcting them, if possible. Precipitating factors can include excessive salt or fluid intake, poor medication compliance, excessive activity, obesity, pulmonary infection or embolism, MI, renal disease, anemia, thyrotoxicosis, or arrhythmias.

Intermittent arrhythmias may seriously compromise ventricular function. Tachyarrhythmias may aggravate ischemia; bradyarrhythmias may decrease cardiac output and blood pressure further. However, antiarrhythmic therapy has been shown to have little benefit in the management of patients with CHF, inasmuch as most of these agents have significant proarrhythmic and negative inotropic properties. However, amiodarone (at low dosage) has proven useful in some patients with recalcitrant atrial fibrillation. In patients with documented *sustained* ventricular tachycardia or fibrillation, ICDs are beneficial. However, the role of ICDs in the therapy for patients with *nonsustained* ventricular tachycardia is still under investigation (see later discussion, Disorders of Cardiac Rhythm). Patients with heart block and other severe bradyarrhythmias may require cardiac pacing.

Patients with a dilated cardiomyopathy and atrial fibrillation should be treated with warfarin (Coumadin) unless specific contraindications exist. Many physicians also prescribe warfarin for patients with a dilated cardiomyopathy, low ejection fraction, and normal sinus rhythm, if no contraindications exist.

Other measures that can assist in the management of CHF are restricting dietary sodium, avoiding fluid overload by carefully monitoring oral and intravenous fluid intake, controlling pain and anxiety, treating concomitant metabolic or pulmonary diseases, and providing supplemental oxygen to hypoxemic patients. Finally, all patients with CHF should receive an influenza vaccination and the pneumococcal vaccine. New agents and devices currently under investigation for the treatment of CHF include etanercept, a recombinant-produced soluble receptor for tumor necrosis factor; angiotensin-receptor antagonists; tezosentan and bosentan, which are endothelin-receptor antagonists; novel inotropic agents; and biventricular pacing devices, which attempt to "resynchronize" the electrical activity of the heart and thereby improve pump function.

Invasive or Surgical Management

Depending on the underlying causes, surgical procedures that may benefit patients with CHF include percutaneous balloon valvuloplasty, mitral commissurotomy, mitral or aortic valve replacement, coronary angioplasty, CABG, left ventricular aneurysmectomy, or pericardectomy. Cardiac transplantation has become an effective surgical treatment for patients with refractory CHF. Many transplant centers have achieved a 5-year survival rate above 75%. The use of corticosteroids and immunosuppressive agents, such as cyclosporine and FK-506, has reduced transplant rejection and mortality.

> Adams KF Jr, Mathur VS, Gheorghiade M. B-type natriuretic peptide: from bench to bedside. *Am Heart J.* 2003;145(2 suppl):S34–S46.
>
> Bradley DJ, Bradley EA, Baughman KL, et al. Cardiac resynchronization and death from progressive heart failure: a meta-analysis of randomized controlled trials. *JAMA.* 2003;289:730–740.
>
> Moller JE, Dahlstrom U, Gotzsche O, et al. Effects of losartan and captopril on left ventricular systolic and diastolic function after acute myocardial infarction: results of the Optimal Trial in Myocardial Infarction with Angiotensin II Antagonist Losartan (OPTIMAAL) echocardiographic substudy. *Am Heart J.* 2004;147(3):494–501.

Disorders of Cardiac Rhythm

Abnormalities of cardiac rhythm can vary widely from asymptomatic premature atrial complexes or mild sinus bradycardia to life-threatening ventricular tachycardia or fibrillation. Disorders of cardiac rhythm can be categorized into several groups:

- bradyarrhythmias and conduction disturbances
- ectopic or premature contractions
- tachyarrhythmias

Although many rhythm and conduction disturbances are caused by underlying IHD, they are also attributable to valvular heart disease, myocarditis, cardiomyopathy, congenital aberrant conduction pathways, pulmonary disease, toxic or metabolic disorders, neurogenic causes, and cardiac trauma.

The electrical impulse that initiates each heartbeat normally begins in the *sinoatrial (SA) node* and is conducted down through the atria and ventricles, resulting in a coordinated series of contractions of these chambers. The SA node is the primary pacemaker of the heart. It controls the heart rate and is influenced by neural, biochemical, and pharmacologic factors. If the SA node function is depressed or absent, secondary pacemakers in the *atrioventricular (AV) junction, the bundle of His,* or the *ventricular muscle* can generate stimuli and maintain the heartbeat. Normally, stimulus formation in these other secondary pacemaker sites is slower than that of the SA node. However, abnormal stimuli can also be generated at any of these sites at a rapid pace, resulting in tachycardia.

Bradyarrhythmias and Conduction Disturbances

A *bradyarrhythmia* is any rhythm resulting in a ventricular rate of less than 60 beats per minute (bpm).

Sinus bradycardia

A sinus rhythm (initiated by the SA node) slower than 60 bpm is called *sinus bradycardia*. Sinus bradycardia is usually innocuous and can occur in healthy persons. Typical causes include increased vagal tone, antiarrhythmic drug effect, ischemia, and primary sinus node disease. Affected persons may be asymptomatic or may complain of fatigue, angina, or syncope. Treatment is almost never indicated.

Sinus arrest

Also called *sinus block* or *SA block,* sinus arrest involves an absence of the entire complex for 1 or more beats. Single or multiple beats may be dropped. If the period of sinus arrest is prolonged, an AV nodal or ventricular escape beat may occur. Sinus arrest may be caused by increased vagal tone, sick sinus syndrome, carotid artery sinus hypersensitivity, hypokalemia, or the same medications that can cause sinus bradycardia. Patients may be asymptomatic if the pause is brief, or they may experience lightheadedness or syncope. If the condition is unstable or syncope develops from a long pause, emergency treatment with intravenous atropine usually increases the heart rate temporarily while definitive treatment is planned. In some cases, a pacemaker may be necessary.

Atrioventricular junctional rhythm

When the sinus node is depressed or nonfunctional, the AV node may take over the pacemaking function. During AV nodal pacing, the atria and ventricles contract independently. The heart rate in an AV junctional rhythm is usually about 30–60 bpm. Periodic prominent pulsations in the neck veins, occurring during systole, are noted. On the ECG, the QRS complex appears normal; however, the P waves are abnormal in shape and may follow the QRS in some leads. No treatment is usually necessary, but evaluating the patient for underlying cardiac disease may be appropriate.

Atrioventricular block

Atrioventricular block is caused by a delay or block in conduction through the AV junction. In first-degree AV block, the PR interval seen on ECG may only be prolonged; in second- or third-degree AV block, ventricular beats may be dropped. Causes of AV block include vagal stimulation, medications, and heart disease.

First-degree AV block is asymptomatic and is diagnosed by the prolongation of the PR interval beyond 0.2 seconds on ECG. There are 2 types of *second-degree AV block*. In the *Wenckebach type,* the ECG reveals progressive PR prolongation prior to a nonconducted P wave, resulting in QRS complexes in regular groupings (grouped beating). In *Mobitz type II* AV block, the QRS complex is dropped at regular intervals, and the QRS complex is usually widened. Patients with second-degree AV block may experience palpitations. The pulse rate is irregular in Wenckebach block and slow and regular in Mobitz type II block. The prognosis is usually worse with Mobitz type II block because it more often heralds underlying cardiac disease and may progress to complete heart block.

Complete, or *third-degree, AV block* is more ominous and usually causes more symptoms. All of the atrial stimuli are blocked at the AV node, so the P waves from the atria and the QRS complexes are completely asynchronous. The rate and width of the QRS complexes depend on whether they originate in the AV node, the bundle of His, or the ventricles. When the stimuli arise in the ventricles, the QRS complex is very wide and aberrant; this is called an *idioventricular escape rhythm.* Patients may be asymptomatic or may become lightheaded if the rate is very slow. If the ventricular rate is profoundly slow or if the beats cease for an interval, syncope may occur. This is known as *Stokes-Adams syndrome.* Atropine or isoproterenol can be given intravenously for immediate management of profound bradycardia or symptomatic heart block. A temporary transvenous pacemaker may be inserted to pace the heart until a permanent programmable pacemaker is implanted.

Intraventricular or fascicular blocks

The bundle of His has 2 main branches, the right and the left. The right branch is composed of a single fascicle, and the left is composed of at least 2. *Left anterior hemiblock (fascicular block)* is characterized by marked left axis deviation on ECG and may result from MI, pulmonary embolism, cardiac surgery, or cardiac catheterization. This condition is insignificant unless it occurs concomitantly with right bundle branch block. *Left posterior hemiblock (fascicular block)* results in right axis deviation on ECG and may be caused by IHD, myocarditis, or valvular heart disease. This type of block is nearly always associated with right bundle branch block, resulting in a bifascicular block. No treatment is required for fascicular blocks.

Complete left bundle branch block (LBBB) LBBB results in a delay in conduction to the left ventricle, causing some asynchrony between the contraction of the 2 ventricles. This condition may be transient or permanent. It is usually secondary to various types of heart disease, but occasionally it is seen in normal hearts. LBBB is asymptomatic; however, it may interfere with the ECG diagnosis of MI by obscuring the Q wave and its secondary ST segment and T wave changes. Most clinicians think that the prognosis is excellent in young patients with LBBB. Older patients with LBBB appear to have a higher risk of cardiac disease and 10-year mortality compared with patients who do not have LBBB. Treatment is not necessary, but an evaluation for underlying heart disease is advised.

Right bundle branch block (RBBB) RBBB delays conduction to the right ventricle but does not cause symptoms. RBBB occurs in healthy persons, but it can also be associated with pulmonary embolism, heart disease, cardiac surgery, chest trauma, cor pulmonale, and congenital heart defects. The ECG shows wide QRS complexes. When RBBB is not associated with pulmonary embolism or MI, prognosis is good. However, significant CAD has been reported in as many as 20% of asymptomatic patients with RBBB.

Premature Contractions

The principal types of premature contractions are

- premature atrial complexes
- premature junctional complexes
- premature ventricular complexes

Premature atrial complexes

Premature atrial complexes (PACs) result from ectopic atrial depolarizations occurring prior to the next depolarization from the sinus node. The resultant P waves usually differ in contour and axis from the normal sinus P wave. Premature atrial complexes may occur in the absence of structural heart disease but are common in the clinical settings of infection, inflammation, myocardial ischemia, drug toxicity, catecholamine excess, electrolyte imbalance, or excessive use of tobacco, alcohol, or caffeine. Symptoms range from none to feelings of "skipped" beats. Premature atrial complexes typically require no therapy. If symptoms are present, therapy should be directed toward correction of underlying abnormalities. β-Adrenergic antagonists or calcium channel antagonists may be useful.

Premature junctional complexes

Premature junctional complexes (PJCs) are premature depolarizations from the AV node or the proximal portion of the His-Purkinje system. Premature junctional complexes usually occur in the absence of structural heart disease but may be seen in clinical settings similar to those surrounding PACs. Premature junctional complexes typically result in a premature, normally conducted QRS. An inverted P wave occurs during or just after the QRS complex, when retrograde AV nodal conduction occurs. The next, normally timed sinus P wave may be delayed or blocked in the AV node because of the retrograde conduction of the PJC. Symptoms and therapy are similar to those pertinent to PACs.

Premature ventricular complexes

Premature ventricular complexes (PVCs) are premature depolarizations that originate from the ventricles and occur prior to the next, normally conducted sinus beat. Premature ventricular complexes often occur in the absence of structural heart disease and are increasingly frequent with age. Potential causes are similar to those for PACs. The ECG reveals a premature QRS complex of bizarre morphology with a T wave polarity opposite to that of the QRS complex. Patients may be asymptomatic or feel "skipped" beats.

Premature ventricular complexes typically require no therapy. When patients are symptomatic, therapy should be directed toward correction of underlying abnormalities. Frequent or complex PVCs in the presence of cardiac disease are markers of an increased risk of SCD. However, a direct causal link between PVCs and the onset of malignant ventricular tachyarrhythmias has never been established. The Cardiac Arrhythmia Suppression Trial showed that suppression of asymptomatic ventricular premature beats with class I antiarrhythmic drugs does not improve mortality in patients who have experienced infarction. In fact, this study showed that class IC drugs (flecainide and encainide) were associated with excessive mortality compared with placebo. The results of other studies also support the conclusion that class I antiarrhythmic drugs should not be used for treatment of PVCs, either asymptomatic or symptomatic, in patients with underlying structural heart disease and IHD.

Tachyarrhythmias

Tachyarrhythmias are defined as a heart rate in excess of 100 bpm. Tachycardias are distinguished as being supraventricular or ventricular, depending on the mechanism and site of origin.

Narrow complex tachycardias are almost exclusively supraventricular in origin.

Sinus tachycardia occurs when the sinus mechanism is accelerated. The pattern of atrial and ventricular activation is normal. Sinus tachycardia may occur in the setting of increased sympathetic or diminished vagal tone, catecholamine excess, pain, hypovolemia, hypoxemia, myocardial ischemia or infarction, pulmonary embolism, fever, and inflammation. The atrial rate is typically between 100 and 160 bpm. The ECG demonstrates P waves with a normal configuration and axis, a normal or slightly shortened PR interval, and a normal QRS pattern. Therapy should be targeted at the underlying pathophysiologic process. Beta-blockers may be used to slow the sinus rate, particularly in the setting of myocardial ischemia.

Supraventricular tachycardias

This category includes paroxysmal atrial tachycardia, AV junctional tachycardia, atrial flutter, and atrial fibrillation. The exact site of the pacing focus may be difficult to determine when the heart rate is very rapid. The prognosis for supraventricular tachycardias is usually better than that associated with ventricular tachycardia. These tachycardias may be paroxysmal or chronic, as with chronic atrial fibrillation. Causes include emotional stress, caffeine, alcohol, drugs, thyrotoxicosis, lung disease, and cardiac disease.

Paroxysmal atrial tachycardia The heart rate in paroxysmal atrial tachycardia (PAT) is often higher than 140 bpm. The P waves have an abnormal configuration and axis, the PR interval depends on the atrial rate, and the QRS pattern may be normal or it may reflect aberrant conduction secondary to the increased rate. If AV block and PAT are observed together, digitalis toxicity should be suspected. Multifocal PAT often is associated with chronic obstructive pulmonary disease and CHF. Clinical manifestations of PAT include palpitations, sensation of a rapid heart rate, lightheadedness, and rarely syncope. Patients with IHD may experience angina or dyspnea. Currently, the treatment of choice for PAT is *intravenous adenosine,* which has a very short half-life and approximately a

90% success rate in yielding normal sinus rhythm. Other therapeutic measures include Valsalva maneuvers, carotid sinus pressure or massage, intravenous verapamil (except in Wolff-Parkinson-White syndrome), digitalis, and beta-blockers. Patients with hemodynamic instability may require DC cardioversion. Precipitating factors should be reduced or eliminated, and any underlying disease should be treated. Unifocal or reentrant atrial tachycardias often can be eliminated permanently via radiofrequency catheter or surgical ablation.

Junctional tachycardia Junctional tachycardia is a rare rhythm disorder due to increased automaticity of the AV node. Junctional tachycardia typically produces heart rates of 60–130 bpm. It occurs in such clinical settings as ischemia, the postoperative state, and myocarditis. If retrograde AV conduction occurs, P waves are inverted and may appear during or immediately after the QRS. Also possible is competitive AV dissociation, wherein normal-appearing nonconducted P waves occur at a rate slower than the ventricular rate. The QRS pattern may be normal or it may reflect rate-related aberrant conduction. Treatment consists of correcting the underlying pathophysiologic process and discontinuing potentially offending agents. If required, lidocaine or beta-blockers may be effective. For patients with competitive AV dissociation and hemodynamic compromise, atrial overdrive pacing may restore AV synchrony.

Wolff-Parkinson-White syndrome The diagnosis of Wolff-Parkinson-White (WPW) syndrome should be considered in patients who present with tachycardia characterized by a widened QRS with an initial up-sloping (delta wave). Wolff-Parkinson-White syndrome is characterized by preexcitation (short PR interval and a delta wave slurring the upstroke of the QRS complex) and supraventricular tachycardia. In this syndrome, the ventricles are stimulated early by preexcitation through accessory fibers. Paroxysmal atrial tachycardia, atrial flutter, or atrial fibrillation may occur with a very rapid rate in WPW syndrome because of a circus movement involving the accessory conduction pathways. The wide QRS complex that accompanies PAT and the WPW syndrome can resemble ventricular tachycardia.

Atrial flutter Atrial flutter is associated with a rapid atrial rate of 200–380 bpm. The ventricular rate is slower, usually with 2:1, 3:1, or 4:1 conduction. Atrial flutter is caused by a macro reentrant circuit isolated in the right atrium. Atrial flutter occurs in some healthy patients, but it is also associated with MI, hyperthyroidism, mitral stenosis, and underlying lung disease. If the ventricular rate is slow, atrial flutter may occur without symptoms. If the rate is very rapid (>200 bpm), the symptoms are similar to those of PAT. The regular, rapid P waves of atrial flutter are called *F (flutter) waves* and have a sawtooth appearance. Some degree of AV block is usually present, resulting in QRS complexes at regular intervals. Atrial flutter may be paroxysmal or persistent. This arrhythmia can be fatal if the ventricular rate is very rapid in the setting of ischemia or heart failure. Conversion of atrial flutter to sinus rhythm should be attempted. Acute treatment measures include both controlling the ventricular response with beta-blockers, calcium channel blockers, and digitalis and attempting to restore sinus rhythm with electrical cardioversion and antiarrhythmic drugs. *Ibutilide* (Corvert) is an agent that rapidly converts recent-onset atrial flutter or fibrillation. Adenosine can be used to confirm the diagnosis of atrial flutter, but its utility as a rate-slowing agent is limited by its very short half-life.

Atrial fibrillation   Atrial fibrillation is caused by multiple simultaneous wavelets occurring in both the right and the left atria. This results in a chaotic electrical rhythm with ineffective atrial contraction. The causes and symptoms are similar to those of atrial flutter. The pulse rate is usually irregular, and characteristic changes—irregular (fibrillation) waves and an irregular ventricular rate—are common on ECG. Occasionally, aberrantly conducted beats result in a wide QRS that can resemble a PVC.

Because atrial contractions are ineffective in atrial fibrillation, cardiac output can be reduced markedly when the ventricular rate is very rapid, possibly resulting in CHF. Atrial thrombi may accumulate from stagnation of blood in the atrial appendages. These thrombi may embolize to the lungs, brain, or other organs. Anticoagulation is indicated for patients with chronic atrial fibrillation associated with valvular disease, cardiomyopathy, or cardiomegaly and before conversion to sinus rhythm is attempted.

Conversion of atrial fibrillation can be attempted with quinidine, procainamide, ibutilide, or DC cardioversion. In many patients with chronic atrial fibrillation, maintenance therapy is often directed toward controlling the ventricular rate. This can usually be accomplished with digitalis, verapamil, or beta-blockers.

Newer curative approaches have been developed for both atrial fibrillation and atrial flutter. These treatments include radiofrequency catheter ablation and the surgical Maze procedure. The Maze procedure interrupts all of the possible reentry circuits to the atrium with multiple incisions. A single uninterrupted pathway is left intact to allow normal conduction from the sinus node to the AV node. Of the 178 patients who underwent the Maze procedure, 93% were free of arrhythmia; the rest were converted to sinus rhythm with medical therapy.

Wide-complex tachycardias   Wide-complex tachycardias may be either supraventricular or ventricular in origin, and correct identification of the origin and mechanism of the tachycardia is critical to the selection of appropriate treatment.

Ventricular tachyarrhythmias

Ventricular tachycardia   Ventricular tachycardia (VT) is defined as a series of 3 or more ventricular complexes occurring at a rate of 100–250 bpm; the origin of activation is within the ventricle. The QRS is wide (usually >120 milliseconds), with T wave polarity opposite to that of the major QRS deflection. *Sustained VT* is defined as tachycardia lasting longer than 30 seconds or associated with hemodynamic collapse. Monomorphic VT has a single QRS morphology throughout the arrhythmia, whereas polymorphic VT is characterized by ever-changing QRS morphology. Underlying causes include CAD, hypokalemia, hypomagnesemia, digitalis, quinidine, and other drugs that are potentially proarrhythmic. A recent study suggests that hearts with low EFs receive markedly increased reflex cardiac sympathetic stimulation, which may play a role in initiating and sustaining ventricular arrhythmias.

Ventricular tachycardia occurs infrequently in young patients with no organic heart disease. Brief episodes of VT cause palpitations; prolonged attacks in patients with organic cardiac disease can lead to heart failure or cardiac shock. If the rate is not very high and there is no significant underlying heart disease, VT may be well tolerated; however, VT may degenerate into ventricular fibrillation, resulting in hemodynamic collapse and death.

Treatment with immediate synchronized DC cardioversion is indicated for sustained VT associated with hemodynamic compromise, severe CHF, or ongoing ischemia or infarction. Pharmacologic cardioversion with IV procainamide or lidocaine and amiodarone may be attempted in patients with clinically stable VT. Amiodarone is probably the agent of choice for recurrent VT if its side effects are tolerated.

Electrophysiologic testing is often performed on patients with suspected or documented ventricular arrhythmias. In this procedure, direct transcatheter electrical stimulation of various sites in the ventricle induces arrhythmias. Given the efficacy and low risk associated with implantation, ICD therapy (often in conjunction with antiarrhythmic drugs) has become the treatment of choice for patients with life-threatening ventricular arrhythmias. Less common therapies include ventricular aneurysmectomy, ventricular electrical mapping and resection of the arrhythmogenic focus, and radiofrequency catheter ablation.

Implantable cardioverter-defibrillators Implantable cardioverter-defibrillators are devices that monitor the heart rhythm and, when a tachyarrhythmia is identified, deliver therapy. Their evolution has been impressive. Initially, a thoracotomy was necessary to implant an epicardial patch or patches. Currently, the overwhelming majority of patients receive a transvenous system, which significantly reduces the morbidity and mortality associated with the implantation of these devices. Current-generation ICDs are generally implanted in the prepectoral region (similar to pacemaker implantation). Although first-generation ICDs delivered only high-energy "defibrillating" shocks, current-generation devices provide tiered therapy, including

- antitachycardia pacing algorithms
- low-energy cardioversion for stable VT
- high-energy cardioversion for VT or ventricular fibrillation
- single-chamber or dual-chamber bradycardic pacing support
- stored diagnostic information for rhythm discrimination

ICDs treat arrhythmias when they occur and do not prevent them. Many patients require concomitant antiarrhythmic therapy to reduce the frequency of device discharges or facilitate antitachycardia pacing by slowing the tachycardia rate. The development of an effective and safe antiarrhythmic prescription may be complex and requires the skills of a trained electrophysiologist. Generally, the acute management of life-threatening ventricular arrhythmias in these patients does not differ from that of other patients with similar rhythm disturbances. If the device fails to terminate an arrhythmia, cardiopulmonary resuscitation and external defibrillation should proceed normally. Three randomized prospective studies have demonstrated that automated ICDs are the preferred first-line therapy for patients who have survived a cardiac arrest or an episode of hemodynamically unstable VT. At 2-year follow-up, the automated ICD was associated with a 20%–30% relative reduction in the risk of death. Other studies have also proven the benefit of ICDs used for primary prevention of sudden death in patients with CAD, reduced EFs, non-sustained VT, and inducible ventricular arrhythmias during electrophysiologic testing. Ongoing trials may expand the role of ICDs in the primary prevention of sudden death.

Torsades de pointes Torsades de pointes is a variant of VT. Specifically, it is a polymorphic VT characterized by QRS complexes that progressively oscillate in amplitude and morphology, giving the appearance of a twisting axis of depolarization. Torsades de pointes is often associated with a prolonged QT interval and may be caused by use of antiarrhythmic drugs, phenothiazines, tricyclic antidepressants, or nonsedating antihistamines (terfenadine or astemizole); or by hypokalemia, hypocalcemia, or hypomagnesemia. Treatment involves replacement of potassium or magnesium and overdrive pacing, if necessary. Therapy for sustained arrhythmia should be immediate DC cardioversion. Quinidine and similar drugs should not be used because they may increase the abnormal QT interval and worsen the arrhythmia. All potentially offending agents should be discontinued.

Ventricular fibrillation Ventricular fibrillation (VF) is the most ominous of all the cardiac arrhythmias because it is fatal when untreated or when refractory to treatment. It is a major cause of SCD outside the hospital. The ventricular contractions are rapid and uncoordinated, resulting in absence of effective ventricular pumping that soon leads to syncope, convulsions, and death if the VF is not interrupted. Ventricular fibrillation often occurs as a terminal rhythm in a dying patient, during or after MI, in patients with complete heart block, or as a result of electrocution, anesthesia, or drug toxicity from digitalis, quinidine, or other antiarrhythmic agents. Ventricular fibrillation rarely occurs spontaneously in an otherwise healthy person. The prognosis is generally poor because each episode can be fatal. However, some patients with complete heart block have recurrent self-limiting episodes of VF for years.

The ECG reveals irregular and rapid oscillations (250–400 bpm) of highly variable amplitude without identifiable QRS complexes or T waves. Emergency cardiopulmonary resuscitation efforts must be initiated right away. Immediate unsynchronized DC cardioversion is the primary therapy. After successful cardioversion, continuous intravenous infusion of effective antiarrhythmic therapy should be maintained until any reversible causes have been corrected. The choice of chronic antiarrhythmic therapy depends on the nature of the conditions responsible for the initial VF episode. Primary VF occurring within the first 72 hours of an acute MI is not associated with an elevated risk of recurrence and does not require chronic antiarrhythmic therapy. However, VF without an identifiable and reversible cause requires chronic therapy in the form of either prophylactic antiarrhythmic drug therapy (eg, amiodarone, sotalol) or implantation of an automatic defibrillator.

> Klein RC, Raitt MH, Wilkoff BL, et al. Analysis of implantable cardioverter defibrillator therapy in the Antiarrhythmics Versus Implantable Defibrillators (AVID) Trial. *J Cardiovasc Electrophysiol.* 2003;14:940–948.
>
> Moss AJ, Zareba W, Hall WJ, et al. Prophylactic implantation of a defibrillator in patients with myocardial infarction and reduced ejection fraction. *N Engl J Med.* 2002;346:877–883.

Pappone C, Santinelli V, Manguso F, et al. A randomized study of prophylactic catheter ablation in asymptomatic patients with the Wolff-Parkinson-White syndrome. *N Engl J Med.* 2003;349:1803–1811.

Ophthalmologic Considerations

Many of the adult patients seen and treated by ophthalmologists are in the age group at risk for IHD and its many complications. These patients often undergo stressful eye surgery under local or general anesthesia. Ophthalmologists need to be cognizant of the risks of myocardial ischemia, infarction, CHF, and arrhythmias in these patients. Similarly, ophthalmologists need to be aware of the association between proliferative diabetic retinopathy and IHD. This information should be given to the patient's primary medical care provider so that appropriate screening tests can be considered.

The cardiac complications of noncardiac surgery are a major cause of perioperative morbidity and mortality. Myocardial infarction remains the most significant complication. Older age, preexisting CAD, and CHF are the principal risk factors for development of MI and other complications.

Finally, ophthalmologists should be aware of the potential ocular side effects associated with some medications commonly used in the treatment of cardiovascular disease. Following are the medications of clinical relevance.

Amiodarone

Corneal microdeposits due to amiodarone probably occur in nearly all patients who use this drug for a long time. The corneal epithelial whorl-like deposition is indistinguishable from that due to chloroquine. Visual changes are unusual and most often consist of complaints of hazy vision or colored halos around lights. Occasionally, a patient may complain that bright lights, especially headlights at night, cause a significant glare problem. A side effect that has been seen secondary to photosensitivity reactions is discoloration (usually slate-gray or blue) of periocular skin. A final adverse effect is amiodarone optic neuropathy, which is characterized by an insidious onset, slow progression, bilateral visual loss, and protracted disc swelling that tends to stabilize within several months of discontinuing the medication.

Guidelines for follow-up of patients using amiodarone are as follows:

1. Patients should have a baseline ophthalmic examination.
2. Because of the strong photosensitizing effects of amiodarone, UV-blocking lenses should be considered in selected cases of chronic lid disease or macular disease.
3. An ophthalmic examination should be scheduled every 6 to 12 months.
4. Patients should see an ophthalmologist if they experience any visual disturbances.

Beta-Blockers

As with other beta-adrenergic blocking agents, there is the possibility of a sicca-like syndrome with use of beta-blockers. There now seem to be enough cases in the literature and in the Registry to implicate beta-blockers in the development of keratoconjunctivitis sicca, probably on the basis of decreased lacrimation. Not all of the listed possible ocular side effects have been reported with each agent; however, in general, these drugs may decrease tear secretion, possibly enhance migraine ocular scotoma, and may decrease ocular pressure. Visual disturbances and vivid visual hallucinations are the most common ocular adverse effects seen with use of these drugs.

Digoxin

The glare phenomenon and disturbances with color vision are the most striking and the most common adverse ocular reactions seen. Following are other possible ocular side effects:

1. Decreased vision
2. Problems with color vision
    a. Color vision defect—blue-yellow defect
    b. Yellow, green, blue, or red tinge to objects
    c. Colored halos (mainly blue) around lights
    d. Decreased color vision
3. Visual sensations
    a. Flickering vision—often yellow or green
    b. Colored borders around objects
    c. Glare phenomenon—objects appear covered with brown, orange, or white snow
    d. Light flashes
    e. Scintillating scotomas
    f. Frosted appearance of objects

Angiotensin-Converting Enzyme Inhibitors

ACE inhibitors have a much higher incidence than most drugs of causing angioedema including the eye and orbit.

CHAPTER 5

Hypercholesterolemia

Recent Developments

- Therapeutic lifestyle changes (TLC) remain an essential modality in the management of hypercholesterolemia.
- More aggressive management of cholesterol and risk factors has been emphasized by the US National Cholesterol Education Program (NCEP).
- Numerous clinical trials have demonstrated that effective low-density-lipoprotein cholesterol (LDL-C) reduction substantially reduces the risk of coronary heart disease (CHD). For every 30-mg/dL change in LDL-C, the CHD risk is changed by 30%. An LDL-C goal of less than 70 mg/dL should be considered for very high risk patients.
- Statin therapy is recommended for the majority of dyslipoproteinemic adult patients with cardiometabolic risk (CMR).
- Apo-B and non-HDL cholesterol levels should be used to guide adjustments of therapy for patients with CMR already on statin therapy.
- Use of statins in acute coronary syndromes reduces the risk of recurrent coronary events.
- There is no definitive evidence that statin use reduces the risk of age-related macular degeneration (AMD).

Ahsan CH, Shah A, Ezekowitz M. Acute statin treatment in reducing risk after acute coronary syndrome: the MIRACL (Myocardial Ischemia Reduction with Aggressive Cholesterol Lowering) Trial. *Curr Opin Cardiol.* 2001;16:390–393.

Grundy SM, Cleeman JI, Merz N, et al. Implications of recent clinical trials for the National Cholesterol Education Program Adult Treatment Panel III guidelines. *Circulation.* 2004;110:227–239.

Sposito AC, Chapman MJ. Statin therapy in acute coronary syndromes: mechanistic insight into clinical benefit. *Arterioscler Thromb Vasc Biol.* 2002;22:1524–1534.

Introduction

Coronary heart disease is the leading cause of death in the United States, accounting for more deaths than all forms of cancer combined. Several major studies have confirmed earlier reports that lowering of elevated LDL-C levels reduces the risk of CHD. The National

Cholesterol Education Program has provided 3 updates for treatment of elevated blood cholesterol levels in adults (Adult Treatment Panel [ATP] I, II, III). ATP I proposed a strategy for primary prevention of CHD in persons with high levels of LDL cholesterol (>160 mg/dL) or borderline high levels of LDL (130–159 mg/dL) and multiple (at least 2) risk factors (discussed later). ATP II added intensive management of LDL cholesterol in persons with established CHD (target cholesterol <100 mg/dL). Table 5-1 lists the guidelines of ATP III, with the most recent (2004) modifications.

Risk Assessment

Approximately half of the US population has a cholesterol level that puts these persons at significant risk. A fasting lipoprotein profile (total cholesterol, LDL cholesterol, high-density-lipoprotein [HDL] cholesterol, and triglyceride levels) determines an individual's risk status and should be obtained in all adults aged 21 and older at least once every 5 years. Table 5-1 shows the ATP III classification of cholesterol levels and triglycerides. According to American Heart Association (AHA) guidelines, the HDL ratio (ratio of total serum cholesterol to HDL cholesterol) should be less than 5. Other CHD risk factors, such as hypertension, should be assessed and managed appropriately in all adults (Table 5-2).

Table 5-1 Adult Treatment Panel III Classification of Triglycerides and LDL, Total, and HDL Cholesterol, mg/dL

Total cholesterol	
<200	Desirable
200–239	Borderline high
≥240	High
LDL cholesterol	
<100	Optimal
100–129	Near or above optimal
130–159	Borderline high
160–189	High
≥190	Very high
HDL cholesterol	
<40	Low: a major risk factor for heart disease
40–59	Borderline high: the higher the better
≥60	High: protective against heart disease
Triglycerides	
<150	Normal
150–199	Borderline high
200–499	High
≥500	Very high

Modified from Executive Summary of the Third Report of the National Cholesterol Education Program (NCEP) Expert Panel on Detection, Evaluation, and Treatment of High Blood Cholesterol in Adults (Adult Treatment Panel III). *JAMA.* 2001;285:2486–2497.

Table 5-2 Major Risk Factors (Exclusive of LDL Cholesterol) That Modify LDL Goals*

Cigarette smoking
Hypertension (blood pressure ≥140/90 mm Hg or on antihypertensive medication)
Low HDL cholesterol (<40 mg/dL)†
Family history of premature CHD (CHD in male first-degree relative <55 yr; CHD in female first-degree relative <65 yr)
Age (men ≥45 yr; women ≥55 yr)

---

*Diabetes is regarded as a CHD risk equivalent.
†HDL cholesterol ≥60 mg/dL counts as a "negative" risk factor; its presence removes 1 risk factor from the total count.

Modified from Executive Summary of the Third Report of the National Cholesterol Education Program (NCEP) Expert Panel on Detection, Evaluation, and Treatment of High Blood Cholesterol in Adults (Adult Treatment Panel III). *JAMA.* 2001;285:2486–2497.

Management

In its simplest terms, the management of hypercholesterolemia consists of matching the intensity of LDL-lowering therapy with absolute risk; the higher the risk, the lower the target level. This approach is based primarily on data from recent clinical trials and epidemiological studies, which have suggested that a direct relationship exists between the level of LDL-C and the risk of CHD (Fig 5-1). The ATP III guidelines suggest the following steps in the management of hypercholesterolemia/hyperlipidemia/hyperlipoproteinemia:

- **Step 1:** Determine lipoprotein levels. Obtain complete lipoprotein profile after 9-hour to 12-hour fast (see Table 5-1).
- **Step 2:** Identify presence of clinical atherosclerotic disease that confers high risk for CHD events (CHD risk equivalent).
  - clinical CHD
  - symptomatic carotid artery disease
  - peripheral arterial disease
  - abdominal aortic aneurysm
- **Step 3:** Determine presence of major risk factors (other than LDL) (see Table 5-2).
- **Step 4:** If 2+ risk factors (other than LDL) are present without CHD or CHD risk equivalent, assess 10-year (short-term) CHD risk.
  - Four levels of 10-year risk:
    1. High risk: >20%—CHD risk equivalent
    2. Moderately high risk: 10%–20%
    3. Moderate risk: <10%
    4. Lower risk: 0–1 risk factor
- **Step 5:** Determine LDL goals based on risk category (Table 5-3).
- **Step 6:** Initiate therapeutic lifestyle changes (TLC) if LDL is above goal.
  - TLC features

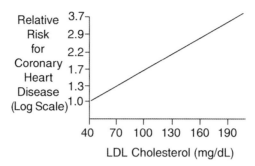

Figure 5-1 Log-linear relationship between LDL-C levels and relative risk for CHD. This relationship is consistent with a large body of epidemiological data and with data available from clinical trials of LDL-lowering therapy. These data suggest that for every 30-mg/dL change in LDL-C, the relative risk for CHD is changed in proportion by about 30%. The relative risk is set at 1.0 for LDL-C = 40 mg/dL. *(Redrawn with permission from Grundy SM, Cleeman JI, Merz N, et al. Implications of recent clinical trials for the National Cholesterol Education Program Adult Treatment Panel III guidelines.* Circulation. *2004;110:231.)*

1. TLC diet (Table 5-4):
   Saturated fat <7% of calories, cholesterol <200 mg/day, carbohydrates 50%–60% of total calories. Consider increased viscous (soluble) fiber (10–25 g/day) and plant stanols/sterols (2 g/day) as therapeutic options to enhance LDL lowering.
2. Weight management
3. Increased physical activity (moderate exercise to expend approximately 200 kcal/day

Step 7: Consider adding drug therapy if LDL exceeds levels shown in Table 5-3.
- Consider drug simultaneously with TLC for high risk and moderately high risk patients.
- Consider adding drug to TLC after 3 months for other risk categories.
- For specific drugs, doses, and side effects, please see Tables 5-5 and 5-6.
- Although statins have few significant side effects, elevated hepatic transaminases, diarrhea, liver failure, polyneuropathy, and myopathy have been noted. The side effects of statin use should be carefully monitored (Table 5-7).

Step 8: Identify metabolic syndrome and treat, if present, after 3 months of TLC (Table 5-8).
- Treatment of the metabolic syndrome (for a person who has any 3 of the risk factors listed in Table 5-8):
   Treat underlying causes (overweight/obesity and physical inactivity):
   - Intensify weight management.
   - Increase physical activity.
   Treat lipid and nonlipid risk factors if they persist despite these lifestyle therapies:
   - Treat hypertension.
   - Use aspirin for CHD patients to reduce prothrombotic state.
   - Treat elevated triglycerides and/or low HDL (Step 9 below).

Step 9: Treat elevated triglycerides.

Table 5-3 ATP III LDL-C Goals and Cutpoints for TLC and Drug Therapy in Different Risk Categories and Proposed Modifications Based on Recent Clinical Trial Evidence

Risk Category	LDL-C Goal	Initiate TLC	Consider Drug Therapy**
High risk: CHD* or CHD risk equivalents† (10-year risk >20%)	<100 mg/dL (optional goal: <70 mg/dL)‖	≥100 mg/dL#	≥100 mg/dL†† (<100 mg/dL: consider drug options)**
Moderately high risk: 2+ risk factors‡ (10-year risk 10% to 20%)§§	<130 mg/dL¶	≥130 mg/dL#	≥130 mg/dL (100–129 mg/dL; consider drug options)‡‡
Moderate risk: 2+ risk factors‡ (10-year risk <10%)§§	<130 mg/dL	≥130 mg/dL	≥160 mg/dL
Lower risk: 0–1 risk factor§	<160 mg/dL	≥160 mg/dL	≥190 mg/dL (160–189 mg/dL: LDL-lowering drug optional)

*CHD includes history of myocardial infarction, unstable angina, stable angina, coronary artery procedures (angioplasty or bypass surgery), or evidence of clinically significant myocardial ischemia.

†CHD risk equivalents include clinical manifestations of noncoronary forms of atherosclerotic disease (peripheral arterial disease, abdominal aortic aneurysm, and carotid artery disease [transient ischemic attacks or stroke of carotid origin or >50% obstruction of a carotid artery]), diabetes, and 2+ risk factors with 10-year risk for hard CHD >20%.

‡Risk factors include cigarette smoking, hypertension (BP ≥140/90 mm Hg or on antihypertensive medication), low HDL cholesterol (<40 mg/dL), family history of premature CHD (CHD in male first-degree relative <55 years of age; CHD in female first-degree relative <65 years of age), and age (men ≥45 years; women ≥55 years).

§§Electronic 10-year risk calculators are available at www.nhlbi.nih.gov/guidelines/cholesterol.

§Almost all people with zero or 1 risk factor have a 10-year risk <10%, and 10-year risk assessment in people with zero or 1 risk factor is thus not necessary.

‖Very high risk favors the optional LDL-C goal of <70 mg/dL, and in patients with high triglycerides, non-HDL-C <100 mg/dL.

¶Optional LDL-C goal <100 mg/dL.

#Any person at high risk or moderately high risk who has lifestyle-related risk factors (eg, obesity, physical inactivity, elevated triglyceride, low HDL-C, or metabolic syndrome) is a candidate for therapeutic lifestyle changes to modify these risk factors regardless of LDL-C level.

**When LDL-lowering drug therapy is employed, it is advised that intensity of therapy be sufficient to achieve at least a 30% to 40% reduction in LDL-C levels.

††If baseline LDL-C is <100 mg/dL, institution of an LDL-lowering drug is a therapeutic option on the basis of available clinical trial results. If a high-risk person has high triglycerides or low HDL-C, combining a fibrate or nicotinic acid with an LDL-lowering drug can be considered.

‡‡For moderately high-risk persons, when LDL-C level is 100 to 129 mg/dL, at baseline or on lifestyle therapy, initiation of an LDL-lowering drug to achieve an LDL-C level <100 mg/dL is a therapeutic option on the basis of available clinical trial results.

Reprinted from Grundy SM, Cleeman JI, Merz N, et al. Implications of recent clinical trials for the National Cholesterol Education Program Adult Treatment Panel III guidelines. *Circulation.* 2004;110:236.

- Determine level of elevated triglycerides (see Table 5-1).
- Treatment of elevated triglycerides (≥150 mg/dL):
  - Primary aim of therapy is to reach LDL goal.
  - Weight management should be intensified.
  - Physical activity should be increased.
  - If triglycerides are ≥200 mg/dL after LDL goal is reached, set secondary goal for non-HDL cholesterol (total − HDL) 30 mg/dL higher than LDL goal.

Table 5-4 Nutrient Composition of the Therapeutic Lifestyle Changes Diet

Nutrient	Recommended Intake
Saturated fat*	<7% of total calories
Polyunsaturated fat	Up to 10% of total calories
Monounsaturated fat	Up to 20% of total calories
Total fat	25%–35% of total calories
Carbohydrate†	50%–60% of total calories
Fiber	20–30 g/d (soluble fiber 10–25 g/d)
Plant stanols/sterols@	2 g/d
Protein	Approximately 15% of total calories
Cholesterol	<200 mg/dL
Total calories‡	Balance energy intake and expenditure to maintain desirable body weight/prevent weight gain

*Trans fatty acids are another LDL-raising fat that should be kept at a low intake.

†Carbohydrates should be derived predominantly from foods rich in complex carbohydrates including grains (especially whole grains), fruits, and vegetables.

@Sitostanol/sterol esters inhibit intestinal absorption of dietary and biliary cholesterol and are available in grocery stores as regular and low-fat margarines.

‡Daily energy expenditure should include at least moderate physical activity (contributing approximately 200 kcal/d).

Modified from Executive Summary of the Third Report of the National Cholesterol Education Program (NCEP) Expert Panel on Detection, Evaluation, and Treatment of High Blood Cholesterol in Adults (Adult Treatment Panel III). *JAMA.* 2001;285:2486–2497.

Special Issues

Use of Statins in Acute Myocardial Syndromes

The Myocardial Ischemia Reduction with Aggressive Cholesterol Lowering (MIRACL) study found that lowering lipids with atorvastatin, 80 mg/day, reduced the number of recurrent ischemic events in patients with acute coronary syndrome in the first 16 weeks. Results from the more recent PROVE IT study suggest that more intensive LDL-cholesterol-lowering therapy reduces the risk of major cardiovascular events in patients with the acute coronary syndrome, compared with less intensive treatment over the first 2 years. Adverse drug effects were rare in both studies.

The Metabolic Syndrome

The so-called metabolic syndrome comprises a constellation of lipid and nonlipid risk factors of metabolic origin. Diagnosis is based on the presence of 3 or more risk determinants (see Table 5-8).

The metabolic syndrome is closely linked to insulin resistance. Excess body fat (particularly abdominal fat) and physical inactivity promote impaired responses to insulin, which may also occur as a genetic predisposition. The risk factors for metabolic syndrome are highly concordant; in aggregate, they increase the risk of CHD at any given LDL level. Management is as outlined previously, with emphasis on increased physical activity and weight reduction.

Table 5-5 Drugs Affecting Lipoprotein Metabolism*

Drug Class	Agents and Daily Doses	Lipid/Lipoprotein Effects	Side Effects	Contraindications	Clinical Trial Results
HMG-CoA reductase inhibitors	Lovastatin (20–80 mg) Pravastatin (20–40 mg) Simvastatin (20–80 mg) Fluvastatin (20–80 mg) Atorvastatin (10–80 mg) Rosuvastatin (5–40 mg)	LDL ↓ 18%–55% HDL ↑ 5%–15% TG ↓ 7%–30%	Myopathy; increased liver enzymes	*Absolute:* active or chronic liver disease *Relative:* concomitant use of certain drugs†	Reduced major coronary events, CHD deaths, need for coronary procedures, stroke, and total mortality
Bile acid sequestrants	Cholestyramine (4–16 g) Colestipol (5–20 g) Colesevelam (2.6–3.8 g)	LDL ↓ 15%–30% HDL ↑ 3%–5% TG no change or increase	Gastrointestinal distress; constipation; decreased absorption of other drugs	*Absolute:* dysbetalipoproteinemia; TG >400 mg/dL *Relative:* TG >200 mg/dL	Reduced major coronary events, CHD deaths
Nicotinic acid	Immediate release (crystalline) nicotinic acid (1.5–3 g); extended release nicotinic acid (Niaspan) (1–2 g); sustained release nicotinic acid (1–2 g)	LDL ↓ 5%–25% HDL ↑ 15%–35% TG ↓ 20%–50%	Flushing; hyperglycemia; hyperuricemia (or gout); upper gastrointestinal distress; hepatotoxicity	*Absolute:* chronic liver disease; severe gout *Relative:* diabetes; hyperuricemia; peptic ulcer disease	Reduced major coronary events and possible total mortality
Fibric acids	Gemfibrozil (600 mg BID) Fenofibrate (200 mg) Clofibrate (1000 mg BID)	LDL ↓ 5%–20% (may be increased in patients with high TG) HDL ↑ 10%–20% TG ↓ 20%–50%	Dyspepsia; gallstones; myopathy; unexplained non-CHD deaths in WHO study	*Absolute:* severe renal disease; severe hepatic disease	Reduced major coronary events

*HMG-CoA indicates 3-hydroxy-3-methylglutaryl coenzyme A; LDL, low-density lipoprotein; HDL, high-density lipoprotein; TG, triglycerides; ↓, decrease; ↑, increase; CHD, coronary heart disease.

†Cyclosporine, macrolide antibiotics, various antifungal agents, and cytochrome P-450 inhibitors (fibrates and niacin should be used with appropriate caution).

Modified from Executive Summary of the Third Report of the National Cholesterol Education Program (NCEP) Expert Panel on Detection, Evaluation, and Treatment of High Blood Cholesterol in Adults (Adult Treatment Panel III). *JAMA.* 2001;285:2486–2497.

Table 5-6 **Doses of Currently Available Statins Required to Attain an Approximate 30% to 40% Reduction of LDL-C Levels (Standard Doses)***

Drug	Dose, mg/d	LDL Reduction, %
Atorvastatin	10†	39
Lovastatin	40†	31
Pravastatin	40†	34
Simvastatin	20–40†	35–41
Fluvastatin	40–80	25–35
Rosuvastatin	5–10‡	39–45

*Estimated LDL reductions were obtained from US Food and Drug Administration package inserts for each drug.

†All of these are available at doses up to 80 mg. For every doubling of the dose above standard dose, an approximate 6% decrease in LDL-C level can be obtained.

‡For rosuvastatin, doses available up to 40 mg; the efficacy for 5 mg is estimated by subtracting 6% from the Food and Drug Administration-reported efficacy at 10 mg.

Reprinted from Grundy SM, Cleeman JI, Merz N, et al. Implications of recent clinical trials for the National Cholesterol Education Program Adult Treatment Panel III guidelines. *Circulation.* 2004;110:233.

Comments on Specific Dyslipidemias

- *Very high LDL-C level (>190 mg/dL).* This condition typically occurs in people with a genetic form of hypercholesterolemia (monogenic or polygenic hypercholesterolemia, familial defective apolipoprotein B). Screening of other family members is important for identification and treatment.
- *Low HDL-C level.* A low HDL level (<40 mg/dL) is a strong independent predictor of CHD.
- *Diabetic dyslipidemia.* Aggressive lowering of the LDL level is recommended.

Ophthalmologic Considerations

Hypercholesterolemia is a significant risk factor for ischemic heart disease, cerebrovascular disease, and peripheral vascular disease. The ophthalmologist may be the first physician to detect or recognize manifestations of atherosclerosis, particularly amaurosis fugax, retinal vascular emboli or occlusions, ischemic optic neuropathy, or cortical visual field deficits from a previous cerebral infarction. Detection of atherosclerosis may initiate a diagnostic evaluation that reveals significant carotid artery stenosis or coronary artery disease.

Patients with ocular hypertension or glaucoma being treated with topical beta-blockers have small but significant changes in the serum levels of HDL and LDL when using these drugs. In a 12-week randomized clinical trial of 112 women aged 60 years and older, topical timolol 0.5% increased LDL-C by 3% and decreased HDL by 6%. In the same trial, topical carteolol 1% had no impact on LDL levels but increased HDL levels by 2%.

The relationship of statin use to AMD is unresolved. Two population-based studies (1 from Melbourne, Australia, and 1 from Sheffield, England) suggest that use of statins is associated with a decreased risk of AMD. However, there are 2 population-based stud-

Table 5-7 Monitoring Parameters and Follow-up Schedule for Patients Using Statins

Monitoring Parameters	Follow-up Schedule
Headache, dyspepsia	Evaluate symptoms initially, 6 to 8 weeks after starting therapy, then at each follow-up visit
Muscle soreness, tenderness, or pain	Evaluate muscle symptoms and CK before starting therapy. Evaluate muscle symptoms 6 to 12 weeks after starting therapy and at each follow-up visit. Obtain a CK measurement when persons have muscle soreness, tenderness, or pain.
ALT, AST	Evaluate ALT/AST initially, approximately 12 weeks after starting therapy, then annually or more frequently if indicated.

ALT = alanine transferase; AST = aspartate transferase; CK = creatine kinase.

Modified from Pasternak RC, Smith SC Jr, Bairey-Merz N, et al. ACC/AHA/NHLBI Clinical Advisory on the Use and Safety of Statins. *Circulation.* 2002;106:1024–1028.

ies (1 from Beaver Dam, Wisconsin, and 1 from Rotterdam, Netherlands) that suggest no similar association. More recently, a retrospective case-series has suggested that therapy with statins is associated with decreased rates of exudative AMD. All of these studies are limited by either small sample size or lack of prospective data on use of statins. Therefore, more data are required to assess the nature of this relationship.

Corneal arcus, a nonreversible lipid deposit at the corneal limbus, is associated with age and hyperlipidemia. In the Blue Mountains Eye Study, a recent population-based study from Australia, the presence of arcus in persons aged 49 years and older was associated with higher total cholesterol and high triglyceride levels.

Finally, clinical experience has revealed that use of lovastatin and other HMG-CoA reductase inhibitors does not significantly increase the risk of cataracts.

> American College of Physicians Clinical Guideline, Part I—Guidelines for using serum cholesterol, high-density lipoprotein cholesterol, and triglyceride levels as screening tests for preventing coronary heart disease in adults. *Ann Intern Med.* 1996;124:515–517.
>
> Binder EF, Williams DB, Schectman KB, et al. Effects of hormone replacement therapy on serum lipids in elderly women: a randomized, placebo-controlled trial. *Ann Intern Med.* 2001;134:754–760.
>
> Eaton CB, Lapane KL, Garber CE, et al. Physical activity, physical fitness, and coronary heart disease risk factors. *Med Sci Sports Exerc.* 1995;27:340–346.
>
> Expert Panel on Detection, Evaluation, and Treatment of High Blood Cholesterol in Adults. Executive Summary of the Third Report of the National Cholesterol Education Program (NCEP) Expert Panel on Detection, Evaluation, and Treatment of High Blood Cholesterol in Adults (Adult Treatment Panel III). *JAMA.* 2001;285:2486–2497. (Full text available online at www.nhlbi.nih.gov.)
>
> Fortmann S, Maron D. Diagnosis and treatment of lipid disorders. In: Dale DC, Federman DD, eds. *Scientific American Medicine.* Vol. 2. New York: Scientific American; 1998:1–20.
>
> Frick MH, Elo O, Haapa K, et al. Helsinki Heart Study: primary prevention trial with gemfibrozil in middle-aged men with dyslipidemia. Safety of treatment, changes in risk factors, and incidence of coronary heart disease. *N Engl J Med.* 1987;317:1237–1245.

Table 5-8 Clinical Identification of the Metabolic Syndrome

Risk Factor	Defining Level
Abdominal obesity* (waist circumference)†	
Men	>102 cm (>40 in)
Women	>88 cm (>35 in)
Triglycerides	≥150 mg/dL
HDL cholesterol	
Men	<40 mg/dL
Women	<50 mg/dL
Blood pressure	≥130/≥85 mm Hg
Fasting glucose	≥110 mg/dL

*Overweight and obesity are associated with insulin resistance and the metabolic syndrome. However, the presence of abdominal obesity is more highly correlated with the metabolic risk factors than is an elevated body mass index (BMI). Therefore, the simple measure of waist circumference is recommended to identify the body weight component of the metabolic syndrome.

†Some male patients can develop multiple metabolic risk factors when the waist circumference is only marginally increased (eg, 94–102 cm [37–40 in]). Such patients may have strong genetic contribution to insulin resistance, and they should benefit from changes in life habits, similar to men with categorical increases in waist circumference.

Geurian KL. The cholesterol controversy. *Ann Pharmacother*. 1996;30:495–500.

Hamilton VH, Racicot FE, Zowall H, et al. The cost-effectiveness of HMG-CoA reductase inhibitors to prevent coronary heart disease. Estimating the benefits of increasing HDL-C. *JAMA*. 1995;273:1032–1038.

Hein HO, Suadicani P, Gyntelberg F. Alcohol consumption, serum low density lipoprotein cholesterol concentration, and risk of ischemic heart disease: six year follow up in the Copenhagen male study. *BMJ*. 1996;312:736–741.

Kreisberg RA, Oberman A. Medical management of hyperlipidemia/dyslipidemia. *J Clin Endocrinol Metab*. 2003;88:2445–2461.

Ozsener S, Sendag F, Koc T, et al. A comparison of continuous combined hormone replacement therapy, HMG-CoA reductase inhibitor and combined treatment for the management of hypercholesterolemia in postmenopausal women. *J Obstet Gynaecol Res*. 2001;27:353–358.

Robins SJ, Collins D, Wittes JT, et al. Relation of gemfibrozil treatment and lipid levels with major coronary events: VA-HIT: a randomized controlled trial. *JAMA*. 2001;285:1585–1591.

Schwartz GG, Olsson AG, Ezekowitz MD, et al. Effects of atorvastatin on early recurrent ischemic events in acute coronary syndromes—the MIRACL study: a randomized controlled trial. *JAMA*. 2001;285:1711–1718.

CHAPTER 6

Pulmonary Diseases

Recent Developments

- The *Global Initiative for Chronic Obstructive Lung Disease (GOLD)*, a collaborative effort of the World Health Organization and the National Heart, Lung, and Blood Institute, offers a framework for the management of chronic obstructive pulmonary disease (COPD). This international consortium on the diagnosis, classification, and management of pulmonary disease publishes a guide that is updated regularly and can be downloaded from the Internet at www.goldcopd.com.

Introduction

The lungs can be affected by numerous pathological processes, including inflammation (allergic, infectious, autoimmune, occupational exposure, toxic), vascular insults, fibrosis, carcinoma, and changes secondary to cardiac or musculoskeletal problems. The functional consequences of the pathological changes can be divided into *obstructive* and *restrictive* limitations of ventilatory functions.

Symptoms of lung disease include dyspnea, cough, and wheezing. *Dyspnea* develops when the demand for gas exchange exceeds the capacity of the respiratory response, as in hypoxemia or hypercapnia. Dyspnea may also reflect the increased work of breathing, as occurs with airway obstruction or reduced compliance of the lung or rib cage. *Cough* develops when mucus, inflammatory debris, or irritants affect the bronchi, causing reflex clearing expectoration, or when the lung parenchyma is infiltrated with fluid, cells, or fibrosis. *Wheezing* occurs when bronchospasm narrows the large airways and exhaled air is forced through the narrowed passages.

Obstructive Lung Diseases

In obstructive lung disease, changes in the bronchi, bronchioles, and lung parenchyma can cause airway obstruction. Obstructive diseases can be separated into reversible and irreversible conditions, although many obstructive lung diseases may have some degree of both reversible and irreversible obstruction.

Reversible obstructive diseases are grouped under the term *asthma*. In asthma, the airways are hyperresponsive and develop an inflammatory response to various stimuli, although the specific cause and duration of the bronchospasm vary. In some persons, allergic IgE-mediated reactions to defined antigens cause bronchospasm. In many patients, however, the cause of abnormal airway reactivity is unknown. Precipitating factors may include exercise, aspirin, sulfites, tartrazine dye, emotional stress, cold air, environmental pollutants, or viral infection. Bronchial smooth muscle constriction, mucosal edema, excess mucus accumulation, and epithelial cell shedding all contribute to airway obstruction. This obstruction may be reversible spontaneously or with treatment.

Irreversible obstructive disease (sometimes referred to as *chronic obstructive pulmonary disease*) comprises a group of conditions in which forced expiratory flow is reduced in either a constant or a slowly progressive manner over months or years. COPD is the fourth leading cause of death in the United States. Some conditions, such as *cystic fibrosis* or *bronchiectasis,* have an identifiable cause. However, most irreversible obstructive diseases, such as *emphysema, chronic bronchitis,* or *peripheral airway disease,* cannot be ascribed to specific conditions; rather, they represent an individual response to cigarette smoking and other airborne pollutants. For example, such responses occur in the setting of either α_1-antitrypsin deficiency (in certain forms of emphysema) or airway hyperactivity and mucus hypersecretion (as in bronchitis). The pathological consequences of the abnormal response result in specific damage to lung tissue. Emphysema is characterized by pathological enlargement of the terminal bronchiole air spaces and by destruction of the alveolar connective tissue septa. Bronchitis is characterized by hypertrophied mucous glands in the bronchi; in peripheral airway disease, only the small airways demonstrate fibrosis, inflammation, and tortuosity.

Two clinical types of patients are seen in the advanced stages of chronic airway obstruction. *Pink puffers* tend to be thin, have hyperinflated lung fields, exhibit dyspnea without significant hypoxemia, and are free of the signs of right-sided heart failure. *Blue bloaters* demonstrate cyanosis, marked hypoxemia, and peripheral edema with right-sided heart failure *(cor pulmonale).*

Restrictive Lung Diseases

The restrictive lung diseases encompass a diverse group of conditions that cause diffuse parenchymal damage. The physiologic consequences of this damage include a reduction in total lung volume, diffusing capacity, and vital capacity. Occasionally, patients without parenchymal involvement who have diseases of the chest wall, respiratory muscles, pleura, or spine may have similarly restricted lung volumes. A *fibrotic* parenchymal response can result from occupational exposure to various substances, including asbestos, silica dust, graphite, talc, coal, and tungsten. A *granulomatous* hypersensitivity reaction can develop in response to moldy hay, grains, birds, humidifiers, and cooling systems. Endogenous pulmonary disease can result from a number of conditions, such as collagen vascular diseases, sarcoidosis, eosinophilic granuloma, Wegener granulomatosis, Goodpasture syndrome, alveolar proteinosis, idiopathic pulmonary hemosiderosis, and idiopathic pulmonary fibrosis. Therapeutic agents such as dilantin, penicillin, gold, methotrexate, or radiation can also cause pulmonary disease.

Evaluation

Although all patients with respiratory problems should be under the care of a capable internist or pulmonologist, ophthalmologists and other physicians should also be aware of the methods used in the diagnosis and evaluation of breathing disorders. The following should be considered:

- *Symptoms:* Symptoms include dyspnea, orthopnea, chronic cough, and chronic sputum production.
- *History:* History may reveal occupational exposure, family history, cigarette use.
- *Signs:* Signs include audible wheezing, cyanosis, finger clubbing, forced expiratory time greater than 4 seconds, and increased anteroposterior diameter of the chest.
- *Laboratory studies:* Results may reveal elevated hematocrit and hypoxia or hypercapnia on arterial blood gas measurement.
- *Chest radiography:* Radiographic findings include parenchymal disease, hyperinflation, diaphragmatic flattening, increased retrosternal lucency, and pleural abnormalities.
- *Computerized tomography* of the chest can detect many abnormalities not seen on chest radiographs such as small areas of adenopathy, pulmonary embolus, small nodules, infiltrative lung disease and bronchiectasis.
- *Pulmonary function tests* measure the mechanical and gas exchange functions of the lungs. The forced expiratory volume in 1 second (FEV_1) represents the volume exhaled in the first second of exhalation; the forced vital capacity (FVC) represents the total volume that the patient can exhale. Both parameters and their serial rate of decline in a patient are objective measures of lung function as well as prognostic indicators of comorbidity and mortality from lung cancer and cardiovascular disease. An FEV_1/FVC ratio less than 70% of predicted suggests obstructive disease; total lung capacity less than 70% of predicted suggests restrictive disease.
- *Bronchoscopy, transbronchial biopsy,* and *bronchial lavage* are used to obtain culture material, cytologic material, and pathological specimens for analysis.

National Heart, Lung and Blood Institute, World Health Organization, The Global Initiative for Chronic Obstructive Lung Disease. A guide for healthcare professionals. Available at www.goldcopd.com. Accessed August 15, 2005.

Treatment

Treatment of pulmonary disease has 2 major goals: first, to favorably alter the natural history of the disease; and second, to improve the patient's symptoms and functional status and minimize associated problems.

Nonpharmacologic Approaches

Smoking cessation is the single most effective and cost-effective intervention to reduce the risk of COPD and to slow COPD progression. Ophthalmologists should not underestimate the impact of even a brief discussion with their patients about the harmful effects of smoking and the benefits of smoking cessation. Similarly, *avoidance of precipitants* of airway obstruction is important in ameliorating asthmatic conditions. In patients with severe pulmonary hypertension and cor pulmonale, use of supplemental oxygen to maintain an arterial oxygen pressure above 60 mm Hg confers a modest reduction in pulmonary hypertension and an improvement in survival rates. However, a patient receiving supplemental oxygen must be carefully monitored because such treatment may decrease the respiratory drive to eliminate carbon dioxide, aggravating the respiratory acidosis that may lead to carbon dioxide narcosis. *Breathing exercises* and *postoperative chest physiotherapy* have demonstrable short-term effects in improving respiratory function.

Noninvasive pressure support ventilation can be used to deliver increased airway pressure. Continuous positive airway pressure (CPAP) provides continuous steady positive airway pressure throughout the ventilation cycle to improve alveolar oxygen exchange. In CPAP a tight, well-fitting mask is placed over the patient's mouth and nose or just over the nose. Noninvasive pressure support ventilation is best applied to patients with respiratory failure who are expected to quickly respond to medical therapy. First described more than 50 years ago, mask CPAP treatment of cardiogenic pulmonary edema has been shown to be a useful adjunct and reduces the need for intubation. Noninvasive pressure support ventilation for acute respiratory failure requires an alert patient capable of protecting the airway and handling secretions. Intubation and standard ventilation are preferred for patients who require total ventilatory support, because the mask may slip and effective ventilation may cease. Nasal CPAP can be used in the management of obstructive sleep apnea. Ophthalmologists should be aware that nasal CPAP has been reported to modestly increase intraocular pressure in patients with glaucoma.

Mojon DS, Hess CW, Goldblum D, et al. Normal-tension glaucoma is associated with sleep apnea syndrome. *Ophthalmologica*. 2002;216(3):180–184.

Pharmacologic Therapy

Pharmacologic approaches include medications that are specific for the particular pulmonary condition and medications that improve the patient's symptoms and functional status. *Specific medications* directly alter the pathophysiologic mechanisms underlying the patient's pulmonary disease. Some examples include cyclophosphamide for treatment of Wegener granulomatosis, steroids for sarcoidosis, and plasmapheresis with immunosuppressive drugs for Goodpasture syndrome.

Symptomatic medications are designed to reduce the obstructive or restrictive components affecting the patient's lung function. Medications used to treat symptomatic bronchospastic airway obstruction include bronchodilators, inhibitors of inflammation, and antibiotics during infection-precipitated airway closure (Table 6-1).

Bronchodilators, which include theophylline, β-adrenergic agonists, and anticholinergics, act primarily by relaxing the tracheobronchial smooth muscle. Although the bronchodilation produced by *theophylline* varies directly with the serum level, theophylline is a weak phosphodiesterase inhibitor whose mechanism of action is unclear. Theophylline has a narrow therapeutic index; thus, serum levels should be measured (reference range 10–20 mg/L) so that toxic effects such as nausea, tachycardia, headache, seizures, and

Table 6-1 **Drugs for the Treatment of Asthma**

Short-acting β_2-selective adrenergic agents
  Albuterol (Proventil, Ventolin)
  Bitolterol mesylate (Tornalate)
  Pirbuterol acetate (Maxair)
  Terbutaline sulfate (Brethaire, Brethine, Bricanyl)
Long-acting β_2-selective adrenergic agents
  Formoterol fumarate (Foradil)
  Salmeterol xinafoate (Serevent)
Anticholinergics
  Ipratropium bromide (Atrovent)
  Oxitropium bromide (Oxivent)
Xanthine derivatives and combinations
  Theophylline (Aerolate, Marax, Quibron, Respbid, Slo-Phyllin, Theo-Dur, Uniphyl)
Combination short-acting β_2-agonist plus anticholinergic
  Fenoterol/ipratropium (Respimat)
  Albuterol/ipratropium (Combivent)
Leukotriene modifiers
  Zafirlukast (Accolate)
  Zileuton (Zyflo)
  Montelukast (Singulair)
Mast cell stabilizers
  Cromolyn sodium (Intal)
  Nedocromil sodium (Tilade)
Corticosteroids
  Beclomethasone dipropionate (Beclovent, Vanceril)
  Budesonide (Pulmicort)
  Flunisolide (AeroBid)
  Triamcinolone acetonide (Azmacort)
  Fluticasone (Flovent)

ventricular arrhythmias can be avoided while efficacy is maintained. For these reasons, theophylline is not frequently used.

β-Adrenergic agonists activate bronchial smooth muscle, resulting in bronchodilation. The selective β_2-adrenergics, which have greater bronchodilatory and less cardiostimulatory effects, are commonly used, often in metered-dose inhalers (they can also be administered orally or parenterally). These drugs have replaced the nonselective β-adrenergic agents such as isoproterenol. The *short-acting β_2-agonists*, which include fenoterol, albuterol, and terbutaline, differ in onset and duration of action. For example, albuterol's onset of action is within 1–3 minutes, and the drug's duration is 60–90 minutes. Common long-acting β_2-agonists include formoterol and salmeterol. Salmeterol, a particularly long-acting β_2-adrenergic, is helpful in maintenance treatment of asthma; it should not be used for acute exacerbations. Although epinephrine causes predominantly β-adrenergic stimulation in the lungs, it also causes peripheral α-adrenergic stimulation, resulting in vasoconstrictive hypertension and tachycardia. Epinephrine is most often administered subcutaneously to help control an acute asthma attack.

Anticholinergic agents directly relax smooth muscle by competing for acetylcholine at muscarinic nerve-ending receptors. Atropine and similar agents have been replaced by poorly absorbing atropinic congeners such as *ipratropium bromide, oxitropium bromide,* and *tiotropium bromide*. These newer inhalation agents have few systemic and minimal cardiac effects. They have an additive bronchodilator effect when combined with submaximal doses of β-adrenergic agonists.

Inhibitors of inflammation include corticosteroids, leukotriene inhibitors, and mast cell stabilizers such as cromolyn sodium. *Corticosteroids* not only suppress inflammation of the bronchioles but also potentiate the bronchodilator response to β-adrenergic receptors. *Inhaled steroids* can be used as long-term therapy for reducing bronchial hyperreactivity; they are not used to manage acute attacks. *Systemic steroids*, however, are highly effective in managing acute episodes. They should be reserved for serious flare-ups. Leukotriene inhibitors suppress the effects of inflammatory mediators. They are especially useful for prophylaxis and as long-term maintenance therapy for asthma. *Cromolyn sodium* prevents the release of chemical mediators from mast cells in the presence of IgE antibody and the specific antigen. *Immunotherapy* has been shown to be helpful for treatment of asthma triggered by a defined antigen.

Asthma treatment should be tailored to disease severity. Medication doses should be adequate to rapidly control symptoms and later reduced to the minimal level required to maintain control. The goals of therapy should include prevention of symptoms, reduction in frequency and severity of exacerbations, maintenance of normal (or near-normal) pulmonary function, maintenance of normal activity levels, and minimization of medication side effects. Maintenance medications include inhaled corticosteroids, chromones, leukotriene modifiers, long-acting $β_2$-agonists, anticholinergic agents, and oral corticosteroids. Appropriately used supplemental oxygen increases survival among patients with chronic respiratory failure and has a beneficial effect on pulmonary arterial pressure, polycythemia, exercise capacity, lung mechanics, and mental state.

Preoperative and Postoperative Considerations

Before undertaking surgery in a patient with lung disease, the surgeon should consult with an internist or pulmonologist to carefully define the patient's functional respiratory status, especially with respect to the supine position. The patient's respiratory function should be maximized through use of medications and by nonpharmacologic means as appropriate. The patient should be sedated only if necessary and, in that case, should be carefully monitored for arterial gas values.

Campos MA, Wanner A. The rationale for pharmacologic therapy in stable chronic obstructive pulmonary disease. *Am J Med Sci.* 2005;329(4):181–189.

Corren J. Asthma in adolescents and adults. In: Rakel RE, ed. *Conn's Current Therapy 2000.* 52nd ed. Philadelphia: Saunders; 2000:730–740.

Fabbri L, Peters SP, Pavord I, et al. Allergic rhinitis, asthma, airway biology, and chronic obstructive pulmonary disease in AJRCCM in 2004. *Am J Resp Crit Care Med.* 2005;171(7): 686–698.

Martinez FJ, Standiford C, Gay SE. Is it asthma or COPD? The answer determines proper therapy for chronic airflow obstruction. *Postgrad Med.* 2005;117(3):19–26.

CHAPTER 7

Hematologic Disorders

Recent Developments

- Iron deficiency anemia remains the most common cause of anemia worldwide. It can be distinguished from anemia of chronic disease by using serum transferrin receptor assays.
- Until recently, iron dextran was the only parenteral iron available. Now, sodium ferric gluconate, which causes fewer anaphylactic reactions, is also available.
- Allogenic bone marrow transplantation has become the treatment of choice for β-thalassemia major and has increased survival rates for this disease.
- The best screening test for paroxysmal nocturnal hemoglobinuria is now flow cytometry, which has largely replaced the classic sucrose hemolysis test.
- Parental diagnosis is now available for couples at risk for producing a child with sickle cell anemia. Genetic counseling should be made available for such couples.
- Additional thrombotic risk factors (eg, factor V and prothrombin gene mutations, hyperhomocysteinemia) have been identified.
- Thrombophilia (the hypercoagulable state) is associated with recurrent fetal loss and preeclampsia.

Ophthalmologic Considerations

Ophthalmologists treat and operate on many patients with coagulation or blood abnormalities. Oftentimes, it is difficult to balance the benefits and risks of maintaining anticoagulation therapy prior to surgery. Many systemic coagulopathies or blood dyscrasias can exhibit ocular findings.

Blood Composition

Formed elements—erythrocytes (red blood cells, or RBCs), white blood cells, and platelets—comprise approximately 45% of the total blood volume. The fluid portion, *plasma,* is about 90% water. The remaining 10% of the plasma consists of proteins (albumin, globulin, fibrinogen, and enzymes), lipids, carbohydrates, hormones, vitamins, and salts. If a blood specimen is allowed to clot, the fibrinogen is consumed and the resultant fluid portion is called *serum.*

Erythropoiesis

All blood cells are thought to originate from an uncommitted pluripotential stem cell, designated the *colony-forming unit–spleen*. This in turn gives rise to (1) the *lymphoid stem cell* and (2) the *myeloid*, or *hematopoietic*, *stem cell* (or *colony-forming unit–culture*). The hematopoietic stem cell is thought to be the common precursor of RBCs, granulocytes, monocytes, and platelets. Stem cells are not morphologically recognizable, but their existence has been shown by various culture techniques.

Red blood cells are formed in the bone marrow in a series of steps. The colony-forming unit–culture gives rise to a *burst-forming unit–erythroid*, which, in response to erythropoietin (discussed next), becomes a *colony-forming unit–erythroid*. This entity differentiates through morphologically identifiable stages, during which the nucleus condenses and the cell gradually shrinks: pronormoblast, basophilic normoblast, polychromatophilic normoblast, and orthochromic normoblast. This phase takes approximately 3 days. The nucleus is then extruded, forming the reticulocyte, which is slightly larger than the normal mature RBC. The reticulocyte remains in the bone marrow 2–3 more days and is then released into the peripheral blood. The mature erythrocyte is round, biconcave, and approximately 7 μm in diameter. Circulating RBCs have a life span of about 120 days.

Erythropoiesis is initiated by *erythropoietin*, a hormone found in the plasma and produced mainly in the kidney. (Some researchers think that erythropoietin is also produced by the liver.) Any reduction in oxygen tension in the kidney (eg, from hypoxemia, low hemoglobin level, arterial insufficiency) stimulates production of erythropoietin, which causes stem cells to differentiate into pronormoblasts, leading to increased production of RBCs. In addition, immature reticulocytes are prematurely released into the peripheral blood. A number of tumors are associated with inappropriate production of erythropoietin, leading to erythrocytosis. These include benign and malignant kidney tumors, cerebellar hemangioblastoma, pheochromocytoma, and adrenal adenoma.

The production of RBCs and hemoglobin requires many substances. Iron is needed for proliferation and maturation of erythrocytes. Folic acid and vitamin B_{12} are necessary for DNA replication and cell division. Also required are manganese; cobalt; copper; vitamins C, E, B_{12}, thiamine, riboflavin, and pantothenic acid; and the hormones erythropoietin, thyroxine, and androgen.

Anemia

Anemia is diagnosed in adults if the hematocrit is less than 13.5 g/dL in males and less than 12 g/dL in females. Congenital anemia is suggested by the patient's personal and family history. Poor diet results in folic acid deficiency and contributes to iron deficiency. Bleeding is commonly the etiology of iron deficiency in adults. If anemia is suspected, a physical examination should concentrate on primary hematologic disease, such as lymphadenopathy or hepatosplenomegaly, and on bone tenderness. Megaloblastic anemia is suggested by mucosal changes such as a smooth tongue.

The usual classification of anemias is based on their pathophysiologic mechanism. Typically, there is either diminished production or accelerated loss of RBCs. The anemias can also be classified according to red blood cell size. If the cell size is very small, *microcytic anemia* is the diagnosis. Possible causes are iron deficiency, thalassemia, and anemia of chronic disease. If the cell size is enlarged, *megaloblastic anemia* is the diagnosis, and possible etiologies are vitamin B_{12} or folate deficiency. Exceptions are the myelodysplastic syndromes.

Iron Deficiency Anemia

By far the most common type of anemia worldwide, *iron deficiency anemia* is diagnosed when serum ferritin is less than 30 µg/L. Every adult with iron deficiency anemia is suspected to be bleeding until proven otherwise. Menstrual blood loss in women plays a major role, as does gastrointestinal bleeding in both men and women. For many patients today, treatment of various conditions includes aspirin, which can cause gastrointestinal bleeding.

The signs and symptoms of iron deficiency anemia are the same as those of the other anemias (pallor, cool skin, exercise intolerance or fatigue at rest, and so forth), but severe iron deficiency can cause mucosal changes, such as a smooth tongue, brittle nails, or cheilosis. Esophageal webs may also occur, as well as pica (which is, most commonly, a craving for ice chips). The most important part of understanding iron deficiency anemia is ensuring that an occult source of blood loss has not been missed. In the absence of this occult source, the preferred therapy is ferrous sulfate (325 mg 3 times daily). Because of the risk of anaphylactic reactions, parenteral iron is reserved for the treatment of persistent anemia, after a reasonable course of oral therapy. Until recently, iron dextran was the only parenteral iron available. Now, sodium ferric gluconate, which causes fewer anaphylactic reactions, is also available.

Anemia of Chronic Disease

A specific type of anemia can occur in chronic conditions such as chronic inflammation, infections, cancer, and liver disease. Chronic renal failure can also cause a more severe type of anemia that is due to the resulting decrease in erythropoietin production. In this case, erythropoietin (epoetin alpha) can be used as treatment.

The Thalassemias

Thalassemia is a hereditary type of anemia characterized by reduction of the synthesis of hemoglobin chains alpha and beta. This leads to reduced hemoglobin synthesis and a microcytic hypochromic anemia. *α-Thalassemia* is due to a gene deletion, which causes reduced alpha hemoglobin chain synthesis. *β-Thalassemia* is caused by a point mutation rather than a deletion. In the absence of beta chains, the excess of alpha chains leads to instability in the RBC and hemolysis. The bone marrow becomes hyperplastic, and in severe cases this may lead to bone deformities and fractures. Transfusion and iron chelation are used for treatment so that iron overload can be minimized. Allogenic bone marrow transplantation has become the treatment of choice for β-thalassemia major, improving the survival rate of these patients to more than 80%.

Sideroblastic Anemia

If the incorporation of heme into protoporphyrin fails, hemoglobin synthesis is reduced; this condition is referred to as *sideroblastic anemia*. (A sideroblast is an erythroblast that has granules of ferritin.) Iron accumulates, particularly in the mitochondria. This may be 1 stage of myelodysplasia leading to leukemia. The causes of sideroblastic anemia are acquired but may also include chronic alcoholism and lead poisoning. The anemia in this case is usually moderate, but transfusions are sometimes required.

Vitamin B_{12} Deficiency

Vitamin B_{12} comes from the diet and is available in all foods of animal origin. To be absorbed, it requires an intrinsic factor produced by the parietal cells. This complex is absorbed in the terminal ileum and stored in the liver. It takes 3 years to deplete the reserves of vitamin B_{12} in the liver. Strict vegetarians (vegans), patients with a history of abdominal surgery or gastrectomy, and persons with parasitic or pancreatic disease are at increased risk for vitamin B_{12} deficiency. *Pernicious anemia* is an autoimmune disease that leads to lack of vitamin B_{12} absorption due to atrophic gastritis. Megaloblastic anemia is the result. Oftentimes, leukopenia and thrombocytopenia may accompany the anemia. Vitamin B_{12} deficiency by itself can cause a neurological syndrome, with peripheral nerves affected first; balance problems and alteration of cerebral function occur in more severe cases (dementia and neuropsychiatric changes). The diagnosis is confirmed by obtaining a serum level of vitamin B_{12} (less than 170 pg/mL). Treatment is with parenteral B_{12} in cases of pernicious anemia. Otherwise, oral B_{12} is adequate.

Folic Acid Deficiency

Folic acid deficiency is another etiology of megaloblastic, or macrocytic, anemia. Macro-ovalocytes and hypersegmented neutrophils are seen on peripheral smear. The serum vitamin B_{12} concentration has to be normal. The most common etiology of folate deficiency is inadequate dietary intake. Treatment is with oral folic acid supplements.

Hemolytic Anemias

In *hemolytic anemia*, the life span of the RBC is reduced. The bone marrow responds to this reduced survival with an increase in production of RBCs; hence, reticulocytosis is an important clue to the presence of hemolysis. The offending factor may be intrinsic or external to the RBC.

Treatment depends on the specific etiology. In hereditary spherocytosis, there is an autosomal dominant membrane abnormality in the RBC, which causes the RBC to acquire a spherical shape. This abnormal shape leads to lack of RBC strength and RBC deformability, trapping of the RBC in the spleen, and hemolysis. The treatment of choice is splenectomy, which eliminates the site of hemolysis. Uninterrupted supplementation of folic acid is also needed.

In paroxysmal nocturnal hemoglobinuria, the RBC membrane is sensitive to lysis by complement. The best screening test is flow cytometry, which has largely replaced the classic sucrose hemolysis test. Prednisone is helpful in decreasing the hemolysis. In glucose-6-phosphate dehydrogenase (G6PD) deficiency, a hereditary enzyme defect causes hemolytic anemia due to decreased ability of the RBC to deal with oxidative stresses. Oxidized hemoglobin precipitates and forms precipitants called *Heinz bodies*. The RBC is then removed by the spleen. The triggering factor is usually an infection or exposure to a specific drug. Specific G6PD assays are available. Treatment consists of avoiding known oxidant drugs.

Sickle cell disease

In *sickle cell anemia*, an abnormal hemoglobin leads to chronic hemolytic anemia, an autosomal recessive disorder causing an amino acid substitution on the beta chain. The new hemoglobin is called *hemoglobin S*. This in turn damages the RBC membrane and leads to sickling. Parental diagnosis is now available for couples at risk for producing a child with sickle cell anemia. Genetic counseling should be made available for such couples. One out of 400 blacks born in the United States has sickle cell anemia. Chronic hemolytic anemia can produce jaundice, gallstones, splenomegaly, and poorly healing ulcers over the lower tibia.

Sickle cell disease is manifested by acute painful episodes that are caused by the sickling of the RBCs and that can be precipitated by infection, dehydration, and hypoxia. Vascular occlusion can lead to necrosis of bone and to infection. Hematuria can be caused by infarction of the renal papillae. Ophthalmologists are familiar with sickle cell retinopathy, which can lead to vision loss in severe cases. With improved supportive care, an affected person now has an average life expectancy of between 40 and 50 years. Most clinical laboratories offer a screening test for sickle cell hemoglobin. For patients who have a positive screening test, the diagnosis is confirmed by hemoglobin electrophoresis, which can detect the presence and measure the amount of hemoglobin S. Patients should be given folic acid supplements, pneumococcal vaccination, and, if infections arise, specific treatment for infections. Patients should be kept well hydrated, and they should be given oxygen if they are hypoxic. Allogenic bone marrow transplantation is being studied as a possible curative option for severely affected young patients. See also BCSC Section 12, *Retina and Vitreous*.

Autoimmune hemolytic anemia

In autoimmune hemolytic anemia, an IgG autoantibody is formed and binds to the RBC membrane, leading to formation of a spherocyte and sequestration in the spleen. Half of all cases of autoimmune hemolytic anemia are idiopathic; others are associated with autoimmune diseases such as systemic lupus and chronic leukemia. The Coombs' test is positive. Treatment consists of administration of prednisone and, if the disease is recurrent, splenectomy.

Disorders of Hemostasis

Disorders of hemostasis may be due to defects in either platelet number or function or to problems in formation of a fibrin clot (coagulation). A basic understanding of the hemostatic process and the manifestations associated with specific abnormalities helps the ophthalmologist with both medical and surgical management. (See Fig 7-1 for a diagram

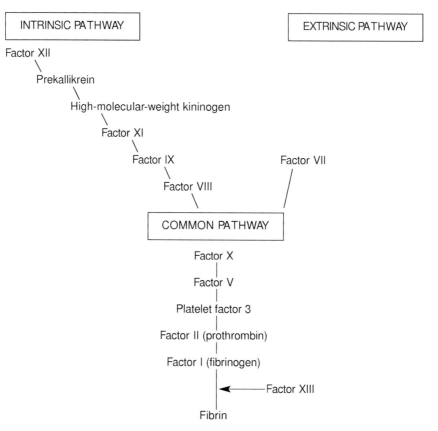

Figure 7-1 Blood-clotting pathways.

of blood-clotting pathways.) For the purpose of laboratory test interpretation, the coagulation cascade can be divided into intrinsic and extrinsic pathways. However, it is now understood that this is an oversimplification. For example, factor IX (an intrinsic factor) can be activated by factor VII (an extrinsic factor).

Hemostasis is initiated by damage to a blood vessel wall. This event triggers constriction of the vessel, followed by accumulation and adherence of platelets at the site of injury. Coagulation factors in the blood are activated, leading to formation of a fibrin clot. Slow fibrinolysis ensues, dissolving the clot while the damage is repaired. Circulating inhibitors are also present, modulating the process by inactivating coagulation factors to prevent widespread clotting. Normal endothelium plays a critical role in naturally anticoagulating blood by preventing fibrin accumulation. The following physiologic antithrombotic components can produce this effect:

- antithrombin III
- protein C and protein S
- tissue factor pathway inhibitor
- the fibrinolytic system

Antithrombin III (AT III) acts to inactivate thrombin. Activated protein C (APC), with its cofactor protein S, functions as a natural anticoagulant by destroying factors Va and VIIa. Thrombin itself activates protein C. Although inherited deficiencies of antithrombin III, protein C, or protein S are associated with a lifelong thrombotic tendency, tissue factor pathway inhibitor deficiency has not yet been related to the hypercoagulable state (see later discussion of thrombotic disorders).

Laboratory Evaluation of Hemostasis and Blood Coagulation

Various techniques are used to assess the status of a patient's hemostatic mechanisms. Following are some of the most common tests:

- *Platelet count.* Minor bleeding may occur at platelet counts below 50,000/μL. Abnormal bleeding at higher platelet counts suggests abnormal platelet function. Below 20,000/μL, spontaneous bleeding may be serious.
- *Bleeding time.* A small dermal wound is created, and the duration of bleeding is recorded. This is a screening test of the vascular and platelet components of hemostasis. Because disorders of blood vessels are rare, the results essentially reflect platelet number and function. Bleeding time is prolonged when platelet counts drop below 50,000–100,000/μL.
- *Partial thromboplastin time (PTT).* The PTT requires all of the coagulation factors involved in the intrinsic and common pathways. The PTT is most commonly used to measure the effect of heparin therapy. Platelet abnormalities do not affect the result of this test.
- *Prothrombin time (PT).* The PT measures the integrity of the extrinsic and common pathways. It requires a 30% concentration of the vitamin K–dependent factors II, VII, and X (though not factor IX, a part of the intrinsic pathway) and therefore is prolonged in conditions affecting these factors (see later discussion). The PT is most commonly used to monitor anticoagulant therapy. The action of heparin may slightly prolong PT.

Efforts have been made to tailor anticoagulation therapy to the problem being treated. For example, treatment or prevention of deep venous thrombosis is thought to require less oral anticoagulation therapy than treatment of endocardial mural thrombi or cardiac replacement valves. However, because of intralaboratory and interlaboratory variation in test results, it has been difficult to standardize therapeutic dosages. To solve this problem, the international normalized ratio (INR) was developed. The INR modifies the standard PT ratio (patient PT/control PT) to reflect the particular thromboplastin reagent used by a laboratory. The resulting reported INR value is an expression of the ratio of the patient's PT to the laboratory's mean normal PT. Thus, for prevention or treatment of deep vein thrombosis, the recommended INR value (comparable to subsequent values measured over time or across different laboratories) is 2.0–3.0; for tissue replacement valves, 2.0–3.0; for mechanical replacement valves, 2.5–3.5.

Clinical Manifestations of Hemostatic Abnormalities

Hemorrhage resulting from hemostatic derangement must be differentiated from hemorrhage caused by localized processes. The presence of generalized or recurrent bleeding suggests abnormal hemostasis. *Petechiae* (small capillary hemorrhages of the skin and mucous membranes) and *purpura* (ecchymoses) are typical of platelet disorders and vasculitis. Subcutaneous hematomas and hemarthroses characterize coagulation abnormalities. Bleeding due to trauma may be massive and life threatening in coagulation disorders, whereas bleeding is more likely to be slow and prolonged when platelet function is impaired.

Vascular Disorders

A number of inherited and acquired disorders of blood vessels and their supporting connective tissues result in pathologic bleeding. *Hereditary hemorrhagic telangiectasia* (Osler-Weber-Rendu disease) is an autosomal dominant condition characterized by localized dilation of capillaries and venules of the skin and mucous membranes. The lesions increase over a period of decades, often leading to profuse bleeding.

Several inherited connective tissue disorders are associated with hemorrhage. *Ehlers-Danlos syndrome* is characterized by hyperplastic fragile skin and hyperextensible joints; it is dominantly inherited. In *osteogenesis imperfecta,* also a dominant trait, bone fractures and otosclerosis (leading to deafness) are common. In both of these conditions, easy bruising and hematomas are common. *Pseudoxanthoma elasticum,* a recessive disorder, is much rarer but is often complicated by gastrointestinal hemorrhage. *Marfan syndrome* is sometimes associated with mild bleeding as well as with aortic dissection.

Scurvy, the result of severe ascorbic acid deficiency, is associated with marked vascular fragility and hemorrhagic manifestations resulting from abnormal synthesis of collagen. In addition to the classic findings of perifollicular petechiae and gingival bleeding, intradermal, intramuscular, and subperiosteal hemorrhages are common. *Amyloidosis* is another acquired disorder in which petechiae and purpura are common.

All of the inherited vascular disorders have associated ocular findings. Conjunctival telangiectasias occur in hereditary hemorrhagic telangiectasia. Blue sclerae are typical of osteogenesis imperfecta. Ocular manifestations of Ehlers-Danlos syndrome include microcornea, myopia, and angioid streaks; retinal detachment and ectopia lentis have also been reported. Angioid streaks also occur in patients with pseudoxanthoma elasticum. Fifty percent of patients with Marfan syndrome have ectopia lentis; severe myopia and retinal detachment are common.

Platelet Disorders

By far the most common cause of abnormal bleeding, platelet disorders may result from an insufficient number of platelets, inadequate function, or both. Mild derangement of platelet function may be asymptomatic or may cause minor bruising, menorrhagia, or bleeding after surgery. More severe dysfunction leads to petechiae, purpura, and gastrointestinal bleeding and other types of serious bleeding.

Thrombocytopenia

The number of platelets may be reduced by decreased production, increased destruction, or abnormal distribution. Production may be suppressed by many factors, including radiation, chemotherapy, alcohol use, malignant invasion of the bone marrow, aplastic anemia, and vitamin B_{12} or folic acid deficiency.

Accelerated destruction may occur through immunologic or nonimmunologic causes. *Idiopathic thrombocytopenic purpura (ITP)* is the result of platelet injury by antiplatelet antibodies. The acute form of ITP usually occurs in children and young adults, often following a viral illness, and commonly undergoes spontaneous remission. Chronic ITP is more common in adults and is characterized by mild manifestations; spontaneous remission is uncommon. Treatment consists of corticosteroid therapy or splenectomy. Danazol is also effective in treating ITP, and when combined therapy is necessary, danazol allows the use of lower doses of corticosteroids. A neonatal form occurs in babies born to women with ITP; this form results from transplacental passage of antiplatelet antibodies. Recovery follows physiologic clearance of the antibodies from the child's circulation.

Many drugs have been implicated as causes of immunologic platelet destruction. Drug-induced thrombocytopenia is rather common. Quinine, quinidine, digitalis, procainamide, thiazide diuretics, sulfonamides, phenytoin, aspirin, penicillin, heparin, and gold can cause it. Another important cause is *posttransfusion isoantibody production,* which occurs predictably after transfusions containing platelets, unless human leukocyte antigen typing is undertaken, and leads to decreasing efficacy of later platelet transfusions.

Nonimmune causes of thrombocytopenia include *thrombotic thrombocytopenic purpura* and the syndromes of intravascular coagulation and fibrinolysis (discussed later). In addition to the symptoms of thrombocytopenia, thrombotic thrombocytopenic purpura is characterized by thrombotic occlusions of the microcirculation and hemolytic anemia. Fever, neurological symptoms, anemia, and renal dysfunction occur with abrupt onset, with death occurring in days to weeks in the majority of untreated cases. Early treatment with exchange plasmapheresis has improved the survival rate to over 80%. Additional treatment includes antiplatelet drugs, corticosteroids, and splenectomy.

Abnormal distribution of platelets is most commonly caused by splenic sequestration. The usual clinical setting is hepatic cirrhosis, and the level of thrombocytopenia is mild. Patients with severely depressed platelet counts probably also have accelerated platelet destruction in the spleen.

Platelet dysfunction

Patients in this category usually come to the physician's attention because of easy bruising, epistaxis, menorrhagia, or excessive bleeding after surgery or dental work. Unlike patients with marked thrombocytopenia, patients with platelet dysfunction rarely have petechiae.

Hereditary disorders of platelet function are rare. Much more important clinically are the acquired forms, of which drug ingestion is the most common cause. As with drugs causing antiplatelet antibodies, the list of causative agents is very long. A single aspirin tablet taken orally irreversibly inhibits platelet aggregation for the life span of the circulating platelets present, causing a modest prolongation of the bleeding time for at least 48–72 hours following ingestion. This reaction has remarkably little effect in normal persons, although intraoperative blood loss may be slightly increased. However, in patients with hemophilia, severe thrombocytopenia, or uremia and in those on warfarin or heparin therapy, bleeding may be significant.

Nonsteroidal anti-inflammatory drugs cause reversible inhibition of platelet function in the presence of the drug; the effect disappears as the drug is cleared from the blood. Other commonly used drugs that may affect platelet function include ethanol, tricyclic antidepressants, and antihistamines.

In addition to uremia, clinical conditions associated with abnormal platelet function include liver disease, multiple myeloma, systemic lupus erythematosus, chronic lymphocytic leukemia, and Hermansky-Pudlak syndrome (an autosomal recessive form of oculocutaneous albinism).

Disorders of Blood Coagulation

Hereditary coagulation disorders
Inherited abnormalities involve all of the coagulation factors except factors III and IV. The most common and most severe is factor VIII deficiency, called *hemophilia A*, or *classic hemophilia*. Typical manifestations of this X-linked disease include severe and protracted bleeding, after even minor trauma, and spontaneous bleeding into joints (hemarthroses), the central nervous system, and the abdominal cavity.

Treatment involves infusion of coagulation factor VIII. Transfusion of pooled human factor VIII, in the past, had always carried a significant risk of transmission of hepatitis B virus; in the 1980s, transmission of the human immunodeficiency virus became a major problem as well. Those risks have now been mostly eliminated with the availability of recombinant factor VIII. Up to 10% of patients with hemophilia A develop antibodies, presumably due to sensitization following administration of factor VIII. These anticoagulants can also develop in healthy elderly patients, in nonhemophiliac patients after drug reactions, and in those with collagen vascular diseases. Clinical manifestations range from mild bleeding to full-blown hemophilia. The result of the PTT is prolonged, and the result of the PT is normal. Treatment involves various regimens of coagulation factor replacement and immunosuppression to try to eliminate the inhibitor. Gene therapy is currently in the developmental phase but could further transform the outlook for these patients.

Von Willebrand disease, another relatively common hereditary disorder, is caused by deficiency or abnormality of a portion of the factor VIII molecule called von Willebrand factor. This deficiency causes platelet adhesion abnormalities, leading to bleeding symptoms that are mild in most cases and may escape detection until adult years.

Acquired coagulation disorders
Vitamin K deficiency Vitamin K is required for the production of factors II (prothrombin), VII, IX, and X in the liver. Normal diets contain large amounts of vitamin K, which is also synthesized by gut flora. Causes of vitamin K deficiency include biliary obstruction and various malabsorption syndromes (including sprue, cystic fibrosis, and celiac disease),

in which intestinal absorption of vitamin K is reduced. Suppression of endogenous gastrointestinal flora, seen commonly in hospitalized patients on prolonged broad-spectrum antibiotic therapy, decreases intestinal production of vitamin K. However, clinical deficiency occurs only if dietary intake is also diminished. Nutritional deficiency is unusual but may occur with prolonged parenteral nutrition. Laboratory evaluation reveals prolongation of both PT and PTT. Most forms of vitamin K deficiency respond to subcutaneous or intramuscular administration of 20 mg of vitamin K_1, with normalization of coagulation defects within 24 hours. Vitamin K_1 should not be given intravenously because of the risk of sudden death from an anaphylactoid reaction. One special form of vitamin K deficiency is *hemorrhagic disease of the newborn,* which is the result of a normal mild deficiency of vitamin K–dependent factors during the first 5 days of life and the absence of the vitamin in maternal milk. This condition is now rare in developed countries because of the routine administration of vitamin K to newborns. Readers are also referred to the antiphospholipid antibodies section in Chapter 8, Rheumatic Disorders.

Liver disease Hemostatic abnormalities of all types may be associated with disease of the liver, the site of production of all the coagulation factors except factor VIII. As liver dysfunction develops, levels of the vitamin K–dependent factors decrease first, followed by factors V, XI, and XII; both PT and PTT are prolonged. Thrombocytopenia, primarily the result of hypersplenism, and a prolonged bleeding time due to platelet dysfunction are common. In addition, intravascular coagulation and fibrinolysis (discussed later) are common, further complicating the clinical picture.

Mild hemorrhagic symptoms are common in patients with significant liver disease. Severe bleeding is usually gastrointestinal in origin, arising from peptic ulcers, gastritis, and esophageal varices. Treatment is difficult at best and consists of blood and coagulation factor replacement. Local measures, such as vasopressin infusion or balloon tamponade of bleeding varices, can sometimes control potentially catastrophic bleeding.

Disseminated intravascular coagulation Disseminated intravascular coagulation (DIC) is a complex syndrome involving widespread activation of the coagulation and fibrinolytic systems within the general circulation. Utilization and consumption of coagulation factors and platelets produce bleeding; formation of fibrin and fibrin degradation products (fibrin split products) leads to occlusion of the microcirculation, various forms of organ failure, and occasionally thrombosis of larger vessels. Laboratory findings may vary but usually include thrombocytopenia, hypofibrinogenemia, and elevated levels of fibrin split products. PT and PTT are usually, though not invariably, prolonged.

Clinically, 2 forms of DIC are recognized. *Acute DIC* is characterized by the abrupt onset of severe, generalized bleeding. The most common causes are obstetrical complications (most notably abruptio placentae and amniotic fluid embolism), septicemia, shock, massive trauma, and major surgical procedures. Treatment, other than specific measures aimed at the underlying disease, is controversial. Among the modalities used are heparinization and replacement of blood, platelets, and fibrinogen.

Chronic DIC is associated with disseminated neoplasms, some acute leukemias, and autoimmune diseases. Laboratory values range from normal to moderately abnormal; levels of coagulation factors may even be elevated. Bleeding and thrombosis (especially leg-vein thrombosis and pulmonary embolism) may occur, but in most patients the syndrome remains undiagnosed unless renal failure results from intravascular coagulation in the kidney. In these patients, the disease has been demonstrated via biopsy to detect fibrin in renal tissue. On occasion, chronic DIC may convert to the acute form.

Thrombotic disorders (thrombophilia)

The "hypercoagulable states" encompass a group of inherited or acquired disorders that increase the risk of thrombosis. The primary hypercoagulable states are caused by abnormalities of specific coagulation proteins involving inherited mutations in 1 of the antithrombotic factors. The trigger for a thrombotic event is often the development of 1 of the acquired secondary hypercoagulable states superimposed on an inherited state of hypercoagulability. The secondary hypercoagulable states cause a thrombotic tendency by complex and often multifactorial mechanisms.

Primary Hypercoagulable States

Antithrombin III deficiency

Antithrombin III deficiency leads to increased fibrin accumulation and a lifelong propensity for thrombosis.

Protein C deficiency

Protein C deficiency leads to unregulated fibrin generation because of impaired inactivation of factors VIIIa and Va, 2 essential cofactors in the coagulation cascade.

Protein S deficiency

Protein S is the principal cofactor of APC, and therefore its deficiency mimics that of protein C.

Activated protein C resistance

Inherited APC resistance causing thrombophilia was originally detected by the finding that the activated PTT of the plasma of affected persons could not be appropriately prolonged by the addition of exogenous APC in vitro. The great majority of these subjects are now recognized to harbor a single specific point mutation in the factor V gene, termed *factor V Leiden*. This mutation is remarkably frequent (3%–7%) in healthy white populations but appears to be far less prevalent or even absent in certain black and Asian populations.

Prothrombin gene mutation

The prothrombin gene mutation has been associated with elevated plasma levels of prothrombin; it is second only to factor V Leiden as a genetic risk factor for venous thrombosis.

Hyperhomocysteinemia

Hyperhomocysteinemia, which is due to elevated blood levels of homocysteine, leads to severe neurologic developmental abnormalities in the homozygous state. Adults with heterozygous deficiency state may have only thrombotic tendencies. Acquired causes of hyperhomocysteinemia in adults commonly involve nutritional deficiencies of pyridoxine, vitamin B_{12}, and folate, all cofactors in homocysteine metabolism. High blood concentrations of homocysteine constitute an independent risk factor for both venous and arterial thrombosis; in contrast, all of the other primary hypercoagulable states are associated only with venous thromboembolic complications, usually involving the lower extremities. The initial treatment of acute venous thrombosis in these patients is not different from treatment in those without genetic defects.

Secondary Hypercoagulable States

Malignancy may stimulate thrombosis directly by elaborating procoagulant substances that initiate chronic DIC. This appears to be most prominent in patients with pancreatic cancer, adenocarcinoma of the gastrointestinal tract or lung, and ovarian cancer. *Myeloproliferative disorders* (polycythemia vera, essential thrombocythemia, chronic myelogenous leukemia, and myelofibrosis) are major causes of thrombosis and paradoxical bleeding, as is the related stem cell disorder *paroxysmal nocturnal hemoglobinuria*. The *phospholipid antibody syndrome* is characterized by both venous and arterial thrombosis, including recurrent spontaneous abortions, deep venous thrombosis, and cerebrovascular arterial thrombotic events. Ophthalmic complications include retinal vein and artery occlusion, retinal vasculitis, choroidal infarction, and anterior ischemic optic neuropathy. Tests for patients with this syndrome include anticardiolipin antibodies, lupus anticoagulants, and biological false-positive VDRL. The hypercoagulability associated with *pregnancy* involves a progressive state of DIC throughout the course of pregnancy, activated in the uteroplacental circulation. *Oral contraceptives* induce similar changes. The *postoperative state* and *trauma* are significant causes of venous thrombosis. Detailed discussion of treatment of these various and complex disorders is beyond the scope of this text.

Therapeutic anticoagulation

Many clinical situations require intentional disruption of the hemostatic process. The effect of aspirin on platelet function has already been discussed.

Heparin is a mucopolysaccharide that binds antithrombin III, inhibiting the formation of thrombin. It is given intravenously or subcutaneously, and therapy is assessed by measuring the PTT. Aspirin should not be given to patients on heparin because the resultant platelet dysfunction may provoke bleeding.

The orally administered warfarin derivatives, of which warfarin sodium (Coumadin) is the most widely used, inhibit the production of normal vitamin K–dependent coagulation factors (II, VII, IX, and X). Therapeutic effect is assessed by measuring the patient's INR. One critical issue is the long list of commonly used drugs that interact with warfarin. These interactions may cause an unintended increase or decrease in the INR, depending on the drug.

Heparin and the warfarin derivatives are used to prevent the formation of new thrombi and the propagation of existing thrombi, but neither affects the original clot.

Thrombolytic agents such as *streptokinase, urokinase,* and *tissue plasminogen activator* are used to dissolve existing thrombi, most notably in the very early stages of myocardial infarction resulting from coronary artery thrombosis. These agents are also currently being used for early treatment of thrombotic stroke; this form of treatment increases the risk of converting a thrombotic stroke into a hemorrhagic stroke.

> Hall CJ, Richards S, Hillmen P. Primary prophylaxis with warfarin prevents thrombosis in paroxysmal nocturnal hemoglobinuria (PNH). *Blood.* 2003;102:3587–3591.
>
> Means RT Jr. Recent developments in the anemia of chronic disease. *Curr Hematol Rep.* 2003;2:116–121.
>
> Provan D, O'Shaughnessy DF. Recent advances in haematology. *BMJ.* 1999;318:991–994.
>
> Schafer A. Approach to the patient with bleeding and thrombosis. In: Goldman L, Bennett JC, eds. *Cecil Textbook of Medicine.* Vol 1. 21st ed. Philadelphia: WB Saunders; 2000:991–995.
>
> Schafer A. Thrombotic disorders: hypercoagulable states. In: Goldman L, Bennett JC, eds. *Cecil Textbook of Medicine.* Vol 1. 21st ed. Philadelphia: WB Saunders; 2000:1016–1021.

CHAPTER 8

Rheumatic Disorders

Recent Developments

- Cyclooxygenase 2 (COX-2) selective nonsteroidal anti-inflammatory drugs were recently introduced to minimize gastrointestinal damage, but recent data have raised a concern that they may have potential cardiovascular risks. Two of the drugs have been removed from the market (rofecoxib [Vioxx] and valdecoxib [Bextra]), and the third now carries warnings regarding its use (celecoxib [Celebrex]).
- Cytokine-based agents such as etanercept (Enbrel) and infliximab (Remicade) are demonstrating efficacy in the treatment of a number of autoimmune diseases. However, there is also increasing recognition of uncommon but significant adverse effects such as opportunistic infections and demyelinating disease that may include optic neuritis.
- Many rheumatologic diseases, such as the spondyloarthropathies and juvenile arthritides, are undergoing reclassification to allow a more uniform approach to defining treatment and prognosis.

Introduction

The rheumatic disorders are a heterogeneous collection of diseases that include rheumatoid arthritis, the spondyloarthropathies, juvenile idiopathic (rheumatoid) arthritis, systemic lupus erythematosus, scleroderma, polymyositis and dermatomyositis, Sjögren syndrome, relapsing polychondritis, Behçet syndrome, and the vasculitides, including polyarteritis nodosa, Wegener granulomatosis, and giant cell arteritis. Ocular involvement is common in the rheumatic diseases but varies among the different disorders.

Rheumatoid Arthritis

Rheumatoid arthritis (RA) is the most common rheumatic disorder, affecting approximately 1% of adults. RA is classically an additive, symmetrical, deforming, peripheral polyarthritis characterized by synovial membrane inflammation. All joints may be involved, but this disorder affects primarily the small joints of the hands and feet. Like all inflammatory arthritides, RA is associated with the *gel phenomenon,* a stiffness at rest that improves with use; patients often complain of morning stiffness, which is a hallmark of inflammatory joint disease.

Approximately 80% of patients with RA are positive for a rheumatoid factor, which is an autoantibody directed against immunoglobulin G (IgG). Seropositive RA aggregates in families. Human leukocyte antigen DR4 (HLA-DR4) is found in 70% of Caucasian seropositive patients. A more recent test involves identification of anticyclic citrullinated peptide antibodies (anti-CCP antibodies), which are antibodies directed toward certain peptides in the skin that contain the amino acid citrulline. Testing for both anti-CCP antibodies and rheumatoid factor increases the sensitivity for detecting early RA, and patients with anti-CCP antibodies may tend to have more erosive disease.

Extra-articular disease in RA may affect a wide variety of nonarticular tissues. Rheumatoid nodules, located subcutaneously on extensor surfaces, occur in approximately 25% of patients with RA. The lungs may be affected with rheumatoid pleural effusions, pleural nodules, pulmonary nodules, and, occasionally, interstitial fibrosis. Cardiac disease includes pericarditis and rheumatoid nodules involving the conducting system, heart valves, or both. Mild anemia of chronic disease is the rule. *Felty syndrome* is a triad of RA, splenomegaly, and neutropenia. Patients with Felty syndrome can also have hyperpigmentation, chronic leg ulcers, and recurrent infections. Rheumatoid vasculitis affects less than 1% of patients with RA. It generally presents either as peripheral polyneuropathy or as refractory skin ulcers. Patients may develop digital gangrene or, occasionally, visceral ischemia. The most common neuropathy is median nerve compression caused by synovitis of the wrist. Ocular manifestations of RA include Sjögren syndrome, scleritis, episcleritis, and marginal corneal ulcers. The ocular manifestations of RA are discussed in BCSC Section 9, *Intraocular Inflammation and Uveitis*.

Therapy

There has been increasing recognition that significant joint damage occurs early in the course of the disease. Thus, the goal is to identify and aggressively treat even subtle evidence of disease activity. A patient's physician can determine disease activity by analyzing a combination of symptoms, clinical findings, laboratory testing, and imaging. Treatment of RA is then approached in a stepwise additive fashion. Nonpharmacologic and preventive measures, such as physical therapy and actions ensuring bone health, form the basis of treatment.

Analgesics and nonsteroidal anti-inflammatory drugs (NSAIDs) are used to control acute symptoms but do not alter disease outcome. Most patients with active disease require at least 1 *slow-acting antirheumatic drug (SAARD)*, also known as *disease-modifying antirheumatic drugs (DMARDs)*. These drugs are capable of reducing or preventing joint damage and include hydroxychloroquine (Plaquenil), methotrexate, and sulfasalazine (Azulfidine). Methotrexate is perhaps the most commonly used DMARD. Depending on disease response and severity, patients may need more aggressive medications such as cyclosporine (Neoral, Sandimmune), cyclophosphamide (Cytoxan), or the various anticytokine drugs. (All of these medications are reviewed at the end of this chapter.) Combination therapy is often used to minimize the toxicity of any one class of medication. Prednisone is often used, ideally at low doses, to increase the patient's mobility and functional capacity. Joint surgery for pain and impaired function may also be necessary.

Spondyloarthropathies

This group of diseases has been referred to as the *seronegative spondyloarthropathies*, with the term *seronegative* referring to a negative rheumatoid factor test. As newer and more specific clinical definitions are created, that term is redundant and less commonly used. The defining clinical term is *spondyloarthropathy*, which refers to a spectrum of diseases that share certain clinical features. There is a predilection for axial (spinal and sacroiliac joint) inflammation, with a hallmark being inflammatory spinal pain. Inflammatory spinal pain is distinguished from more typical low back pain symptoms by the tendency to be worse after rest (morning stiffness) and to improve with activity. Other distinctive features of the various spondyloarthropathies include asymmetric arthritis, genital and skin lesions, eye and bowel inflammation, and an association with previous or ongoing infectious disorders. The presence of these other features is used to distinguish between the various types of spondyloarthropathies, although there may be a great deal of overlap. The spondyloarthropathies are also linked by their statistical association with the antigen type HLA-B27 and by a tendency to have a specific type of joint inflammation known as *enthesitis*. The spondyloarthropathy family consists of undifferentiated spondyloarthropathy, reactive arthritis, Reiter syndrome, and both the juvenile and adult forms of ankylosing spondylitis. Also included are the spondyloarthropathies associated with psoriasis and inflammatory bowel disease (Crohn disease and ulcerative colitis).

Undifferentiated spondyloarthropathy is a newer category created for patients who do not fall into one of the other categories. It was formed with the recognition that for the majority of patients with spondyloarthropathy, there is no apparent antecedent cause. Most patients present primarily with arthritis. Undifferentiated spondyloarthropathy is probably the most common of the spondyloarthropathies, followed by ankylosing spondylitis, with reactive arthritis and Reiter syndrome being much less common. It is hoped that this newer categorization of the spondyloarthropathies will eventually lead to better understanding and management of this subset of rheumatologic diseases.

Awareness of these various entities is important for the ophthalmologist because they all share the potential to develop acute HLA-B27–associated anterior uveitis. At times the characteristic uveitis may be the presenting feature of a spondyloarthropathy, and the ophthalmologist may therefore be crucial in suggesting the diagnosis. See BCSC Section 9, *Intraocular Inflammation and Uveitis*, for further discussion of the ophthalmic manifestations.

Ankylosing Spondylitis

Ankylosing spondylitis (AS) is characterized by involvement of the axial skeleton and by bony fusion (ankylosis). Inflammation occurs particularly at the enthesis (enthesitis), a complex structure that extends into bone at the point where ligaments and tendons are attached. The cause is unknown, but the strong association with HLA-B27 (90% of patients) suggests a genetic predisposition. Men are affected 3 times more often than women are, and the radiographic features seem to evolve more slowly in women.

The classic features of ankylosing spondylitis are inflammatory low back pain, fusion of the axial skeleton (spinal ankylosis), and sacroiliitis on x-ray examination. The last stage of this process is a completely fused and immobilized spine, also known as a *bamboo* or *poker spine*. In addition to the spinal arthritis that is the hallmark of the disease, patients may develop arthritis of peripheral joints, limited chest expansion, and restrictive lung disease. Other extra-articular features include apical pulmonary fibrosis, ascending aortitis, aortic valvular incompetence, and heart block. Ankylosing spondylitis is surprisingly resistant to the usual rheumatologic therapeutics. The most effective agents seem to be sulfasalazine and tumor necrosis factor alpha inhibitors.

The primary ocular manifestation of ankylosing spondylitis is recurrent, acute, nongranulomatous iridocyclitis, which occurs in approximately 25% of these patients and does not seem to be correlated with the activity of the joint disease. Conversely, a study of patients presenting with HLA-B27 uveitis showed that approximately 45% either were known to have or ultimately developed AS. A rheumatologic evaluation of patients with HLA-B27 uveitis should be considered, because early diagnosis and treatment of AS with physical therapy may slow disease progression.

   Monnet D, Breban M, Hudry C, et al. Ophthalmic findings and frequency of extraocular manifestations in patients with HLA-B27 uveitis: a study of 175 cases. *Ophthalmology*. 2004;111(4):802–809.

Reactive Arthritis

In the broadest sense, the term *reactive arthritis* implies an autoimmune response to some sort of antecedent infection that usually involves the genitourinary or gastrointestinal system. Reiter syndrome—which features the classic triad of arthritis, urethritis, and conjunctivitis—can be considered to be a subset of reactive arthritis, although different authors may use the 2 terms interchangeably because the classification of the various spondyloarthropathies is in flux. Like ankylosing spondylitis, reactive arthritis has a clear genetic predisposition in that 63%–95% of patients are positive for HLA-B27. The male-female ratio is at least 5:1. Precipitating agents include *Chlamydia trachomatis* in the genitourinary tract, and *Salmonella, Shigella, Yersinia,* or *Campylobacter* organisms in the gastrointestinal tract. Fragments of *Yersinia, Salmonella,* and *Chlamydia* organisms have been identified in the synovial tissues of patients with reactive arthritis, but intact organisms have not been cultured—hence the designation "reactive" and not "infective."

The arthritis of reactive arthritis typically appears within 1–3 weeks of the inciting urethritis or diarrhea. It is an asymmetrical, episodic oligoarthritis affecting primarily the lower extremities, in particular the large joints such as the knees or ankles. Other features include inflammatory spinal pain, enthesitis, interphalangeal arthritis of the toes and fingers producing "sausage digits," and sacroiliitis. Mucocutaneous lesions include urethritis in men and cervicitis in women, shallow ulcers on the glans penis (circinate balanitis), painless oral ulcers, nail lesions, and skin lesions on the soles and palms (keratoderma blennorrhagicum). Patients may also have systemic symptoms, including fever and weight loss. The disease tends to follow an episodic course, and most patients go into remission within 2 years, although some may develop long-term disease. Systemic treatment includes use of NSAIDs and sulfasalazine in addition to appropriate antibiotic therapy if an active infection is still present after initial treatment.

Ophthalmic considerations

Conjunctivitis is one of the most common ophthalmic manifestations of the disease and is part of the original triad described by Reiter. It tends to be mild and bilateral with a mucopurulent discharge. There may be follicular or papillary changes. Cultures are negative, and the conjunctivitis typically resolves within 10 days without treatment. A more serious ocular manifestation is uveitis, which occurs in 15%–25% of patients with reactive arthritis. It is often the acute, nongranulomatous, recurrent iridocyclitis that is characteristic of HLA-B27 disease. The uveitis may also be chronic, and some patients may even require long-term immunosuppressive therapy.

The conjunctivitis and urethritis of Reiter syndrome are by definition sterile autoimmune phenomena that can occur after either gastrointestinal tract or genital infections. Confusion occurs because *Chlamydia trachomatis* can cause both conjunctivitis and urethritis, and a *Chlamydia* infection can stimulate a genetically predisposed individual to develop Reiter syndrome. It is important to rule out an infectious cause in a patient with presumed Reiter syndrome, especially because chlamydial urethritis may be asymptomatic. Most of the time, however, the precipitating infection will have resolved by the time the reactive autoimmune response supervenes. See BCSC Section 9, *Intraocular Inflammation and Uveitis,* for additional information on Reiter syndrome.

> Kiss S, Letko E, Qamruddin S, et al. Long-term progression, prognosis, and treatment of patients with recurrent ocular manifestations of Reiter's syndrome. *Ophthalmology.* 2003;110(9):1764–1769.

Other Spondyloarthropathies

Spondyloarthropathy may also occur in association with ulcerative colitis or with Crohn disease. *Ulcerative colitis* is an inflammatory disorder of the gastrointestinal mucosa with diffuse involvement of the colon. *Crohn disease* is a focal granulomatous disease involving all areas of the bowel and affecting both the large and the small intestine. Crohn disease is also known as *regional enteritis, granulomatous ileocolitis,* and *granulomatous colitis.* Symptoms of inflammatory bowel disease include diarrhea, bloody diarrhea, and cramping abdominal pain.

Extraintestinal manifestations of inflammatory bowel disease include dermatitis, mucous membrane disease, ocular inflammation, and arthritis. Arthritis associated with inflammatory bowel disease is referred to as *enteropathic arthritis* and may include a peripheral arthritis or a spondyloarthropathy or both. Multiple series have shown that 50% to 75% of patients with inflammatory bowel disease–associated spondyloarthropathy are positive for HLA-B27, which also predisposes them to iridocyclitis. The activity of the spondyloarthropathy is unrelated to the activity of the bowel disease. Enteropathic arthritis that involves the peripheral joints is not associated with HLA-B27, and disease activity tends to parallel the activity of the bowel disease.

Psoriasis is another systemic disease that may be associated with spondyloarthropathy. Psoriatic arthritis may have multiple presentations, including an oligoarthritis, a distal polyarthritis, and a destructive arthritis known as *arthritis mutilans*. Spondyloarthropathy is often seen in psoriatic arthritis, and there is an increased frequency of HLA-B27 in these patients, although the frequency of HLA-B27 in psoriatic arthritis is not as high as it is in ankylosing spondylitis or Reiter syndrome. Uveitis in patients with psoriatic arthritis tends to be more insidious in onset, smoldering, posterior, and bilateral compared with more typical HLA-B27–associated anterior uveitis.

Spondyloarthropathies may occur in childhood, although their occurrence is rare before the second decade. The diagnosis may be difficult to make because the recurrent arthritis may be initially misdiagnosed as being caused by multiple injuries. Patients may develop all the features of ankylosing spondylitis (juvenile ankylosing spondylitis), or they may have systemic diseases similar to those of the adults (eg, inflammatory bowel disease, reactive arthritis, or psoriasis). Many patients may not meet the criteria for any 1 particular type of spondyloarthropathy and are therefore considered to have undifferentiated disease. As in adults, the majority of young patients are HLA-B27 positive. There tends to be a preponderance of males, and these patients may develop acute uveitis characteristic of HLA-B27–associated uveitis. These juvenile onset spondyloarthropathies should not be confused with the various subsets of juvenile idiopathic (rheumatoid) arthritis.

Paiva ES, Macaluso DC, Edwards A, et al. Characterisation of uveitis in patients with psoriatic arthritis. *Ann Rheum Dis.* 2000;59(1):67–70.

Juvenile Idiopathic Arthritis

The older term *juvenile rheumatoid arthritis (JRA)* is being replaced by the term *juvenile idiopathic arthritis (JIA)* or *juvenile chronic arthritis*. The term *rheumatoid* is not considered accurate because for most children, these entities have no relationship to adult onset RA. The juvenile arthritides have, classically, been divided into 3 subsets based on associated symptoms and the number of joints involved. (Juvenile spondyloarthropathy is sometimes included as a fourth entity but is discussed separately in the previous section.)

Pauciarticular (or *oligoarticular*) *onset JIA* includes those patients with involvement of fewer than 5 joints after 6 months of illness. It accounts for approximately 50% of JIA cases. The antinuclear antibody (ANA) test is positive in many of these patients, and there is a strong predilection for females. The arthritis tends to remit, but 10%–50% of patients may develop chronic iridocyclitis. Thus, periodic eye examinations are important in order to detect occult ocular inflammation. (See BCSC Section 6, *Pediatric Ophthalmology and Strabismus;* and Section 9, *Intraocular Inflammation and Uveitis.*)

Responsible for 30%–40% of JIA cases, *polyarticular onset arthritis* is defined by the involvement of more than 4 joints after 6 months of illness. As with pauciarticular onset JIA, there is a female preponderance. The arthritis tends to be severe, but uveitis is rare.

Responsible for approximately 10%–15% of JIA cases, *systemic onset arthritis* (formerly called *Still disease*) refers to patients with fever, rash, and arthritis of any number of joints. Patients may also have hepatosplenomegaly and lymphadenopathy. The male-female ratio for systemic onset arthritis is approximately 1:1, in contrast with that of the other variants. Ocular disease is generally not associated with this variant.

This classification is now considered insufficient to reflect the many subgroups that exist within each category. Recently proposed criteria for classification of the idiopathic arthritides of childhood attempt to define these diseases in a way that will allow differentiation of etiologic mechanisms, prognostication, and response to therapy. This newer classification system includes systemic arthritis, polyarthritis, pauciarthritis, psoriatic arthritis, and enthesitis-related arthritis (the last category includes spondyloarthropathies). Each category then has various subcategories, such as ANA positivity and the presence of uveitis. However, because there is currently no universal agreement regarding this approach, several different classification systems are still in use. It is therefore likely that the older terminology will persist at the interface between pediatric rheumatology and ophthalmology, at least for now, simply because the screening and treatment guidelines for uveitis are based on the classic categories.

Systemic Lupus Erythematosus

Systemic lupus erythematosus (SLE) is generally regarded as the prototypical autoimmune disease. The cause of SLE is unknown, but familial aggregation of autoimmune diseases and association with the HLA types DR2 and DR3 suggest a genetic predisposition. Pathogenically, SLE is characterized by B-cell hyperreactivity, polyclonal B-cell activation, hypergammaglobulinemia, and a plethora of autoantibodies. These autoantibodies include antinuclear antibodies, antibodies to DNA, and antibodies to cytoplasmic components. SLE classically has been considered an immune complex disease in which immune complexes incite an inflammatory response and lead to tissue damage.

Women, especially in their 20s and 30s, are affected more frequently than men. Patients with SLE are subject to myriad symptoms and to inflammation that can affect virtually every organ. Although multiple system involvement is typical, patients may also present with single organ involvement such as nephritis or cytopenias. Cutaneous disease, which occurs in approximately 70%–80% of patients, is most often manifested by the characteristic butterfly rash across the nose and cheeks, also known as a *malar rash*. Other cutaneous manifestations include discoid lesions, vasculitic skin lesions such as cutaneous ulcers or splinter hemorrhages, purpuric skin lesions, and alopecia. Mucosal lesions, characteristically painless oral ulcers, occur in 30%–40% of patients. Photosensitivity occurs in many patients with SLE.

Approximately 80%–85% of patients with SLE experience articular disease at some point, either polyarthralgias or a nondeforming, migratory polyarthritis. Systemic features—including fatigue, fever, and weight loss—occur in more than 80% of patients with lupus. Renal disease is present in approximately 50%–75% of patients with SLE, presenting, clinically, as either proteinuria with nephrotic characteristics or glomerulonephritis with an active urinary sediment. Lupus nephritis is a major cause of the morbidity and mortality of SLE.

Raynaud phenomenon occurs in 30%–50% of SLE patients (Fig 8-1). Cardiac disease includes pericarditis, occasionally myocarditis, and Libman-Sacks endocarditis.

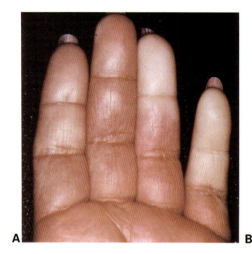 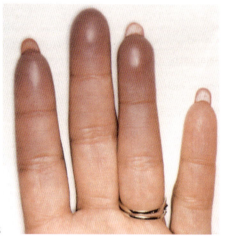

Figure 8-1 Raynaud phenomenon. **A,** Sharply demarcated pallor resulting from the closure of digital arteries. **B,** Digital cyanosis of the fingertips in a patient with primary Raynaud phenomenon. *(Reproduced with permission from Wigley FM. Raynaud's phenomenon. N Engl J Med. 2002 Sep 26;347(13):1001. Copyright ©2002 Massachusetts Medical Society. Images from UpToDate.)*

Pleuropulmonary lesions include pleuritic chest pain and, less commonly, pneumonitis. Hepatosplenomegaly and adenopathy occur in more than 50% of patients with SLE.

Central nervous system (CNS) involvement occurs in more than 35% of patients with SLE, and manifestations are typically transient. The most common manifestations of CNS lupus are headache, seizures, an organic brain syndrome, and psychosis. Transverse myelitis is an uncommon manifestation in patients with SLE, but it can occur in association with optic neuritis in active disease. Pseudotumor cerebri also can be associated with SLE.

SLE frequently affects the hematologic system. Patients often have an anemia of chronic disease but may also develop an autoimmune hemolytic anemia. Leukopenia, in particular lymphopenia, is a characteristic feature. Thrombocytopenia occurs in approximately one third of patients.

Diagnosis

Because of the protean manifestations of SLE, a list of diagnostic criteria has been established (Table 8-1). Four or more of these criteria must be met for a diagnosis of definite SLE; patients with fewer criteria may be labeled *probable* or *possible SLE*. These criteria were developed for investigational purposes, but they have been useful clinically.

The ANA test is the best diagnostic test for SLE and should be performed whenever SLE is suspected. The result of the ANA test is positive in significant titer (usually 1:160 or higher) in virtually all patients with SLE. A positive test at lower titers is not as specific because many diseases other than SLE may be ANA positive. However, if the ANA test result is negative, then it is very unlikely that a patient has SLE.

In the past, diagnostic significance was assigned to the pattern of antibody staining demonstrated by the ANA test (ie, homogeneous, peripheral, speckled, nucleolar).

Table 8-1 ARA Criteria for Diagnosis of Systemic Lupus Erythematosus

Criterion	Definition
Malar rash	Fixed erythema, flat or raised, over the malar eminences, tending to spare the nasolabial folds
Discoid rash	Erythematosus raised patches with adherent keratotic scaling and follicular plugging; atrophic scarring may occur in older lesions
Photosensitivity	Skin rash as a result of unusual reaction to sunlight, by patient history or physician observation
Oral ulcers	Oral or nasopharyngeal ulceration, usually painless, observed by a physician
Arthritis	Nonerosive arthritis involving 2 or more peripheral joints, characterized by tenderness, swelling, or effusion
Serositis	Pleuritis—convincing history of pleuritic pain or rub heard by a physician or evidence of pleural effusion **OR** pericarditis—documented by EKG, rub, or evidence of pericardial effusion
Renal disorder	Persistent proteinuria greater than 0.5 gram per day or greater than 3+ if quantitation not performed **OR** cellular casts—may be red cell, hemoglobin, granular, tubular, or mixed
Neurologic disorder	Seizures **OR** psychosis—in the absence of offending drugs or known metabolic derangements (uremia, ketoacidosis, or electrolyte imbalance)
Hematologic disorder	Hemolytic anemia—with reticulocytosis **OR** leukopenia—less than 4000/mm^3 total on two or more occasions **OR** lymphopenia—less than 1500/mm^3 on two or more occasions **OR** thrombocytopenia—less than 100,000/mm^3 in the absence of offending drugs
Immunologic disorders	Positive antiphospholipid antibody **OR** anti-DNA—antibody to native DNA in abnormal titer **OR** anti-Sm—presence of antibody to Sm nuclear antigen **OR** false-positive serologic test for syphilis known to be positive for at least six months and confirmed by *Treponema pallidum* immobilization or fluorescent treponemal antibody absorption test
Antinuclear antibody	An abnormal titer of antinuclear antibody by immunofluorescence or an equivalent assay at any point in time and in the absence of drugs known to be associated with "drug-induced lupus" syndrome

From Schur PH. Diagnosis and differential diagnosis of systemic lupus erythematosus in adults. In: *UpToDate*, Rose BD (Ed), Waltham, MA. Available at http://www.uptodate.com. Accessed March 1, 2005.

Because the interpretation of these patterns may be subjective, greater emphasis is now placed on assays that look for the specific type of autoantibody that is causing the staining. Two such autoantibodies that are highly specific for SLE are anti-double-stranded DNA (dsDNA) antibodies and anti-Smith (anti-Sm) antibodies. There are also a host of additional specific antinuclear and cytoplasmic antibodies (anti-Ro, or anti–SS-A; anti-La, or anti–SS-B; anti-RNP; and anti-RA33, to name a few) that may indicate a predisposition to specific SLE manifestations or suggest the presence of another autoimmune disease (for instance, Sjögren syndrome is associated with anti–SS-A and anti–SS-B).

Unfortunately, ANA testing is often done to screen for disease in patients with little likelihood of having SLE (such as uveitis patients with no systemic symptoms). The test is very nonspecific under these circumstances. False-positive ANAs are commonly found in the normal population; 1 study found that 32% of individuals without SLE had an ANA titer above 1:40. The combination of very low titers of antibody (<1:80) and no signs or symptoms of disease suggests that the patient should simply be monitored.

SLE can run a varied clinical course, ranging from a relatively benign illness to fulminant organ failure and death. Most patients have a relapsing and remitting course that requires frequent titration of medications. Treatment depends on disease severity and may include NSAIDs, hydroxychloroquine (Plaquenil), glucocorticoids, and immunosuppressive drugs. Refractory cases may require high-dose pulse therapy with glucocorticoids and cyclophosphamide (Cytoxan). Experimental treatments include immunoablation, with or without hematopoetic stem cell transplantation, and anti–B-cell antibodies. Such treatments are reserved for life-threatening disease that is unresponsive to standard measures.

Ophthalmic Considerations

The major ocular manifestations of SLE include discoid lesions of the skin of the eyelids, keratitis sicca from secondary Sjögren syndrome, and retinal and choroidal microvascular lesions. Retinal lesions include cotton-wool spots, hemorrhages, vascular occlusions, and neovascularization. The prevalence of retinal vascular manifestations varies from 3% of outpatients with mild disease to 29% of hospitalized patients with more active disease. The inflammatory vasculopathy of SLE should be distinguished from vascular damage due to secondary problems such as hypertension from renal disease or occlusions due to embolic disease or antiphospholipid antibodies. Typical anterior or intermediate uveitis is not a common feature of SLE. Neuro-ophthalmic involvement in SLE includes cranial nerve palsies, lupus optic neuropathy, and central retrochiasmal disorders of vision. The cerebral disorders of vision include hallucinations, visual field defects, and cortical blindness.

Antiphospholipid Antibody Syndrome

The *antiphospholipid antibody syndrome (APS)* is a potential cause of vascular thrombosis. The diagnosis of APS requires the presence of both clinical and laboratory findings, specifically, by fulfilling 1 of the clinical and 1 of the laboratory criteria. The clinical features include 1 or more episodes of arterial and/or venous thrombosis or complications of pregnancy such as fetal death, spontaneous abortions without a maternal cause, and premature births. Laboratory criteria include anticardiolipin IgG or IgM antibodies present at moderate to high levels and/or lupus anticoagulant activity. Abnormalities in lab tests must be detected on at least 2 different occasions at least 12 weeks apart.

Antiphospholipid antibody syndrome can occur in association with SLE and other rheumatic diseases, and it can be caused by certain infections and drugs. It is referred to as the *primary antiphospholipid antibody syndrome* when it occurs alone. The main clinical manifestation is venous and arterial thrombosis. Deep venous thrombosis is the most common type of thrombosis, occurring in approximately one third of patients. Patients may also have pulmonary embolism and superficial thrombophlebitis. Central nervous system disease can include strokes, transient ischemic attacks, dementia, and even psychosis. Antiphospholipid antibody syndrome should be considered when cerebrovascular disease occurs in a young patient without other risk factors for stroke.

Ophthalmic Considerations

Ocular manifestations of scleroderma include eyelid involvement resulting in tightness and blepharophimosis (but only rarely corneal exposure); conjunctival vascular abnormalities, including telangiectasia and vascular sludging; and keratoconjunctivitis sicca. Patchy choroidal nonperfusion can be seen on fluorescein angiography as part of the diffuse microvascular damage caused by scleroderma. Occasionally, a patient develops retinopathy of malignant hypertension, with cotton-wool spots, intraretinal hemorrhages, and optic disc edema, as a result of scleroderma renal crisis.

Sjögren Syndrome

Sjögren syndrome was originally described as a triad of dry eyes, dry mouth, and RA. Subsequently, it became apparent that Sjögren syndrome could coexist with a variety of other connective tissue diseases, including SLE and scleroderma (secondary Sjögren syndrome) or without a definable connective tissue disease (primary Sjögren syndrome).

The dry eyes and dry mouth in patients with Sjögren syndrome is the result of an inflammatory mononuclear infiltrate involving the lacrimal and salivary glands that causes glandular destruction and dysfunction. Several studies have demonstrated the usefulness of minor salivary gland biopsy in documenting the presence of such an inflammatory infiltrate. Patients with Sjögren syndrome often have autoantibodies known as anti–SS-A and anti–SS-B. Criteria for the diagnosis of Sjögren syndrome have been published, including parameters referring to oral and ocular symptoms, ocular signs, salivary gland involvement, histopathologic features, and the presence of autoantibodies anti–SS-A and anti–SS-B (Table 8-2). The presence of 4 of 6 items confers high sensitivity and specificity. Patients with primary Sjögren syndrome may have a number of possible systemic manifestations that extend far beyond dry eyes and mouth, including upper-airway dryness and mucous plugs, purpuric vasculitis, hyperglobulinemia, CNS inflammation that may mimic multiple sclerosis, psychiatric problems, and an increased risk of lymphoma. Treatment is aimed at symptomatic relief and substitution of the missing secretions, although immunosuppression may be necessary for patients with systemic manifestations. (See also BCSC Section 8, *External Disease and Cornea*.)

Polymyositis and Dermatomyositis

Polymyositis and dermatomyositis are inflammatory diseases of skeletal muscle characterized by pain and weakness in the involved muscular groups. Typically, weakness begins insidiously and involves the proximal muscle groups, particularly those of the shoulders and hips. *Dermatomyositis* is distinguished from *polymyositis* by the presence of cutaneous lesions. These skin lesions are an erythematous to violaceous rash variably affecting the eyelids (heliotrope rash), cheeks, nose, chest (V-neck sign), and extensor surfaces (Gottron sign). Pathogenically, dermatomyositis is associated with immune complex deposition in the vessels; whereas polymyositis appears to reflect direct T cell–mediated muscle injury. Laboratory findings include elevated serum levels of skeletal muscle enzymes and abnormal electromyography results; also, muscle damage and inflammation may be re-

Scleroderma

Scleroderma, also known as *progressive systemic sclerosis,* is a rheumatic disease characterized by fibrous and degenerative changes in the viscera, skin, or both. The disease seems to be mediated by the activation of fibroblasts that produce excessive fibrosis, but the mechanism by which this occurs is not understood. Scleroderma is much more common in women and rare in childhood. The disorder may be localized (confined to the skin, subcutaneous tissue, and muscle) or systemic (which may be diffuse or limited). Localized scleroderma is not a severe illness and may allow a normal life span. The limited form of systemic scleroderma, known as *CREST* (*c*alcinosis, *R*aynaud phenomenon, *e*sophageal involvement, *s*clerodactyly, and *t*elangiectasias), involves internal organs less frequently and therefore carries a better prognosis than does the diffuse form.

In addition to the thickening and fibrous replacement of the dermis, scleroderma is characterized by vascular insufficiency and vasospasm. The hallmark of scleroderma is the skin change, which consists of thickening, tightening, and induration, with subsequent loss of mobility and contracture. The disease most characteristically begins peripherally and involves the fingers and hands, with a subsequent centripetal spread up the arms to involve the face and body. Telangiectasia and calcinosis (calcium phosphate nodules under the skin) are common. More than 95% of scleroderma patients experience Raynaud phenomenon (see Fig 8-1). Although Raynaud phenomenon usually represents reversible vasospasm, in scleroderma, episodes may be prolonged, and the structure of vessels is permanently altered, possibly leading to digital ulcers or infarcts.

Organ involvement is common and includes esophageal dysmotility with gastroesophageal reflux in more than 90% of patients. The small and large intestines may be involved, with decreased motility, malabsorption, and diverticulosis. Cardiopulmonary disease is manifested primarily by pulmonary fibrosis, which results in restrictive lung disease with a decreased diffusing capacity. The consequences of the interstitial fibrosis include pulmonary hypertension and right-sided heart failure. Conduction abnormalities and arrhythmias result from cardiac fibrosis. Musculoskeletal features include polyarthralgias, tendon friction rubs, and occasionally myositis. There is no known cure for the disease, and treatment is largely directed toward controlling problems related to the organ systems that are involved.

Most patients with scleroderma have positive ANA test results. It was thought that certain antinuclear staining patterns were fairly specific for scleroderma (such as the nucleolar pattern), but it is now recognized that these are not especially sensitive or specific. Instead, testing is done looking for specific ANAs such as anti-centromere, anti-topoisomerase I (anti-Scl-70), and anti-RNA polymerase. These tests can help with the diagnosis and may help identify various syndromes that overlap with scleroderma. The best-known overlap syndrome is *mixed connective tissue disease,* which has features of SLE, systemic sclerosis, and myositis. This syndrome is characterized by autoantibodies directed at U1-ribonucleoprotein complex.

Renal disease is a major cause of mortality and is often associated with the onset of malignant hypertension and a rapid progression to renal failure *(scleroderma renal crisis).* This complication was uniformly fatal until the late 1970s, when aggressive antihypertensive therapy was found to be able to sometimes reverse the scleroderma renal crisis.

coagulation system is demonstrated by the apparent paradox of lupus anticoagulants. The in vitro effect of these substances results in inhibition of clotting, yet in vivo the effect is to enhance thrombosis. A number of mechanisms have been postulated for the procoagulant effect. One possibility is that antiphospholipid antibodies may interfere with the normal anticoagulant effect of beta 2-glycoprotein I and lead to spontaneous thrombosis.

Ophthalmic Considerations

Ophthalmic manifestations of APS include amaurosis fugax, ischemic optic neuropathy, and retinal and choroidal vascular occlusion. Visual field loss, diplopia, and even proliferative retinopathy have also been reported. Some studies have suggested that the prevalence of antiphospholipid antibodies is increased in patients with retinal vaso-occlusive disease, but it is difficult to assign a definite causative etiology, given the prevalence of antiphospholipid antibodies in the population without APS. Furthermore, in a study looking for ophthalmic findings in a population of patients with known APS, there were no patients with definite vaso-occlusive disease, and only 13% of patients had identifiable changes, which largely consisted of mild retinopathy. Patients in this series were more likely to have visual symptoms from neurologic disease.

Although a high index of suspicion for APS should be maintained, it should be recognized that testing for this entity may lead to false-positive results and it may be difficult to determine if a cause-and-effect relationship truly exists. This is important because treatment of APS may include long-term anticoagulation, which carries a significant risk, and it may be very difficult for a consulting specialist to determine if an isolated ophthalmic vascular occlusion represents the type of thrombotic episode that warrants such treatment. In such cases, it has been proposed that repeatedly positive levels of antiphospholipid antibodies suggest the presence of APS. More studies are needed to determine the prevalence of ophthalmic disease in APS, as well as the significance of positive lab test results in patients with ocular vaso-occlusive disease without systemic features of APS.

Treatment

Therapy for thrombosis usually consists of heparin, followed by warfarin (Coumadin). The optimal duration of treatment is not known. Some experts feel that anticoagulation can be discontinued if the antiphospholipid antibody titers decrease, but lifelong treatment is recommended for patients with recurrent disease. Treatment of the pregnant patient remains controversial and may include some combination of heparin or low-molecular-weight heparin and aspirin (warfarin is teratogenic). Patients with antiphospholipid antibodies but no prior history of thrombosis may benefit from prophylactic aspirin.

Behbehani R, Sergott RC, Savino PJ. The antiphospholipid antibody syndrome: diagnostic aspects. *Curr Opin Ophthalmol.* 2004;15(6):483–485.

Episodes of thrombosis can be recurrent, and this recurrence may be more likely in patients with high antiphospholipid antibody titers. Additional manifestations of APS include thrombocytopenia, hemolytic anemia, and livedo reticularis. Cardiac manifestations include valvular thickening and vegetations, both of which are caused by thrombotic endocardial deposits. This syndrome can also cause significant problems with pregnancy. Patients may have multiple first-trimester abortions and premature births due to pre-eclampsia or placental insufficiency, and fetal death may occur after 10 weeks. Rarely, a severe form of APS can occur with multiple vessel occlusion and multiorgan failure. This is referred to as *catastrophic antiphospholipid syndrome* and carries a mortality rate of 48%.

Diagnosis

Testing for antiphospholipid antibodies can be divided into 2 broad categories: tests for anticardiolipin antibodies and tests for lupus anticoagulants. Anticardiolipin antibodies are 1 type of antiphospholipid antibody; usually both IgG and IgM antibodies are looked for in testing, with medium to high levels being more clinically significant. Perhaps 5%–10% of blood donors without APS may have some level of positive anticardiolipin antibodies, and this percentage can be higher among elderly donors. However, repeatedly positive results are required for the diagnosis of APS, and less than 2% of the normal population remained positive for a period of 9 months in 1 study. Antiphospholipid antibodies also occur in association with other conditions, such as infections or cancer, and with the use of some drugs. In these cases, the antibodies are present at low levels and are not usually associated with thrombotic events.

In addition to tests for anticardiolipin antibodies, other tests for antiphospholipid antibodies include a false-positive serology for syphilis, tests for antiphosphatidylserine antibodies, and tests for antibodies to the plasma protein beta 2-glycoprotein I, which is a phospholipid-binding inhibitor of coagulation. The risk of thrombosis may increase with both the absolute level of antiphospholipid antibodies and the number of different antibodies. There is an ongoing effort to standardize the various assays between labs and to identify the most clinically relevant types of antiphospholipid antibodies.

Testing for lupus anticoagulant activity involves looking for evidence of a functional inhibition of clotting. In other words, testing for antiphospholipid antibodies will simply indicate that such antibodies are present. Testing for lupus anticoagulant activity determines if the antibodies have an identifiable effect on phospholipid-dependent clotting pathways. With lupus anticoagulant positivity, there seems to be a somewhat greater risk for thrombosis than with isolated antiphospholipid positivity. Lupus anticoagulants will prolong in vitro clotting assays such as the activated partial thromboplastin time (aPTT), the dilute Russell viper venom time (dRVVT), the kaolin plasma clotting time (KCT), and rarely the prothrombin time. More than 1 test for lupus anticoagulant is often needed because patients with negative test results for one test may have positive results for another.

The antibodies detected by assays for antiphospholipid antibodies may or may not be the same antibodies responsible for lupus anticoagulant activity—hence the need to perform both types of testing when the disease is suspected. The remarkable complexity of the

Table 8-2 Preliminary Criteria for the Classification of Sjögren Syndrome*

1. Ocular symptoms
   A positive response to at least 1 of the following 3 questions:
   (a) Have you had daily, persistent, troublesome dry eyes for more than 3 months?
   (b) Do you have recurrent sandy or gravelly feeling in the eyes?
   (c) Do you use tear substitutes more than 3 times a day?
2. Oral symptoms
   A positive response to at least 1 of the following 3 questions:
   (a) Have you had a daily feeling of dry mouth for more than 3 months?
   (b) Have you had recurrent or persistently swollen salivary glands as an adult?
   (c) Do you frequently drink liquids to aid in swallowing dry foods?
3. Ocular signs
   Objective evidence of ocular involvement determined on the basis of a positive result on at least 1 of the following 2 tests:
   (a) Schirmer-1 test (≤5 mm in 5 minutes)
   (b) Rose bengal score (≥4, according to the van Bijsterveld scoring system)
4. Salivary gland involvement
   Objective evidence of salivary gland involvement, determined on the basis of a positive result on at least 1 of the following 3 tests:
   (a) Salivary scintigraphy
   (b) Parotid sialography
   (c) Unstimulated salivary flow (≤1.5 mL in 15 minutes)
5. Histopathologic findings
   Focus score ≥1 on minor salivary gland biopsy
   (focus defined as an agglomeration of at least 50 mononuclear cells, focus score defined as the number of foci/4 mm^2 of glandular tissue)
6. Autoantibodies
   Presence of at least 1 of the following autoantibodies in the serum: Antibodies to Ro (SS-A) or La (SS-B) antigens or antinuclear antibodies or rheumatoid factor

*A patient is considered as having probable Sjögren syndrome if 3 of 6 criteria are present, and as definite if 4 of 6 criteria are present.

vealed by muscle biopsy. These entities may be primary, or they may arise in association with a malignancy. They may also overlap with other connective tissue diseases, such as in mixed connective tissue disease, which has features of scleroderma, SLE, and myositis.

Ocular involvement is relatively uncommon in inflammatory myositis, other than the heliotrope rash of dermatomyositis, which is very specific but not often present (Fig 8-2). Occasionally, ophthalmoplegia may occur because of involvement of the extraocular muscles, which myositis can provoke.

Relapsing Polychondritis

Relapsing polychondritis is an episodic autoimmune disorder characterized by recurrent, widespread, potentially destructive inflammation of cartilage, the cardiovascular system, and the organs of special sense. The most common clinical features are auricular inflammation, arthropathy, and nasal cartilage inflammation. Auricular chondritis and nasal chondritis are the features that most often suggest the diagnosis. Laryngotracheobronchial disease may lead to a fatal complication from laryngeal collapse. Involvement of the internal ear, cardiovascular system, and skin is less common. Cardiovascular lesions

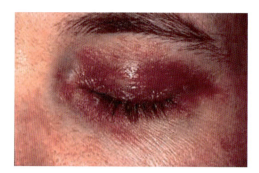

Figure 8-2 Heliotrope rash in dermatomyositis. A reddish-purple eruption on the upper eyelid (the heliotrope rash), accompanied by swelling of the eyelid in a patient with dermatomyositis. This is the most specific rash in DM, although it is only present in a minority of patients. *(Reproduced with permission from Miller ML, MD. Clinical manifestations and diagnosis of adult dermatomyositis and polymyositis. Image from UpToDate.)*

include aortic insufficiency (due to progressive dilation of the aortic root) and vasculitis. Skin lesions are most often due to cutaneous vasculitis.

This disease can be associated with other autoimmune diseases such as SLE or RA or with any of the systemic vasculitides, such as Wegener granulomatosis, polyarteritis nodosa, and Behçet disease. Other associations include Sjögren syndrome, Graves disease, and myelodysplastic syndromes (dysplastic and ineffective blood cell production due to malignant stem cells). Ocular manifestations occur in approximately 50% of patients with relapsing polychondritis. The most common ocular conditions are conjunctivitis, scleritis, uveitis, and retinal vasculitis.

Vasculitis

The primary systemic vasculitides are a group of diseases whose principal pathology involves autoimmune damage to blood vessels. The classification of these entities is largely based on the size of the vessel involved and the various clinical features. Table 8-3 outlines the definitions created by the Chapel Hill Consensus Conference on these diseases. A number of other diseases are capable of causing vasculitis as part of their clinical spectrum, and these are considered to be secondary vasculitides. Secondary causes of vasculitis include exogenous factors such as infections, neoplasia, or use of certain drugs. Secondary vasculitis can also occur as part of other autoimmune disorders such as SLE or Behçet's disease. This section will emphasize the primary vasculitides that are more likely to have ophthalmic involvement.

Large Vessel Vasculitis

Giant cell (temporal) arteritis
Giant cell arteritis (GCA) has been described in all races, although whites are most often affected. It is a disease of the elderly, rarely occurring in patients younger than age 50. It is particularly common in northern European countries, such as Scandinavia, and in the

Table 8-3 **Names and Definitions of Vasculitides Adopted by the Chapel Hill Consensus Conference on the Nomenclature of Systemic Vasculitis**

Name	Definition
Large vessel vasculitis[a]	
Giant cell (temporal) arteritis	Granulomatous arteritis of the aorta and its major branches, with a predilection for the extracranial branches of the carotid artery. *Often involves the temporal artery. Usually occurs in patients older than 50 and often is associated with polymyalgia rheumatica.*
Takayasu arteritis	Granulomatous inflammation of the aorta and its major branches. *Usually occurs in patients younger than 50.*
Medium-sized vessel vasculitis	
Polyarteritis nodosa[b]	Necrotizing inflammation of medium-sized or small arteries without glomerulonephritis or vasculitis in arterioles, capillaries, or venules.
Kawasaki disease	Arteritis involving large, medium-sized, and small arteries, and associated with mucocutaneous lymph node syndrome. *Coronary arteries are often involved. Aorta and veins may be involved. Usually occurs in children.*
Small vessel vasculitis	
Wegener granulomatosis[c]	Granulomatous inflammation involving the respiratory tract, and necrotizing vasculitis, affecting small to medium-sized vessels. *Necrotizing glomerulonephritis is common.*
Churg-Strauss syndrome[c]	Eosinophil-rich and granulomatous inflammation involving the respiratory tract, and necrotizing vasculitis affecting small to medium-sized vessels, and associated with asthma and eosinophilia.
Microscopic polyangiitis[b] (microscopic polyarteritis)[c]	Necrotizing vasculitis, with few or no immune deposits, affecting small vessels (ie, capillaries, venules, or arterioles). *Necrotizing arteritis involving small and medium-sized arteries may be present. Necrotizing glomerulonephritis is very common. Pulmonary capillaritis often occurs.*
Henoch-Schönlein purpura	Vasculitis, with IgA-dominant immune deposits, affecting small vessels (ie, capillaries, venules, or arterioles). *Typically involves skin, gut, and glomeruli, and is associated with arthralgias or arthritis.*
Essential cryoglobulinemic vasculitis	Vasculitis, with cryoglobulin immune deposits, affecting small vessels (ie, capillaries, venules, or arterioles), and associated with cryoglobulins in serum. *Skin and glomeruli are often involved.*
Cutaneous leukocytoclastic angiitis	Isolated cutaneous leukocytoclastic angiitis without systemic vasculitis or glomerulonephritis.

[a]Large vessel refers to the aorta and the largest branches directed toward major body regions (eg, to the extremities and the head and neck); medium-sized vessel refers to the main visceral arteries (eg, renal, hepatic, coronary, and mesenteric arteries); small vessel refers to venules, capillaries, arterioles, and the intraparenchymal distal arterial radicals that connect the arterioles. Some small and large vessel vasculitides may involve medium-sized arteries, but large and medium-sized vessel vasculitides do not involve vessels smaller than arteries. Essential components are represented by normal type; italicized type represents usual, but not essential, components.
[b]Preferred term.
[c]Strongly associated with antineutrophil cytoplasmic autoantibodies.

Reprinted with permission from Jennette JC, Falk RJ, Andrassy K, et al. Nomenclature of systemic vasculitides. Proposal of an international consensus conference. *Arthritis Rheum.* 1994;37(2):187–192.

northern United States. Autopsy studies in Scandinavia have estimated the prevalence of GCA at 1.1% of the population.

The clinical features of GCA include headache, polymyalgia rheumatica, jaw claudication, constitutional symptoms such as fever and malaise, and ophthalmic symptoms. The signs of GCA include tenderness over the temporal artery, a pulseless temporal artery, scalp tenderness, fever, and loss of vision. Polymyalgia rheumatica is a symptom complex of proximal muscle pain and weakness that may occur by itself without overt GCA.

The most common abnormal laboratory result in GCA is an elevated erythrocyte sedimentation rate (ESR). C-reactive protein (CRP) is another acute phase reactant that appears to have a strong predictive value in identifying patients with GCA. A common formula to determine the upper normative value for the ESR is [age]/2 for males and [age + 10]/2 for females. Unfortunately, studies suggest that perhaps 15% of patients with GCA may have a normal ESR; obtaining both an ESR and CRP may be more sensitive, but at times the diagnosis may depend largely on clinical suspicion. Other laboratory findings that may occur include anemia and elevated fibrinogen and plasma factor VIII levels. Reactive thrombocytosis can also be seen in GCA, and an elevated platelet count greater than $400 \times 10^3/\mu L$ is predictive of positive results for a temporal artery biopsy.

Even with strongly supportive lab work, a temporal artery biopsy is suggested for all cases of suspected GCA because it is the definitive test for this disease. Treatment should not be delayed pending biopsy results, however. It is acceptable to obtain a biopsy within a week of starting treatment because the characteristic pathologic findings persist. A specimen at least 3–6 cm long should be obtained to minimize the risk of a false-negative result. A contralateral biopsy may be necessary if the clinical suspicion is high but the result of the first biopsy is negative.

If untreated, GCA can cause blindness. Thus, treatment with systemic corticosteroids should be initiated as soon as the diagnosis is suspected. The initial oral prednisone dosage is approximately 1 mg/kg/day (60–80 mg daily), although some experts feel that an intravenous methylprednisolone dosage of 1 gram a day for 3–5 days should be used initially in cases of vision loss. There are as yet no prospective controlled trials to define whether oral or IV treatment is best. Generally, the symptoms respond promptly within several days. Alternate-day steroids are ineffective in the initial treatment of GCA.

Some studies have suggested that GCA is a self-limited disease that will run its course in 1–2 years. These studies recommend continuing therapy for 1–2 years. Treatment is generally instituted at the initial high dose. Using the ESR and clinical symptoms to monitor disease, the physician may taper the corticosteroid dose. Patients may require extended treatment and the use of other immunosuppressive agents to minimize the complications of long-term corticosteroid use.

Ophthalmic considerations   The most frequent ocular manifestation of GCA is ischemic optic neuropathy. Other ocular manifestations include amaurosis fugax, ischemic retinopathy, ocular ischemic syndrome, choroidal ischemia, and cortical blindness. Diplopia, ophthalmoplegia, or both may occur because of ischemia of the extraocular muscles. (Ocular involvement with GCA is discussed in BCSC Section 5, *Neuro-Ophthalmology*.)

Takayasu arteritis

Takayasu arteritis affects large arteries, particularly branches of the aorta. It occurs primarily in children and young women. The disease is rare in the West but common in the Far East, particularly Japan. Other names for Takayasu arteritis include *aortic arch arteritis, aortitis syndrome,* and *pulseless disease.*

The disease may involve the entire aorta or be localized to any segment of the aorta or its primary branches. The inflammatory process is characterized by a panarteritis with a granulomatous inflammation. The involved vessels may ultimately become narrowed or obliterated, resulting in ischemia to the supplied tissues. Areas of weakened vascular wall may develop dissections or aneurysms.

Systemic features such as fatigue, weight loss, or low-grade fever are common. Evidence of vascular insufficiency due to large-artery narrowing leads to the characteristic pulseless phase. The disease is most often diagnosed via arteriography. Treatment is generally with systemic corticosteroids, which may successfully suppress the disease. Cyclophosphamide or methotrexate is added in resistant cases. Surgical reconstruction of damaged vessels may be necessary.

Ophthalmic considerations Patients may report transient visual disturbances and blindness due to decreased perfusion. The most characteristic ocular findings are retinal arteriovenous anastomoses, best demonstrated by fluorescein angiography. Earlier in the course of the disease, milder changes are small-vessel dilation and microaneurysm formation; more severe ischemia may result in peripheral retinal nonperfusion, iris and retinal neovascularization, and vitreous hemorrhage.

Medium-sized Vessel Vasculitis

Polyarteritis nodosa

Classic *polyarteritis nodosa (PAN)* is characterized by necrotizing vasculitis of the medium-sized and small muscular arteries. The lesions are segmental, and aneurysms may develop, which can be detected by angiography. One of the most common presenting symptoms is mononeuritis multiplex, which is simultaneous or sequential ischemic damage to anatomically unrelated peripheral nerves. Central nervous system lesions can also occur. Renal involvement is common, and hypertension develops as a consequence of the renal disease. Gastrointestinal disease with infarction of the viscera is also common. Polyarteritis nodosa may be limited to a single organ such as the appendix, uterus, or testes. It may be triggered by hepatitis B.

The mean age of onset of PAN is 40–50 years, and men are affected more often than women. Survival in patients with untreated PAN is poor. However, most patients are now treated with a combination of corticosteroids and an immunosuppressive drug such as cyclophosphamide, and this therapy appears to improve disease control and long-term outcome.

Ocular manifestations occur in approximately 10%–20% of patients with PAN and include hypertensive retinopathy, retinal vasculitis, and visual field loss from CNS lesions. Cranial nerve palsies can occur, as well as scleritis and marginal corneal ulceration.

Choroidal vasculitis is often overlooked in PAN and may cause transient visual symptoms, exudative retinal detachments, and pigment changes. Fluorescein angiography may be necessary to identify choroidal involvement. *Cogan syndrome,* manifested by interstitial keratitis, hearing loss, tinnitus, and vertigo, may be associated with PAN (see also BCSC Section 8, *External Disease and Cornea*). There is no specific test to diagnose PAN. Rather, the diagnosis depends on characteristic clinical features, angiographic findings, and biopsy results. Results of hepatitis B studies may be positive in a subset of patients.

Small Vessel Vasculitis

Wegener granulomatosis

Wegener granulomatosis was originally described as the classic triad of necrotizing granulomatous vasculitis of both the upper respiratory tract and the lower respiratory tract and focal segmental glomerulonephritis. The clinical features of Wegener granulomatosis include granulomatous inflammation of the paranasal sinuses in 90% of cases, nasopharyngeal disease in 63%, cutaneous vasculitis in 45%, and vasculitis affecting the nervous system in 25%. Ocular disease occurs in up to 60% of patients with Wegener granulomatosis and may be the presenting feature. Ocular findings include scleritis with or without peripheral keratitis, orbital pseudotumor, and vasculitis-mediated retinal vascular or neuro-ophthalmic lesions. Limited forms of the disease may occur without significant systemic involvement and may be difficult to diagnose. Approximately 80% of patients with Wegener granulomatosis are serum positive for a cytoplasmic pattern of antineutrophil cytoplasmic antibodies (c-ANCA). As this cytoplasmic pattern is usually caused by the presence of autoantibodies to proteinase 3, the specificity of positive findings for c-ANCA may be enhanced by testing for these antibodies. (See also BCSC Section 7, *Orbit, Eyelids, and Lacrimal System,* and BCSC Section 9, *Intraocular Inflammation and Uveitis.*)

Before immunosuppressive drugs were used as treatment of Wegener granulomatosis, the disease was uniformly fatal, with a mean untreated survival rate of 5 months. With corticosteroid treatment, the mean survival time increased to 12.5 months; long-term survival occurred only in patients with limited disease. However, the use of cytotoxic drugs, especially cyclophosphamide (Cytoxan), has dramatically improved the outcome for patients with Wegener granulomatosis. Once the disease is controlled, it may be possible to switch to safer immunosuppressive agents such as methotrexate. Trimethoprim-sulfamethoxazole (Bactrim, Septra) may also be helpful in preventing relapses.

Microscopic polyangiitis is a systemic necrotizing vasculitis affecting small vessels and associated with necrotizing glomerulonephritis. It is felt by some investigators to be part of a spectrum of Wegener granulomatosis. Characteristic features include constitutional symptoms, renal disease, pulmonary involvement, arthralgias, rash, and neuropathy. Patients with microscopic polyangiitis often have positive findings for ANCA, with peripheral staining around the nucleus (p-ANCA). This particular staining pattern is nonspecific and needs to be confirmed by testing for autoantibodies to myeloperoxidase (MPO-ANCA). Peripheral ulcerative keratitis may be a presenting feature of this entity.

Churg-Strauss syndrome

An allergic diathesis, particularly asthma, is present in Churg-Strauss syndrome (CSS) (allergic granulomatosis and angiitis). Eosinophilia is generally present, often before the disease manifests, and pathological examination often shows granulomas with eosinophilic tissue infiltration of smaller vessels. The disease tends to overlap both PAN and Wegener granulomatosis. Asthma is the principal feature of the disease, and the systemic vasculitis may, in addition, involve the heart, skin, kidneys, and gastrointestinal tract. Central nervous system disease may also occur, and mononeuritis multiplex is common. Ophthalmic manifestations include conjunctival granulomas, retinal vasculitis and occlusion, uveitis, and cranial nerve palsies. The diagnosis depends on the presence of several criteria, including asthma, eosinophilia, eosinophilic vasculitis, transient pulmonary infiltrates, and neuropathy. Patients with CSS may also have positive p-ANCA titers.

Behçet Syndrome

Behçet syndrome was initially described as a triad of oral ulcers, genital ulcers, and uveitis with hypopyon. It is now recognized as a multisystem vasculitis of unknown etiology with various clinical manifestations. The disease is most common in the Middle East and Far East, particularly Japan. Oral ulcers are the most common clinical feature, affecting 98%–99% of patients. Genital ulcers occur in 80%–87%; skin disease occurs in 69%–90% and includes erythema nodosum, superficial thrombophlebitis, and pyoderma. Pathergy (pustular response to skin injury) and dermatographism can also be seen. Some 44%–59% of patients have asymmetrical, nondeforming, large-joint polyarthritis that frequently responds to steroids.

Vascular disease, which occurs in 10%–35% of patients, can present as migratory superficial thrombophlebitis, major vessel thrombosis, arterial aneurysms, or even peripheral gangrene. Central nervous system disease, found in 10%–30% of patients, classically has been divided into 3 types: brain stem syndrome, meningoencephalitis, and confusional states. Most often, patients present with combinations of the three. The major cause of mortality in Behçet syndrome is CNS involvement or large vessel disease.

A number of nonspecific abnormalities in laboratory findings may be seen in these patients, including an elevated ESR, C-reactive protein, and circulating immune complexes. Patients may also have serologic evidence of a hypercoagulable state and elevated levels of intracellular adhesion moleclule-1. The prevalence of HLA-B51 is also greater in some populations with Behçet syndrome. However, there are no specific laboratory tests that define Behçet disease. The diagnosis is based on the patient's meeting clinical criteria that include oral ulcers and any 2 of the following: uveitis, genital ulcers, skin involvement, or pathergy. Other criteria may be used, depending on regional differences in disease presentation.

Treatment

The clinical impression of most authors is that the use of corticosteroids alone may control acute exacerbations but does not seem to alter the ultimate outcome of this disease. As a result, 1 or more immunosuppressive agents are usually used as therapy, in addition to the corticosteroids. Unfortunately, there are many small studies that suggest but do not prove the effectiveness of various agents, and there is a paucity of large well-controlled trials to guide the choice of therapy. Common treatments include use of drugs such as azathioprine (Imuran) and cyclosporine (Neoral, Sandimmune), although there may be an increased risk of inducing CNS disease with use of cyclosporine. Alkylating agents such as cyclophosphamide (Cytoxan) and chlorambucil (Leukeran) may be used in refractory cases, although these drugs may have significant toxicity. Newer agents that may hold promise include infliximab (Remicade) and interferon alfa-2a (Roferon-A), especially for treatment of ophthalmic disease.

Ophthalmic Considerations

Ophthalmic disease is a significant cause of morbidity in Behçet syndrome, with the most common ocular manifestations being iridocyclitis, with or without hypopyon, and retinal vasculitis. The natural history of retinal vasculitis in Behçet syndrome is poor. The majority of untreated patients lose all or part of their vision within 5 years of onset. See also BCSC Section 9, *Intraocular Inflammation and Uveitis*.

Medical Therapy for Rheumatic Disorders

Medications are used for analgesia, an anti-inflammatory effect, and immunosuppression. These drugs and their use in treating ocular inflammatory diseases are also discussed in BCSC Section 9, *Intraocular Inflammation and Uveitis*.

Corticosteroids

Although the overall anti-inflammatory effect of glucocorticoids is the result of a number of mechanisms, one important action involves the inhibition of prostaglandin synthesis. This inhibition results from preventing the release of the prostaglandin precursor arachidonic acid from membrane phospholipids. Glucocorticoids have a variety of other effects in addition to their anti-inflammatory activity. Gluconeogenesis is promoted, with a concomitant negative nitrogen balance and reduction in protein production. Fat oxidation, synthesis, storage, and mobilization are also affected. The number of circulating neutrophils increases because mature neutrophils are released from bone marrow and their movement from blood to other tissues decreases, while the number of other circulating leukocytes decreases after glucocorticoid administration. Associated mineralocorticoid activity increases sodium retention and potassium excretion.

The molecular structure of the steroid nucleus can be modified to dissociate glucocorticoid from mineralocorticoid activity. Unfortunately, the goal of dissociating beneficial anti-inflammatory effects from the harmful side effects of glucocorticoid activity has not been achieved. The ophthalmologist must be aware of both ocular and systemic toxicity in patients who are receiving systemic steroids. Ocular adverse effects of systemic steroids include posterior subcapsular cataracts, glaucoma, mydriasis, ptosis, papilledema associated with pseudotumor cerebri, reactivation or aggravation of ocular infection, and delay of wound healing. Systemic complications may include peptic ulceration, osteoporosis, aseptic necrosis of the femoral head, and muscle and skin atrophy. Hyperglycemia, hypertension, edema, weight gain, and changes in body fat distribution resulting in cushingoid habitus can occur. Other adverse effects include hyperosmolar nonketotic coma, hypokalemia, and growth retardation in children. Mental changes are a common problem and may range from mild mood alterations to severe psychological reactions. Psychological dependence may also occur with use of glucocorticoids, particularly in those patients who have been given repeated courses of therapy for recurring problems such as asthma or certain dermatologic conditions.

Osteoporosis is a particularly insidious problem that may increase the risk of fractures as early as a few months after beginning treatment with steroids. In the past, little could be done to prevent this, but today, there are several approaches that can help minimize the risk: Bone mineral density testing can be done to assess the degree of osteoporosis. Patients can be treated with calcium and vitamin D supplementation. More sophisticated interventions include hormone replacement therapy or use of nasal calcitonin supplements or bisphosphonates. Specialty consultation should be obtained to optimize the identification and management of this disease.

Another frequently overlooked complication of systemic steroid therapy is rapid withdrawal. The rate of steroid withdrawal should be determined by the degree of hypothalamic-pituitary-adrenal (HPA) suppression, which, in turn, is related to dose and duration of therapy, as well as by the response of the underlying disease to the steroid withdrawal. A variety of schedules have been suggested. Glucocorticoids given in large doses for 1–3 days probably suppress HPA function only temporarily, so they can be withdrawn suddenly or gradually over 1 week. After 1 or more months of treatment, a dosage-reduction protocol is usually followed. Otherwise, sudden withdrawal of steroid therapy may result in adrenal insufficiency, with symptoms such as fatigue, weakness, arthralgias, nausea, orthostatic hypotension, and hypoglycemia. In severe cases, adrenal suppression may be fatal. After steroid therapy has been discontinued, adrenal function may not return to normal for 1 year or more; thus, supplementary steroids may be needed if the patient has a serious illness or undergoes surgery during this recovery period. Because of the likelihood of withdrawal symptoms, even physiologic doses of long-term steroids (5 mg of prednisone a day) should be gradually reduced.

Ophthalmologists may have occasion to initiate steroid therapy for ophthalmic diseases, and ideally they should do so with the assistance of their patients' general medical doctors, given the need to monitor patients for these potential problems. It is easy for the physician to become complacent with the use of corticosteroids because of their effectiveness and relative ease of use to control symptoms. However, studies have shown that a dosage as low as 5 mg a day is associated with increased adverse events over time. For patients who seem to require high or extended doses of steroids, clinicians should strongly consider early use of other immunosuppressive medications, which can decrease patient dependency on steroids. The ophthalmologist may need to be responsible for initiating this discussion if the steroids are being used to treat localized ocular disease. The other physicians involved in the patient's care may be unaware of or uninterested in making relatively onerous changes in the management of a disease viewed as being in the ophthalmologist's "turf."

Cervantes RA, Kump LI, Neer RM, et al. Glucocorticoid-induced osteoporosis: considerations in ophthalmology. *Ophthalmology.* 2004;111(8):1437–1438.

Nonsteroidal Anti-inflammatory Drugs

A wide variety of nonsteroidal anti-inflammatory drugs (NSAIDs) have been developed in recent years to treat RA and other rheumatic diseases. The names of and starting dosages for some of these agents are listed in Table 8-4. All of these agents decrease synthesis of inflammatory mediators such as the prostaglandins by inhibiting the enzyme cyclooxygenase (COX), and all of them are analgesic, antipyretic, and anti-inflammatory. Their relative efficacy remains largely untested, and individual patients vary in their responsiveness to these drugs.

Complications from NSAID use result in approximately 100,000 hospitalizations and 10,000 to 20,000 deaths per year. The most significant adverse effects from use of oral nonsteroidal anti-inflammatory agents are gastrointestinal bleeding, renal failure, worsening hypertension, and heart failure, as well as onset of asthma in aspirin-sensitive individuals. Oral NSAIDs can interfere with platelet function and clotting and can cause bone marrow suppression, hepatic toxicity, and CNS symptoms, including headache, dizziness, and confusion. On rare occasion, the NSAIDs have been associated with ocular adverse effects such as nonspecific blurred vision or diplopia. There have also been reports of possible optic neuropathy and macular edema, especially with use of ibuprofen (Motrin).

There are 2 isoforms of the COX enzyme. COX-1 is present in most cells and appears to be involved in various aspects of cellular metabolism, such as gastric cytoprotection, platelet aggregation, and renal function. COX-2 is present in some tissues, such as brain and bone, but it also is expressed in other sites in response to inflammation. The traditional NSAIDs inhibit both forms, but in 1999 selective COX-2 inhibitors were introduced. The benefit of the selectivity is that the risk of gastrointestinal damage is lessened, and there is also less effect on platelet function. Unfortunately, 2 of the drugs (rofecoxib [Vioxx] and valdecoxib [Bextra]) have been removed from the market because an excessive number of adverse cardiovascular events were identified in various studies. Similar concerns have been raised about celecoxib (Celebrex), and although it is still available, this drug now carries significant warnings. It has been proposed that the selective blocking of COX-2 decreases the production of prostacyclins, which cause vasodilation and inhibit platelet aggregation, leading to increased prothrombotic activity. Ophthalmologists should be aware that conjunctivitis, temporary blindness, and vague visual blurring have been reported with use of COX-2 inhibitors.

The exact role of oral nonsteroidal agents in treating ocular inflammation remains uncertain. For instance, systemic NSAIDs may be useful in some patients with uveitis or scleritis in at least partially controlling the disease. In general, however, these drugs are not as effective as corticosteroids. Several topical nonsteroidal anti-inflammatory agents have been approved for ocular use. *Flurbiprofen* (Ocufen) is used primarily to control intraoperative miosis during anterior segment surgery. *Diclofenac* (Voltaren) has been approved for the treatment of postoperative inflammation following cataract surgery. *Ketorolac tromethamine* (Acular) is approved for treating the symptoms of allergic conjunctivitis but

Table 8-4 The Nonsteroidal Anti-inflammatory Drugs

NSAID	Trade Name	Usual Dose
Carboxylic acids		
Aspirin (acetylsalicylic acid)		2.4–6 g/24 h in 4–5 divided doses
Buffered aspirin	Multiple	Same
Enteric-coated salicylates	Multiple	Same
Salsalate	Disalcid	1.5–3.0 g/24 h BID
Diflunisal	Dolobid	0.5–1.5 g/24 h BID
Choline magnesium trisalicylate	Trilisate	1.5–3 g/24 h BID-TID
Proprionic acids		
Ibuprofen	Motrin, Rufen, OTC	OTC: 200–400 mg QID Rx: 400–800 mg; max 3200 mg/24 h
Naproxen; Enteric	Naprosyn, Anaprox OTC: Alleve	250, 375, 500 mg BID 225 mg BID
Fenoprofen	Nalfon	300–600 mg QID
Ketoprofen	Orudis; Oruvail	75 mg TID; q day
Flurbiprofen	Ansaid	100 mg BID-TID
Oxaprozin	Daypro	600 mg; 2 tabs per day
Acetic acid derivatives		
Indomethacin	Indocin, Indocin SR	25, 50 mg TID-QID; SR: 75 mg BID; rarely >150 mg/24 h
Tolmetin	Tolectin	400, 600, 800 mg; 800 to 2400 mg/24 h
Sulindac	Clinoril	150, 200 mg BID; some increase to TID
Diclofenac	Voltaren; Cataflam;	50, 75 mg BID-QID
(plus misoprostol)	(Arthrotec)	(50 mg BID)
Etodolac	Lodine	200, 300 mg BID-QID Max: 1200 mg/24 h
Fenamates		
Meclofenamate	Meclomen	50–100 mg TID-QID
Mefenamic acid	Ponstel	250 mg QID
Enolic acids		
Piroxicam	Feldene	10, 20 mg q day
Phenylbutazone	Butazolidin	100 mg TID up to 600 mg/24 h
Naphthylkanones		
Nabumetone	Relafen	500 mg BID up to 1500 mg/24 h
Selective COX-2 inhibitors		
Celecoxib	Celebrex	100, 200 mg q day-BID

Modified with permission from Simon LS. NSAIDs: overview of adverse effects. In: *UpToDate*, Rose BD (Ed), Waltham, MA. Available at http://www.uptodate.com. Accessed March 1, 2005.

has also been studied for the treatment of cystoid macular edema and for the relief of pain following corneal injuries. Both ketorolac and diclofenac are used to relieve postoperative pain following excimer laser photorefractive keratectomy. Two new topical nonsteroidal drugs have recently been released. *Bromfenac* (Xibrom) is indicated for the treatment of postoperative inflammation. *Nepafenac* (Nevanac) is a prodrug designed to enhance penetration of the active metabolite into the eye.

Severe corneal problems associated with the use of topical NSAIDs have been reported, including keratitis and corneal perforations. Most of the cases involved a generic formulation of diclofenac that is no longer available, but problems have also been reported with nongeneric ketorolac and diclofenac. The problems appear to occur in patients with predisposing conditions such as RA, dry eye, or epithelial defects, and with concomitant topical steroid use. Patients should be warned about the possibility of complications, and these drugs should be used cautiously when confounding conditions exist.

> Guidera AC, Luchs JI, Udell IJ. Keratitis, ulceration, and perforation associated with topical nonsteroidal anti-inflammatory drugs. *Ophthalmology.* 2001;108(5):936–944.

Methotrexate

Methotrexate, a structural analogue of folic acid, interferes with folate-dependent metabolic pathways such as purine and with pyrimidine metabolism. Its disease-modifying effect may in part be mediated via increased extracellular adenosine, which has intrinsic anti-inflammatory activity. Methotrexate is given weekly, usually beginning at a dose of 7.5–10 mg, and gradually increasing to a maximum dose of 25 mg depending on disease response. All patients are supplemented with folic acid. Major adverse effects include hepatic fibrosis, interstitial lung disease, marrow toxicity, and sterility. Minor problems include gastric upset, stomatitis, and rash.

Hydroxychloroquine

Hydroxychloroquine (Plaquenil) is an antimalarial compound commonly used to treat rheumatologic diseases (chloroquine [Aralen] is a related drug that has an increased risk of retinal toxicity and is rarely used). The drug seems to work by slightly raising the pH of various cellular compartments. This has multiple subtle effects that include decreased cytokine production and decreased lymphocyte proliferation. The response to treatment may take weeks to months, in part because of the drug's half-life (1–2 months) and the time required to achieve steady state levels.

Hydroxychloroquine is one of the safest immunomodulating drugs. Gastrointestinal symptoms may occur and, rarely, a myopathy. When the drug is first started, patients may complain of a self-limited decrease in accommodation, which is probably mediated by transient effects on ciliary muscle function. Retinopathy (bull's-eye maculopathy) due to use of hydroxychloroquine is relatively unusual. A screening protocol has been developed that assigns a patient's level of risk for retinopathy based on factors such as duration of drug use, age, the presence of preexisting retinal disease, and the presence of renal or liver disease. Dosing >6.5 mg/kg/day also increases the risk. It should be remembered that this drug is not retained in fatty tissues, so the dosage limit refers to lean body weight—not the patient's actual weight. In other words, a short obese patient may actually be at greater risk for toxicity than a taller, leaner patient of similar weight. Higher risk patients should have annual examinations that include, at a minimum, Amsler grid testing and/or central visual field tests. Patients should be given an Amsler grid for self-monitoring at home because subtle paracentral changes may be the earliest sign of toxicity. Retinopathy is discussed more fully in BCSC Section 12, *Retina and Vitreous.*

> Marmor MF, Carr RE, Easterbrook M, et al. Recommendations on screening for chloroquine and hydroxychloroquine retinopathy: a report by the American Academy of Ophthalmology. *Ophthalmology.* 2002;109(7):1377–1382.

Sulfasalazine

Sulfasalazine (Azulfidine) is effective in treating RA, although the exact mechanism of action is unclear. As they are with other sulfa drugs, side effects can be due to idiosyncratic hypersensitivity (skin reactions, aplastic anemia) or may be dose-related (gastrointestinal tract symptoms, headache). Sulfasalazine is often used in combination with other drugs such as hydroxychloroquine and methotrexate.

Gold Salts

Gold salts are rarely used because of modest efficacy and a high side-effect profile involving hematologic, renal, and dermatologic reactions.

Anticytokine Therapy and Other Immunosuppressive Agents

More detailed understanding of the immune response has allowed the development of drugs targeting specific mediators. Cytokines, which are compounds generated by activated immune cells, can enhance or inhibit the immune response. Tumor necrosis factor α (TNF α) is a major proinflammatory cytokine involved in the pathogenesis of RA and other inflammatory diseases. Three TNF-α antagonists are currently available. *Etanercept* (Enbrel) is a recombinant TNF-α receptor protein fused to the Fc portion of an IgG molecule. It works by binding free TNF α and preventing it from attaching to cell membrane receptors. *Infliximab* (Remicade) and *adalimumab* (Humira) are different types of antibodies that directly target TNF α. Etanercept and adalimumab are given approximately once a week as subcutaneous injections. Infliximab is given as an IV infusion every 4 to 8 weeks.

The drugs are usually well tolerated, but there is a potential for severe side effects. These include the development of opportunistic infections such as tuberculosis or atypical mycobacteria, a possible association with demyelinating disease, and a possible association with lymphoma. Other associations include cytopenias, heart failure, antibodies to the drugs, and a lupus-like syndrome. Ophthalmologists should be aware that these drugs have been reported to cause optic neuritis due to demyelinization and, rarely, to exacerbate uveitis. The drugs are also very expensive; for instance, the cost of infliximab is approximately $12,000 per year based on an average of 8 treatments. In spite of these problems, these drugs can be very effective medications in the treatment of autoimmune diseases, and they herald the onset of immunomodulatory therapies that target specific aspects of the immune response.

Anakinra (Kineret) is another anticytokine drug that inhibits interleukin 1 (IL-1) by binding to IL-1 receptors on the cell surface. It works best when combined with other disease-modifying agents such as methotrexate. Abatacept (Orencia) has recently been approved for the treatment of rheumatoid arthritis that is poorly responsive to other therapies. This drug blocks the T-cell receptor CD28, which is involved in T-cell activation and can be very effective in refractory disease. Rituximab (Rituxan) is a B-cell–depleting monoclonal antibody used for chemotherapy that is also being used in rheumatoid arthritis unresponsive to other agents.

Leflunomide (Arava) is a relatively new drug that inhibits pyrimidine synthesis, targeting rapidly dividing cell populations such as activated lymphocytes. Potential adverse effects include liver toxicity, neuropathy, and birth defects. This drug is approximately as effective as methotrexate, and the two are often combined when methotrexate is ineffective alone.

Cyclophosphamide (Cytoxan) and *chlorambucil* (Leukeran) are alkylating agents that are very potent immunosuppressive agents. Their primary mechanism of action involves the cross-linking of DNA molecules, which halts cellular processes. They also have the potential for severe adverse effects that include infertility, bone marrow suppression, increased risk of infection, and late malignancy (particularly bladder cancer with use of cyclophosphamide). Consequently, these drugs are saved for very resistant or life-threatening diseases for which the benefits are worth the substantial risk, such as Wegener granulomatosis. Cyclophosphamide is the most commonly used drug, and it may be given as a daily oral dose or as intermittent IV pulse therapy.

Azathioprine (Imuran) is an antimetabolite that ultimately interferes with purine metabolism. The most common adverse effects are gastrointestinal tract symptoms, infection, and bone marrow suppression. Up to 10% of the population may have decreased levels of the enzyme thiopurine methyltransferase (TPMT), which is important in the metabolism of this drug. As decreased levels of TPMT may lead to more pronounced bone marrow suppression and toxicity, measuring the levels of this enzyme may help identify patients at risk.

Cyclosporine (Neoral, Sandimmune) and *tacrolimus* (Prograf) are drugs that inhibit the transcription of interleukin-2 and other cytokines, primarily in T-helper cells. They are used primarily in transplant patients to prevent rejection, but there is increasing recognition of their usefulness in treating autoimmune diseases. The chief adverse effects of both drugs are nephrotoxicity and hypertension. Other potential problems include neurologic symptoms, infections, and malignancy. Because of such risks, these agents are reserved for recalcitrant cases that do not respond to standard therapies. Though rare, ophthalmic adverse effects reported with use of systemic cyclosporine include disc edema, hallucinations, and unexplained eye pain.

Mycophenolate mofetil (CellCept) inhibits the production of guanosine in lymphocytes and thereby decreases cellular proliferation and antibody production. It is another drug that was initially used in transplant patients and is increasingly used in patients with immunologic diseases. Primary adverse effects include gastrointestinal symptoms, bone marrow suppression, and increased risk of infection. Overall, the drug seems to be well tolerated by patients and may serve as an adjunct to other medications. As this drug is relatively new, its role in the treatment of autoimmune disease is not yet well defined.

Cush JJ, Kavanaugh A, Stein CM. *Rheumatology: Diagnosis and Therapeutics.* 2nd ed. Philadelphia: Lippincott Williams & Wilkins; 2005.

Fraunfelder FT, Fraunfelder FW. *Drug-Induced Ocular Side Effects.* 5th ed. Boston: Butterworth-Heinemann; 2001.

Harris ED, Jr, et al, eds. *Kelley's Textbook of Rheumatology.* 7th ed. St Louis: Elsevier; 2005.

UpToDate Web site. Available at http://www.uptodate.com.

The authors would like to thank Karen Ringwald, MD, and Susan Ballinger, MD, for their contributions to this chapter.

CHAPTER 9

Endocrine Disorders

Recent Developments

- Simple measures such as moderate exercise and weight loss can prevent the onset of type 2 diabetes in patients at risk for developing the disease. Early pharmacologic intervention may also delay the onset of diabetes in prediabetic patients and may help prolong pancreatic function in patients with type 2 diabetes.
- Although careful glucose control is the mainstay of diabetic therapy, newer treatments are being developed that target downstream mechanisms of diabetic pathophysiology in order to help prevent complications. Examples of these treatments include protein kinase C inhibitors, drugs that decrease advanced glycosylation end products, and inhibitors of growth factors such as vascular endothelial growth factor.
- There is increasing use of glargine (Lantus) and detemir (Levemir), long-acting insulins with constant absorption characteristics that allow more physiologic dosing of insulin when combined with intermittent short-acting insulin.
- There has been heightened recognition that poor glucose control is only 1 of several risk factors contributing to the complications of diabetes and that equal attention must be paid to other factors such as hypertension and lipid abnormalities.
- Current cigarette smoking in patients with Graves disease is associated with an increased incidence of ophthalmopathy that parallels the number of cigarettes smoked per day.

Diabetes Mellitus

The prevalence of diabetes in the United States is estimated at 8% of the population. Obesity is a major contributing factor and continues to increase in prevalence yearly. In 2007, the total economic impact of diabetes in the United States was $174 billion, because of both the direct medical costs and costs related to work loss, disability, and early mortality. New diabetes is diagnosed in more than 1 million people each year, a number expected to increase 165% by 2050. Annual spending is increasing by 14.5% for diabetes treatment and will be the fastest-growing therapeutic category by 2009. As diabetes is still the leading cause of new cases of blindness among adults 20–74 years old, the ophthalmologist plays a crucial role as part of a multidisciplinary team involved in prevention, treatment, and management of this disease.

Basics of Glucose Metabolism

The plasma glucose level is reduced by a single hormone, insulin. In contrast, there are 6 hormones that increase the plasma glucose level: somatotropin, adrenocorticotropin, cortisol, epinephrine, glucagon, and thyroxine. All of these hormones are secreted as needed to maintain normal serum glucose levels in the face of extremely variable degrees of glucose intake and utilization. In the fed state, *anabolism* is initiated by increased secretion of insulin and growth hormone. This leads to conversion of glucose to glycogen for storage in the liver and muscles, synthesis of protein from amino acids, and combining of fatty acid and glucose in adipose tissue to form triglycerides.

In the fasting state, *catabolism* results from the increased secretion of hormones that are antagonistic to insulin. In this setting, glycogen is reduced to glucose in the liver and muscles; proteins are broken down into amino acids in muscles and other tissues and transported to the liver for conversion to glucose or ketoacids; and triglycerides are degraded into fatty acids and glycerol in adipose tissue for transport to the liver for conversion to ketoacids and glucose (or for transport to muscle for use as an energy source).

The normal lean adult secretes approximately 33 units of insulin per day. If the pancreatic beta cell mass is reduced (as it is in type 1 diabetes), then insulin production falls. The relative excess of catabolic hormones results in fasting hyperglycemia, and persistent catabolism may lead to fatal diabetic ketoacidosis if insulin therapy is not started. This disastrous chain of events explains why type 1 diabetes was uniformly fatal before the development of insulin. It also explains why insulin-dependent diabetic patients require a continuous baseline dose of insulin, even in the fasting state: some level of insulin is needed to offset the effect of all the other hormones.

In the obese overfed adult, insulin secretion can increase almost 4-fold to approximately 120 units per day. In this state, the plasma glucose level may rise only slightly, but pancreatic beta cell mass increases. When serum insulin levels are elevated, the number of insulin receptors on the surface of insulin-responsive cells actually decreases, and formerly insulin-sensitive tissues become resistant to the glucose-lowering effects of both endogenous and exogenous insulin. This condition may progress to fasting hyperglycemia and type 2 diabetes. The risk of hyperglycemia is 2 times as great in persons who are 20% above ideal body weight, compared with persons at ideal body weight; 4 times as great at 40% above; 8 times as great at 60% above; 16 times as great at 80% above; and 32 times as great at 100% above.

Definition

The definition of diabetes mellitus has changed considerably in recent years. *Diabetes mellitus* is now defined as a group of metabolic diseases characterized by hyperglycemia resulting from defects in insulin secretion, insulin action, or both. The American Diabetes Association Expert Panel recommends a diagnosis of diabetes when 1 of the 3 criteria shown in Table 9-1 is met (and confirmed with retesting by any of the 3 methods on a subsequent day).

Table 9-1 American Diabetes Association Plasma Glucose Diagnostic Criteria for Diabetes Mellitus

Diagnosis	Test Condition Plasma Glucose, mg/dL	
	Fasting ≥8 hr	2 hr after 75 g oral glucose
Normal	<110	<140
Impaired glucose tolerance (IGT)	<126	≥140–<200
Impaired fasting glucose (IFG)	≥110–<126	<200
Diabetes mellitus	≥126	—
Diabetes mellitus	<126	≥200
Diabetes mellitus (Classic symptoms + casual plasma glucose, ≥200 mg/dL)	—	—

	Plasma Glucose, mg/dL	
Gestational diabetes mellitus (GDM)	Fasting	After 100 g oral glucose
	>105*	1 hr ≥190*
	>105*	2 hr ≥165*
	>105*	3 hr ≥145*

Note: The Fourth International Workshop–Conference on Gestational Diabetes Mellitus has proposed lower criteria, which would increase the percentage of cases from 4% to 7% in white women. These criteria are fasting, 95; 1 hour, 180; 2 hours, 155; and 3 hours, 140, after 100 g oral glucose.
*Two of these four criteria must be met for diagnosis of GDM.

Reproduced with permission from Genuth S. Diabetes mellitus. [ACP Medicine Web site]. May 2004 Update. Available at http://www.acpmedicine.com. Accessed March 1, 2005.

Classification

Diabetes can be caused by a number of different mechanisms, as outlined in Table 9-2. This chapter will emphasize types 1 and 2, which are most frequently seen in clinical practice, but it is important to remember that many diseases and drugs can be associated with diabetes (eg, onset of diabetes in association with use of synthetic glucocorticoids to treat ophthalmic diseases).

Type 1 diabetes

Type 1 diabetes was previously called *insulin-dependent diabetes mellitus* or *juvenile-onset diabetes*. Although type 1 diabetes does have a peak incidence around the time of puberty, approximately 25% of cases present after 35 years of age. This form of diabetes is due to a deficiency in endogenous insulin secretion secondary to destruction of insulin-producing beta cells in the pancreas.

Most type 1 diabetes is due to immune-mediated destruction characterized by the presence of various autoantibodies. The rate of destruction varies, but it is usually rapid in children and slow in adults. One or more autoantibodies are present in 90% of patients at initial presentation of fasting hyperglycemia. Studies have shown that patients newly diagnosed with type 1 diabetes can avoid the use of insulin if they are placed on systemic immunosuppressive agents to prevent further beta cell destruction. Unfortunately, this treatment is too toxic to be practical. There are strong human leukocyte antigen (HLA)

Table 9-2 Etiologic Classification of Diabetes Mellitus

I. Type 1 diabetes* (β-cell destruction, usually leading to absolute insulin deficiency)
   A. Immune mediated
   B. Idiopathic
II. Type 2 diabetes* (may range from predominantly insulin resistance with relative insulin deficiency to a predominantly secretory defect with insulin resistance)
III. Other specific types
   A. Genetic defects of β-cell function
      1. Chromosome 12, HNF-1α (MODY3)
      2. Chromosome 7, glucokinase (MODY2)
      3. Chromosome 20, HNF-4α (MODY1)
      4. Mitochondrial DNA
      5. Others
   B. Genetic defects in insulin action
      1. Type A insulin resistance
      2. Leprechaunism
      3. Rabson-Mendenhall syndrome
      4. Lipoatrophic diabetes
      5. Others
   C. Diseases of the exocrine pancreas
      1. Pancreatitis
      2. Trauma/pancreatopathy
      3. Neoplasia
      4. Cystic fibrosis
      5. Hemochromatosis
      6. Fibrocalculous pancreatopathy
      7. Others
   D. Endocrinopathies
      1. Acromegaly
      2. Cushing syndrome
      3. Glucagonoma
      4. Pheochromocytoma
      5. Hyperthyroidism
      6. Somatostatinoma
      7. Aldosteronoma
      8. Others
   E. Drug- or chemical-induced
      1. Vacor
      2. Pentamidine
      3. Nicotinic acid
      4. Glucocorticoids
      5. Thyroid hormone
      6. Diazoxide
      7. β-Adrenergic agonists
      8. Thiazides
      9. Dilantin
     10. α-Interferon
     11. Others
   F. Infections
      1. Congenital rubella
      2. Cytomegalovirus
      3. Others
   G. Uncommon forms of immune-mediated diabetes
      1. "Stiff-man" syndrome
      2. Anti-insulin receptor antibodies
      3. Others

(Continued)

Table 9-2 *(continued)*

    H. Other genetic syndromes sometimes associated with diabetes
        1. Down syndrome
        2. Klinefelter syndrome
        3. Turner syndrome
        4. Wolfram syndrome
        5. Friedreich ataxia
        6. Huntington chorea
        7. Laurence-Moon-Biedl syndrome
        8. Myotonic dystrophy
        9. Porphyria
     10. Prader-Willi syndrome
     11. Others
IV. Gestational diabetes mellitus (GDM)

*Patients with any form of diabetes may require insulin treatment at some stage of the disease. Such use of insulin does not, of itself, classify the patient's condition.

Modified from American Diabetes Association. Clinical practice recommendations 2001. *Diabetes Care.* 2001;24(suppl).

associations with and multiple genetic predispositions related to type 1 diabetes. These patients are also prone to other autoimmune disorders, such as Graves disease, Hashimoto thyroiditis, Addison disease, vitiligo, and pernicious anemia. However, environmental factors may also play a role, as studies of monozygotic twins have shown that both twins develop diabetes only 30%–50% of the time.

Type 2 diabetes

Type 2 diabetes was formerly known as *non–insulin-dependent* or *adult-onset diabetes mellitus*. This group accounts for 90% of Americans with diabetes and also has a strong genetic predisposition. Type 2 patients are usually, but not always, older than age 40 at presentation. Obesity is a frequent finding and, in the United States, is present in 80%–90% of these patients. Other risk factors for type 2 diabetes include hypertension, gestational diabetes, physical inactivity, and low socioeconomic status. This form of diabetes is frequently undiagnosed for years because the hyperglycemia develops slowly and symptoms are not severe enough to warrant attention. Although symptoms may initially be minimal, these patients are at increased risk for microvascular and macrovascular complications.

In spite of the fact that there is a strong genetic tendency for developing type 2 diabetes, no specific genetic locus has been uniquely associated with the disease. It is likely that the disease is a function of a variable number of abnormal genes that combine to create a tendency for obesity and abnormal glucose metabolism, as well as a predisposition for developing complications.

Autoimmune destruction of beta cells does not usually occur in type 2 diabetes. The beta cells continue to function at first, but their ability to control hyperglycemia gradually diminishes, in part owing to a process known as *glucose toxicity*, which is basically a positive feedback loop involving glucose metabolism. Glucose toxicity occurs when elevated glucose levels result in increasing insulin resistance in target tissues and a gradual loss of compensatory insulin production by the beta cells. The result is a vicious cycle, as elevated glucose levels lead to even higher glucose levels. It is therefore crucial to encourage the patient to try to break this cycle by decreasing the glucose level. In a significant number of these patients, the elevated plasma glucose level can revert to normal simply with caloric restriction and weight loss.

Although gestational diabetes is a separate entity (see Table 9-1), it is metabolically similar to type 2 disease. In 30%–50% of affected women, type 2 diabetes develops within 10 years of initial diagnosis. Defined as any degree of glucose intolerance with onset or first recognition during pregnancy, gestational diabetes complicates approximately 4% of all pregnancies in the United States. It is also significant for the risk it poses to the fetus, including intrauterine mortality, neonatal mortality, metabolic problems, and macrosomia.

Approximately 10% of patients presenting with type 2 diabetes may also have serum islet cell autoantibodies typical of type 1 diabetes. This combination of disease types is referred to as *latent autoimmune diabetes in adults (LADA)*. These patients are more likely to need insulin therapy than are the more typical type 2 diabetic patients.

Prediabetic disorders

Impaired glucose tolerance and impaired fasting glucose   *Impaired glucose tolerance (IGT)* is defined as a standard 75 g oral glucose tolerance test yielding a 2-hour plasma glucose level of ≥140 mg/dL to <200 mg/dL. A new category, *impaired fasting glucose (IFG)*, requires a fasting plasma glucose level of ≥110 mg/dL to <126 mg/dL (see Table 9-1). Both conditions can be considered early stages of type 2 diabetes and are often referred to as *prediabetic states*. For instance, 30%–50% of patients with IGT develop type 2 diabetes within 10 years of diagnosis. Although there is a great deal of overlap, IFG and IGT are not identical states.

These patients do not yet appear to be at risk for retinopathy or nephropathy, but they do have an elevated risk of macrovascular disease, compared with persons who have normal glucose tolerance.

Metabolic syndrome

Closely associated with type 2 diabetes, the metabolic syndrome (formerly known as *metabolic syndrome X* or the *insulin resistance syndrome*) is not a disease but a collection of disorders. The definition of this syndrome includes a significant degree of obesity, lipid abnormalities, hypertension, and some type of glucose intolerance (see Table 5-8 in Chapter 5, Hypercholesterolemia)—risk factors for both diabetes and cardiovascular disease. Thus, awareness of this syndrome is becoming increasingly important. There is a significant prevalence in the United States, with the metabolic syndrome being present in 44% of those older than 50 years. Men with a majority of the features of the syndrome have 3.7 times the risk of coronary heart disease and 24.5 times the risk of diabetes compared with those without these abnormalities. The metabolic syndrome represents a profound public health risk, and treatment of the syndrome may have a significant impact on preventing diabetes and cardiovascular diseases.

Clinical Presentation of Diabetes

The classic findings of diabetes mellitus are polyuria, polydipsia, and polyphagia. Type 1 diabetes tends to present more acutely than type 2, and the diagnosis is usually made based on the presence of these classic symptoms in association with an elevated plasma glucose level. The diagnosis of type 2 diabetes is often more dependent on lab testing, because patients may have abnormal glucose metabolism long before overt symptoms develop. Other important historical findings that suggest the diagnosis of diabetes include complications during pregnancy or giving birth to large babies, reactive hypoglycemia, family history, advanced vascular disease, impotence, leg claudication, and neuropathy symptoms.

Physical findings, particularly in type 2 diabetes, may include obesity, hypertension, arteriopathy, neuropathy, genitourinary tract abnormalities (especially recurrent *Candida* infections or bacterial bladder or kidney infections), periodontal disease, foot abnormalities, skin abnormalities, and unusual susceptibility to infections.

Diagnosis and Screening

Table 9-1 lists the criteria for diagnosing diabetes mellitus. The preferred test for type 2 diabetes is a fasting plasma glucose test (FPG). Although the oral glucose tolerance test (OGTT) is more sensitive than the FPG, it is not recommended for routine use because it is more costly, inconvenient, and difficult to reproduce. Note that hemoglobin A_{1c} (HbA_{1c}) measurement is not currently recommended for diagnosing diabetes, although this may change when the test is more standardized. Criteria for diabetes testing in asymptomatic persons are given in Table 9-3.

Prevention of Diabetes

Several clinical trials have recently demonstrated that the risk of progression from IGT to type 2 diabetes can be markedly reduced—approximately 50% over several years—with relatively simple lifestyle modifications such as a combination of diet and exercise therapy. The amount of weight loss and exercise required to achieve this result is surprisingly modest. For instance, in the Diabetes Prevention Program, patients who were asked to perform only 150 minutes of brisk walking a week (a little over 20 minutes a day) on average lost only about 12 pounds of weight but reduced their risk by 50%. Other studies have suggested that early pharmacologic intervention with oral hypoglycemic agents also decreases the risk of progression to diabetes. There are, as yet, no known ways to prevent type 1 diabetes, although trials looking at potential interventions for high-risk individuals such as first-degree relatives of type 1 diabetic patients are under way.

Management

Diet and exercise

Adherence to nutrition and meal planning principles is a challenging but essential component of successful diabetes management. Diet planning should include lifestyle and nutrition goals as well as specific biochemical and other physiologic parameters for the individual. Insulin requirements are then matched to the patient's diet, not vice versa. Although the "one type fits all" diabetic diet is no longer recommended, meals should be consistent, regularly spaced, and low in cholesterol, with less than 10% of calories coming

Table 9-3 Criteria for Testing for Diabetes Mellitus in Asymptomatic Patients in Whom Diabetes Has Not Been Diagnosed

1. Testing for diabetes should be considered in all persons at age 45 years and older; if results are normal, testing should be repeated at 3-yr intervals.
2. Testing should be considered at younger ages or performed more frequently in persons who
   - are obese (≥120% desirable body weight or a BMI ≥25 kg/m^2)*
   - have a first-degree relative with diabetes
   - are members of a high-risk ethnic population (eg, African American, Hispanic American, Native American, Asian American, Pacific Islander)
   - have delivered a baby weighing >9 lb or have a diagnosis of gestational diabetes mellitus
   - are hypertensive (≥140/90 mm Hg)
   - have an HDL cholesterol level ≤35 mg/dL (0.90 mmol/L) and/or a triglyceride level ≥250 mg/dL (2.82 mmol/L)
   - were shown to have impaired glucose tolerance or impaired fasting glucose
   - have polycystic ovary syndrome
   - have history of vascular disease
   - are habitually physically inactive

*May not be correct for all ethnic groups.

Modified from American Diabetes Association. Screening for type 2 diabetes. *Diabetes Care.* 2004; 27(suppl 1):S12.

from saturated fat and 10%–20% of calories derived from protein, depending on the patient's renal function.

If type 2 diabetes is diagnosed and the patient is overweight, a diet (prudent low fat, low cholesterol) is begun and an exercise routine is initiated with the goal of approaching ideal weight. This goal is often not realized, but even a modest weight loss of 10 to 20 lbs may ameliorate or cause a remission of the diabetes. Extensive and continuing counseling on weight reduction may be necessary. A good exercise program aids with the weight-loss program and improves fitness. Before an exercise program is prescribed for anyone older than age 35, a determination must be made that the heart is normal and that there are no contraindications. Anyone who has been sedentary or who is out of condition should start slowly and work up to more demanding activities.

Unfortunately, it may be difficult for patients with type 2 diabetes to maintain these lifestyle changes, especially those involving weight loss. This difficulty should not simply be attributed to a lack of willpower on the part of the patient, as it may well represent a central nervous system manifestation of the multifactorial genetics of this disease. Psychiatric counseling also seems to be an important part of treating type 2 diabetic patients. Studies suggest that efforts directed toward treating the stress and depression often associated with this disease may help improve glucose control.

Bariatric surgery is becoming a more popular option for very obese individuals who are unresponsive to other forms of therapy. The National Institutes of Health recommend consideration of bariatric surgery in well-informed and motivated patients with severe obesity for whom conventional treatment modalities have failed or for those who have multiple comorbidities or severe lifestyle limitations. Although bariatric surgery may be advertised as the only "cure" for type 2 diabetes, there is potential for both morbidity and mortality.

There are several different techniques that involve either restricting stomach volume (restrictive surgery) or minimizing the ability of the GI tract to absorb nutrients (malabsorptive surgery). Combined restrictive and malabsorptive approaches are also performed. There is approximately a 1% risk of mortality, and morbidity can include venous thrombosis, infection, nutritional complications, and complications related to the surgical approach. The surgery is not universally effective, with perhaps 50%–70% of patients actually losing about half of their weight and maintaining the weight loss. Significant counseling and lifestyle changes are still required, and patients can potentially overcome the eating limitations imposed by the surgery by eating small amounts of food very frequently—especially high carbohydrate liquids such as milkshakes.

Insulin therapy

Approximately 1 million North Americans require insulin therapy. Such therapy is indicated in diabetic patients who are pregnant or at or below ideal body weight with sustained hyperglycemia, ketoacidosis, or a hyperosmotic state. The use of insulin in type 2 diabetes actually decreases the number of target-cell insulin receptors, increases food intake, and promotes weight gain. Therefore, patients who are above ideal body weight, who have not experienced ketoacidosis, and who are not pregnant should not be treated with insulin initially.

The goal of therapy is to simulate the physiologic changes in insulin levels that would normally occur in response to food intake and activity level. This therapy usually involves use of a longer-acting insulin to maintain a baseline level, and then use of a rapid-acting insulin to cover meals. As insulins can be created with different rates of absorption by substituting amino acids or complexing with zinc, patients can fine-tune glucose control (Table 9-4). In the past, most insulin was derived from animals, but currently, recombinant human insulin is used almost exclusively.

Regular insulin is the traditional rapid-acting agent used for short-term coverage; however, the development of very rapid-acting insulins allows diabetic patients the convenience of timing injections just a few minutes before meals. Very rapid-acting insulins include insulin lispro (Humalog), insulin aspart (Novolog), and insulin glulisine (Apidra). Intermediate-acting insulins are insulin zinc suspension (Lente) or isophane insulin suspension (NPH insulin). Ultralente is a long-acting insulin made of extended insulin zinc

Table 9-4 Pharmacokinetics of Most Commonly Used Insulin Preparations

Insulin Type	Onset of Action	Time to Peak Effect	Duration of Action
Lispro (Humalog), aspart (Novolog), glulisine (Apidra)	5 to 15 min	45 to 75 min	2 to 4 h
Regular	About 30 min	2 to 4 h	5 to 8 h
NPH or Lente	About 2 h	6 to 10 h	18 to 28 h
Ultralente	About 4 h	10 to 20 h	12 to 20 h
Insulin glargine (Lantus)	About 2 h	No discernible peak	20 to >24 h
Insulin detemir (Levemir)	About 2 h	No discernible peak	10 to 24 h

Modified with permission from McCulloch DK. Insulin therapy in type 1 diabetes mellitus. In: *UpToDate*, Rose BD (Ed), Waltham, MA. Available at http://www.uptodate.com. Accessed August 1, 2007.

preparations. Glargine (Lantus) and detemir (Levemir) are newer long-acting insulins with very stable absorption characteristics that result in a constant level of basal insulin.

Sophisticated patients can adjust each injection using formulas that depend on preprandial glucose level, activity level, and amount of food to be ingested, provided they have extensive knowledge of the carbohydrate types and overall nutritional value of each meal. Intensive insulin therapy requires that patients become very involved with their own management and, ideally, almost as familiar with the disease pathophysiology as their health care professionals are. Premixed combinations of various insulins are also available for patients less able to work with all these variables.

In addition to exercise and intake, 2 physiologic phenomena may need to be accounted for with insulin therapy. The *Somogyi phenomenon* is the occurrence of posthypoglycemic rebound hyperglycemia. Hypoglycemia as mild as 50–60 mg/dL of plasma glucose (which may be asymptomatic) can activate counterregulation. Current evidence indicates that catecholamines and growth hormone are the major factors involved. Recognition of this process is important because patients may incorrectly decide to increase their longer-acting insulin dose to treat the hyperglycemia and thereby increase the hypoglycemia that precipitated the problem. The incidence of the Somogyi phenomenon is not known, but it is probably not frequent.

The second phenomenon is the *dawn phenomenon,* which occurs when a normal physiologic process is exaggerated, resulting in substantial hyperglycemia. Characterized by early morning hyperglycemia not preceded by hypoglycemia or waning of insulin, this phenomenon is thought to be caused by a surge of growth hormone secretion shortly after the patient falls asleep. It can occur with equal frequency in type 1 and type 2 diabetes, but its severity varies, making this condition difficult to treat. Management consists of increasing a patient's before-supper intermediate-acting insulin or delaying insulin administration until just before bedtime.

Continuous subcutaneous insulin infusion (CSII) pumps allow even more physiologic levels of insulin than do traditional injections. For instance, CSII pumps can be programmed to increase the basal insulin level during the latter half of the night in anticipation of the dawn effect. CSII is not a simple treatment, however, as patients must be able to understand the more sophisticated demands of using a pump, and improvement in glucose control is not automatic. In the Diabetes Control and Complications Trial (DCCT), the overall rate of control was not better in patients using the pump than in patients using multiple injections, although more recent studies using very rapid-acting insulins do demonstrate slightly better control with a pump compared with multiple injections.

The pump tends to be used when multiple-injection therapy fails, although some endocrinologists will consider using it with motivated patients who understand the nuances of living with the pump because it can provide greater lifestyle flexibility. Disadvantages include a higher cost, infection at the infusion site, and infusion failure. Infusion failure is significant, because patients can develop diabetic ketoacidosis if the pump fails for as little as 4 to 6 hours. The pump delivers a low dose of rapid-acting insulin that quickly disappears if the infusion is stopped. The patient may be unaware of a failure at first (in contrast to a multi-injection regimen in which the patient is absolutely aware of giving a dose). A state of hypoinsulinemia develops with resulting hyperglycemia and possible ketoacidosis if pump failure is not recognized. Finally, because patients need to wear the pump on an almost constant basis, some patients discontinue use simply because it interferes with activities such as bathing or sex. CSII technology is continually improving, however, and for many patients the pump is becoming a preferred option over multiple injections.

Complications of insulin therapy *Hypoglycemia* is the most significant complication of insulin therapy. Stimulation of the adrenal medulla with resulting hyperepinephrinemia may result in anxiety, palpitations, perspiration, pallor, tachycardia, hypertension, and dilated pupils. Neurologic dysfunction is manifested as headache, paresthesia, blurred vision, drowsiness, irritability, bizarre behavior, mental confusion, combativeness, and a variety of other symptoms. Short-term hypoglycemia can lead to accidental injury and even criminal behavior. Prolonged hypoglycemia can result in irreversible brain damage or death. Unfortunately, the epinephrine response to hypoglycemia can diminish over time, often in association with the global autonomic neuropathy that occurs in diabetes. As a result, patients have fewer warning symptoms of hypoglycemia, as well as a decreased ability to metabolically respond to the hypoglycemia. Thus, the first clinical manifestation of a hypoglycemic episode is CNS dysfunction, and by then it may be too late for the patient to recognize and self-treat the episode. This is the clinical syndrome of *hypoglycemia unawareness*. The result may be a very rapid deterioration from normal functioning to dangerous hypoglycemia in patients with long-standing diabetes.

Hypoglycemia is usually caused by inadequate carbohydrate intake secondary to a missed or delayed meal, vigorous exercise, decreased hepatic gluconeogenesis, or an excessive dose of insulin. The condition needs to be promptly verified by testing for a venous plasma glucose level of lower than 50 mg/dL. Patients who are still able to swallow should be given candy, soft drinks, orange juice, food, or glucose. For those unable to swallow, 25 g of intravenous glucose or 1 mg of subcutaneous or intramuscular glucagon is administered. The patient needs to be observed until recovery is complete, and the plasma glucose test is repeated with additional food given.

Other complications of insulin include lipoatrophy (loss of fat) or lipohypertrophy (accumulation of fat) at sites of insulin injection. Local insulin allergy can occur and usually clears as therapy continues. Generalized anaphylaxis, hives, and angioedema may also develop and may need to be treated with desensitization techniques. Immunologic insulin resistance may occur because of production of insulin-neutralizing antibodies. All of these immunologic phenomena have become much less frequent with the use of human insulins.

Oral agents (Table 9-5)
Sulfonylureas The sulfonylureas have been widely used in the United States and Canada since 1967 for treatment of type 2 diabetes. Their major mechanism of action is stimulation of pancreatic insulin secretion, although some studies have suggested a peripheral augmentation of insulin action.

The major problem with sulfonylurea therapy is that approximately one third of patients who begin therapy do not become normoglycemic ("primary failures"). Further-

Table 9-5 Pharmacokinetics of Oral Hypoglycemic Drugs

Drug	Usual Daily Dose, mg	Dosing per Day
First-generation sulfonylureas		
Acetohexamide	500 to 750	Once or divided
Chlorpropamide	250 to 500	Once
(Diabinese)		
Tolbutamide	1000 to 2000	Once or divided
(Orinase)		
Second-generation sulfonylureas		
Glipizide	2.5 to 10	Once or divided
(Glucotrol)		
(Glucotrol XL)	5 to 10	Once
Glyburide	2.5 to 10	Once or divided
(DiaBeta)		
(Micronase)		
(Glynase)		
Glimepiride (Amaryl)	2 to 4	Once
Biguanides		
Metformin (Glucophage)	1500 to 2550	Twice to three times
(Glucophage XR)		
Alpha-glucosidase inhibitors		
Acarbose (Precose)	150 to 300	Three times
Miglitol (Glyset)	150 to 300	Three times
Thiazolidinediones		
Rosiglitazone (Avandia)	4 to 8	Once or divided
Pioglitazone (Actos)	15 to 45	Once
Other		
Repaglinide (Prandin)	2 to 16	Three times
Nateglinide (Starlix)	360	Three times
Sitagliptin (Januvia)	100	Once

Modified with permission from McCulloch DK. Treatment of blood glucose in type 2 diabetes mellitus. In: *UpToDate*, Rose BD (Ed), Waltham, MA. Available at http://www.uptodate.com. Accessed March 1, 2005.

more, during a 5-year period, 85% of those who initially respond to the drug experience secondary failure to control blood glucose. The sulfonylureas are also contraindicated in diabetic patients who are pregnant or in those who have had ketoacidosis.

The most significant adverse effect of the sulfonylureas is hypoglycemia, which though infrequent may be severe and prolonged, depending on the half-life of the specific drug. Sulfonylureas compete for carrier protein-binding sites with many other drugs, including sulfonamides, salicylates, and thiazides. Because the pharmacologic effect of the sulfonylureas may be increased when they are displaced from their albumin-combining sites, combination drug therapy may have unforeseen toxic consequences. It is also difficult to maintain stable anticoagulation therapy in a patient taking sulfonylureas, because anticoagulants and sulfonylureas compete for the same binding sites. In addition, the effects of alcohol are potentiated by sulfonylureas.

Second-generation sulfonylurea agents *glipizide* (Glucotrol, Glucotrol XL), *glyburide* (DiaBeta, Micronase, Glynase), and *glimepiride* (Amaryl) differ from the first-generation agents in structure and potency. On a weight-for-weight basis, the newer sulfonylureas are approximately 50–100 times more potent than first-generation agents, and these drugs generally need to be given only once daily. Complications are less frequent with the second-generation agents because of their nonionic binding to albumin and patients may be less susceptible to drug interactions. Although these newer agents are more potent than the first-generation sulfonylureas in facilitating insulin release, this enhanced beta-cytotrophic effect is not associated with better control of hyperglycemia. As a result, in most cases the choice of initial sulfonylurea depends on cost and availability; the efficacy of the various agents tends to be similar.

Meglitinides *Repaglinide* (Prandin) and *nateglinide* (Starlix) are meglitinides whose mechanism of action and side effect profile are similar to those of the sulfonylureas. However, they are more expensive and generally no more efficacious than the sulfonylureas. Because of their rapid onset of action and short duration, these agents are taken 2 to 4 times daily with meals. They can be used as single agents or in combination therapy with other oral hypoglycemic agents.

Biguanides A major advance occurred with the development of *metformin* (Glucophage, Glucophage XR), currently the only available biguanide. Metformin improves insulin sensitivity, unlike the sulfonylureas and meglitinides, which enhance insulin secretion. Also, it may lead to modest weight loss or at least stabilization (in contrast to the weight gain that may occur with use of insulin or sulfonylureas). In addition, it is less likely to cause hypoglycemia and can be used in nonobese patients. Metformin can be used as either first-line therapy or in combination with other hypoglycemic agents.

Although metformin is generally very safe, patients may complain of gastrointestinal tract symptoms, including a metallic taste, nausea, and diarrhea. A more severe potential problem is lactic acidosis. Though rare, this problem is more likely to occur in patients with renal insufficiency. Metformin should therefore not be prescribed to patients with elevated serum creatinine levels, and the drug should also be discontinued before any studies involving iodinated contrast materials, given the risk of renal failure. The same precaution should be taken before major surgery when there is a possibility of circulatory compromise and secondary renal insufficiency. Metformin is also available as a combination pill with glyburide (Glucovance), glipizide (Metaglip), and rosiglitazone maleate (Avandamet).

α-Glucosidase inhibitors *Acarbose* (Precose) and *miglitol* (Glyset) are administered with meals to delay digestion and absorption of carbohydrates by inhibiting the enzymes that convert complex carbohydrates into monosaccharides. Although relatively safe, these agents often cause flatulence, which limits patient compliance, and they are to be avoided in patients with intestinal disorders.

Thiazolidinediones This new class of orally active drugs, represented by *rosiglitazone* (Avandia) and *pioglitazone* (Actos) is thought to increase insulin sensitivity in muscle and adipose tissue and to inhibit hepatic gluconeogenesis, thereby increasing glycemic control while reducing circulating insulin levels. These drugs also act to increase insulin secretion. The first available agent of this class, *troglitazone* (Rezulin), was withdrawn from the market in 2000, when the FDA noted that this drug had a higher rate of liver toxicity than did rosiglitazone and pioglitazone. Both rosiglitazone and pioglitazone can cause weight gain, in part owing to proliferation of new adipocytes. Fluid retention is another problem that can occur, and there have now been case reports of macular edema associated with this side effect. Recent studies also suggest a possible increased incidence of myocardial infarction with rosiglitazone.

The general approach to treating type 2 diabetes is to begin with diet and exercise modifications. If this does not work, then 1 of the oral agents is started, usually metformin or a sulfonylurea. If this is insufficient, then a second agent with a different mechanism is usually added. If better control is required, then insulin is usually added, in addition to either 1 or 2 agents, because triple drug oral therapy is both more expensive and less effective than the addition of insulin. Insulin may need to be started earlier in the course if patients are underweight or ketotic at any point, or if they are losing weight.

Other therapies

Incretins are gut-derived factors that are released when nutrients enter the stomach; they help to stimulate postprandial insulin release. Incretin mimetics improve glycemic control by enhancing pancreatic secretion of insulin in response to nutrient intake, inhibiting glucagon secretion and promoting early satiety. Two recently approved injectable drugs are *exenatide* (Byetta), an incretin mimetic used as adjunctive therapy for type 2 diabetic patients inadequately controlled on oral agents, and *pramlintide* (Symlin), a synthetic analog of amylin, used in patients treated with mealtime insulin. Sitagliptin (Januvia) is an oral incretin mimetic that requires only once a day dosing.

For type 1 diabetic patients, pancreas transplantation can be performed in conjunction with renal transplantation. With modern techniques and immunosuppression, there is a high survival rate of the transplant, and the majority of patients become euglycemic without the need for insulin. Although a patient's quality of life is usually improved, he or she faces the risks of both surgery and long-term immunosuppression. The use of pancreas transplantation alone is therefore saved for special situations, such as patients with frequent metabolic complications or patients for whom standard insulin therapy consistently fails to control disease. When pancreas transplantation is combined with renal transplantation in a patient with end-stage renal disease, however, the benefits of surgery far outweigh the risks.

Islet cells can be injected directly into the liver without the need for formal transplantation. This procedure has been attempted in humans, but there is a high failure rate because of rejection. Ongoing studies are under way to identify effective immunosuppressive regimens and other sites for cell placement. Islet cell–producing stem cell research is also being done, although this is still at the basic research stage.

The Importance of Glucose Control

The Diabetes Control and Complications Trial showed that intensive therapy aimed at maintaining near-normal glucose levels had a large and beneficial effect on delaying the development and retarding the progression of long-term complications for type 1 diabetic patients. These levels were obtained either by 3 or more daily self-administered insulin in-

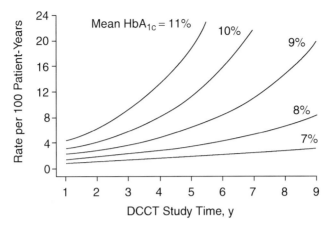

Figure 9-1 Rate of retinopathy progression relative to mean hemoglobin A_{1c}. *(Redrawn with permission from the DCCT Research Group. The relationship of glycemic exposure (HbA$_{1c}$) to the risk of development and progression of retinopathy in the Diabetes Control and Complications Trial. Diabetes. 1995;44:968–983.)*

jections or via a battery-powered insulin pump. Intensive therapy decreased the risk of the development and progression of retinopathy, nephropathy, and neuropathy by 40%–76%. The beneficial effects increased over time but came with a 3-fold increased risk of hypoglycemia. Thus, intensive therapy is recommended for most patients with type 1 disease, but with careful self-monitoring of blood glucose levels to prevent hypoglycemic episodes. A related study, the United Kingdom Prospective Diabetes Study (UKPDS), was designed to assess the effect of intensive control on patients with type 2 diabetes. The UKPDS used a combination of diet, sulfonylureas, and insulin to achieve a median HbA_{1c} of 7.0 in the intensive care group and also showed a reduction in complications.

Tight control has a tremendous effect on the development of complications. As Figure 9-1 shows, the risk of retinopathy progression rises almost exponentially as the hemoglobin A_{1c} increases. The risk of retinopathy decreases approximately 30% for every 1% decrease in the HbA_{1c}, and this benefit seems to be true for all diabetic complications. Every health care provider involved in the care of a diabetic patient needs to emphasize this fact to the patient and encourage the patient to achieve good control.

Glucose Surveillance

Probably the most important advance in glycemic control is self-monitoring of blood glucose. Newer blood-testing devices require smaller amounts of blood than do older units; they are also less painful. The glucose values are stored in memory and are downloaded to give an accurate assessment of the glucose control without depending on the patient to recall or reconstruct the data. Having patients maintain a glucose log is still useful, however, because it can serve as an important reminder of their progress. The development of implantable devices that not only measure glucose levels but also release the appropriate amount of insulin would be another major advance in glycemic control.

Although reliable long-term in-dwelling glucose sensors have been developed and are being investigated, the success of such devices is limited by problems with obstruction of insulin delivery.

In recent decades, the ability to measure *glycosylated hemoglobin levels* has significantly improved long-term glucose-control surveillance. All serum-bound and membrane-bound proteins are exposed to glucose, and these proteins undergo a nonenzymatic postsynthetic modification that results in the attachment of glucose to the protein (glycosylation). Higher concentrations of glucose and longer periods of exposure result in a higher concentration of glycosylated proteins. The time period reflected by the glycosylated protein concentration depends on the particular protein's turnover rate. Red blood cells and hemoglobin have a half-life of 60 days. Thus, the glycosylated hemoglobin level reflects the mean blood glucose concentration during the preceding 2 months.

Hemoglobin A_{1c}, the most abundant of the glycosylated hemoglobins, is the assay most commonly performed. The amount of glycosylated hemoglobin is expressed as a percentage of total hemoglobin. The HbA_{1c} assay is used to monitor the level of long-term glucose control in both type 1 and type 2 disease and is especially useful in uncooperative or unreliable patients. The American Diabetes Association recommends measuring levels at least twice a year for well-controlled diabetic patients and quarterly for those with less-optimal control. Nondiabetic values are less than 6, goal values in persons with diabetes are less than 7, and levels greater than 8 warrant further interventions.

Acute Complications of Diabetes

The acute complications of diabetes are *nonketotic hyperglycemic-hyperosmolar coma* and diabetic *ketoacidosis*. Either of these, if not recognized promptly and treated aggressively, can lead to death. These complications should be considered part of a continuum of hyperglycemia rather than separate entities; the main difference between the two is whether ketoacids accumulate. Both are often precipitated by some sort of stress, such as infection, that results in the increased production of glucagon, catecholamines, and cortisol, which in turn enhances gluconeogenesis. If insufficient amounts of insulin or oral hypoglycemic agents are used, then the resulting elevated glucose level will lead to osmotic diuresis and volume depletion. If insulin levels are extremely low or absent (such as in a type 1 diabetic patient), then catabolic processes prevail (such as the conversion of lipids to ketones), and ketoacids are produced, superimposing severe metabolic acidosis on the hyperosmotic volume-depleted state.

The treatment of both these entities involves correcting any precipitating factors such as infection and addressing metabolic abnormalities, which includes reversing the hypovolemia, hyperglycemia, or metabolic acidosis and correcting electrolyte abnormalities such as hypokalemia. The treatment is complex and usually involves admission to an intensive care unit and careful monitoring of all metabolic parameters.

Long-Term Complications of Diabetes

The long-term complications of diabetes are usually secondary to vascular disease. Nephropathy, neuropathy, peripheral vascular disease, coronary atherosclerosis, secondary cerebral thrombosis, cardiac infarction, and retinopathy are all important causes of morbidity and mortality. (Diabetic retinopathy is discussed in BCSC Section 12, *Retina and Vitreous*.)

The precise mechanism for the development of diabetic complications is elusive, but hyperglycemia plays some central role by triggering a number of different mechanisms. These mechanisms include toxicity from elevated sorbitol due to activation of the enzyme aldose reductase by hyperglycemia. An elevated glucose level also results in increased activity of the enzyme protein kinase C (PKC), which in turn results in phosphorylation of various proteins (reversible phosphorylation of proteins is the principal means of governing protein activity within cells). The resultant imbalance of enzymatic activity ultimately causes vascular damage from processes such as excessive endothelial cell basement membrane formation.

Another mechanism involved in diabetic pathophysiology is the formation of advanced glycosylation end products due to nonenzymatic attachment of glucose to various proteins (hemoglobin A_{1c} is an example of such an end product). These advanced glycosylation end products interfere with a number of metabolic processes and have been implicated in the development of all major complications of diabetes. In the retina, all of these mechanisms may in turn stimulate production of vascular endothelial growth factor (VEGF), the compound that appears to be associated with the development of vascular leakage and with the proliferation seen in diabetic retinopathy.

Although careful glucose control is the mainstay of diabetic therapy, the recognition of these additional pathways has led to research into treatments targeting these more distal processes. Potential new treatments include aldose reductase inhibitors, protein kinase C inhibitors, drugs that prevent the formation of advanced glycosylation end products, and inhibitors of VEGF. Clinical studies are under way, and it is hoped that such treatments can be added to the armamentarium in the near future.

Glucose control is not the only risk factor that can be modified to minimize the development of complications. In particular, hypertension and lipid abnormalities seem to be inextricably intertwined with glucose control. Thus, any attempt to minimize complications must include aggressive control of these other factors. Additional risk factors for diabetic complications include duration of disease, smoking, pregnancy, and a genetic predisposition for the disease and for specific complications. Risk factors that seem to exacerbate diabetic retinopathy in particular include early renal disease and anemia.

Nephropathy

Approximately 40% of patients who have had diabetes mellitus for 20 or more years have nephropathy. Albuminuria >300 mg/24 hours is the hallmark of diabetic nephropathy, which is about the level at which a standard urine dipstick test becomes positive. The disease can be diagnosed clinically if diabetic retinopathy is also present and there is no other kidney or renal tract disease. Renal failure eventually occurs in approximately 50% of patients who develop diabetes before age 20 and in 6% of those with onset after age 40. Diabetic nephropathy is the leading cause of end-stage renal disease, and the 5-year survival rate of diabetic patients on maintenance dialysis is less than 20%. Almost invariably, nephropathy and retinopathy develop within a short time of each other.

The progression of diabetic nephropathy is as follows: microalbuminuria (urine albumin levels of 30–300 mg/24 hours), macroalbuminuria (urine albumin levels of over 300 mg/24 hours), nephrotic syndrome, and finally end-stage renal disease. Tight control of blood glucose can delay and perhaps prevent the development of microalbuminuria. Controlling hypertension (particularly with angiotensin-converting enzyme inhibitors) and adhering to low-protein diets may help decrease the rate of decline in glomerular filtration rate.

Neuropathy

Diabetic neuropathy is a common problem. After 30 years of diabetes mellitus, 45%–50% of diabetic patients have signs of neuropathy, and 15%–20% have symptoms of distal symmetrical polyneuropathy. Changes in nerve metabolism and function are thought to be mediated in part through increased aldose reductase activity; Schwann cell synthesis of myelin is impaired, and axonal degeneration ensues. In addition, microangiopathy of the endoneural capillaries leads to vascular abnormalities and microinfarcts of the nerves, with multifocal fiber loss. Symptoms in the feet and lower legs are most common. Foot pain, paresthesias, and loss of sensation occur frequently and probably result from both ischemic and metabolic abnormalities of nerves. Weakness may occur as part of mononeuritis or a mononeuritis multiplex and is usually associated with pain. Cranial neuropathies may also occur (see BCSC Section 5, *Neuro-Ophthalmology*). Significant morbidity can also occur from neuropathy affecting the autonomic nervous system. Problems can include male and female sexual dysfunction, impaired urination, delayed gastric emptying, orthostatic hypotension, and tachycardia due to loss of vagal tone.

There is no specific treatment for diabetic neuropathy. Aldose reductase inhibitors (not yet commercially available) may improve nerve conduction slightly but do not result in major clinical improvement. The pain may respond to tricyclic antidepressants or capsaicin cream (capsaicin, a component of hot peppers, causes analgesia through local depletion of substance P). Anticonvulsant drugs such as carbamazepine (Tegretol) and gabapentin (Neurontin) may also be useful.

Large vessel disease

In diabetic patients, the risk of coronary artery disease is 2–10 times higher than that of the general population, and the mortality rate in diabetic patients with an anterior myocardial infarction is twice that of nondiabetic patients. Because myocardial infarction in patients with diabetes may present without the classic symptom of chest pain, an increased index of suspicion is required to make the diagnosis. Hypertension adds significantly to the risk of cardiovascular disease for persons with diabetes. Cerebral thrombosis is approximately twice as prevalent in the diabetic population as it is in the nondiabetic population, and peripheral vascular disease is 40 times more prevalent in the diabetic population.

Ophthalmologic Considerations

Many times, the ophthalmologist is the physician responsible for identifying and managing what is often the first apparent complication related to a patient's diabetes, whether it is the transient refractive change due to glucose elevation or actual diabetic retinopathy. The ophthalmologist may therefore represent the only regular contact a patient has with the health care system, especially if there are financial or compliance issues that have kept the patient away from other doctors. Efforts should be made to make sure that the patient is seeing the general physician on a regular basis, in the same way that ophthalmologists expect primary care physicians to make timely referrals for patients with diabetes.

In the past, it was considered sufficient for ophthalmologists to simply ask the patient about his or her glucose control and accept an answer such as "good" or "bad." This approach is no longer sufficient. Both the patient and the ophthalmologist should be aware of the patient's HbA_{1c} level, which is a specific and objective measure of glucose control. Patients who do not know about the test should be educated about it, and follow-up with their primary care physicians should be secured, as studies have shown that patients who are knowledgeable about their HbA_{1c} tend to have better control. Unfortunately, even with this knowledge, a patient may still be being managed in a less-than-optimal fashion. A population-based study of more than 7200 patients with type 2 diabetes demonstrated that many patients have HbA_{1c} levels which are higher than ideal for years because changes in therapy to improve glycemic control were not made or were only made slowly. Input from the ophthalmologist may be valuable in nudging the patient, as well as the patient's other health care providers, to be more aggressive about control.

From a purely ophthalmic standpoint, awareness of a patient's control is important because it may affect the rate of retinopathy progression (and thereby affect decisions regarding treatment and frequency of follow-up). Studies have shown that poor control can increase the rate of retinopathy progression after cataract surgery and blunt the treatment response to laser for diabetic macular edema. Educating poorly controlled patients about their prognosis prior to surgical intervention may facilitate more realistic expectations. A recent study suggests yet another reason to be aware of a patient's glucose control at the time of cataract surgery. Although the goal with diabetic patients should always be to improve control, attempting to improve glucose control rapidly in a patient with poor control at the same time that cataract surgery is performed may actually contribute to retinopathy progression and a poorer visual outcome.

It is also important to remember that glucose control is only 1 of many modifiable risk factors for retinopathy progression. Patients should be reminded that diabetic retinopathy is also affected by other problems, including hypertension, lipid abnormalities, early renal failure, and anemia. The importance of these other issues should also be conveyed to the patient's medical doctor so that all potential exacerbating factors are controlled as much as possible. The ophthalmologist should strive to be aware of how well these issues are being controlled, because a patient with significant problems in any of these areas is likely to have less-than-optimal results with any ophthalmic surgical intervention.

Do DV, Shah SM, Sung JU, et al. Persistent diabetic macular edema is associated with elevated hemoglobin A_{1c}. *Am J Ophthalmol.* 2005;139(4):620–623.

Hauser D, Katz H, Pokroy R, et al. Occurrence and progression of diabetic retinopathy after phacoemulsification cataract surgery. *J Cataract Refract Surg.* 2004;30(2):428–432.

Suto C, Hori S, Kato S, et al. Effect of perioperative glycemic control in progression of diabetic retinopathy and maculopathy. *Arch Ophthalmol.* 2006;124:38–45.

Surgical Considerations in Diabetes

Surgery poses additional problems for the diabetic patient. These include the perioperative management of glucose and the risk of systemic complications. A thorough preoperative history should be taken and a careful physical should be performed. Ideally, the patient's primary care physician should be involved in the perioperative management to both anticipate and treat problems related to diabetes. Of particular importance is the increased risk for cardiovascular complications that exists for these patients. Postoperative gastroparesis and problems related to autonomic neuropathy are other potential complications. The stress of both surgery and general anesthesia can result in poor glucose control, because of the release of hormones that act to counteract the effects of insulin. This problem is complicated by the variable amount of oral intake in the perioperative period.

Both severe hyperglycemia and hypoglycemia should be avoided, and fluid and electrolyte balance need to be maintained. There is a tendency to allow the glucose level to run higher at the time of surgery simply to avoid the more devastating acute problems associated with hypoglycemia. However, some studies suggest that an elevated glucose level increases the risk of wound infections and impairs polymorphonuclear leukocyte function. Accordingly, there is general agreement that the perioperative glucose level should ideally range between 120 and 200 mg/dL.

Unfortunately, there are no perioperative guidelines that work for every patient, and both the patient's medical doctor and the anesthesiologist should be involved in management. Frequent blood glucose monitoring is also an important part of the perioperative period. It is best if surgeries for diabetic patients can be scheduled for early in the morning so that these patients' usual schedules can be maintained, especially if a brief surgery such as cataract extraction is planned.

In general, type 2 diabetic patients who are treated with diet alone do not require any specific treatment, although they may require short-acting insulin in the postoperative period to control spikes in glucose levels. Type 2 patients treated with oral agents should hold their drugs on the morning of surgery to avoid hypoglycemia; they can be supplemented with insulin following surgery, if necessary.

For type 1 patients and those type 2 patients who are dependent on insulin, it is usually possible to use subcutaneous injections rather than insulin infusions for brief ophthalmic procedures. It is important to remember that patients who are dependent on insulin require a baseline amount of the drug to avoid developing ketoacidosis, even if their blood glucose level is normal and they are not eating. Depending on the time of surgery, these patients may need to decrease their dose of long-acting insulin the day before surgery and perhaps decrease the nighttime dosing of any intermediate-acting agents. If an early-morning procedure of brief duration is planned, patients may simply delay their usual morning short-acting insulin until they begin to eat after surgery. If the procedure is scheduled for later in the day, approximately half of the usual morning intermediate-acting dose may be used, although the actual recommendations will vary depending on the patient's usual insulin regimen. Additional factors are whether the IV infusion includes glucose and what the infusion rate is. Patients on continuous insulin infusion pumps should simply continue their usual basal infusion rate, making adjustments as needed to allow for varying glucose levels. Finally, patients undergoing longer surgeries may need IV insulin and glucose infusions, and management of these more complex situations should be individualized with input from the patient, the doctor, and the anesthesiologist.

> American Diabetes Association National Institute of Diabetes and Digestive and Kidney Diseases. The prevention or delay of type 2 diabetes. *Diabetes Care.* 2004;27 suppl 1:S47–S54.
> Genuth S. Diabetes mellitus. [ACP Medicine Web site]. May 2004 Update. Available at http://www.acpmedicine.com.
> Henderson KE, Baranski TJ, Bickel PE, eds. *The Washington Manual Endocrinology Subspecialty Consult.* Philadelphia: Lippincott Williams & Wilkins; 2005.
> Larsen PR, ed. *Williams Textbook of Endocrinology.* 10th ed. Philadelphia: Saunders; 2003.

Thyroid Disease

Physiology

Functionally, the thyroid gland can be thought of as having 2 parts. The *parafollicular* (or C) cells secrete calcitonin and do not play a role in thyroid physiology. Thyroid *follicles* are made up of a single layer of epithelial cells surrounding colloid, which consists mostly of thyroglobulin, the storage form of the thyroid hormones T_4 and T_3.

T_4 (thyroxine), the main secretory product of the thyroid gland, contains 4 iodine atoms. Deiodination of T_4, which occurs mainly in the liver and kidney, gives rise to T_3, the metabolically active form of thyroid hormone. Eighty percent of serum T_3 is derived through deiodination; the remainder is secreted by the thyroid. Only a small fraction of the hormones circulate free in the plasma (0.02% of total T_4 and 0.3% of total T_3); the remainder is bound to the proteins thyroxine-binding globulin (TBG), transthyretin, and albumin.

Thyroid function is regulated by the interrelationships of hypothalamic, pituitary, and thyroid activity. Thyrotropin-releasing hormone (TRH) is secreted by the hypothalamus, causing the synthesis and release of thyrotropin (or thyroid-stimulating hormone, TSH) from the anterior pituitary. TSH, in turn, stimulates the thyroid, leading to release of T_4 and T_3. T_4 and T_3 inhibit the release of TSH and the TSH response to TRH at the level of the pituitary.

The main role of the thyroid hormones is regulation of tissue metabolism through their effects on protein synthesis. Normal development of the central nervous system requires adequate amounts of thyroid hormone during the first 2 years of life. Hypothyroidism results in irreversible mental retardation (cretinism). Normal growth and bone maturation also depend on sufficient hormone levels.

Testing for Thyroid Disease

Detection of thyroid disease and evaluation of the efficacy of therapy require the use of various combinations of laboratory tests. Increased availability of direct measurement of free T_4 and the "sensitive" TSH test have greatly simplified the testing process.

Measurement of serum T_4

Total serum T_4 is composed of 2 parts: the protein-bound fraction and the free hormone. Total T_4 levels can be affected by changes in serum TBG levels while euthyroidism is maintained and free T_4 levels remain normal. Levels of TBG and total T_4 are elevated in pregnancy and with use of oral contraceptives, while free T_4 levels remain normal. Low TBG and total T_4 levels are associated with chronic illness, protein malnutrition, hepatic failure, and use of glucocorticoids.

For many years, laboratory determination of total T_4 by radioimmunoassay was the most commonly used direct measurement of thyroid function. Free T_4 was then calculated indirectly via multiplication of total T_4 by the T_3 resin uptake (itself an indirect determination of the fraction of unbound thyroid hormone in the serum). Direct determination of free T_4 has become widely available, however, improving the accuracy of thyroid function testing.

Measurement of serum T_3

Serum T_3 levels may not accurately reflect thyroid gland function for 2 reasons: first, because T_3 is not the major secretory product of the thyroid; and second, because many factors influence T_3 levels, including nutrition, medications, and mechanisms regulating the enzymes that convert T_4 to T_3. Determination of T_3 levels is indicated in patients who may have T_3 thyrotoxicosis, an uncommon condition in which clinically hyperthyroid patients have normal T_4 and free T_4 but elevated T_3 levels.

Measurement of serum TSH

TSH secretion by the pituitary is tightly controlled by negative feedback mechanisms regulated by serum T_4 and T_3 levels. TSH levels begin to rise early in the course of hypothyroidism and fall early in hyperthyroidism, even before free T_4 levels are outside the reference range. Therefore, the serum TSH level is a sensitive indicator of thyroid dysfunction.

The concentration of TSH is very low and, until recently, available tests were not sensitive enough to differentiate between the normal and reduced TSH levels seen in hypothyroidism. In recent years, extremely sensitive assays of TSH have been developed that can detect levels down to 0.005 mU/L, making it possible to differentiate low normal values from abnormally low levels. The TSH test is useful for (1) screening for thyroid disease, (2) monitoring replacement therapy in hypothyroid patients (TSH levels respond 6–8 weeks after changes in hormone replacement dosage), and (3) monitoring suppressive therapy for thyroid nodules or cancer. In screening for thyroid disease, the combination of free T_4 and sensitive TSH assays has a sensitivity of 99.5% and a specificity of 98%. As a result, the combination of both TSH and free T_4 is used for screening in most situations. There is presently some controversy about the upper limit of normal for TSH, and endocrinologic consultation is indicated in borderline cases.

Serum thyroid hormone–binding protein tests

TBG concentrations can be measured directly by immunoassay. However, it is rarely necessary to determine the levels of circulating TBG and transthyretin in the clinical setting. The T_3 resin uptake test can be used to estimate thyroid hormone–binding.

Radioactive iodine uptake

A 24-hour test of the thyroid's ability to concentrate a dose of radioactive iodine, radioactive iodine uptake (RAIU) is not always accurate enough to assess thyroid metabolic status. The RAIU test is used mainly to determine whether a patient's hyperthyroidism is due to Graves disease (elevated RAIU, >30%–40%), toxic nodular goiter (normal to elevated), or subacute thyroiditis (low to undetectable, <2%–4%).

Testing for antithyroid antibodies

Several antibodies related to thyroid disease can be detected in the blood. The most common is *thyroid microsomal antibody,* found in about 95% of patients with Hashimoto thyroiditis, 55% of those with Graves disease, and 10% of adults with no apparent thyroid disease. Antibodies to thyroglobulin are also found in thyroid disease of various causes, including Hashimoto thyroiditis, Graves disease, and thyroid carcinoma. Patients with Graves disease usually have antibodies directed at TSH receptors. These antibodies generally stimulate the release of thyroid hormone, although rare patients may have antibodies that block thyroid hormone release. High serum levels of thyroid stimulating immunoglobulin and the absence of antithyroperoxidase antibody are both risk factors for ophthalmopathy in Graves disease. Assays are being developed to detect antibodies against antigens present on extraocular muscles in Graves ophthalmopathy.

Thyroid scanning

Scanning with iodine 123 reveals concentration and binding, whereas using technetium 99m demonstrates iodide-concentrating capacity. Thyroid scanning is useful in distinguishing functioning (hot) from nonfunctioning (cold) thyroid nodules and in evaluating chest and neck masses for metastatic thyroid cancer.

Thyroid ultrasonography

Ultrasonography is used to establish the presence of cystic or solid thyroid nodules when palpation is inconclusive in suspicious cases. This modality detects nodules as small as 1 mm, although nodules of this size are not of clinical significance. Thyroid ultrasonography is also useful in assessing the effectiveness of suppressive therapy for reduction of thyroid nodule size.

Biopsy or fine-needle aspiration biopsy

These techniques are used to obtain tissue samples for the evaluation of thyroid nodules. Fine-needle aspiration specimens require interpretation by an experienced cytopathologist. Needle aspiration is also used to drain fluid from cystic thyroid nodules.

Hyperthyroidism

Hypermetabolism caused by excessive quantities of circulating thyroid hormones results in the clinical syndrome of *hyperthyroidism (thyrotoxicosis)*. This syndrome can be caused by a number of diseases. Graves hyperthyroidism accounts for approximately 85% of cases of thyrotoxicosis. Toxic nodular goiter and thyroiditis account for most of the remaining cases. *Thyroid storm*, a potentially fatal complication seen in some patients with hyperthyroidism, is a medical emergency. It is often precipitated by stress or infection in a patient with otherwise mild hyperthyroidism; modern treatments aimed at controlling the process have dramatically reduced mortality.

Graves hyperthyroidism

Patients with Graves hyperthyroidism (also known as *diffuse toxic goiter*) exhibit various combinations of hypermetabolism, diffuse enlargement of the thyroid gland, ophthalmopathy (or orbitopathy), and infiltrative dermopathy. Although the exact cause is not known, Graves hyperthyroidism is thought to be an autoimmune disorder: 85%–90% of patients have circulating TSH receptor antibodies. Patients with ophthalmopathy usually have high titers of antibodies against the TSH receptors; antibodies to soluble human eye muscle antigens have also been found in these patients but not in patients with Graves hyperthyroidism without eye involvement. Graves hyperthyroidism and Graves ophthalmopathy can be considered separate diseases that share a common autoantibody—the actual clinical presentation is determined by the response of the target tissue (either thyroid or retro-orbital connective tissue) to the autoantibody.

Graves hyperthyroidism is common, with a 10:1 female preponderance. The incidence peaks in the third and fourth decades of life; there is a strong familial component, and stress may also play a role. Current smoking is associated with an increased incidence of ophthalmopathy that parallels the number of cigarettes smoked per day.

The clinical syndrome is well known, consisting of nervousness, tremor, weight loss, palpitations, heat intolerance, emotional lability, muscle weakness, and gastrointestinal hypermotility. Clinical signs include tachycardia or atrial fibrillation, increased systolic and decreased diastolic blood pressure (widened pulse pressure), and thyroid enlargement. Infiltrative dermopathy—brawny, nonpitting swelling of the pretibial area, ankles, or feet—may be present and is almost always associated with orbitopathy. *Infiltrative dermopathy* was known as *pretibial myxedema* in the past. The terminology has changed to avoid confusion with the term *myxedema,* which refers to the diffuse accumulation of glycosaminoglycans and fluid in hypothyroidism.

Approximately 20%–40% of patients with Graves hyperthyroidism have clinically obvious Graves ophthalmopathy at the time of diagnosis of the hyperthyroidism. However, if imaging techniques such as CT or MRI are used, subtle evidence of ophthalmopathy can be seen in many patients with Graves hyperthyroidism who do not have clinically obvious eye changes. The ophthalmopathy may appear before the onset of hyperthyroidism in approximately 20% of patients, concurrently in about 40%, and in the 6 months after diagnosis, in about 20%. The eye disease may also first become apparent after treatment of the hyperthyroidism, especially if radioiodine is used. Graves disease can also occur in approximately 5% of patients with myasthenia gravis, which can complicate the clinical findings.

One notable situation for the ophthalmologist is *euthyroid* Graves ophthalmopathy, which occurs in perhaps 10% of patients with eye disease. These patients present with ophthalmopathy but without coexisting hyperthyroidism, although they often have elevated levels of serum antithyroid antibodies. Patients may eventually develop manifest thyroid disease months to years later. In some cases, however, patients have ophthalmic manifestations without ever demonstrating thyroid abnormalities.

Treatment of Graves hyperthyroidism is aimed at returning thyroid function to normal. A significant proportion of patients (30%–50%) experience remission in association with drug treatment directed at the thyroid. Later in the course of the disease, patients may experience relapse, hypothyroidism, or both.

The first step in treatment is to control symptoms, if necessary, with a beta-blocker. In addition, thyroid secretion is suppressed using 1 of the thiourea derivatives, propylthiouracil or methimazole *(Tapazole)*. The drugs work by inhibiting the organification of iodine by the gland. Treatment is continued until clinical and laboratory indices show improvement. Adverse effects include rash (common), liver damage (rare), vasculitis (rare), and agranulocytosis (0.02%–0.05% of patients).

There are several options for long-term treatment of Graves hyperthyroidism: the aforementioned antithyroid drugs can be continued for 12–24 months in hopes of a remission; part of the gland can be surgically removed, an option that is frequently successful, although approximately half of such patients eventually become hypothyroid; or radioactive iodine can be used, which is the third and most common choice. Iodine 131 is highly effective, resulting in hypothyroidism in 80% of patients within 6–12 months; some require a second treatment. Side effects are minimal, although use of iodine 131 may be associated with worsening of the ophthalmopathy. Steroids may be useful in preventing progression of ophthalmopathy related to this treatment.

The optimal management of Graves ophthalmopathy is variable. Control of the thyroid disease is the first step, and patients who smoke should be urged to stop smoking. Prednisone may be useful in treating inflammatory exacerbations. Investigators have recently questioned the benefit of orbital radiotherapy for Graves ophthalmopathy. Surgical decompression is an option when involvement is more severe. (Graves hyperthyroidism and Graves ophthalmopathy are discussed extensively in BCSC Section 7: *Orbit, Eyelids, and Lacrimal System.*)

Toxic nodular goiter

In this condition, thyroid hormone–producing adenomas (either single or multiple) make enough hormone to cause hyperthyroidism. Hot nodules (those shown to be functioning on thyroid scan) are almost never carcinomatous and often result in hyperthyroidism. Toxic nodules may be treated with radioactive iodine or surgery.

Hypothyroidism

Hypothyroidism is a clinical syndrome resulting from a deficiency of thyroid hormone. *Myxedema* is the nonpitting edema caused by subcutaneous accumulation of mucopolysaccharides in severe cases of hypothyroidism; the term is sometimes used to describe the entire syndrome of severe hypothyroidism.

Primary hypothyroidism accounts for more than 95% of cases and may be a congenital condition or it may be acquired. Most primary cases are due to Hashimoto thyroiditis (discussed next), "idiopathic" myxedema (thought by many to be end-stage Hashimoto thyroiditis as well), and iatrogenic causes (after iodine 131 or surgical treatment of hyperthyroidism). *Secondary hypothyroidism,* caused by hypothalamic or pituitary dysfunction (usually after pituitary surgery), is much less common. As in hyperthyroidism, the female preponderance among adults with hypothyroidism is significant. *Subclinical hypothyroidism* is defined as a normal T_4 concentration and a slightly elevated TSH level. These patients may or may not have symptoms suggestive of hypothyroidism, and there is some controversy about whether such patients should be treated.

Clinically, the patient with hypothyroidism presents with signs and symptoms of hypometabolism and accumulation of mucopolysaccharides in the tissues of the body. Many of the symptoms are nonspecific, and their relationship to thyroid dysfunction may not be recognized for some time: weakness, fatigue, lethargy, decreased memory, dry skin, deepening of the voice, weight gain (despite loss of appetite), cold intolerance, arthralgias, constipation, and muscle cramps. Clinical signs include bradycardia, reduced pulse pressure, myxedema, loss of body and scalp hair, and menstrual disorders. In severe cases, personality changes ("myxedema madness") and death (following "myxedema coma") may occur.

Treatment of hypothyroidism is straightforward, consisting of oral thyroid replacement medication to normalize circulating hormone levels. Levothyroxine is the most commonly used preparation. Serum T_4 and TSH levels are monitored at regular intervals to ensure that euthyroidism is maintained.

Thyroiditis

Thyroiditis may be classified as acute, subacute, or chronic. *Acute thyroiditis,* caused by bacterial infection, is extremely rare. *Subacute thyroiditis* occurs in 2 forms: granulomatous and lymphocytic. Hashimoto thyroiditis is the most common type of *chronic thyroiditis.*

Patients with *subacute granulomatous thyroiditis* present with a painful, enlarged gland associated with fever, chills, and malaise. Thyroid function tests may be helpful because they may reveal the unusual combination of an elevated T_4 level and a low RAIU. Patients may be hyperthyroid because of release of hormone from areas of thyroid destruction; pathologic examination reveals granulomatous inflammation. The disease is self-limited, and treatment is symptomatic, with use of either analgesics or, in severe cases, oral corticosteroids. After resolution, transient hypothyroidism, which becomes permanent in 5%–10% of patients, may occur.

Patients with *subacute lymphocytic thyroiditis* ("painless" thyroiditis), which commonly occurs 2–4 months postpartum in mothers but may occur in isolation, present with symptoms of hyperthyroidism and a normal or slightly enlarged but nontender thyroid gland. Pathologic investigation shows lymphocytic infiltration resembling Hashimoto thyroiditis, suggesting an autoimmune cause. This disease is also self-limited, generally lasting less than 3 months. Hypothyroidism may ensue. Treatment is symptomatic.

An autoimmune disease that appears to be closely related to Graves hyperthyroidism, Hashimoto thyroiditis is the most common cause of goitrous hypothyroidism in iodine-sufficient areas of the world. Patients have antibodies to 1 or more thyroid antigens and an increased incidence of other autoimmune diseases, such as Sjögren syndrome, systemic lupus erythematosus, idiopathic thrombocytopenic purpura, and pernicious anemia.

Rarely, other endocrine organs—the adrenals, parathyroids, pancreatic islet cells, pituitary, and gonads—may be involved as well.

Patients with Hashimoto thyroiditis may present with hypothyroidism, an enlarged thyroid, or both. Pathologic examination reveals lymphocytic infiltration. Treatment is aimed at normalizing hormone levels with thyroid replacement therapy. Patients with enlarged glands and airway obstruction that do not respond to TSH suppression may require surgery. The risk of primary thyroid lymphoma is slightly increased in patients with Hashimoto thyroiditis.

Postpartum thyroiditis occurs in approximately 5% of women after delivery (often in subsequent pregnancies) and can cause hyperthyroidism or hypothyroidism (or first one problem and then the other). Postpartum thyroiditis is usually painless and self-limited and is often associated with antimicrosomal antibodies.

Thyroid Tumors

Virtually all tumors of the thyroid gland arise from glandular cells and are, therefore, adenomas or carcinomas. Functioning adenomas have been discussed previously (see the discussion of toxic nodular goiter).

On thyroid scan, 90%–95% of thyroid adenomas are nonfunctioning ("cold" nodules) and come to attention only if large enough to be physically apparent. Diagnostic testing involves a combination of approaches, including ultrasonography (cysts are benign and simply aspirated), fine-needle aspiration, and surgery, depending on the clinical situation. Treatment options for benign cold nodules are suppressive therapy, in which thyroid hormone replacement is used to suppress TSH secretion and its stimulatory effect on functioning nodules, and surgery.

Carcinomas of the thyroid are of 4 types: papillary, follicular, medullary, and anaplastic (undifferentiated). *Papillary carcinoma* is the most common form of thyroid tumor. Tumors removed prior to extension outside the capsule of the gland appear to have no adverse effect on survival. *Follicular carcinoma* may also be compatible with a normal life span if it is identified before it becomes invasive, although late metastases can occur. *Medullary carcinoma* arises from the C cells and produces calcitonin. The lesion can occur as a solitary malignancy or as part of the multiple endocrine neoplasia syndrome type 2 (discussed later). *Anaplastic carcinoma*, though rare, is the most malignant tumor of the thyroid gland and is found mainly in patients older than age 60. With the giant cell form, the survival time is less than 6 months from time of diagnosis; with the small cell form, the 5-year survival rate is 20%–25%.

The Hypothalamic-Pituitary Axis

The hypothalamus is the coordinating center of the endocrine system. It consolidates signals from upper cortical inputs, the autonomic nervous system, the environment, and systemic endocrine feedback. The hypothalamus then delivers precise instructions to the pituitary gland, which releases hormones that influence most endocrine systems in the body. The hypothalamic-pituitary axis directly affects the thyroid gland, the adrenal gland, and the gonads, and it influences growth, milk production, and water balance.

Table 9-6 shows the various hypothalamic and anterior pituitary hormones involved in this system. The hypothalamic hormones are released directly into a primary capillary plexus that empties into the portal venous circulation, travels down the pituitary stalk, and bathes the anterior pituitary gland in a secondary capillary plexus. The hormones released by the hypothalamic neurons therefore reach their target cells rapidly and in high concentrations. This proximity allows a rapid, pulsatile response to signals between the hypothalamus and the anterior pituitary. The posterior pituitary is controlled by direct neuronal innervation from the hypothalamus rather than by blood-borne hormones. The main products of the posterior pituitary are vasopressin and oxytocin. Vasopressin (antidiuretic hormone) is primarily involved in controlling water excretion by the kidneys. Oxytocin produces uterine contractions required for delivery.

Pituitary Adenomas

Pituitary tumors constitute 10% of intracranial tumors. They are classified as *microadenomas* (<10 mm in widest diameter) or *macroadenomas* (>10 mm in widest diameter). Typically benign, these tumors arise from hormone-producing cells and may be functionally active (ie, producing usually large amounts of hormones) or inactive. The clinical presentation depends on what type of cell the tumor is derived from and whether there is hormone production. Any type of tumor may be clinically nonfunctioning and therefore will become apparent only when it has enlarged enough to cause symptoms, at which time patients may present with headaches, visual symptoms due to chiasmal compression, cranial neuropathies and/or hypopituitarism from compression of normal pituitary tissue. (The visual effects of pituitary adenomas and other parasellar lesions are discussed in BCSC Section 5, *Neuro-Ophthalmology*.)

Accounting for approximately 15% of pituitary tumors, *somatotroph adenomas* produce growth hormone and cause acromegaly in adults and gigantism in prepubertal patients. Acromegaly often develops insidiously over several years. Patients may present with headaches and visual symptoms due to enlargement of the adenoma before the diagnosis is recognized. The characteristic findings are an enlarged jaw, coarse facial features, and enlarged and swollen hands and feet. Patients may also have cardiac disease and diabetes mellitus in addition to the typical bone and soft tissue changes.

Lactotroph adenomas (prolactinomas) account for approximately 25% of symptomatic pituitary tumors. Hyperprolactinemia produces amenorrhea and galactorrhea in women and decreased libido and impotence in men. The symptoms tend to be gradual in males, and patients may present with compression symptoms due to tumor enlargement before the hormonal effects are recognized.

Thyrotroph adenomas are rare, accounting for less than 1% of pituitary tumors. They may cause hyperthyroidism, hypothyroidism, or no change in thyroid function depending on how the TSH subunits are processed in the tumor cells. These tumors tend to be large macroadenomas, and patients may present with compressive symptoms in addition to any thyroid changes.

Corticotroph adenomas account for approximately 15% of pituitary tumors. They are associated with Cushing syndrome, which includes the classic features of centripetal obesity, hirsutism, and plethora. Patients develop fat deposits over the thoracocervical spine

Table 9-6 Major Hypothalamic Hormones and Their Effect on Anterior Pituitary Hormones

Corticotropin-releasing hormone releases adrenocorticotropic hormone (ACTH).
Growth hormone–releasing hormone releases growth hormone.
Somatostatin inhibits growth hormone release.
Gonadotropin-releasing hormone releases luteinizing hormone (LH) and follicle-stimulating hormone (FSH).
Thyrotropin-releasing hormone (TRH) releases thyrotropin (TSH).
Prolactin-releasing factors (including serotonin, acetylcholine, opiates, and estrogens) release prolactin.
Prolactin-inhibiting factors (including dopamine) inhibit the release of prolactin.
Melanocyte-stimulating hormone-releasing factor releases melanocyte-stimulating hormone.

Reproduced with permission from Martin KA. Hypothalamic-pituitary axis. In: *UpToDate*, Rose BD (Ed), Waltham, MA. Available at http://www.uptodate.com. Accessed March 1, 2005.

(buffalo hump) and temporal regions (moon facies). Psychiatric abnormalities occur in 50% of patients, and long-standing Cushing disease can produce osteoporosis. Patients bruise easily and have violet striae on the abdomen, upper thighs, and arms. Hypertension and glucose intolerance leading to diabetes can also occur. Cushing syndrome can also occur because of adrenal gland neoplasms and, most commonly, because of iatrogenic administration of glucocorticoids.

Gonadotroph adenomas (approximately 10% of pituitary tumors) may produce serum follicle-stimulating hormone and, rarely, luteinizing hormone. Affected patients present with hypogonadism related to gonadal down-regulation. Gonadotropin-producing pituitary tumors may also be clinically nonfunctioning, and patients may present with compression symptoms.

Accounting for approximately 15% of pituitary tumors, *plurihormonal adenomas,* as the name implies, produce more than 1 type of hormone. Common combinations include elevated growth hormone with prolactin, and growth hormone with TSH.

Null-cell adenomas (approximately 20% of pituitary tumors) do not have any pathologic markers to suggest a certain cell type and do not produce hormone excess. The majority of tumors that present with signs of enlargement and compression are gonadotroph or null cell adenomas.

Tumors of the pituitary gland are best diagnosed with MRI focused on the pituitary region. Endocrinologic testing is warranted when hypersecretion syndromes are suspected or when the patient has evidence of hypopituitarism due to compression of the normal pituitary by a nonfunctioning adenoma. The treatment approach is complex and depends on a number of factors, including the size of the tumor and the nature of the hormonal activity. Treatment is discussed further in BCSC Section 5, *Neuro-Ophthalmology.*

Pituitary Apoplexy

Pituitary apoplexy results from hemorrhage in a pituitary adenoma that can occur spontaneously or after head trauma. In its most dramatic presentation, apoplexy causes the sudden onset of excruciating headache, visual field loss, diplopia due to pressure on the oculomotor nerves, and hypopituitarism. All pituitary hormonal deficiencies can occur, but cortisol deficiency is the most serious because it can cause life-threatening hypotension. Imaging of the pituitary reveals intra-adenomal hemorrhage and deviation of the pituitary stalk. Most patients recover but experience long-term pituitary insufficiency. Signs of reduced visual acuity and altered mental status are indications for transsphenoidal surgical decompression. Ophthalmologists need to be aware of this entity because of the high incidence of visual symptoms on presentation.

Multiple Endocrine Neoplasia Syndromes

Multiple endocrine neoplasia (MEN) syndromes are rare hereditary syndromes of benign and malignant endocrine neoplasms. There are 2 syndromes, MEN type I and MEN type II, both of which are inherited in an autosomal dominant fashion. MEN II is further divided into types IIA and IIB.

The most common features of MEN type I are parathyroid, enteropancreatic, and pituitary tumors. Hyperparathyroidism is the most common endocrine abnormality. Enteropancreatic tumors include gastrinomas, which cause increased gastric acid output (Zollinger-Ellison syndrome), and insulinomas, which cause fasting hypoglycemia. Pituitary adenomas can be present and are usually prolactinomas, though other types can also occur. Carcinoid and adrenal tumors can develop as well.

MEN types IIA and IIB are characterized by medullary thyroid cancer, which occurs in 90%–100% of patients and is the main cause of morbidity. Pheochromocytoma occurs with an incidence of approximately 50%. Hyperparathyroidism is seen in approximately 20%–30% of patients with MEN type IIA, but is rarely seen in type IIB.

MEN type IIB is characterized by ganglioneuromas, which occur in 95% of patients. They can occur in the lips, eyelids, and tongue, giving these patients a characteristic phenotype that can be apparent at birth. Patients with MEN type IIB may also have marfanoid features but do not have lens subluxation or aortic disease. The eyelid margins may be nodular because of the presence of multiple small tumors (Fig 9-2), and neuromas have also been reported subconjunctivally. Perhaps the most striking ophthalmic finding is the presence of prominent corneal nerves in a clear stroma; this is reported to occur in 100%

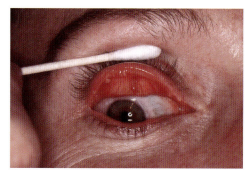

Figure 9-2 Eyelid nodules in MEN type IIB. *(Photograph courtesy of Jason M. Jacobs, MD, and Michael J. Hawes, MD.)*

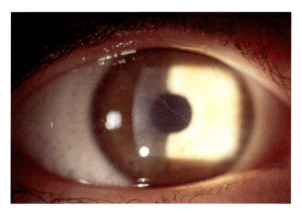

Figure 9-3 Enlarged corneal nerves in MEN type IIB. *(Photograph courtesy of Jason M. Jacobs, MD, and Michael J. Hawes, MD.)*

of cases (Fig 9-3). Because the medullary thyroid cancer may not appear until the patient's second or third decade, the ophthalmic manifestations may be the initial indication that a patient has MEN type IIB, making ophthalmologists potentially instrumental in diagnosing this disease.

The management of MEN depends on the nature of the tumor and usually involves medical treatment to control hormonal effects and/or surgical excision when possible. The genes that cause all types of MEN have been located, and genetic testing can identify patients at risk. Identification of involved family members is particularly useful in MEN type II because prophylactic thyroidectomy can decrease the risk of death from medullary thyroid cancer. Screening for pheochromocytoma is also warranted in order to identify problems before complications such as hypertension develop. Ophthalmologists have a critical role to play in recognizing the findings associated with MEN type IIB, because early diagnosis of this syndrome may be lifesaving.

> Henderson KE, Baranski TJ, Bickel PE, eds. *The Washington Manual Endocrinology Subspecialty Consult*. Philadelphia: Lippincott Williams & Wilkins; 2005.
> Jacobs JM, Hawes MJ. From eyelid bumps to thyroid lumps: report of a MEN type IIb family and review of the literature. *Ophthal Plast Reconstr Surg*. 2001;17(3):195–201.
> Larsen PR, ed. *Williams Textbook of Endocrinology*. 10th ed. Philadelphia: Saunders; 2003.
> UpToDate Web site. Available at http://www.uptodate.com.

The authors would like to thank David A. Sorg, MD, for his contributions to this chapter.

CHAPTER 10

Geriatrics

The expanding percentage of elderly persons in the United States presents a growing challenge to primary care physicians and medical subspecialists. With increasing life expectancies (a record high of 76.9 years in 2000) and the aging of the post–World War II baby boomers, the population older than age 65 has grown from 4% at the turn of the 20th century to 12.35% in 2002. By some projections, in the year 2030, 20% of Americans will be older than age 65, and by the year 2010 the number of seniors older than age 85 will have increased to 6.1 million. In addition, this subpopulation accounts for a disproportionately large share (one third) of the US health care dollar.

Ophthalmology is one specialty that will be significantly affected by this demographic shift. Although ophthalmologists already care for elderly patients, there will be an increasing need for geriatric expertise in all the medical subspecialties, including ophthalmology. In addition, cataracts, age-related macular degeneration (AMD), ischemic optic neuropathy, giant cell arteritis, diabetic retinopathy, and glaucoma are all diseases that disproportionately affect older persons. These eye conditions are discussed elsewhere, but the ophthalmologist needs to consider the impact of visual loss on activities of daily living (ADL) and functional outcome.

Ophthalmologists may be expert in dealing with ophthalmic problems in the geriatric population, but they may lack experience in identifying and managing geriatric problems in general. In the past, most medical specialties (including ophthalmology) have followed the traditional medical paradigm of diagnosis of illness, treatment of disease, and measurement of objective outcomes (usually vision parameters such as visual acuity or visual field). The relatively new subspecialty of geriatrics emphasizes a different medical paradigm of functional assessment and a more holistic approach to patient care. For example, rather than measuring visual acuity as an independent and isolated outcome, a functional approach might incorporate improvement in ADL and independence.

Geriatricians have developed validated instruments for assessment of ADL. Practicing ophthalmologists probably would not use these instruments daily, but they must recognize the potential impact of visual loss on ADL, as well as the importance of joining the geriatrician or primary care physician in complete evaluation and management of their elderly patients. The paradigm involves a multidisciplinary history and comprehensive physical examination incorporating measures of physical health (including visual function), psychosocial assessment (including mental health, social support), and functional assessment.

These goals were summarized by the National Institutes of Health Development Conference on Geriatric Assessment: "The multiple problems of older persons are uncovered, described, and explained, if possible, and the resources and strengths of the person are catalogued, the need for services assessed, and a coordinated care plan developed to focus interventions on the person's problems."

The ophthalmologist's role in this multidisciplinary evaluation is to communicate the visual limitations and visual needs of the older patient to the geriatrician and contribute to the integrated goals of the care plan. The role of the ophthalmologist is not to provide a comprehensive geriatric assessment but to screen for and identify particular geriatric conditions (eg, depression, dementia).

Lee and coworkers have shown that, in an ophthalmology practice, screening for depression, dementia, and functional impairment can be accomplished quickly (less than 5 minutes) and easily with a geriatric screening tool that they developed. Their investigation selected elements from more comprehensive established tests (clock drawing, Instrumental Activities of Daily Living) and from a depression screening. Questions taken from *Modules in Clinical Geriatrics* and incorporated into the screening related to using the telephone, traveling, shopping, preparing meals, doing housework, taking medication, and managing money. To screen for depression, they asked, "Do you often feel sad or depressed?" By incorporating questions from accepted geriatric screening tests into their newly devised test, Lee and colleagues were able to screen, in a relatively short time, a selected group of geriatric patients before their eye examination. They demonstrated that 20% of patients studied were depressed or showed early signs of dementia and 6% of these patients had a functional impairment. Using this tool, the ophthalmologist would be able to identify patients at risk and refer them to appropriate resources.

The psychosocial assessment recognizes the age-related role changes and identifies and coordinates available services. The goals are to increase the level of functioning but maintain patient self-determination. The ophthalmologist should recognize the need for psychosocial assessment when there is a change in the patient's cognitive, affective, or functional abilities (eg, loss of visual function, new signs or symptoms of depression or dementia, inability to drive).

Appropriate referral and coordination of care with the geriatrician or primary care physician should accomplish the following:

- Identify the strengths and weaknesses of patients in their environment.
- Assess cognitive, affective, functional, environmental, and economic issues.
- Include any appropriate changes in social support, and identify caregiver stress.
- Explore possible placement issues and options.

The ophthalmologist, though generally not the primary clinician involved in placement, should be aware of the placement options and refer appropriately. The ophthalmologist should also be able to assess the effect of vision loss on function. A final role of the ophthalmologist is to provide low-vision rehabilitation or to refer patients for such care when needed. Low-vision rehabilitation can significantly improve the patient's quality of life. A successful program can ameliorate depression and enhance independence, potentially avoiding the need for institutionalization.

Physiologic Aging and Pathologic Findings of the Aging Eye

Aging changes of the eye occur naturally but with marked variability among individuals. The periorbital and eyelid skin and soft tissues atrophy with age. Dermatochalasis and levator dehiscence may produce secondary ptosis. Lid laxity may cause entropion, ectropion, and trichiasis. Lacrimal gland dysfunction, decreased tear production, meibomian gland disease, and goblet cell dysfunction may cause dry eye symptoms. As a person ages, the conjunctiva undergoes atrophic changes, and corneal sensitivity is reduced. The pupils become progressively miotic and less reactive to light. There is an increasing incidence of presbyopia, cataract, glaucoma, AMD, and diabetic retinopathy. Contrast sensitivity and visual field sensitivity are reduced. In addition, refractive error (of some type) is present in more than 90% of older patients and remains a significant cause of visual disability in the nursing home patient.

The 4 leading causes of visual loss in the elderly are AMD, glaucoma, cataract, and diabetic retinopathy. It is estimated that more than 1,070,000 patients older than age 65 will have neovascular AMD. Glaucoma becomes more common with increasing age, and screening is recommended for patients older than age 50. By 2020, 30.1 million Americans will have cataracts—an increase of 50%. The number of Americans with pseudophakia/aphakia, by 2020, is estimated to be 9.5 million, an increase of 60%.

Pharmacology

Medication use and the number and frequency of medications, adverse reactions to medicines, and drug interactions increase with advancing age. Ophthalmologists need to be aware that, in elderly patients, ophthalmic medications may have adverse effects or may interact with other medications. Age-related pharmacokinetic changes include changes in drug absorption, distribution, metabolism, and elimination. Caution is needed when using new agents, which are often less tested and proven in the elderly. A complete medication history including prescription medications, over-the-counter drugs, herbal agents, vitamins and supplements, and topical agents is mandatory in all patients. As some elderly patients are unaware of or do not remember their medication allergies, verifying this information with the family or primary medical doctor would be prudent. See also BCSC Section 2, *Fundamentals and Principles of Ophthalmology,* Chapter 17.

The ophthalmologist should regularly review all of the patient's medications (including topical antibiotics, steroids, and antiglaucoma medications). Elderly patients (especially nursing home patients) often take multiple medications whose indications expired long ago. Review of the indications for current ophthalmic medications and discontinuation of unnecessary medications should reduce ophthalmology's contribution to polypharmacy. In addition, ophthalmologists should be familiar with all of the agents that they prescribe, their side effects in the elderly, and their potential interactions with other medications used by the elderly patient. For example, the long-term use of systemic steroids in the elderly patient may cause proximal muscle wasting and may exacerbate osteoporosis. Finally, if medical therapy is needed, the ophthalmologist should recognize that compliance issues are often more complex in elderly persons. Considerations include dosing frequency, difficulty in applying the medication or remembering complex dosing regimens (because of dementia, arthritis, poor vision), the number of agents, and expense. A list of prescribed eye medications that includes the dose and frequency of administration (preferably printed in large type and color coded to match the caps on the bottles) helps to ensure compliance.

Outpatient Visits

Ophthalmology is largely an outpatient specialty. Access to the ophthalmologist's office can be a major physical barrier to eye care for the elderly. The ideal outpatient office should be designed to accommodate geriatric patients with various disabilities. The geriatric-friendly office environment should include the following:

- a safe, well-lit office that is close to drop-off areas and parking
- automatic or assisted doors (doorways with pull levers or handles)
- large-print, legible, and well-placed signs
- wheelchair-accessible entranceways and waiting rooms
- obstacle-free and well-lit, high-contrast walkways, hallways, and waiting areas (free of rugs, electrical cords, and hazards for falls, such as toys)
- accessible bathrooms with elevated toilet seat, grab bars, and wheelchair-accessible sink
- trained staff to assist the patient with a disability to and from the examination room
- a private area where patients with decreased hearing and vision can receive assistance from staff in completing forms

Elder Abuse

The ophthalmologist may be the first or only physician to see an elderly patient suffering from maltreatment. The signs of elder abuse (a form of domestic violence) may be subtle, and early recognition is key. The national prevalence of elder maltreatment is between 2% and 10% and may affect 1.5 to 2 million older adults per year. The actual numbers are probably significantly higher because of underreporting of cases. Major risk factors for elder maltreatment include external stresses due to marital, financial, and legal difficulties; dependent relationships (eg, the abuser may be dependent on the elderly patient for finances or housing); mental illness and substance abuse; social isolation; and misinformation about normal aging or about the patient's medical or nutritional needs. Maltreatment can occur at home, in assisted living, or in nursing homes. It can take the form of physical or psychological abuse, material misappropriation, neglect, or sexual attack.

Physical neglect includes withholding of food or water, medical care, medication, or hygiene. Neglect may be intentional or unintentional and may be fostered by financial constraints or other lack of resources (eg, transportation, supervision). Elder maltreatment also includes financial abuse or exploitation, and deprivation of basic rights (eg, decision making for care, privacy).

The ophthalmologist should suspect elder maltreatment ("red flags") in the following circumstances:

- repeated visits to the emergency room or office
- conflicting or noncredible history from caregiver or patient
- unexplained delay in seeking treatment
- unexplained, inconsistent, vague, or poorly explained injuries
- history of being "accident-prone"
- expressions of ambivalence, anger, hostility, or fear by the patient toward the caregiver
- poor compliance with follow-up or care instructions
- evidence of physical abuse (eg, skin bruises, lacerations, wounds in various stages of healing, unusually shaped bruises, burns, welts, patches of hair loss, or unexplained subconjunctival, retinal, or vitreous hemorrhage)

Sometimes it is necessary to obtain the history with the caregiver absent. Directed questions for the patient include "Has anyone at home tried to harm you?" "Has anyone tried to make you do things that you don't wish to do?" "Has anyone taken anything from you without your consent?"

Any suspected case of elder neglect or abuse should prompt a complete written report. Documentation of any suspicious injuries is mandatory, including type, size, location, and characteristics of injury and stage of healing. Mandatory reporting of elder abuse varies from state to state, and many localities have abuse hotlines for reporting maltreatment. The physician should be aware of local services for adult protection, community social service, and law enforcement agencies.

Surgical Considerations

The ophthalmologist should be aware of how preoperative and perioperative evaluation and management differ for the elderly patient. Loss of visual acuity alone may not be an appropriate sole indication for surgical intervention (eg, cataract surgery). Functional assessment includes determining how visual loss affects ADL (eg, reading, driving, glare). Documentation of these functional impairments is important for preoperative assessment. In addition, issues of informed consent are important in patients with mild dementia or in those who have legal guardians or caregivers.

The ophthalmic surgeon should know some general principles regarding the preoperative assessment of elderly patients. Delirium and confusion affect up to 25% of elderly patients in the postoperative period. There are numerous causes for confusion in this setting, but many are preventable. Minimization of preoperative sedation or psychotropic medications, appropriate patient and family orientation by nursing or ancillary staff, and careful supervision and reassurance in the postoperative period can decrease postoperative confusion. Often, a confused elderly patient simply needs a familiar face or reassurance to regain calm. The use of restraints should be minimized.

Confusion may be exacerbated in patients with visual loss or in those who require visual rehabilitation. In monocular elderly patients, patching of the eye after surgery may aggravate confusion and disorientation. Having a family member in the recovery room can be very helpful. The patch should be removed as soon as possible, and patients should be provided with appropriate eye protection. Topical anesthesia may not be indicated because of comorbidities such as cognitive impairment and inability to cooperate during surgery. In addition, patients with decreased vision following intraocular surgery may experience decreased mobility or be at increased risk for falls. Bed rest and immobilization can lead to disuse, pressure ulcers, and other problems. Active rehabilitation should be encouraged as soon as possible ("Bed is bad").

Although rare in outpatient ophthalmic surgery, surgical or anesthesia complications may produce life-threatening problems. The surgeon must pay careful attention to any preexisting directives (eg, do not resuscitate orders or living wills) prior to any surgical intervention (including laser treatments and periocular injections or anesthesia). By discussing possible treatment decisions early on—preferably before any serious illness arises or, if a serious illness is present, early in its course—the surgeon can avoid emergency decisions.

Some potential issues for discussion include limits of treatment, feeding tubes, antibiotics, and changes in living situation. Candidly and openly discussing these important issues with the patient and the family (especially in cases of dementia) in the preoperative period allows them to consider these matters in the context of their belief systems and without the disorientation and confusion created by an emergency. The content, context, time, and date of such discussions should be well documented in the medical record and communicated to the patient, the family, and the primary care physician or geriatrician.

When difficult decisions do need to be made, the physician should not merely set forth a menu of possible choices but should provide information on probable outcomes (such as survival with cardiopulmonary resuscitation, which patients and family members tend to overestimate). Treatments that are futile need not be offered, but the question of what constitutes medical futility is complex.

Psychology of Aging

The psychology of aging is influenced by a wide range of factors, including physical changes, adaptive mechanisms, and psychopathology. Each elderly patient has a unique psychological profile and social life history. Deleterious changes are not universal; in fact, in the absence of disease, growth of character and the ability to learn continue throughout life.

As we age, the issue of loss becomes more prevalent. Losses—of status, physical abilities, loved ones, and income—become more frequent. A fear of loss of social and individual power, and with it an attendant loss of independence, is common. In addition, the reality of death has increasing influence on a person's psychological status.

Normal Aging Changes

Age-related changes in sensation and perception can have great influence, isolating an individual from the surrounding environment and requiring complex psychological reactions. There may be diminution of hearing and vision (see Ophthalmologic Considerations, later in this chapter), slowing of intellectual and physical response time, and increasing difficulty with memory.

Many physical and intellectual abilities, however, are retained throughout life, and their loss should not be assumed to be part of the normal aging process. These include the senses of taste and smell, intelligence, the ability to learn, and sexuality. Any change in physical, intellectual, or emotional capabilities may reflect underlying organic or psychological disease.

Psychopathology

Functional disorders

Depression is the most frequent psychiatric problem in the elderly. The prevalence of clinical depression in primary care settings varies between 17% and 37%. The incidence of depression in elderly patients with other illness is even greater. The suicide rate in white American men older than age 65 is 5 times greater than that of the general population. Loneliness is the main reason cited, along with financial problems and poor health. Successful suicide is much less common in older American women, but older women attempt suicide more often than do men.

Major depressive disorder is characterized by episodes of at least 2 weeks of depressed mood or loss of interest with 4 or more of the following symptoms:

- loss of appetite
- significant weight loss or gain
- sleep disturbance, agitation, or retardation
- loss of energy
- feelings of worthlessness or guilt
- difficulties in concentration and decision making
- recurrent thoughts of suicide or death

The signs and symptoms of depression are similar to those seen in younger age groups, although elderly depressed patients are *more likely* than younger patients to express somatic or hypochondriacal complaints, minimize depression symptoms (masked depression), and have psychotic delusional disease but *less likely* to report symptoms of guilt. The most frequent presentations of subclinical depression include new medical complaints, fatigue, poor concentration, exacerbation of existing symptoms and medical problems, preoccupation with health, and diminished interest in pleasurable activities.

The ophthalmologist's role is to recognize and refer the patient with depression. In particular, loss of function such as moderate or severe visual loss can precipitate depression. So can recent death of a spouse. In addition to the signs of depression listed previously, other red flags may be frequent visits to the ophthalmology office and unexplained visual loss. Early recognition may be crucial because elderly patients, particularly men older than age 65, are at highest risk for suicide. Further, most elderly patients who commit suicide have communicated suicidal ideation to family or friends. There is no evidence that questions about suicide increase the likelihood of suicide attempts.

Another disorder seen in elderly persons is *paranoia*, which is usually the result of social isolation or reduced cognitive and sensory capabilities rather than the severe personality disorganization seen in younger patients. For example, a hearing-impaired person may have difficulty understanding what is being said and may imagine hostile motivations on the part of others. Although it may begin in adolescence, *hypochondriasis* more often begins in middle to late adulthood and is relatively common in the older population.

Organic disorders/dementia

Dementia is a collection of multiple, chronic, and acquired neurocognitive deficits (eg, memory, calculation, orientation, language, construction, purposeful activity, executive planning, or complex behavior control). Acute confusion (ie, delirium), focal deficits (eg, aphasia), and congenital defects (eg, mental retardation) should be excluded. The most common causes of dementia are Alzheimer disease, vascular (multi-infarct) disease, depression (pseudodementia), and frontal lobe disease. (Alzheimer disease is discussed at length in Chapter 12.) Although less than 15% of dementias are due to reversible causes, these should be ruled out (eg, vitamin B_{12} or folate deficiency, alcohol abuse, normal-pressure hydrocephalus, drug toxicity, thyroid disease, syphilis, seizure, central nervous system infection, tumor).

Some elderly depressed patients may have pseudodementia. These patients manifest prominent symptoms resembling dementia, with several important differences. Impairment of memory and orientation in pseudodementia has a sudden onset and rapid progression. There is often a prior history of depression, and depressive symptoms are present. Most important, the intellectual deficits are relieved by successful treatment of the depression.

Treatment

Functional disorders in the elderly are as amenable to treatment as they are in younger patients. Psychotherapy and pharmacologic therapy are effective and should be offered to all patients. Acute mental disorders due to a general medical condition (organic brain syndromes) may also be treatable and thus should be thoroughly worked up.

Ophthalmologic Considerations

Diminishing visual capabilities of any cause can contribute to behavioral disorders in the elderly. Depression, paranoia, and organic brain syndromes may be exacerbated. Optimizing visual function through optical correction, medical therapy for vision-impairing disorders, surgical correction of cataract, and low-vision rehabilitation can reduce symptoms of behavioral disorders and greatly improve the quality of life.

Osteoporosis

Osteoporosis is a condition of varied etiology involving a decrease in the mass of bone per unit volume (reduced bone density), leading to increased bone fragility and risk of fracture. It is the most common bone disorder confronting the clinician.

Osteoporosis is a significant, worldwide public health problem whose prevalence seems to be increasing. The disease is rare among black women and females of southern

European ancestry. Approximately 25% of white women older than age 60 have documented spinal compression fractures in association with osteoporosis. As many as 50% of women develop vertebral fractures by age 75. After age 45, the incidence of distal forearm fractures increases markedly. By age 60, there are 10 times as many forearm fractures in women as in men of comparable age. The risk of hip fractures increases with age and, among women, reaches 20% by age 90; 80% of hip fractures are associated with preexisting osteoporosis. Approximately 17% of women with hip fractures die within 3 months of the fracture. In the United States, it is estimated that osteoporosis causes 1.5 million fractures each year at a cost of $14 billion.

Bone Physiology

Bone is a 2-component system, with an organic and an inorganic phase. The organic phase *(osteoid)* consists of a matrix of collagen, glycoproteins and phosphoproteins, mucopolysaccharides, and lipids. The inorganic phase *(hydroxyapatite)* consists of an insoluble calcium-phosphate mineral. There are 3 types of bone cells: *osteoclasts,* which resorb bone; *osteoblasts,* which form bone; and *osteocytes,* which maintain bone structure and function. The outer portion of bone *(cortical bone)* comprises 80% of total bone volume and consists of less than 5% soft tissue. The inner portion of bone *(trabecular bone)* is more porous and includes 75% soft tissue.

Bone is metabolically active and continually remodels throughout life along lines of mechanical stress. During late adolescence, bone mineral content increases rapidly. Bone mass peaks in the third decade of life. With age, the balance between bone resorption and bone formation is altered, and bone mass decreases. By age 60, skeletal mass may be as little as 50% of that at age 30.

Risk Factors

Many risk factors are associated with osteoporosis, some of which are modifiable (Table 10-1). Peak bone mass (the maximum bone density reached by an individual, normally in young adulthood) appears to be the strongest correlate to lifetime fracture risk. Racial and sexual differences in peak bone mass at skeletal maturity may explain the high relative risk in white women compared with black women and white men (intermediate peak density and risk) and black men (highest peak bone density and lowest risk).

Sex hormones play a significant role: rates of osteoporosis are high in women after menopause or oophorectomy, in girls with gonadal dysgenesis, and in female long-distance runners with functional hypogonadism. Age-related factors include decreased formation of new bone, impaired calcium absorption (with secondary hyperparathyroidism and increased bone loss), and nutritional vitamin D deficiency. Other associated factors include insufficient dietary calcium intake, sedentary lifestyle, nulliparity, alcohol abuse, and cigarette smoking.

In addition, glucocorticoid excess, thyrotoxicosis of Graves disease, acromegaly, diabetes mellitus, and a variety of other systemic diseases and drugs are all associated with bone loss.

Table 10-1 Risk Factors for Osteoporotic Fracture

Nonmodifiable	Personal history of fracture as an adult
	History of fracture in first-degree relative
	Caucasian
	Advanced age
	Female
	Dementia
Potentially modifiable	Current cigarette smoking
	Low body weight (<127 lb)
	Estrogen deficiency:
	Early menopause (age <45) or bilateral oophorectomy
	Prolonged premenopausal amenorrhea (>1 yr)
	Low calcium intake
	Alcoholism
	Impaired eyesight despite adequate correction
	Recurrent falls
	Inadequate physical activity
	Vitamin D deficiency
	Poor health, frailty

Clinical Features

The typical clinical picture in osteoporosis includes back pain, spinal deformity, loss of height, and fractures of the vertebrae, hips, and (less commonly) other bones. Multiple vertebral fractures over a period of years can lead to severe kyphosis, with a loss of height of 4–8 inches, and cervical lordosis ("dowager's hump").

Diagnostic Evaluation

Radiographic evaluation

Patients at risk with a history of back pain are evaluated for radiographic evidence of vertebral fracture. Radiographic changes become visible only when at least 30% of bone mass has been lost. The changes may be subtle because osteoporosis involves a generalized reduction in bone mass. The amount of loss necessary for detection by conventional radiography depends on the bone involved. The spinal column exhibits the most characteristic radiographic features of osteoporosis, with accentuation of the vertebral end plates, anterior wedging in the thoracic spinal column, biconcave compression ("ballooning," or "codfish vertebrae") in the lumbar region, and disc herniation into the vertebral body. The long bones exhibit cortical thinning with irregularity of endosteal surfaces. Osteoporosis caused by glucocorticoid excess presents a somewhat different picture, with radiographic changes in the skull, ribs, and pelvic rami.

    Several other techniques allow more accurate measurement of bone density than can be obtained through conventional radiography. All of these methods measure the degree of attenuation of a beam of photons from an x-ray tube by targeted bones and surrounding soft tissues. Measurements of the spine are used to predict vertebral fractures, of the femoral neck to predict hip fractures, and of the wrist or heel to predict peripheral fractures. Results are compared with mean bone mineral density (BMD) values in young adults, the normal for women being within 1 standard deviation (SD) of this reference mean (the *T score*). The risk of fractures increases with age and with each SD below the mean; below 2 SD, the risk rises exponentially. *Osteoporosis* is defined as values more than 2.5 SD below the mean, whereas *osteopenia* is a value 2.0 SD below the mean. The *Z score* represents a patient's BMD compared with the mean value for persons of the same age and sex. A Z score less than 2.0 SD below the mean suggests accelerated bone loss and warrants further evaluation of a secondary cause (Table 10-2).

Dual-photon x-ray absorptiometry is currently the technique of choice because it allows for shorter examination time (a few minutes with current machines), greater accuracy, improved resolution, and longer source life. The radiation dose of this test is less than 5 millirem (mrem).

Dual-energy quantitative computed tomography scans the lower thoracic and upper lumbar vertebral bodies in cross section at numerous levels, and the computed tomographic values obtained are compared with standards for soft tissue, fat, and mineral. Dual-energy quantitative computed tomography is highly accurate but is more expensive than dual-photon x-ray absorptiometry and may be less reproducible. The x-ray dose is less than 3 mrem.

Who Should Be Tested?

- all postmenopausal women younger than age 65 who have 1 or more risk factors for osteoporotic fractures (besides menopause)

Table 10-2 Causes of Secondary Osteoporosis

Primary osteoporosis
  Juvenile
  Idiopathic (young adults)
  Involutional
Endocrine
  Hypogonadism
  Ovarian agenesis
  Glucocorticoid excess
  Hyperthyroidism
  Hyperparathyroidism
  Diabetes mellitus
  Acromegaly
  Addison disease
Gastrointestinal
  Subtotal gastrectomy
  Malabsorption syndromes
  Chronic obstructive jaundice
  Primary biliary cirrhosis
  Severe malnutrition
  Hemochromatosis
  Parental nutrition

Bone marrow disorders
  Multiple myeloma
  Systemic mastocytosis
  Disseminated carcinoma
  Lymphoma and leukemia
  Pernicious anemia
  Hemophilia
  Thalassemia
Connective tissue diseases
  Osteogenesis imperfecta
  Homocystinuria
  Ehlers-Danlos syndrome
  Marfan syndrome
  Ankylosing spondylitis
  Rheumatoid arthritis
Miscellaneous
  Immobilization
  Chronic obstructive pulmonary disease
  Chronic alcoholism
  Sarcoidosis
  Chronic heparin administration
  Chronic use of anticonvulsant drugs
  Lithium use
  Tamoxifen (premenopausal use)

- all women aged 65 and over
- postmenopausal women who present with fractures
- women who are considering therapy for osteoporosis (if BMD testing would facilitate the decision)
- women who have been on hormone replacement therapy for prolonged periods

Clinical Evaluation

If densitometric studies confirm the diagnosis of osteoporosis, a medical evaluation should be undertaken to rule out secondary causes (see Table 10-2). Serum calcium and phosphorus levels are usually normal, although slight hyperphosphatemia may be present in postmenopausal women. The alkaline phosphatase level is usually normal but may be slightly elevated following a fracture. Sustained elevation of alkaline phosphatase in the absence of liver disease suggests osteomalacia or skeletal metastasis.

Treatment

General considerations

All patients with osteoporosis should adhere to a diet that supplies adequate amounts of calcium, protein, and vitamins. Weight-bearing exercise (eg, walking, jogging, and weight lifting) is important in the maintenance of bone mass. Limitation of alcohol intake and cessation of smoking are also beneficial. Back pain is treated with analgesics and physical therapy.

Calcium and vitamin D

Ingestion of elemental calcium is important for the maintenance of bone mass. The incidence of hip fractures appears to be significantly less in female populations wherein dietary calcium and vitamin D intake is high. The recommended daily intake is at least 1200 mg/day of calcium (roughly the equivalent of four 8-ounce glasses of milk) and vitamin D (400–800 IU per day for persons at risk of deficiency), but the average calcium intake in American women is only about 375 mg/day. During pregnancy and lactation, women may need much more calcium. This calcium may be obtained from dietary as well as pharmacologic sources. Calcium and vitamin D supplementation is recommended in patients on long-term steroid therapy to treat an underlying disease. Calcium is available in a variety of preparations, including calcium carbonate, citrate, gluconate, lactate, and phosphate. Calcium carbonate and phosphate have the highest concentration of elemental calcium, which is approximately 40%; calcium citrate has 21%; lactate, 13%; and gluconate, 9%. Calcium therapy may cause constipation, nausea, flatulence, bloating, hypercalcuria, and renal stones. Hypercalcemia does not occur in patients with normal renal function. However, massive doses of vitamin D can lead to dangerous hypercalcemia.

Pharmacologic therapy

Five medications are approved by the US Food and Drug Administration for prevention or treatment of osteoporosis (Table 10-3). They are estrogen, alendronate, risedronate, raloxifene, and calcitonin.

Table 10-3 FDA-Approved Drugs for Osteoporosis Prevention and Treatment

Name	Dosage	Indications	Side Effects and Risks	Estimated Reduction for Fracture
Estrogen	Depends on formulation of estrogen (eg, conjugated equine estrogen, 0.625 mg daily)	Prevention	Vaginal bleeding, breast tenderness, gallbladder disease; risk of breast cancer, deep vein thrombosis, pulmonary embolism; increased risk of heart disease and stroke	Vertebral, 50%–80% Nonvertebral, 25%
Alendronate	5 mg/day 10 mg/day	Prevention Treatment	Gastrointestinal disturbances (abdominal pain, nausea, dyspepsia), esophageal ulcer (rare)	Vertebral, 50% Nonvertebral, 50%
Risedronate	5 mg/day	Treatment	Same as alendronate	Vertebral, 40% Nonvertebral, 40%
Raloxifene	60 mg/day 60 mg/day	Prevention Treatment	Deep vein thrombosis or pulmonary embolism, hot flashes, leg cramps	Vertebral, 40% Nonvertebral*
Calcitonin	200 IU intranasal/day (alternating nostrils)	Treatment	Nasal irritation, rhinitis	Vertebral, 40% Nonvertebral*

*No studies thus far have demonstrated benefit for nonvertebral fracture rate.

Adapted from McGarry KA, Kiel DP. Postmenopausal osteoporosis. Strategies for preventing bone loss, avoiding fracture. *Postgrad Med.* 2000;108:79–88.

Estrogen Numerous clinical studies have established that estrogens help to prevent osteoporosis. Estrogens produce significant calcium retention, decrease the imbalance between bone formation and resorption, and tend to decrease the progression of osteoporosis by slowing bone turnover. One study showed an increase in BMD in women taking estrogen or combination estrogen-progestin treatment (discussed later) compared with those taking placebo.

Estrogen therapy may preserve height and reduce the rate of vertebral and hip fracture (by 70% and 25%, respectively, in some studies), prevent vertebral deformity, and stabilize bone loss in postmenopausal women, amenorrheic premenopausal women, and patients who have undergone oophorectomy. When estrogen therapy is combined with calcium supplementation or calcitonin therapy, its effectiveness may be enhanced. The benefit of estrogen treatment appears to be maximized when therapy is started at the onset of menopause and continued for at least 7–10 years, although such therapy has also been shown to have some benefit in older women with established osteoporosis.

Unopposed estrogen treatment increases the risk of endometrial carcinoma, but concurrent progestin therapy reduces this risk to that of the general population. The Women's Health Initiative randomized trial demonstrated an increased risk of breast cancer, ovarian cancer, heart disease, hypertension, thromboembolic diseases, ischemic stroke, and dementia in women taking hormone replacement therapy (HRT). In view of these findings, patients should be advised of the risks of HRT before starting this treatment for osteoporosis.

Bisphosphonates Alendronate and risedronate are second-generation bisphosphonates, a class of drugs that bind strongly to hydroxyapatite crystals, are adsorbed onto new bone matrix, and prevent bone resorption by inhibiting osteoclast activity. Bisphosphonates shift the balance between bone formation and resorption toward formation. High doses, however, interfere with the process of bone mineralization. The main side effects of bisphosphonates are gastrointestinal. As with other therapies for osteoporosis, treatment with bisphosphonates requires adequate calcium and vitamin D intake.

Raloxifene Raloxifene is an agent in a class of compounds called *selective estrogen receptor modulators,* which have estrogen-agonistic effects on bone, lipids, and blood clotting and estrogen-antagonistic effects on the breast and uterus. Raloxifene has been shown to increase BMD and reduce the risk of vertebral fractures by 30%–50%.

Calcitonin Calcitonin is a hormone that interferes with osteoclast function and inhibits bone resorption. Derived from salmon, it has been used in the treatment of osteoporosis for many years but could be given only by subcutaneous or intramuscular injection. Calcitonin nasal spray *(Miacalcin)* is also available. It is well tolerated and has shown some effectiveness in increasing bone density and reducing fractures. Adequate concomitant intake of calcium and vitamin D is necessary.

Osteoporosis in Men

Osteoporosis is perceived primarily as a disease of postmenopausal women. It should be noted, however, that women have only twice the incidence of hip fracture as men. Cigarette smoking, alcohol consumption, steroid therapy, and hypogonadism are associated with an increased incidence of osteoporosis in men, who also seem to benefit from the previously cited protective measures (with the exception of estrogen therapy).

Falls

The incidence and severity of falls increases with increasing age. Fall-related expenses for persons older than age 65 totaled $27.3 billion in 1994, according to the Centers for Disease Control. Accidental death is the fifth-leading cause of death in the elderly, and two thirds of these deaths are due to falls. Three fourths of these fall-related deaths occur in the 13% of the population older than 65 years. In the community-living elderly patient population, 33% of patients will fall, and 5% of these falls will result in a fracture or hospitalization. Falls were the single largest cause of restricted activity in the elderly (18%). The hospital mortality rate of relatively isolated hip fracture is 6%; with multiple medical problems, the mortality rate may be as high as 22%. The incidence rate is much higher among patients in nursing homes or hospitals: up to 10%–20% of these patients experience a serious fall that causes fracture or hospitalization. Each year, 1800 fatal falls occur in nursing homes in the United States.

In addition to serious injury or death, falls have a significant psychosocial impact on patients (eg, fear of falling, postfall anxiety, depression, social isolation, and loss of mobility, self-confidence, independence, and function). The 3 most common risk factors for falls are gait or balance disorder, dizziness, or environment-related. Visual disorders, however, account for up to 4% of falls. The ophthalmologist's role in fall prevention includes recognition and treatment of visual disorders (including refractive error), multifactorial and multidisciplinary risk reduction, and preventive targeting of risk factors (eg, postural hypotension, multiple medications, and impairments in transferring, strength, balance, and gait). If the ophthalmologist recognizes that a patient is at risk for falls (due to visual disorders or other risk factors), appropriate referral can lead to help in establishing safety and preventive measures in the home (eg, increasing lighting, removing obstacles from the environment, eliminating slippery surfaces, removing loose rugs and electrical cords, and using high-contrast colors, handrails, better-fitting and nonskid footwear, and assistive devices) (Table 10-4).

Systemic Diseases

Ophthalmologists should be aware of the increased incidence of systemic disease in the elderly. The prevalence of anemia due to vitamin B_{12} deficiency increases with age. In patients with low to normal serum vitamin B_{12} levels, increased excretion of serum and urinary methylmalonic acid and homocysteine may assist with the diagnosis. In addition, 30% of patients with early vitamin B_{12} deficiency have anemia, but 59% may have reversible memory deficits. For the ophthalmologist, patients with vitamin B_{12} deficiency may present with painless, bilateral, progressive visual loss; a central or cecocentral scotoma on visual field testing; and optic atrophy (temporal pallor). Concomitant alcohol and tobacco use should be discontinued.

Table 10-4 Interior Safety Checks

Living room	Are scatter rugs firmly anchored with rubber backing?
	Are electrical cords in good repair, especially on heating pad?
	Light, heat, and ventilation
	Is there adequate night lighting?
	Are stairways continually illuminated?
	Is temperature within comfortable range (70°–75°F)?
	Is the heater vented properly?
	Is there cross ventilation?
	Is furniture sturdy enough to give support?
	Is there a minimum of clutter, allowing enough room for easy mobility as well as lower fire hazard?
	Are emergency telephone numbers posted in a handy place and easily read, such as doctor, fire department, ambulance, paramedics, nearest relative?
	If the person has limited vision, does phone have enlarged dial?
Kitchen	Stove, refrigerator, and sink
	Is the stove free of grease and flammable objects?
	Is baking soda available in case of fire?
	Are matches used or is there a pilot light?
	Is the refrigerator working properly?
	Is sink draining well?
	Is food being stored properly?
	Is trash taken out daily?
	Is there a sturdy stepping stool in evidence?
	Are there skid-proof mats on the floor?
	In the bathroom, are safety measures observed?
	Are there handrails beside the tub and toilet?
	Are there skid-proof mats in the bathtub and/or shower?
	Are electrical outlets a safe distance from the tub?
Outside the home	Walks and stairs
	Are there raised or uneven places on the sidewalks?
	Are stairs in good repair?
	Are the top and bottom stairs painted white or a bright contrasting color to improve visibility?
	Are handrails securely fastened?
	Are screens on doors and windows in good repair?
	Is there an alternate exit for the house?

From Hypertext modules in geriatric medicine. Computer-based self-instruction modules. Baylor College of Medicine, 1998.

The prevalence of hypertension, cardiovascular disease, cerebrovascular disease, and diabetes mellitus increases with age; these conditions may affect the eye (eg, homonymous hemianopsia, hypertensive or diabetic retinopathy, amaurosis fugax). Pulmonary diseases such as tuberculosis are more frequent in elderly persons (who account for 25% of active cases; 60% of deaths related to pulmonary disease occur in patients older than 65 years). Tuberculosis may cause anterior or posterior uveitis or present with neuro-ophthalmic manifestations. Antituberculosis therapy (eg, ethambutol and isoniazid) may produce toxic optic neuropathy.

Herpes zoster affects 10% of patients older than age 80 (who have decreased cell-mediated immunity). Herpes zoster ophthalmicus may produce uveitis or central nervous system manifestations (including ophthalmoplegia) in addition to vesicular dermatomal skin eruption and postherpetic neuralgia (which occurs in 10%–15% of patients). The early use of antiviral agents (eg, acyclovir, famciclovir) may reduce the duration of pain with herpes zoster and the development of postherpetic neuralgia.

Hyperthyroidism and Graves ophthalmopathy may occur in elderly persons (up to 25% of patients are older than 65 years). Thyroid disease may be iatrogenically precipitated by iodine-containing contrast (eg, contrast-enhanced computed tomography). Elderly patients with a particular form of hyperthyroidism—apathetic thyrotoxicosis—may present with depression and apathy.

Cauley JA, Robbins J, Chen Z, et al. Effects of estrogen plus progestin on risk of fracture and bone mineral density: the Women's Health Initiative randomized trial. *JAMA*. 2003;290:1729–1738.

Congdon N, O'Colmain B, Klaver CC, et al. Causes and prevalence of visual impairment among adults in the United States. *Arch Ophthalmol*. 2004;122(4):477–485.

Congdon N, Vingerling R, Klein BE, et al. Prevalence of cataract and pseudophakia/aphakia among adults in the United States. *Arch Ophthalmol*. 2004;122(4):487–494.

Katz PR, Grossberg GT, Potter JF, et al. *Geriatrics Syllabus for Specialists*. New York: American Geriatrics Society; 2002:chapters 11, 19, 36, 39.

Kempen JH, Mitchell P, Lee KE, et al. The prevalence of refractive errors among adults in the United States, Western Europe, and Australia. *Arch Ophthalmol*. 2004;122(4):495–505.

Lachs MS, Pillemer K. Elder Abuse. *Lancet*. 2004;364:1263–1272.

Lee AG, Beaver HA, Jogerst G, et al. Screening elderly patients in an outpatient ophthalmology clinic for dementia, depression, and functional impairment. *Ophthalmology*. 2003;110(4):651–657.

McGarry KA, Kiel DP. Postmenopausal osteoporosis. Strategies for preventing bone loss, avoiding fracture. *Postgrad Med*. 2000;108:79–88.

National Center for Health Statistics/CDC Web site. Available at http://209.217.72.34/aging/ReportFolders/reportfolders.aspx. Accessed September 15, 2005.

Physician's Guide to Prevention and Treatment of Osteoporosis. Washington, DC: National Osteoporosis Foundation; 1998.

Reuben DB, Herr KA, Pacala JT, et al. *Geriatrics at Your Fingertips: 2005, 7th Edition*. New York: The American Geriatrics Society; 2005.

Rovner BW, Shmuely-Dulitzki Y. Screening for depression in low-vision elderly. *Int J Geriatr Psychiatry*. 1997;12:955–959.

CHAPTER 11

Cancer

Recent Developments

- More precise molecular targets for anti-cancer drugs are increasing the effectiveness and reducing the toxicity of chemotherapy.
- Biological therapies utilizing the immune system continue to play a major role in the treatment of cancer.
- Angiogenesis inhibitors may prove to be a significant form of cancer therapy in humans.
- The genetic profiling of tumors may contribute significantly to their potential treatment.

Incidence

Cancer is the second-leading cause of death in the United States, with about 23% of all deaths in the United States due to this disease. Each year, approximately 2 million new cases are diagnosed, and some 550,000 deaths occur. More than 3 million Americans have survived cancer, and in more than 2 million of these cases, the diagnosis was established longer than 5 years ago.

Cancer is actually many different diseases; questions of etiology, cancer prevention, and cancer cure must address the specific types of tumors. Nonmelanotic skin cancers are the most common tumors in adult Americans, but these cancers rarely produce major clinical problems. After these types, the most common forms of cancer in adult Americans (in decreasing order of incidence) are lung, breast, prostate, and colorectal. Approximately 80% of adult cancers arise from the epithelial tissues; leukemias and sarcomas are relatively rare in adults.

Cancer is the leading cause of death by disease in children younger than age 15 in the United States. The number of children diagnosed with cancer each year has risen from 12 per 100,000 in the early 1970s to 14 per 100,000 today. At the same time, death rates have dropped and survival rates have risen. The 5-year survival rate for all childhood cancers is now 71%, compared with approximately 51% in 1973. Cancer is diagnosed in more than 8500 children each year: 30% with leukemia, 12% with Hodgkin and non–Hodgkin lymphoma, and the remainder with solid tumors.

Etiology

Cancer is caused by mutations in genes that control cell division. Some of these genes, called *oncogenes,* stimulate cell division; others, called *tumor-suppressor genes,* slow this process. In the normal state, both types of genes work together, enabling the body to replace dead cells and repair damaged ones. Mutations in these genes cause cells to proliferate out of control. Such mutations can be inherited or acquired through environmental insults. Cancer causes, therefore, are explained on the basis of chemical, radiation-related, or viral causes that occur in a complex milieu, including host genetic composition and immunobiological status. Between 60% and 90% of cases are understood on the basis of environmental origin. Several examples of environmental causes are cigarette smoking (lung cancer), asbestos (lung cancer and mesothelioma), vinyl chloride (hepatic angiosarcoma), benzidine (leukemia), dietary nitrates (gastrointestinal carcinoma), and lye injury (esophageal carcinoma).

Carcinogenic Factors

Chemical

Since the 1950s, definite changes have occurred in the cancer mortality rates in the United States. For example, lung cancer death rates have increased markedly in both men and women. This increase parallels the rise in cigarette smoking, but the higher death rate lags about 20 years behind the increase in smoking. The increased incidence of and mortality from lung cancer are particularly striking in women, in whom the mortality rate is increasing approximately 6% per year. Even though breast cancer remains more prevalent, lung cancer kills more women than does breast cancer. Most cases of lung cancer can be attributed to cigarette smoking. One promising development in lung cancer is the drop in the number of new cases diagnosed each year in men. Lung cancer deaths among men dropped nearly 7% between 1991 and 1995 and continued to decline in 2000. Lung cancer deaths in women had increased in 1995 but leveled off in 2000. The mortality rates from breast, colon, and rectal cancer have remained essentially unchanged since about 1960.

Stomach cancer has become fairly rare in the United States, presumably because of a decrease in human exposure to exogenous agents such as dietary nitrates. In the United States and Western Europe, mortality from lung, colon, and breast cancer is high, and mortality from stomach cancer is low. In Japan, stomach cancer predominates, and colon and breast cancer are relatively rare. After several generations, descendants of Japanese persons who migrated to the United States show a decreased incidence of stomach cancer and acquire the high incidence of colon cancer characteristic of the United States. Similarly, Japanese in Japan who adopt a Western diet and lifestyle have an increased rate of colon cancer and a decreased rate of stomach cancer, whereas people of Japanese ancestry in the United States who marry Japanese citizens and do not adopt a Western diet continue to show high stomach cancer and low colon cancer rates. These examples support the argument for the predominant role of environmental factors as opposed to genetic or inborn factors in the etiology of most human cancers.

The incidence of specific cancers in different subsets of the American population varies considerably. For example, the black population has a higher incidence of cancer of the prostate, uterine cervix, lung, esophagus, and oropharynx than does the white population; however, the black population also has a lower incidence of cancer of the breast and corpus uteri than does the white population.

Epidemiologic data suggest that as much as 80% of human cancer may be due to exogenous chemical exposure. If these chemicals could be properly identified, then host exposure could be reduced or the host could be protected, thus preventing a major proportion of human cancers. A number of industrial processes or occupational exposures and numerous chemicals or groups of chemicals have been implicated in various forms of human cancer. Specific causes of major cancers, such as large bowel and breast cancer, have not been identified with certainty.

Carcinogenesis

Cancer arises from genetic mutations that cause a cell to grow and divide without regard for cell death. There is failure of differentiation resulting in altered cell position and the capacity to proliferate while cut off from normal cell regulatory signals. The cell cycle is regulated biochemically, and one very important group of enzymes involved in this regulation is the cyclin-dependent kinases (CDKs). One example of CDK function is *p53*, the tumor suppressor gene that up-regulates another protein, *p21*, which inhibits CDK function. When p21 is bound to CDK, the cell does not progress through the cell cycle. Defective p53 results in decreased levels of p21 and uncontrolled cell cycling.

Radiation in carcinogenesis

In 1927, American geneticist and educator Hermann J. Muller demonstrated that x-rays caused inheritable genetic damage, a discovery for which he received the Nobel Prize. This discovery led to our understanding of the role of radiation in carcinogenesis.

The general population is exposed to both naturally occurring ionizing radiation and man-made ionizing radiation. Man-made sources deliver an average of 106 mrem per year to each person. These sources include medical diagnostic equipment, technologically altered natural sources (such as phosphate fertilizers and building materials containing small amounts of radioactivity), global fallout from atmospheric testing of atomic weapons, nuclear power, high-altitude jet flight, occupational exposure, and consumer products such as color television sets, smoke detectors, and luminescent clocks and instrument dials.

The carcinogenic effects of radiation exposure result from molecular lesions caused by random interactions of radiation with atoms and molecules. Most molecular lesions induced in this way are of little consequence to the affected cell. However, DNA is not repaired with 100% efficiency, and mutations and chromosomal aberrations accrue with increasing radiation dose. Although these changes in genes and chromosomes have been postulated to account for the carcinogenic effect of radiation, the precise molecular mechanisms are unknown. Parameters that influence response of the target tissue include the total radiation dose, the dose rate, the quality of the radiation source, the characteristics of certain internal emitters (such as radioiodine), and individual host factors.

Viral carcinogenesis

Viruses play a role in the etiology of cancer, and this has been studied extensively. The inoculation of animals with specific viruses may produce tumors. Several human cancers (Burkitt lymphoma, nasopharyngeal carcinoma, carcinoma of the cervix, and hepatocellular carcinoma) show a definite correlation with viral infection, as well as reveal the presence and retention of specific virus nucleic acid sequences and virus proteins in the tumor cells.

All of the DNA virus groups, except for the parvovirus family, have been associated with cancer. This exception is notable because all the DNA viruses associated with cancer contain double-stranded DNA, whereas the parvoviruses contain only single-stranded DNA.

There are 9 RNA virus groups, but only 1 is associated with oncogenicity: the retrovirus group. The retroviruses differ from all other RNA viruses in that they require a DNA intermediate to replicate. Retroviruses contain and specify an enzyme called *reverse transcriptase*. In the presence of the 4 nucleoside triphosphates, reverse transcriptase can synthesize DNA complementary to the single-stranded RNA contained in the virion, producing an RNA-DNA hybrid. The RNA in this RNA-DNA hybrid is then degraded, and a double-stranded linear DNA molecule forms. This double-stranded DNA molecule moves into the cell nucleus and is integrated into the cellular DNA as a provirus.

The papillomavirus of the papovavirus group has been associated with squamous cell carcinoma and laryngeal papilloma in humans. The hepatitis B virus has been associated with primary hepatocellular carcinoma in humans.

The human herpesviruses that are associated with disease include Epstein-Barr virus, herpes simplex virus type 1, herpes simplex virus type 2, cytomegalovirus, and varicella-zoster virus. The Epstein-Barr virus, which causes infectious mononucleosis, has been associated with Burkitt lymphoma and nasopharyngeal carcinoma. The herpes simplex virus type 1, which causes gingivostomatitis, encephalitis, keratoconjunctivitis, neuralgia, and labialis, has been associated with carcinoma of the lip and oropharynx. The herpes simplex virus type 2, which causes genital herpes, disseminated neonatal herpes, encephalitis, and neuralgia, has been associated with cancer of the uterine cervix, vulva, kidney, and nasopharynx. The cytomegalovirus, which causes cytomegalovirus disease, transfusion mononucleosis, interstitial pneumonia, and congenital defects, has been associated with prostate cancer, Kaposi sarcoma, and carcinoma of the bladder and uterine cervix. The varicella-zoster virus, which causes chickenpox, shingles, and varicella pneumonia, has not yet been associated with specific human cancers.

Genetic and familial factors

Host susceptibility is an established but poorly defined concept in human carcinogenesis. A heritable component may be more important in some forms of cancer (eg, colon cancer) and less important in others (eg, esophageal cancer). Certain cancers show an ethnic predilection.

Cancers may aggregate in a nonrandom manner in certain families. These cancers may be of the same type or dissimilar. Such cancer-cluster families may have several children with soft tissue sarcoma and relatives with a variety of cancers, especially of the breast in young women. Multiple endocrine neoplasia (types I and II) is yet another example of familial cancers. The recognition of family cancer syndromes permits early detection that may be lifesaving.

Therapy

Radiation

Radiation dose for clinical purposes is frequently measured in energy absorbed. The *rad* (R, roentgen), a metric unit equivalent to 100 erg per gram and used for measuring radiation dose, is the term found in older literature. However, the SI unit of radiation dose, the gray (Gy), equal to 1.0 J per kg of mass, is now used almost exclusively. One Gy is equal to 100 rad.

Ionizing radiation interacts with host tissues and malignant tumors by an energy transfer and a chemical reaction, with the release of free radicals and the decomposition of water into hydrogen, hydroxyl, and perhydroxyl ionic forms. These ionic forms probably react with DNA and RNA in vital enzymes, producing biological injury.

The injuries noted to date include mitotic-linked death and chromosomal aberrations such as breakage, sticking, and cross-bridging. Consequent cell death occurs in both normal tissue and malignant lesions. In radiotherapy, biochemical recovery and biological repair occur in the normal host, maintaining the integrity of vital systems.

The poorly differentiated lymphoid cells, intestinal epithelium, and reproductive cells are more readily damaged and recover more quickly than do the highly differentiated normal cells. Lymphocytes are damaged by 1 Gy, and central nervous system tissue by 50 Gy. Surface irradiation of approximately 10 Gy produces skin erythema. The most serious damage is the late development of postradiation malignant changes in as many as 21% of patients, manifesting as squamous cell carcinoma and basal cell carcinoma. Bone absorption can produce osteogenic sarcomas and fibrosarcomas.

Ocular manifestations of fetal irradiation in the first trimester include microphthalmos, congenital cataracts, and retinal dysplasia. A 0.5 Gy dose may cause congenital anomalies in a fetus. Fetal exposure to approximately 0.30–0.80 Gy doubles the incidence of congenital defects; 5 Gy (the LD_{50} for a human fetus) generally induces an abortion.

Effects of irradiation on the eye and adnexa

The ocular effects of irradiation depend not only on total dose, fractionation, and treatment portal size, but also on associated systemic diseases such as diabetes mellitus and hypertension. Concomitant chemotherapy has an additive effect.

The lens is the most radiosensitive structure in the eye, followed by the cornea, the retina, and the optic nerve. The orbit is completely included in the treatment portal in diseases such as large retinoblastomas, and it is partially included in tumors of adjacent structures, such as the maxillary antrum, nasopharynx, ethmoid sinus, and nasal cavity. Usual doses range from 20 to 100 Gy. The total dose is usually fractionated during the treatment. With brachytherapy, a low-energy isotope such as radioactive iodine delivers a high dose of radiation within a few millimeters of the tumor but does not penetrate deep into it, thus allowing for radioactive episcleral implants to deliver a dose of 100 Gy to the apex of a tumor but much less to the rest of the eye. The sclera can tolerate doses up to 400–800 Gy.

Doses to the lens as low as 2 Gy in one fraction may cause a cataract. However, cataracts caused by low doses may be asymptomatic and may not progress. Cataracts caused by higher doses (7–8 Gy) may continue to progress, resulting in considerable visual loss. The average latent period for the development of radiation-induced cataracts is 2–3 years.

The clinical picture of radiation retinopathy resembles that of diabetic retinopathy. Radiation retinopathy is very rare below the fractionated dose of 50 Gy administered over 5–6 weeks. At higher fractionated doses (70–80 Gy), most patients develop radiation retinopathy. The usual interval between radiation exposure and the development of radiation-induced retinopathy is 2–3 years. Radiation retinopathy may develop earlier in patients who have diabetes or who are on chemotherapy. The earliest clinical manifestation of radiation retinopathy is usually cotton-wool spots, which fade away after several months, leaving large areas of capillary nonperfusion. Into these areas of capillary nonperfusion, telangiectatic vessels grow in the retina. Microaneurysms may also develop. These ischemic changes may cause rubeosis iridis, which in turn may lead to neovascular glaucoma.

Histologically, the capillary endothelial cell is the first type of cell to be damaged by radiation, followed closely by the pericytes and then the endothelial cells of the larger vessels. The new intraretinal telangiectatic vessels have thick collagenous walls. There may be spotty occlusion of the choriocapillaris.

Doses to the optic nerve in the range of 60–70 Gy cause some injury in a small number of patients. Damage to the distal end of the optic nerve is called *radiation optic neuropathy*. Clinically, these patients have disc pallor with splinter hemorrhages. If the damage occurs to the more proximal part of the optic nerve, the injury resembles retrobulbar optic neuropathy. Affected patients may complain of unilateral headaches and ocular pain; the disc may not reveal edema or hemorrhage. The effect of radiation on lacrimal tissue depends on the total dose. Permanent damage is not common below 50 Gy. With doses of 60–70 Gy, a dry eye syndrome sometimes develops. This syndrome usually develops within a year of irradiation and occasionally progresses to corneal ulceration and severe pain.

Chemotherapy

The goal of cancer chemotherapy is to damage or destroy cancer cells without killing normal cells. The first candidate drugs to selectively target rapidly dividing cells were sulfur and nitrogen mustards that were noted to suppress bone marrow when used in warfare. These compounds bound covalently to DNA, and thus DNA was the first molecular target of chemotherapy. In the 1950s, attention was directed to the precursors of DNA, and folate analogues such as methotrexate were found effective. The recognition that some tumors were hormonally dependent led to hormonal therapy or suppression as a means of treating cancer. More recently, a whole class of drugs derived from bacteria that inhibit mitotic spindle formation has been developed.

Chemotherapeutic agents can be divided into the following basic groups: natural products, angiogenesis inhibitors, and biological therapies.

Natural products

Natural products include a wide variety of agents, the most common of which are vinca alkaloids, podophyllin derivatives, paclitaxel, antitumor antibiotics, and related drugs (Table 11-1). Vinca alkaloids are derived from the periwinkle plant and include vincristine (Oncovin), vinblastine (Velban), and several investigational agents. These agents block incorporation of orotic acid and thymidine into DNA and cause arrest and inhibition of mitosis. Podophyllin derivatives and semisynthetic plant derivatives arrest cells in the G2 phase. Two examples of these derivatives are VP-16 (etoposide) and VM-26 (teniposide), both of which are gaining acceptance in many treatment protocols.

Paclitaxel (Taxol) is a compound originally isolated from the bark of the Pacific yew tree. It has been approved by the FDA to treat breast, ovarian, and lung cancers as well as AIDS-related Kaposi sarcoma. Paclitaxel stops microtubules from breaking down. In normal cell growth, microtubules are formed when a cell starts dividing. Once the cell stops dividing, the microtubules are broken down or destroyed. With paclitaxel, cancer cells become clogged with microtubules and cannot grow and divide.

Antitumor antibiotics are compounds produced by species of *Streptomyces* in culture. These agents interfere with the synthesis of nucleic acid. Following is a partial list:

- anthracyclines (doxorubicin and derivatives), which interfere with template function of DNA (a unique adverse effect is cardiac muscle degeneration leading to cardiomyopathy)
- bleomycin, which causes DNA-strand scission
- dactinomycin (actinomycin D), which inhibits DNA-directed RNA synthesis
- mitomycin, which impairs replication by causing cross-linking between DNA strands

The major dose-limiting toxicity of mitomycin is myelosuppression. Mitomycin has also been implicated as a cause of the hemolytic-uremic syndrome.

Angiogenesis inhibitors

Angiogenesis is important to the growth and spread of cancers. New blood vessels are critical in the formation of tumors. In animal studies, angiogenesis inhibitors have successfully stopped the formation of new blood vessels, causing the tumor to shrink and die. Currently, various angiogenesis inhibitors are being evaluated in human clinical trials. These studies include patients with cancers of the breast, prostate, brain, pancreas, lung, stomach, ovary, and cervix; some leukemias and lymphomas; and AIDS-related Kaposi sarcoma.

Antibodies against vascular endothelial growth factor have proven effective. Aptamers are a new class of drugs consisting of oligonucleotides that bind to specific proteins to inactivate these growth factors much the way that a monoclonal antibody would without the problems inherent in injecting foreign protein into a patient.

Biological therapies

Biological therapies (sometimes called *immunotherapy, biotherapy,* or *biological response modifier therapy*) use the immune system, either directly or indirectly, to fight cancer or to lessen the side effects that may be caused by some cancer treatments. Further, cancer may

Table 11-1 Antineoplastic Drugs

Drugs by Class	Mechanism of Action	Tumors Commonly Responsive	Toxicity and Remarks
Alkylating agents Mechlorethamine (nitrogen mustard) Chlorambucil (Leukeran) Cyclophosphamide (Cytoxan) Melphalan (Alkeran) Ifosfamide (Ifex)	Alkylation of DNA with restriction of strands' uncoiling and replication	Hodgkin, malignant lymphoma, small cell lung Ca, Ca of breast and testis, CLL	Alopecia with high IV dosage; nausea and vomiting; myelosuppression; hemorrhagic cystitis (especially with ifosfamide), which can be ameliorated with mesna; muto- and leukemogenic; aspermia; permanent sterility possible
Antimetabolites Folate antagonist methotrexate (MTX)	Folate antagonist with binding to dehydrofolate reductase and interference with (pyrimidine) thymidylate synthesis	Choriocarcinoma (female), Ca of head and neck, ALL, Ca of ovary, malignant lymphoma, osteogenic sarcoma	Mucosal ulceration; bone marrow suppression; toxicity increased with renal function impairment or ascitic fluid (with pooling of drug). Leucovorin rescue can reverse toxicity at 24 h (10–20 mg q 6 h × 10 doses).
Purine antagonist 6-mercaptopurine (6-MP)	Blocks de novo purine synthesis	Acute leukemia	Myelosuppression, alopecia
Pyrimidine antagonist 5-fluorouracil (5-FU)	Interferes with thymidylate synthase to reduce thymidine production	GI neoplasms, Ca of breast	Mucositis, alopecia, myelosuppression, diarrhea and vomiting, hyperpigmentation. When given after MTX, synergistic effect is significant.
Cytarabine (Ara-C)	DNA polymerase inhibition	Acute leukemia (especially nonlymphocytic), malignant lymphoma	Myelosuppression, nausea and vomiting, cerebellar and conjunctival toxicities at high dosage, skin rash

ALL = acute lymphocytic leukemia; Ca = cancer; CLL = chronic lymphocytic leukemia; CML = chronic myeloid leukemia; IFN = interferon; SIADH = syndrome of inappropriate antidiuretic hormone secretion.

Plant alkaloids
Vincas

Vinblastine (Velban)	Mitotic arrest by alteration of microtubular proteins	Lymphomas, leukemias, Ca of breast, Ewing sarcoma, Ca of testis	Alopecia, myelosuppression, peripheral neuropathy, ileus
Vincristine (Oncovin)	As above	As above, plus retinoblastoma	Peripheral neuropathy, SIADH. Dose commonly "capped" at total of 2 mg in adults.
Paclitaxel (Taxol)	Promotes assembly of microtubules	Ca of breast, lung, ovary, head, neck, and bladder; Kaposi sarcoma	Myelosuppression, alopecia, myalgia, arthralgia, neuropathy
Podophyllotoxins			
Etoposide (VePesid, VP-16)	Inhibition of mitosis by unknown mechanisms	Retinoblastoma, lymphoma, Hodgkin, Ca of testis, Ca of lung (especially small cell), acute leukemia	Nausea, vomiting, myelosuppression, peripheral neuropathy. Etoposide cleared by liver (teniposide by kidney); increased toxicity in renal failure.
Teniposide (VM-26)	As above	Acute lymphoblastic leukemia, non-Hodgkin lymphoma, neuroblastoma	Nausea, vomiting, alopecia

Antibiotics

Doxorubicin (Adriamycin)	Intercalation between DNA strands inhibits uncoiling of DNA	Acute leukemia, Hodgkin, other lymphomas, Ca of breast, Ca of lung	Nausea and vomiting, myelosuppression, alopecia. Cardiac toxicity at cumulative dosage >500 mg/m^2. Higher dosage tolerated when given by continuous IV.
Bleomycin	Incision of DNA strands	Squamous cell Ca, lymphoma, Ca of testis, Ca of lung	Anaphylaxis, chills and fever, skin rash; pulmonary fibrosis at dosage >200 mg/m^2; requires renal excretion
Mitomycin	Inhibits DNA synthesis by acting as a bifunctional alkylator	Gastric adenocarcinoma; colon, breast, and lung Ca; transitional cell Ca of the bladder	Local extravasation causes tissue necrosis; myelosuppression, with leukopenia and thrombocytopenia 4–6 wk after treatment; alopecia; lethargy; fever; hemolytic-uremic syndrome
Dactinomycin (actinomycin-D)	Inhibits DNA synthesis by intercalating with guanine residues	Wilms tumor, rhabdomyosarcoma, Ewing sarcoma	Rash, nausea, vomiting, myelosuppression

ALL = acute lymphocytic leukemia; Ca = cancer; CLL = chronic lymphocytic leukemia; CML = chronic myeloid leukemia; IFN = interferon; SIADH = syndrome of inappropriate antidiuretic hormone secretion.

(Continued)

Table 11-1 *(continued)*

Drugs by Class	Mechanism of Action	Tumors Commonly Responsive	Toxicity and Remarks
Nitrosoureas			
Carmustine (BiCNU)	Alkylation of DNA with restriction of strands' uncoiling and replication	Brain tumors, lymphoma	Myelosuppression, pulmonary toxicity (fibrosis), renal toxicity
Lomustine (CeeNU)	Carbamoylation of amino acids in proteins	As above	As above
Inorganic ions			
Cisplatin (Platinol)	Intercalation and intracalation between DNA strands inhibits uncoiling of DNA	Ca of lung (especially small cell), testis, breast, and stomach; lymphoma	Anemia, ototoxicity, peripheral neuropathy, myelosuppression, nausea, vomiting
Biologic response modifiers			
IFN (Intron-A, Roferon-A)	Antiproliferative effect	Hairy cell leukemia, CML, lymphomas, Kaposi sarcoma (AIDS), renal cell Ca, melanoma	Fatigue, fever, myalgias, arthralgias, myelosuppression, nephrotic syndrome (rarely)
Enzymes			
Asparaginase (Elspar)	Depletion of asparagine, on which leukemic cells depend	ALL	Acute anaphylaxis, hyperthermia, pancreatitis, hyperglycemia, hypofibrinogenemia
Hormones			
Tamoxifen (Nolvadex)	Places cells at rest: binding of estrogen receptor	Ca of breast	Hot flushes, hypercalcemia, deep vein thrombosis
Flutamide (Eulexin)	Binding of androgen receptor	Ca of prostate	Decreased libido, hot flushes, gynecomastia

ALL = acute lymphocytic leukemia; Ca = cancer; CLL = chronic lymphocytic leukemia; CML = chronic myeloid leukemia; IFN = interferon; SIADH = syndrome of inappropriate antidiuretic hormone secretion.

Adapted from *The Merck Manual of Diagnosis and Therapy*. 17th ed. Rahway, NJ: Merck Research Laboratories; 1999:990–993.

develop when the immune system breaks down or when it is not functioning adequately. Biological therapies are designed to repair, stimulate, or enhance the immune system's responses.

Cells in the immune system secrete 2 types of proteins: antibodies and cytokines. Cytokines are substances produced by some immune system cells to communicate with other cells. Types of cytokines include lymphokines, interferons, interleukins, and colony-stimulating factors. Some antibodies and cytokines can be used to treat cancer. These substances are called *biological response modifiers*. Other biological response modifiers include monoclonal antibodies and vaccines.

Interferons are types of cytokines that occur naturally in the body. There are 3 major types of interferons: interferon-α, interferon-β, and interferon-γ. Interferon-α is the type most widely used in cancer treatment. Interferons can improve the way a cancer patient's immune system acts against cancer cells. Furthermore, interferons may act directly on cancer cells by slowing their growth or promoting their development into cells with more normal behavior. Interferons may also stimulate natural killer cells, T cells, and macrophages, boosting the immune system's anticancer function. The FDA has approved the use of interferon-α for the treatment of hairy cell leukemia, melanoma, chronic myeloid leukemia, and AIDS-related Kaposi sarcoma.

Interleukins, like interferons, are cytokines that occur naturally in the body. They can also be made in the laboratory. Many interleukins have been identified; interleukin-2 (IL-2) has been the most widely studied in cancer treatment. Interleukin-2 stimulates the growth and activity of many immune cells, such as lymphocytes, that can destroy cancer cells. The FDA has approved IL-2 for the treatment of metastatic kidney cancer and metastatic melanoma.

Colony-stimulating factors (sometimes called *hematopoietic growth factors*) usually do not directly affect tumor cells but instead stimulate bone marrow production. Colony-stimulating factors allow doses of anticancer drugs to be increased without increasing the risk of infection or need for transfusion.

The fact that a patient has a cancer suggests that there has been a failure in that patient's immune system. This makes reconstituting the immune system an attractive approach for treating metastatic tumors.

Monoclonal antibodies (MOABs) are produced by a single type of cell and are specific for a particular antigen. Researchers are examining ways to create MOABs that are specific to the antigens found on the surface of cancer cells being treated.

Monoclonal antibodies are made by injecting human cancer cells into mice, stimulating an antibody response. The cells producing antibodies are then removed and fused with laboratory-grown cells to create hybrid cells called *hybridomas*. Hybridomas can indefinitely produce large quantities of these MOABs.

Monoclonal antibodies have many potential uses in cancer treatment. One such treatment is to link MOABs to anticancer drugs, radioisotopes, other biological response modifiers, or other toxins. When the antibodies attach to cancer cells, they can deliver these poisons directly to the cells. Monoclonal antibodies carrying radioisotopes may also prove useful in the diagnosis of certain cancers, such as colorectal, ovarian, and prostate cancer.

Cancer vaccines are being developed to assist the immune system in recognizing cancer cells. These vaccines, designed to be injected after the disease is diagnosed rather than before it develops, may help the body reject tumors and prevent cancer from recurring. Vaccines are being studied in the treatment of melanomas, lymphomas, and cancers of the kidney, breast, ovaries, prostate, colon, and rectum.

In the future, other biological approaches to cancer therapy may include *genetic profiling* of certain tumors. Genetic profiling may prove more helpful and effective than classifying tumors by their organ of origin. Tumors with a specific genetic profile may be more sensitive to chemotherapy.

Ophthalmic Considerations

The eye and its adnexa are frequently involved in systemic malignancies as well as in extraocular malignancies that extend into ocular structures (including local malignancies of skin, bone, and sinuses). Breast and lung cancers are common intraocular tumors in adults. Acute myelogenous and lymphocytic leukemias frequently have uveal and posterior choroidal infiltrates as part of their generalized disease. In children, these manifestations are often signs of central nervous system involvement, and they suggest a poor prognosis. Although malignant lymphomas do not usually involve the uveal tract, histiocytic lymphoma is one type that often involves the vitreous and presents as uveitis. The retina and choroid may also be involved. Tumors of the eye and adnexa are discussed in several other BCSC sections, including Section 4, *Ophthalmic Pathology and Intraocular Tumors;* Section 6, *Pediatric Ophthalmology and Strabismus;* Section 7, *Orbit, Eyelids, and Lacrimal System;* and Section 8, *External Disease and Cornea.*

CHAPTER **12**

Behavioral and Neurologic Disorders

Recent Developments

- Newer therapeutic agents for psychiatric diseases allow more effective treatment with generally fewer side effects compared with older agents.
- Progress continues to be made concerning the etiology of neurodegenerative disorders such as Alzheimer disease and Parkinson disease, but therapeutic options are still primarily palliative and of limited benefit.
- The antiepileptic medications topiramate (Topamax) and vigabatrin (Sabril) are associated with ophthalmic side effects. Topiramate can cause angle-closure glaucoma, and vigabatrin can cause visual field loss.
- Atypical antipsychotic agents are increasingly used both for the treatment of schizophrenia and for off-label uses such as therapy for major depression, anxiety disorders, and Alzheimer disease. The FDA recently issued a warning that such off-label use has been associated with increased mortality. Ophthalmologists should be aware that this class of drugs has also been associated with an increased risk for diabetes mellitus.

Introduction

Since the 1980s, the World Health Organization (WHO) has focused its efforts on behavioral and neurologic disorders that occur frequently, cause substantial disability, and create a burden on individuals, families, communities, and societies. The WHO approach has been based on epidemiologic evidence: the assessment of disease burden using disability-adjusted life years. This approach has emphasized the public health importance of behavioral and neurologic disorders, which in 1990 accounted for 10.5% of the worldwide disease burden. It is estimated that such disorders will account for 15% of disability-adjusted life years in 2030.

In addition to behavioral disorders, the neurologic disorders that significantly affect this disease burden include epilepsy, dementias (in particular, Alzheimer disease), multiple sclerosis, Parkinson disease and other motor system disorders, stroke, pain syndromes, and brain injury.

Behavioral Disorders

Behavioral disorders encompass a wide variety of conditions in which the common factor is disordered functioning of personality. These disturbances range from mild reactions to the events or circumstances of a person's life to debilitating, life-threatening illnesses. Although the practicing ophthalmologist will not be called on to treat mental illness, such disease may profoundly affect the diagnosis and treatment of ocular diseases. In addition, some of the medications used to treat psychiatric disorders may have significant ophthalmic side effects.

Mental Disorders Due to a General Medical Condition

Formerly called *organic mental syndromes,* this category was renamed in the *Diagnostic and Statistical Manual of Mental Disorders,* better known as *DSM-IV*. The essential feature of mental disorders due to a general medical condition is a psychological or behavioral abnormality associated with transient or permanent dysfunction of the brain. Causes include any disease, drug, or trauma that directly affects the central nervous system (CNS), and systemic illnesses that indirectly interfere with brain function; Alzheimer disease is included in this category. Orientation, memory, and other intellectual functions are impaired. Psychiatric symptoms may occur, including hallucinations, delusions, depression, obsessions, and personality changes.

Patients with a mental disorder due to a general medical condition with or without cognitive impairment are often unable to remember instructions and therefore unable to comply with treatment regimens. This global inability to understand instructions, integrate information, and perform tasks is referred to as *executive function deficit*. Depression, which frequently accompanies the syndrome, can complicate the situation. Medications with CNS side effects, such as beta-blockers and carbonic anhydrase inhibitors, must be used with care because often these patients are sensitive to these agents. See also the discussion of dementia in Chapter 10, Geriatrics.

Schizophrenia

The term *schizophrenia* actually encompasses a group of disorders with similar features. These are some of the most devastating mental illnesses in terms of personal and societal cost. Schizophrenia usually begins when patients are young and continues to a greater or lesser extent throughout their lives. The hallmarks of schizophrenia include "positive" psychotic symptoms such as hallucinations (usually auditory) and delusions, as well as "negative" symptoms such as emotional and cognitive blunting and poor social and occupational functioning. The incidence is estimated at 0.5%–1.0% of the population.

The classic manifestations are delusions, hallucinations, and disorganized speech and behavior. *Delusions* are disturbances in thought: firmly held beliefs that are untrue. Other thought abnormalities include loosening of associations and tangential thinking. *Hallucinations* are abnormal perceptions, experienced without any actual external stimulus. The patient's affect is often flattened or inappropriate.

Motor disturbances range from uncontrolled, aimless activity to catatonic stupor, in which the patient may be immobile, mute, and unresponsive yet fully conscious. Repetitive, purposeless mannerisms and inability to complete goal-directed tasks are also common. Associated illnesses include *schizophreniform disorder,* in which schizophrenic manifestations occur for less than 6 months, and *brief psychotic disorder,* which lasts less than 1 month. *Schizoaffective disorder* refers to patients who have a significant mood disorder, such as depression, that manifests itself independently of the psychotic disorder.

Mood Disorders

Also known as *affective disorders,* mood disorders range from appropriate reactions to negative life experiences to severe, recurrent, debilitating illnesses. Common to all of these disorders is depressed mood, elevated mood (mania), or alternations of the two.

Major depression is far more common than mania and therefore has a greater impact on all aspects of society. The lifetime risk for major depressive disorder is 7%–12% for men and 20%–25% for women. Major depression may occur at any age, but it is most common in middle-aged and elderly persons. Affective changes include a feeling of sadness, emptiness, and nervousness. Thought processes are typically slowed and reflect low self-esteem, pessimism, and feelings of guilt. Social withdrawal and psychomotor retardation are seen, although agitation also occurs. Basic physical functions are impaired, as manifested by sleep disturbances, changes in appetite with associated weight loss or gain, diminished libido, and an inability to experience pleasure *(anhedonia)*. Common somatic complaints are fatigue, headache, and other nonspecific symptoms. Up to 15% of seriously depressed patients may commit suicide. The term *major depressive disorder* is used to describe patients who have major depressive episodes without any manic symptoms. *Dysthymic disorder* refers to patients with chronic, less severe depressive symptoms that do not meet the criteria for major depression.

Mania is a period of abnormally and persistently elevated or irritable mood sufficiently severe to cause impairment in social or occupational functioning. Typical symptoms include euphoria or irritability, grandiosity, decreased need for sleep, increased talkativeness, flight of ideas, and increased goal-directed activity. The classic term *manic depression* has been replaced by *bipolar disorder.* Bipolar I disorder describes any illness in which mania is present, whether or not depression occurs. Bipolar II disorder refers to patients with major depressive episodes and at least 1 mild manic episode (hypomania). *Cyclothymic disorder* describes cyclical episodes of mild depression and mania.

For the nonpsychiatric clinician, depression creates a number of problems. In some patients, mood change may not be apparent, and the illness is manifested in somatic complaints leading to time-consuming, expensive workups. Conversely, in patients known to be depressed, an organic disease may be overlooked as psychosomatic. Appropriate recommendations for psychotherapeutic intervention may be met with resistance, anger, or denial, disrupting the patient-physician relationship. Compliance with diagnostic and treatment regimens for medical disorders and surgical procedures can be problematic. A screening study of elderly patients attending an ophthalmology clinic showed that 1 in 5 patients suffered from depression. It is estimated that up to 30% of patients with macular degeneration have depression, and it is likely that other causes of vision loss contribute to the presence of significant depression in many patients.

Casten RJ, Rovner BW, Tasman W. Age-related macular degeneration and depression: a review of recent research. *Curr Opin Ophthalmol.* 2004;15(3):181–183.

Lee AG, Beaver HA, Jogerst G, et al. Screening elderly patients in an outpatient ophthalmology clinic for dementia, depression, and functional impairment. *Ophthalmology*. 2003; 110(4):651–657.

Somatoform Disorders

The essential feature of these disorders is the presence of symptoms suggesting physical disease in the absence of physical findings or a known physiologic mechanism to account for the symptoms. The symptoms in somatoform disorders are considered to be outside the patient's voluntary control. The practicing physician should be aware of these syndromes because encounters with these patients are common.

Several somatoform disorders are recognized. *Conversion disorders* are characterized by temporary and involuntary loss or alteration of physical functioning due to psychosocial stress. Symptoms are typically neurologic and include functional visual loss ("hysterical blindness"). In *somatoform pain disorder,* prolonged, severe pain is the only symptom. Psychotherapy is the primary therapeutic modality.

Somatization disorder is most common in women and consists of multiple somatic complaints. Patients are often histrionic in describing their symptoms and may have undergone multiple hospitalizations and surgery. The incidence of associated psychiatric illness is high. Treatment is aimed at providing psychological support and minimizing the expenditure of medical resources. Psychotherapy is typically met with resistance and is therefore usually unsuccessful. Psychopharmacologic treatment of underlying psychiatric disorders may help.

Hypochondriasis is a preoccupation with the fear of having or developing a serious disease. Physical examination fails to support the patient's belief, and reassurance by the examining physician fails to allay the fear. Treatment principles are the same as for somatization disorder. In *body dysmorphic disorder,* the patient believes that his or her body is deformed, even though there is no physical defect, or the patient has an exaggerated concern about a mild physical anomaly. Ophthalmologists performing reconstructive and cosmetic surgery should be aware of this disorder because surgical repair of the "defect" is rarely successful in the patient's mind.

Two other conditions that are not actually somatoform disorders bear mentioning here. *Factitious disorders* are characterized by willful production of physical or psychological signs or symptoms in the absence of external incentives. It is thought that these patients feign illness solely because of a psychological need to assume the role of a sick person. Treatment requires discovery of the true nature of the physical illness, a carefully planned confrontation, and psychotherapy. Prognosis for recovery is guarded. Chronic conjunctivitis, keratitis, and even scleritis are the usual ophthalmic presentations of factitious disease. *Malingering* is the intentional production of physical or psychological symptoms for the purpose of identifiable secondary gain. Malingering is not considered a primary psychiatric illness.

Ophthalmologists should be familiar with techniques for detecting malingerers who feign loss of vision, because such persons are occasionally encountered in practice. (See BCSC Section 5, *Neuro-Ophthalmology,* for some of these techniques.)

The anxiety disorders represent another group of diseases that can significantly interfere with normal functioning. *Generalized anxiety disorder (GAD)* is the most common anxiety disorder and is characterized by unrealistic or excessive anxiety and worry about 2 or more life circumstances. Generalized anxiety disorder is also correlated with depression. Pharmacologic therapy and psychotherapy may be very successful in treating this disease.

Patients with *panic disorder* report discrete periods of intense terror and impending doom that are almost intolerable. These episodes can occur abruptly, either in certain predictable situations or without any situational trigger. Mild disease can be treated with psychotherapy, but more significant disease is often treated with antidepressant medication, especially the selective serotonin reuptake inhibitors (SSRIs).

Post-traumatic stress disorder (PTSD) occurs after an individual has been exposed to a dramatic event that is associated with intense fear. When exposed to reminders of the event, the patient then persistently re-experiences the event through intrusive recollections, nightmares, flashbacks, or distress. The prevalence of PTSD is 8% in the general population and increases to 60% in combat soldiers and assault victims. Treatment usually includes psychotherapy and use of antidepressants. Other anxiety-related conditions that may require pharmacologic intervention include obsessive-compulsive disorder and social phobia.

The various personality disorders merit recognition because of the potential for associated problems to arise, such as poor compliance and substance abuse. Personality disorders are diagnosed when personality traits become inflexible and maladaptive to the point where they create significant dysfunction. Patients usually have little or no insight into their disorder. The personality disorders include *cluster A personality disorders,* which are related to a tendency to develop schizophrenia and include paranoid, schizotypal, and schizoid disorders. *Cluster B personality disorders* include antisocial, borderline, histrionic, and narcissistic personality disorders. These patients may display dramatic or irrational behavior and may be very disruptive in clinical settings. *Cluster C personality disorders* often stem from maladaptive attempts to control anxiety and include avoidant, dependent, and obsessive-compulsive personality disorders. Psychotherapy tends to be the treatment of choice for all of these entities. There is no specific pharmacotherapy, although medication may be used to treat certain symptoms or coexisting mood disorders.

Substance Abuse Disorders

Drug dependence is the abuse of a drug to the point that one's physical health, psychological functioning, or ability to exist within the demands of society is threatened. Common to all types of drug dependence is *psychic dependence*—that is, a psychic drive or a feeling of satisfaction requiring periodic or continuous drug administration in order to avoid discomfort, produce pleasure, relieve boredom, or facilitate social interaction. *Physical dependence* occurs when repeated administration of a drug causes an altered physiologic state in the central nervous system so that sudden cessation of the drug causes an *abstinence syndrome* (a physical illness whose symptoms are determined by the specific drug). *Tolerance* occurs when increasing amounts of a drug are necessary to achieve the same desired effect. The drugs causing dependence fall into several groups, as listed in Table 12-1.

Table 12-1 Classification of Dependence-Producing Drugs

Class I—Drugs producing both psychic and physical dependence
A. Opiate type
   1. Morphine group: opium, morphine, diacetylmorphine (heroin), hydromorphone (Dilaudid), codeine, dihydrohydroxycodeinone
   2. Morphinans: oxycodone (Percodan)
   3. Benzomorphans: phenazocine (Prinadol)
   4. Meperidine group: meperidine (Demerol)
   5. Methadone group: methadone, propoxyphene (Darvon)
B. Alcohol-barbiturate type
   1. Ethyl alcohol
   2. Barbiturates
   3. Paraldehyde
   4. Chloral hydrate
   5. Meprobamate (Miltown, Equanil)
   6. Piperidinediones: glutethimide, methyprylon (Noludar)
   7. Benzodiazepines: chlordiazepoxide (Librium), diazepam (Valium), alprazolam (Xanax)
   8. Tertiary carbinols: methylpentynol (Dormison), ethchlorvynol (Placidyl)
C. Opiate agonist-antagonist type
   1. Nalorphine
   2. Levallorphan
   3. Cyclazocine
   4. Pentazocine (Talwin)
D. Amphetamine type
   1. dl-amphetamine (Benzedrine), dextroamphetamine (Dexedrine)
   2. Phenmetrazine (Preludin)
   3. Methylphenidate (Ritalin)
   4. Diethylpropion (Tenuate)
   5. Pipradrol (Meratran)
E. Cocaine type: coca leaf, cocaine

Class II—Drugs producing psychic dependence but not physical dependence
A. Hallucinogens
   1. Lysergic acid diethylamide (LSD)
   2. Mescaline
   3. Tryptamines: psilocybin, dimethyltryptamine, diethyltryptamine
   4. Hallucinogenic amphetamines
B. Cannabis type: cannabis leaf (marijuana), hashish
C. Bromides

Drug abuse and addiction are often viewed as strictly social problems. Some believe that drug abusers and addicts should be able to stop taking drugs if they are willing to change their behavior. Recent scientific research provides overwhelming evidence that in addition to short-term effects, drugs also have long-term effects on brain metabolism and activity. At some point, changes occur in the brain, turning drug abuse into the illness of addiction. Those addicted to drugs have a compulsive drug craving and frequently are unable to quit by themselves. Treatment is necessary to end the compulsive behavior.

Opiates

Heroin is the most commonly abused nonprescription opiate in the United States. Diagnosis of heroin use is made by history, and findings may include miotic pupils and puncture sites on the skin. Symptoms of abstinence include restlessness, yawning, rhinorrhea, pupillary mydriasis, hyperthermia (38°–40°C), vomiting, and diarrhea. Withdrawal, although not fatal to people with no other serious illness, can be dangerous in ill or elderly people. A plan of complete withdrawal as well as full support (economic, social, and psychiatric) must be employed to prevent the patient from returning to drug dependence. Because many former heroin abusers are unable to remain drug-free, methadone maintenance is sometimes used. Methadone, which is absorbed orally, prevents drug craving and abstinence symptoms for 24–36 hours and causes tolerance (blockage of other opiates). Unfortunately, drug-free status is difficult to maintain for long periods; 90% of patients who leave methadone treatment programs will be incarcerated, deeply involved in drugs, readmitted to the program, or dead within 1 year.

Sedative-hypnotics

Sedative-hypnotic drugs include benzodiazepines, barbiturates, and other sleeping pills. These drugs elevate the threshold of excitation of neurons, thereby resulting in lethargy, ataxia, nystagmus, impaired judgment, and emotional lability. Cessation of the drug causes anxiety, restlessness, convulsions, delusions, and hyperthermia; cessation may even be fatal. Diagnosis of drug abuse is made from history and confirmed by a blood or urine level of the drugs. Abuse of hypnotic drugs should be suspected in anyone appearing drunk without evidence of alcohol ingestion. Treatment consists of a monitored hospital withdrawal, with posthospital support.

Flunitrazepam (Rohypnol) is a benzodiazepine that has been of particular concern the last few years because of its abuse in date rape. When mixed with alcohol, it can incapacitate victims, preventing them from resisting sexual assault. It can also produce anterograde amnesia and has the potential to be lethal when combined with alcohol or other sedatives. Illicit use of flunitrazepam started in the United States in the early 1990s, even though the drug is not approved for use in the United States and its importation is banned.

Alcohol

Alcohol is also considered a sedative-hypnotic and is by far the most commonly abused drug, owing to its widespread availability. It is estimated that 7% of adults in the United States are alcohol-dependent. Although multiple factors contribute to alcoholism, twin and adoption studies have shown a genetic influence. According to several studies, approximately 25% of fathers and brothers of alcohol-dependent persons are themselves alcohol-dependent.

Like hypnotic drugs, alcohol depresses the CNS and leads to similar clinical findings; blood levels of ethyl alcohol should be obtained in suspicious cases. The *alcohol abstinence syndrome* consists of restlessness, hallucinations, and even seizures 72–96 hours after cessation of drinking. Awareness of this syndrome is important when patients are admitted, for instance, for an eye-related injury. Treatment consists of a supported, controlled withdrawal using a different sedative-hypnotic drug. In addition, the patient needs long-term support, which may be obtained by joining groups such as Alcoholics Anonymous.

Alcohol crosses the placental barrier, and children born to alcoholic mothers may be affected by fetal alcohol syndrome. Some of the ocular manifestations of this syndrome are blepharophimosis, telecanthus, ptosis, optic nerve hypoplasia or atrophy, and tortuosity of the retinal arteries and veins. (See also BCSC Section 6, *Pediatric Ophthalmology and Strabismus.*)

Amphetamines

Amphetamine-type drugs are sympathomimetic amines that are widely abused. Acute use produces hyperactivity, euphoria, a heightened sense of effectiveness, tachycardia, and paranoia. The use of methamphetamine in particular is increasing because of the relative ease with which it can be made in illegal laboratories. Treatment consists of hospital observation until the abstinence syndrome, especially depression, passes.

Chemically similar to the stimulant methamphetamine and the hallucinogen mescaline, *MDMA* (3,4-methylenedioxymethamphetamine, or *ecstasy*) is a synthetic, psychoactive drug that is gaining in popularity in a number of groups, especially on college campuses, because of its euphoric and hallucinogenic effects. Animal studies have clearly shown that the drug is neurotoxic, and human studies suggest but so far have not conclusively proven that it has similar effects in humans. There is the added potential for drugs sold as ecstasy to be contaminated with other toxic chemicals. Although not physically addicting, MDMA has significant potential for experimental use because the demographics at greatest risk perceive the drug to be short-acting and harmless. Ecstasy may also be associated with severe acute toxicity, including fulminant hyperthermia, seizures, disseminated intravascular coagulation, rhabdomyolysis, acute renal failure, and hepatotoxicity.

Cocaine

Cocaine has become an increasingly abused drug in the United States since the mid-1970s. It is a powerfully addictive drug, and a person who tries cocaine cannot predict or control the extent to which he or she will continue to use the drug.

Cocaine hydrochloride is a white crystal powder derived from coca leaves, which can be taken intranasally or intravenously. Intranasal cocaine has a half-life of less than 90 minutes, its euphoric effects lasting 15–30 minutes. Removal of the hydrochloride salt produces freebase cocaine, an 80% pure alkaloid form of cocaine. "Crack," or "rock," cocaine is a freebase derivative that is smoked, producing intense euphoria within seconds. The widespread availability of inexpensive crack has dramatically increased the scope of the cocaine abuse problem.

The symptoms of cocaine abstinence are not as stereotypical as those of opiate withdrawal. In general, there is a dysphoric state consisting of depression, anhedonia, insomnia, and anxiety lasting about 3 days. As these symptoms wane, cocaine craving persists, often leading to binge cycles at intervals of 3–10 days. If the cycle of abuse can be broken, craving tends to wane over a 3-week period. Symptoms of major depression are common during this period but eventually clear.

Cocaine addiction among pregnant women is a growing problem. Premature labor, abruptio placentae, and fetal asphyxia may occur. "Crack babies" are associated with intrauterine growth retardation, microcephaly, seizures, sudden infant death syndrome (SIDS), rigidity, developmental delay, and learning disabilities. Crack babies also have an increased risk of strabismus, and neonatal retinal hemorrhages have been reported.

Ophthalmic considerations

Substance abuse is associated with an increased incidence of ocular trauma. Toxic optic neuropathy is seen in alcohol-dependent patients as a direct effect of the disease or in association with the malnutrition that often accompanies alcoholism. Vascular occlusion and endophthalmitis can occur in association with intravenous drug abuse. Optic neuropathy can occur in association with cocaine-induced nasal and sinus pathology. Crack cocaine use in particular should be considered in young patients who present with corneal ulcers or epithelial defects without an obvious cause. Marijuana has a transient lowering effect on intraocular pressure; thus, many patients assume that marijuana is good for treating or relieving the symptoms of glaucoma and other eye problems. In fact, marijuana has only a temporary effect on ocular pressure (3–4 hours), and the response diminishes with time. Furthermore, the ocular hypotensive effect cannot be isolated from the psychological effect, making this drug clinically useless in ophthalmology.

Pharmacologic Treatment of Psychiatric Disorders

Antipsychotic Drugs

The antipsychotics may be broadly divided into 2 groups, namely, "first generation," or "typical," drugs, and "second generation," or "atypical," drugs. The older term "major tranquilizer" is no longer used. The distinction between the first-generation and the second-generation antipsychotics is based on differences in receptor activity, side effects, and overall efficacy. The first-generation drugs are primarily dopamine receptor blockers; by contrast the second-generation antipsychotics have an inhibitory effect on serotonin receptors, as well as dopamine-blocking activity. With regard to side effects, most of the second-generation drugs are better tolerated than the first-generation ones are. Commonly used first-generation antipsychotics include haloperidol (Haldol), fluphenazine (Prolixin), and chlorpromazine (Thorazine). The number of second-generation drugs is continually growing, and these are listed in Table 12-2. Clozapine (Clozaril), risperidone (Risperdal), and olanzapine (Zyprexa) are superior to the first-generation agents; whether the other second-generation drugs share this superiority has not yet been demonstrated in controlled trials. Clozapine has an increased risk of agranulocytosis and is reserved for patients with refractory disease. The atypical antipsychotics are also increasingly administered for off-label uses such as treatment of major depression, anxiety disorders, and Alzheimer disease. The FDA recently issued a warning that such off-label use has been associated with increased mortality, due usually to heart-related events or infections.

These medications effectively reduce many of the symptoms of acute and chronic psychoses and have allowed many more patients to function outside the walls of psychiatric institutions. A wide range of side effects may occur with these agents, including

Table 12-2 Antipsychotic Medications
First generation (typical or neuroleptic)
Aripiprazole (Abilify)
Chlorpromazine (Thorazine)
Fluphenazine (Prolixin)
Haloperidol (Haldol)
Loxapine (Loxitane)
Mesoridazine (Serentil)
Molindone (Moban)
Perphenazine (Trilafon)
Pimozide (Orap)
Thioridazine (Mellaril)
Thiothixene (Navane)
Second generation (atypical)
Clozapine (Clozaril)
Olanzapine (Zyprexa)
Quetiapine (Seroquel)
Risperidone (Risperdal)
Ziprasidone (Geodon)
Anticholinergic agents used to minimize extrapyramidal side effects
Benztropine (Cogentin)
Biperiden (Akineton)
Diphenhydramine (Benadryl)
Trihexyphenidyl (Artane)

extrapyramidal reactions, drowsiness, orthostatic hypotension, anticholinergic effects, and tardive dyskinesia. Less common problems include cholestatic jaundice, blood dyscrasias, photosensitivity, and a rare idiosyncratic reaction known as *neuroleptic malignant syndrome (NMS)*. Neuroleptic malignant syndrome is characterized by "lead pipe" muscle rigidity and hyperthermia and can lead to death if not recognized and treated. The atypical antipsychotics are far less likely to cause these side effects, although problems may still occur to some extent at higher doses. Some patients may be maintained on first-generation drugs, however, for reasons of cost, effectiveness, and familiarity.

There are some specific issues of concern to ophthalmologists. The atypical agents—especially olanzapine (Zyprexa) and clozapine (Clozaril)—may be associated with initiating or worsening diabetes, and the possibility of secondary refractive and retinal vascular changes should be considered in this patient population. Because of the results of animal studies, the atypical agent quetiapine (Seroquel) was thought to increase the risk of cataracts. For this reason, psychiatrists are instructed to obtain twice-yearly examinations for this patient population. But because a true causal relationship is unlikely, annual screening examinations are sufficient. Anticholinergic problems such as dry eye symptoms, accommodative symptoms, and precipitation of angle-closure glaucoma are possible, especially with use of the first-generation agents and the newer drugs olanzapine and clozapine. These problems may be exacerbated because patients may be placed on additional anticholinergic medications to minimize extrapyramidal side effects of the antipsychotics (see Table 12-2). Potential ocular side effects of the first-generation drugs include corneal deposition, lens pigmentation, and vision loss from retinal pigmentary degeneration. These adverse effects are most common with use of thioridazine and are more likely to occur with long-term use at high doses (usually higher than 800 mg/day). Blepharospasm and other ocular motility problems can occur in association with extrapyramidal side effects.

> Fraunfelder FW. Twice-yearly exams unnecessary for patients taking quetiapine. *Am J Ophthalmol*. 2004;138(5):870–871.

Antianxiety and Hypnotic Drugs

Benzodiazepines

The benzodiazepines are usually the drugs of choice when an antianxiety, sedative, or hypnotic action is needed. Other indications for selected benzodiazepines include preanesthetic medication, alcohol withdrawal, seizures, spasticity, localized skeletal muscle spasm, and nocturnal myoclonus. The benzodiazepines have distinct advantages over other agents, with respect to adverse reactions, drug interactions, and lethality. The pharmacokinetics of these medications greatly affects their efficacy and adverse reactions and thus influences drug selection (Table 12-3). Because of their enhanced safety profile, benzodiazepines have largely supplanted the use of barbiturates when antianxiety or hypnotic drugs are required. Barbiturates have been relegated to treatment of seizure disorders and use in anesthesia.

All benzodiazepines alleviate the uncomplicated anxiety of generalized anxiety disorder and improve symptoms of situational anxiety. Long-acting agents such as diazepam (Valium) are useful for patients requiring chronic treatment. The treatment of insomnia is another common indication for these drugs. Short-acting agents such as temazepam (Restoril), estazolam (Prosom), and triazolam (Halcion) are preferred for this purpose because there is less residual somnolence. Zolpidem (Ambien) and zaleplon (Sonata) are newer short-acting non-benzodiazepine hypnotic agents that are increasingly used in the treatment of insomnia. All of these drugs, however, have the potential to cause retrograde amnesia and rebound insomnia.

Sedation is the most common initial untoward effect of the benzodiazepines. Other common dose-related adverse effects with oral use include dizziness and ataxia. Respiratory depression can occur, especially if these agents are combined with alcohol. Products available in parenteral form, such as diazepam (Valium) and midazolam (Versed), must be administered with careful monitoring because of an increased risk for apnea and cardiac arrest.

The abuse potential of benzodiazepines is mild compared with that of drugs such as hydromorphone (Dilaudid) and cocaine. Nevertheless, long-term administration of these agents can cause physical dependence. Once physical dependence is established, withdrawal reactions may occur if the drugs are discontinued abruptly. Psychological dependence is more common than physical dependence and can occur with any dose. This type of drug reliance is difficult to distinguish from a recurrence of the original anxiety disorder. Consequently, good medical practice demands that these agents be prescribed initially only when a disorder known to respond to such therapy can be diagnosed with reasonable assurance, and that their use be continued only for the shortest time required.

Table 12-3 Antianxiety and Hypnotic Drugs

Benzodiazepines
  Compounds with active metabolites
    Chlordiazepoxide (Librium)
    Clorazepate (Tranxene)
    Diazepam (Valium, Valrelease)
    Flurazepam (Dalmane)
    Halazepam (Paxipam)
  Compounds with weakly active, short-lived, or inactive metabolites
    Alprazolam (Xanax)
    Clonazepam (Klonopin)
    Estazolam (Prosom)
    Lorazepam (Ativan)
    Midazolam (Versed)
    Oxazepam (Serax)
    Quazepam (Doral)
    Temazepam (Restoril)
    Triazolam (Halcion)

Barbiturates
  Amobarbital (Amytal)
  Mephobarbital (Mebaral)
  Phenobarbital (Solfoton)
  Pentobarbital (Nembutal)
  Secobarbital (Seconal)

Nonbenzodiazepine-nonbarbiturates
  Antianxiety agents
    Buspirone (BuSpar)
    Hydroxyzine (Atarax, Vistaril)
    Meprobamate (Equanil, Miltown)
  Hypnotic agents
    Chloral hydrate
    Ethchlorvynol (Placidyl)
    Paraldehyde
    Zaleplon (Sonata)
    Zolpidem (Ambien)

Ocular side effects can occur, although they tend to be dose-related and transient. Decreased accommodation and diplopia from increased phorias have been reported. Transient allergic conjunctivitis with benzodiazepine use has also been seen.

Antidepressants

Psychotherapy, either alone or in combination with antidepressant medication, is the first line of intervention in mild to moderate depression. In patients with major depression, antidepressants can improve symptoms, increase the chances and rate of recovery, reduce the likelihood of suicide, and help social and occupational rehabilitation.

In general, antidepressants take 3–6 weeks to show significant effect. A summary of studies concluded that antidepressants are associated with a 50%–60% response rate among patients with major depression in the primary care setting. These drugs can result in mood elevation, improved appetite, better sleep, and increased mental and physical activity. Treatment is usually necessary for 3–6 months after recovery is apparent.

Table 12-4 Pharmacology of Antidepressants

Tricyclics and tetracyclics
  Amitriptyline (Elavil)
  Amoxapine (Asendin)
  Clomipramine (Anafranil)
  Desipramine (Norpramin)
  Doxepin (Adapin, Sinequan)
  Imipramine (Tofranil)
  Maprotiline (Ludiomil)
  Nortriptyline (Pamelor)
  Protriptyline (Vivactil)
  Trimipramine (Surmontil)
Selective serotonin reuptake inhibitors
  Citalopram (Celexa)
  Escitalopram (Lexapro)
  Fluoxetine (Prozac)
  Fluvoxamine (Luvox)
  Paroxetine (Paxil)
  Paroxetine CR (Paxil CR)
  Sertraline (Zoloft)
Dopamine-norepinephrine reuptake inhibitors
  Bupropion (Wellbutrin)
  Bupropion SR (Wellbutrin SR)
  Bupropion XL (Wellbutrin XL)
Serotonin-norepinephrine reuptake inhibitors
  Venlafaxine (Effexor)
  Venlafaxine XR (Effexor XR)
  Duloxetine (Cymbalta)
Serotonin modulators
  Nefazodone (Serzone)
  Trazodone (Desyrel)
Noradrenergic and specific serotonergic antidepressant
  Mirtazapine (Remeron)
Monoamine oxidase inhibitors
  Phenelzine (Nardil)
  Tranylcypromine (Parnate)

Modified from Paulsen RH, Katon W, Ciechanowski P. Treatment of depression. In: *UpToDate*, Rose BD (Ed), Waltham, MA. Available at http://www.uptodate.com. Accessed March 1, 2005.

Table 12-4 shows the various classes of antidepressants. The selective serotonin reuptake inhibitors (SSRIs) were developed in response to research that implicated specific monoamines such as serotonin in the etiology of depression. They are the most commonly prescribed agents, although a meta-analysis suggested that they are no more efficacious than older tricyclic or heterocyclic antidepressants. The most compelling reason for using SSRIs, however, is lower severity of side effects due to their more targeted mechanism of action. SSRIs are also less dangerous than other antidepressants if an overdose occurs. Common adverse effects that can occur with use of the SSRIs include restlessness, insomnia, headache, gastrointestinal symptoms, mild sedation, and sexual dysfunction. SSRIs may cause inhibition of platelet function that can increase the risk of GI bleeding and possibly increase the risk for transfusions with major surgery. It is not known if this effect is clinically significant in ophthalmic surgery.

The SSRIs can also cause nonspecific visual symptoms such as blurred vision in 2%–10% of patients. In addition, patients may complain of "tracking" difficulties; this is more common in younger patients than in older persons and tends to occur upon withdrawal of the drug. The SSRIs can also cause mydriasis, and rare cases of angle-closure glaucoma have been reported with use of these drugs, most commonly with paroxetine (Paxil), which tends to have a stronger anticholinergic effect.

Recently, there has been a concern that the SSRIs may initially increase the risk of suicide in some patients, especially in adolescents and children, although the data are controversial. Careful monitoring of patients is recommended when treatment is initiated. Abrupt cessation of SSRIs may result in a "discontinuation syndrome," characterized by dizziness, nausea, fatigue, muscle aches, chills, anxiety, and irritability. This syndrome may be problematic, but it is much more benign than the severe side effects that can occur if heterocyclic or monoamine oxidase inhibitor drugs are abruptly discontinued.

The other major class of antidepressants is the *heterocyclics,* of which the tricyclic antidepressants were the first described. These drugs tend to have more pronounced side effects than the SSRIs, including anticholinergic symptoms such as dry eye and mouth, accommodative changes, constipation, urinary retention, tachycardia, and confusion or delirium. Sedation, weight gain, and orthostatic hypotension may also occur. Most concerning is the toxicity of these medications in overdose. In contrast to the SSRIs, the cyclic antidepressants can be fatal in doses as little as 5 times the therapeutic dose. Mortality is usually due to arrhythmias, although anticholinergic toxicity and seizures can also occur. Sudden cessation may cause pronounced changes in affect, cognition, and cardiac dysrhythmias.

The *monoamine oxidase (MAO) inhibitors* have long been considered second-line drugs in the treatment of mood disorders; however, it has been recognized that they can be useful in the treatment of refractory and atypical depression. The significant risk of hypertensive crisis caused by interactions between MAO inhibitors and various foods and drugs must be accounted for when they are prescribed. When combined with food and beverages of high tyramine content, these drugs may produce severe hypertension that can lead to subarachnoid or cerebral hemorrhage. Foods to be avoided include cheese, herring, chicken liver, yeast, and yogurt. Red wine and beer also have high tyramine content. Because MAO inhibitors prevent catabolism of catecholamines, patients taking these substances have exaggerated hypertensive responses to drugs containing vasopressors, such as cold remedies, nasal decongestants, and even topical or retrobulbar epinephrine.

There are other agents that have variable effects on other neurotransmitters and do not fall into specific categories. These include bupropion (Wellbutrin), venlafaxine (Effexor), duloxetine (Cymbalta), trazodone (Desyrel), and nefazodone (Serzone). The side effect profile for each of these drugs, as well as the SSRIs and heterocyclics, is slightly different from that of the others, thus allowing the selection of an agent that seems to best fit a given patient's constellation of symptoms.

Mood stabilizers

This is a heterogeneous group of medications that do not clearly share a common mechanism of action. These are the drugs of choice for treatment of mania, bipolar disorder, schizoaffective disorder, and cyclothymia. They may also be used for impulse control disorders, symptoms associated with mental retardation, and aggressive behavior. This class consists essentially of lithium carbonate (Eskalith, Lithonate) and various antiepileptic medications. Valproic acid (Depakote) and carbamazepine (Tegretol) are the most commonly used antiepileptic drugs, but many others have been studied and prescribed. The antiepileptic medications are discussed in the section on epilepsy later in this chapter.

Lithium carbonate is effective in the treatment of bipolar disorder and in some patients with recurrent unipolar depression. It has a very narrow therapeutic ratio, making close monitoring of plasma levels mandatory. Adverse effects include renal, thyroid, parathyroid, cardiac, and neurologic toxicity. Weight gain and gastrointestinal upset are common. Toxic plasma levels due to renal dysfunction, concurrent use of diuretics, or overdose can lead to persistent nausea and vomiting, coma, circulatory failure, and death. Ocular side effects include blurred vision, ocular irritation due to secretion in tears, nystagmus (usually downbeating), and exophthalmos that is often associated with lithium-induced changes in thyroid function.

Ophthalmologic Considerations

Although behavioral disorders do not directly affect the eye, a number of related issues are important to the ophthalmologist. For example, awareness of the potential ocular side effects of the various psychiatric medications is important. Patient education and reassurance may be required because the underlying psychopathology may make anticholinergic ophthalmic side effects such as dry eye and accommodative changes much more frightening and less tolerable for patients with behavioral disorders than for those without such disorders. Noncompliance is another common problem among patients with psychiatric illness, dementia, and depression. Malingering and functional visual loss require a high index of suspicion and special diagnostic skills on the part of the clinician. Some medications used to treat eye disease, including carbonic anhydrase inhibitors, oral corticosteroids, and possibly beta-blockers, may induce or exacerbate depression.

> Costagliola C, Parmeggiani F, Sebastiani A. SSRIs and intraocular pressure modifications: evidence, therapeutic implications and possible mechanisms. *CNS Drugs.* 2004;18(8):475–484.
> Fraunfelder FT, Fraunfelder FW. *Drug-Induced Ocular Side Effects.* 5th ed. Boston: Butterworth-Heinemann; 2001.
> Hahn RK. *Current Clinical Strategies: Psychiatry.* Laguna Hills, CA: Current Clinical Strategies Publishing; 2003.
> Moore DP, Jefferson JW. *Handbook of Medical Psychiatry.* 2nd ed. Philadelphia: Elsevier/Mosby; 2004.
> National Institute on Drug Abuse Web site. Available at http://www.drugabuse.gov. Accessed March 1, 2005.

Neurologic Disorders

Parkinson Disease

Parkinson disease belongs to a group of conditions known as *bradykinetic movement disorders*. These disorders are usually associated with rigidity, postural instability, and loss of automatic associated movements. Parkinson disease strikes men and women in almost equal numbers, usually affecting people older than age 50. The average age of onset is 60 years. In recent years, however, the number of reported cases of "early-onset" Parkinson disease has increased; it is estimated that 5%–10% of patients are now younger than age 40, and there is also a juvenile form that presents before age 20.

Etiology

The basal ganglia are a complex of deep nuclei that consist of the corpus striatum, globus pallidus, and substantia nigra. These structures regulate the initiation and control of movement. Parkinson disease occurs when neurons in the substantia nigra die or become impaired. Normally, these neurons produce dopamine, a neurotransmitter responsible for transmitting signals between the substantia nigra and the corpus striatum to produce smooth, purposeful muscle activity. Loss of dopamine causes the nerve cells of the striatum to fire out of control, leaving patients unable to direct or control their movements normally. Patients with Parkinson disease have lost 80% or more of dopamine-producing cells in the substantia nigra. An associated pathologic finding is the presence of eosinophilic cytoplasmic inclusion bodies in the substantia nigra that are known as *Lewy bodies*.

The cause of this cell impairment and death is not known. One theory suggests that Parkinson disease may occur when either an external or an internal toxin selectively destroys dopaminergic neurons. For instance, methylphenyltetrahydropyridine is a specific toxin that can produce Parkinson disease in humans and animals. Another theory focuses on the possibility that the normal protein degradation pathways in the substantia nigra may be impaired in Parkinson patients, leading to abnormal protein aggregation. Normal and abnormal proteins then accumulate and form Lewy bodies, which in turn lead to neurodegeneration. Free radicals and increased oxidative stress also seem to play a role. The metabolic pathways for dopamine generate numerous by-products that include hydrogen peroxide, superoxide anions, and hydroxy-radicals. Interaction between these chemicals and membrane lipids leads to lipid peroxidation, membrane disruption, and even cell death.

Genetic factors are also implicated. In 15%–20% of patients, a close relative has experienced parkinsonian symptoms. At least 5 possible causative genes have been identified, and the number of Parkinson-like disorders associated with specific genetic defects is growing. Many of these defects appear to be involved in cellular protein metabolism. Overall, Parkinson disease seems to have a multifactorial etiology that includes genetic predisposition, environmental factors, and age-related changes in neuron metabolism. Interestingly, there are reports suggesting that the frequency of Parkinson disease is actually decreased in patients with a history of cigarette smoking and caffeine consumption.

Symptoms

Usually the first symptom of Parkinson disease is tremor of a limb, especially at rest. The tremor often begins on 1 side of the body, frequently in the hand. Other common symptoms include bradykinesia, rigidity, a shuffling gait, and stooped posture. People with Parkinson disease often show reduced facial expression and speak in a soft voice. The disease can also cause depression, personality changes, sexual difficulties, hallucinations, loss of olfactory functioning, and dementia.

Treatment

There is currently no cure for Parkinson disease. The main treatment is levodopa (L-dopa), and treatment is generally initiated when symptoms begin to become significant. Neurons use L-dopa to make dopamine and replace the brain's diminishing supply.

Dopamine itself cannot be given because it does not cross the blood–brain barrier. Although levodopa helps at least three fourths of Parkinson cases, not all symptoms respond equally to the drug. Bradykinesia and rigidity respond best; tremor may be only marginally reduced. Problems with balance and other symptoms may not be alleviated at all. Usually, patients are given levodopa combined with carbidopa (Lodosyn), often as a combined pill (Sinemet). When added to levodopa, carbidopa delays the conversion of levodopa into dopamine until it reaches the brain, diminishing some of the side effects that often accompany levodopa therapy.

After years of therapy, patients can become acutely aware of a "wearing off" effect that occurs about 4 hours after a dose of levodopa, when their symptoms return. Alterations in dosing or absorption do not seem to help, although more frequent dosing may decrease symptoms initially. Catechol O-methyltransferase inhibitors such as entacapone (Comtan) provide a new method of extending the duration of L-dopa effect and reducing the "off" time by inhibiting the methylation of L-dopa and dopamine. Long-term levodopa use can also be associated with drug-related dyskinesias and dystonias that may require changes in dosing and additional medications. In addition, there is ongoing controversy about whether long-term use of levodopa may actually increase the rate of progression of Parkinson disease. A trial is under way to address this issue, but for now levodopa remains the mainstay of treatment.

Bromocriptine (Parlodel), pergolide (Permax), pramipexole (Mirapex), and ropinirole (Requip) are 4 drugs that stimulate dopamine receptors in the brain. These drugs can be given alone or in combination with levodopa. They are generally less effective than levodopa in controlling rigidity and bradykinesia, but they may have a neuroprotective effect that may delay the need for levodopa. Trials are under way to evaluate this possibility. Selegiline (Eldepryl) inhibits the activity of the enzyme monoamine oxidase B, which metabolizes dopamine in the brain. Selegiline may delay the need for levodopa or, when given in combination with levodopa, may enhance and prolong the response of levodopa, although the beneficial effect of this drug appears to be mild and short-lived.

Anticholinergic drugs such as trihexyphenidyl (Artane) and benztropine (Cogentin) were the main treatment for Parkinson disease before the introduction of levodopa. Although their benefit is limited and their effect is usually short-lived, anticholinergics may help control tremor and rigidity. Only about half of patients respond to anticholinergics, and the typical anticholinergic side effects can be problematic.

Amantadine (Symmetrel), an antiviral drug, is often used in the early stages of the disease either alone or in combination with anticholinergics or levodopa. After several months, the effectiveness of amantadine wears off in a third to a half of patients taking the drug.

Modern surgical treatments consist primarily of pallidotomy and deep brain stimulation. The dopamine deficiency in Parkinson disease results in excitation of the globus pallidus, which in turn inhibits thalamic activity. Both surgical techniques serve to suppress this excessive globus pallidus activity. Pallidotomy carries the risk of complications such as stroke and hemorrhage, as well as the risk of irreversible side effects. Deep brain stimulation is safer than pallidotomy initially but requires intensive adjustments and lifelong maintenance, with the risk of hardware complications and infection. Trials are under way to define the role for these therapies.

Experimental transplantation of embryonic dopamine neurons has been attempted with little or no success. A potential complication is "runaway dyskinesia," possibly due to excessive dopaminergic stimulation. Direct brain infusion of glial cell line–derived neurotrophic factor is another approach that is under investigation and may have some utility.

Ophthalmic considerations

There are numerous ophthalmologic findings in patients with Parkinson disease. These findings can be divided into eyelid disorders and ocular motor abnormalities.

Eyelid disorders include seborrheic dermatitis and blepharitis, apraxia of eyelid opening, lid retraction, decreased blinking (with secondary dry eye), and blepharospasm. Ocular motor abnormalities include convergence insufficiency, limitation of upgaze, hypometric saccades, saccadic ("cogwheel") pursuit, square wave jerks, and oculogyric crisis. Trouble with reading is a common initial complaint, and the ocular surface abnormalities and motor abnormalities may synergize with other ophthalmic and neurologic problems to increase visual difficulties.

Drug-related side effects may also be superimposed, especially for patients on anticholinergic medications, which may exacerbate dry eyes and cause accommodative changes or precipitate angle-closure glaucoma. Visual hallucinations may occur as a result of both the disease and its treatment; this adverse effect has been reported in particular with use of levodopa and anticholinergic agents. Amantadine has been reported to cause corneal infiltrates and edema, though these complications are rare.

Multiple Sclerosis

See BCSC Section 5, *Neuro-Ophthalmology*.

Epilepsy

Epileptic seizures result from synchronized electrical activity of neuronal networks in the cerebral cortex. Epilepsy is characterized by recurrent epileptic seizures due to a genetically determined or acquired brain disorder. More than 2 million people in the United States—

approximately 1 in 100—have experienced an unprovoked seizure or been diagnosed with epilepsy. Patients with relatively controlled epilepsy may still have problems with depression, driving, employment, and insurance. In 1 survey, 31% of respondents with 1 seizure or fewer per year reported that epilepsy had a great impact on their lives; more than 40% of college-educated people with "well-controlled" seizures were unemployed.

Etiology

Epilepsy is a disorder with many possible causes. Any disturbance of normal neuronal activity, including injury, infection, and abnormal brain development, can lead to seizures. Approximately half of all seizures have no known cause. Seizures may develop because of an abnormality in brain wiring, an imbalance of neurotransmitters, or some combination of these factors.

Epilepsy can result from brain damage that can be caused by numerous disorders. Head injury, prenatal injury, developmental problems, and exposure to lead, carbon monoxide, and other poisons have all been associated with seizures. Brain tumors, alcoholism, and Alzheimer disease frequently lead to epilepsy. Strokes and myocardial infarctions that produce cerebral ischemia may account for as much as 32% of all newly developed epilepsy in elderly persons. Meningitis, AIDS, viral encephalitis, and other infectious diseases can lead to epilepsy. Epilepsy can also be part of a set of symptoms in a variety of developmental and metabolic disorders, including cerebral palsy, neurofibromatosis, tuberous sclerosis, and autism.

Certain types of epilepsy have been shown to be caused by mutations in specific genes. It is likely that genetics plays a more indirect role for many patients, perhaps by increasing a person's susceptibility to seizures that are triggered by an environmental factor or by having subtle effects on neuronal development or physiology that predispose to seizure activity.

Epileptic seizures are distinguished from *nonepileptic seizures (NES)*, which are sudden changes in behavior that resemble epileptic seizures but are not associated with the typical neurophysiological changes characterizing epileptic seizures. Nonepileptic seizures are often caused by medical problems such as hypoglycemia, electrolyte abnormalities, and cerebral anoxia; treatment of the underlying problem controls the seizure activity.

More than 30 types of seizures have been described. Typically, seizures are divided into 2 major categories: *partial seizures* and *generalized seizures.* Partial seizures occur in just 1 part of the brain, and are further divided into simple (without impairment of consciousness) and complex (with impairment of consciousness). Symptoms of simple partial seizures (also called *auras*) will depend on the part of the brain that they originate from and include motor symptoms, sensory symptoms, or even autonomic symptoms. Complex partial seizures (previously called *temporal lobe seizures* or *psychomotor seizures*) are the most common type of seizure in epileptic adults. During the seizure, patients appear to be awake but do not interact with others in their environment and do not respond normally to instructions or questions. They often stare into space and either remain motionless or engage in repetitive behaviors, called *automatisms,* such as facial grimacing or gesturing.

Generalized seizures, of which there are 6 main types, almost always produce impaired consciousness and demonstrate abnormal activity in both hemispheres at the onset of the seizure. They may be nonconvulsive (absence, or "petit mal") or convulsive (tonic-clonic or variations of tonic-clonic). Absence seizures almost always begin in childhood or adolescence and are frequently familial, suggesting a genetic cause. Some patients may make purposeless movements during their seizures, such as jerking an arm or rapidly blinking their eyes. Others have no noticeable symptoms except for brief periods when they are "out of it." Childhood absence epilepsy usually stops when the child reaches puberty. A generalized tonic-clonic ("grand mal") seizure is the most dramatic type of seizure. It begins with an abrupt loss of consciousness, often in association with a scream or shriek. All of the muscles then become stiff and the patient may become cyanotic during the tonic phase. After approximately 1 minute, the muscles begin to jerk and twitch for an additional 1 to 2 minutes, and then the patient remains in a deep sleep.

The end of a seizure is referred to as the *postictal period* and signifies the recovery period for the brain. This period may last several seconds up to a few days, depending on factors such as the severity of the seizure and the patient's age. Postictal paresis (Todd's paralysis) is a transient focal motor deficit that lasts for hours or, rarely, days after an epileptic convulsion and is thought to be related either to neuronal exhaustion (from electrical overactivity during the seizure) or to active inhibition.

Diagnosis

The EEG is the most common diagnostic test for epilepsy. In most patients with epilepsy, the EEG appears abnormal, although provocative testing (such as sleep deprivation) may need to be done to demonstrate the abnormality. A normal EEG does not rule out epilepsy, however. Computed tomography and magnetic resonance imaging (MRI) are useful tools to determine structural abnormalities in the brain that cause epilepsy. More sophisticated modalities are being developed that allow imaging of abnormal physiology in addition to anatomy. *Magnetoencephalography (MEG)* detects magnetic fields associated with the intracellular current flow within neurons and can detect signals from deeper in the brain than an EEG can. *Magnetic source imaging (MSI)* is an advanced technique that combines MEG and MRI to measure the magnetic field generated by a series of neurons. Magnetic source imaging is particularly useful for the investigation of patients who may be candidates for epilepsy surgery. Positron emission tomography (PET) and single-photon emission computed tomography (SPECT) are related functional imaging techniques that are also used to locate seizure foci.

Treatment

Currently available treatments control seizure activity at least some of the time in 80% of patients with epilepsy. Twenty percent experience intractable seizures or obtain inadequate relief from available treatment. The primary form of treatment for epilepsy is the use of antiepileptic drugs, and the choice of drug is determined by the type of epilepsy. In recent years, a number of new drugs have become available (Table 12-5). The drug dose is titrated up until the disease is controlled or toxic side effects occur; a second agent may be added if necessary, but monotherapy is preferred, if possible, to minimize side effects.

Table 12-5 Mechanisms of Action of Antiepileptic Drugs

Drug	Mechanism of Action
Carbamazepine (Tegretol, Tegretol-XR, Carbatrol)	Blocks voltage-dependent sodium channels
Ethosuximide (Zarontin)	Modifies low-threshold T-type calcium currents
Felbamate (Felbatol)	Blocks NMDA receptor; potentiates GABA-mediated inhibition
Gabapentin (Neurontin)	Exact mechanism unknown; GABA analog
Lamotrigine (Lamictal)	Blocks voltage-dependent sodium channels
Levetiracetam (Keppra)	Exact mechanism unknown
Oxcarbazepine (Trileptal)	Blocks voltage-dependent sodium channels
Phenobarbital, mysoline, benzodiazepines	Accentuate GABA-mediated chloride channel openings
Phenytoin (Dilantin)	Blocks voltage-dependent sodium channels
Fosphenytoin (Cerebyx)	Water soluble prodrug of phenytoin
Tiagabine (Gabitril)	Inhibits GABA uptake in neurons and glia
Topiramate (Topamax)	Blocks voltage-dependent sodium channels; inhibits kainate/AMPA receptor; enhances GABA-mediated inhibition at GABA (A) receptors
Valproate (Depakene capsules and syrup, Depakote sprinkle capsules, Depakote delayed-release tablets, Depakote ER, Depacon)	Blocks voltage-dependent sodium channels; enhances postsynaptic GABA-mediated inhibition
Zonisamide (Zonegran)	Blocks voltage-dependent sodium and T-type calcium channels

Reprinted with permission from Schachter SC. Pharmacology of antiepileptic drugs. In: *UpToDate*, Rose BD (Ed), Waltham, MA. Available at http://www.uptodate.com. Accessed March 1, 2005.

There are 2 main categories of side effects for the antiepilepsy drugs: systemic and neurotoxic. Systemic side effects generally include variable problems such as nausea, rash, and anorexia. Neurotoxic effects include somnolence, dizziness, and confusion. The neurotoxic effects seem to be an inevitable consequence of the mechanism of action of these drugs and often become the dose-limiting factor.

When medications inadequately control seizures, surgery is a potential option. The most commonly performed surgery for epilepsy is the removal of a seizure focus. This procedure, called *lobectomy* or *lesionectomy*, is appropriate for partial seizures that originate in a single area of the brain. Temporal lobe resection is the most commonly performed type of lobectomy and is successful in 70%–90% of patients. Other surgical procedures for epilepsy include multiple subpial transection, corpus callosotomy, and hemispherectomy. In patients with seizures poorly controlled by medications or surgery, vagus nerve stimulation may be used. The vagal nerve stimulator is a battery-powered device that is surgically implanted under the skin of the chest and is attached to the vagus nerve in the lower neck. The device delivers short bursts of electrical energy to the brain via the vagus nerve. On average, the device reduces seizures by 20%–40%.

Ophthalmic considerations

Transient unilateral mydriasis can occur as an expression of minor or major seizure activity, during or after the event. This phenomenon is most common in children. In some patients, the dilated pupil reacts poorly to light. In children, the eyes may deviate to the side of the dilated pupil. Horizontal or vertical gaze deviations are commonly associated with seizure activity. The gaze tends to be directed away from the side of the cortical lesion during a seizure and then toward the side of the lesion after the seizure. Some patients experience conjugate, convergent, or monocular nystagmus during the clonic stage of a seizure. Clonic lid retraction has also been described in patients with petit mal or myoclonic seizures.

Certain antiepileptic drugs have the potential for characteristic ocular side effects. Phenytoin (Dilantin) can cause dose-related nystagmus, and maternal use of this medication can cause the fetal hydantoin syndrome (which includes hypertelorism, epicanthal folds, glaucoma, optic nerve hypoplasia, and retinal colobomas). Topiramate (Topamax) has been associated with acute angle-closure glaucoma, anterior chamber shallowing, acute myopia, and choroidal effusions, usually within the first 2 weeks of therapy. These effects may be an idiopathic response related to the presence of sulfa in topiramate. Treatment of the glaucoma includes cessation of the drug and use of cycloplegics and topical hypotensives.

Vigabatrin (Sabril) is licensed in Canada and in many countries of Europe and Asia but is not available in the United States. As many as 30%–50% of patients with long-term exposure to vigabatrin have developed irreversible concentric visual field loss of varying severity that is often asymptomatic. Visual field testing should be performed before starting therapy and repeated every 6 months.

Stroke

See Chapter 3, Cerebrovascular Disease.

Pain Syndromes

See BCSC Section 5, *Neuro-Ophthalmology*.

Alzheimer Disease and Dementia

Dementia is a disorder characterized by a general decrease in the level of cognition and memory and usually includes behavioral disturbances and inability to remain independent. Dementia is not a specific disease. Although it is common in very elderly persons, dementia is not a normal part of the aging process. Dementia also differs from delirium. Delirium, or an acute confusional state, is an acute or subacute onset of disorientation with alterations in levels of awareness. The major difference between dementia and delirium is that demented patients are alert and without the disturbance of consciousness characteristic of delirious patients.

Alzheimer disease is the most common cause of dementia in people older than age 65, but there are a number of other causes of dementia. Other major dementia syndromes include vascular dementia (previously known as *multi-infarct dementia*), Lewy body dementia, and Parkinson disease with dementia. Most elderly patients with chronic dementia have Alzheimer disease (approximately 60%–80%). The vascular dementias account for 10%–20%; dementia associated with Parkinson disease about 5%. Dementia can be associated with trauma (eg, dementia pugilistica, or boxer's syndrome) and with infections such as neurosyphilis and AIDS. Metabolic problems such as diabetes mellitus, electrolyte disturbances, and hypothyroidism can cause dementia. Nutritional causes include thiamine deficiency (Wernicke-Korsakoff syndrome) or vitamin B_{12} deficiency, and toxic dementia can occur, for instance, with heavy metal exposure or chronic alcoholism. Other causes include drug use, depression, subdural hematomas, and normal pressure hydrocephalus. A crucial part of the evaluation of a patient with dementia is looking for any potentially treatable factors that may help reverse the problem.

Vascular dementia is associated with findings on neurologic examination consistent with prior strokes, and patients will often have evidence of multiple infarcts on cerebral imaging. Patients may have abrupt onset of symptoms followed by stepwise deterioration, unlike the gradual progression that occurs with neurodegenerative conditions such as Parkinson disease. Vascular dementia may also present subsequent to a stroke (poststroke dementia). The incidence of vascular dementia is relatively high in blacks, hypertensive persons, and patients with diabetes or dyslipidemias. Other causes of vascular dementia include vasculitis, profound hypotension, and lesions caused by cerebral hemorrhages. The term *mixed dementia* refers to patients who have a combination of vascular dementia and Alzheimer disease.

Lewy body dementia (LBD) is the second most common form of neurodegenerative dementia after Alzheimer disease. Lewy body dementia is characterized neuropathologically by the presence of Lewy bodies in the brain stem and cortex (Lewy bodies are intracytoplasmic inclusions that are also seen in the substantia nigra in Parkinson disease). There may be considerable clinical and neuropathologic overlap between LBD, Parkinson disease, and Alzheimer disease, and the clinical distinction between these entities may be difficult at times. Ophthalmologists should be aware of LBD, however, because patients with this syndrome often present with complex formed visual hallucinations. With treatment, patients who have LBD can have marked improvements in cognition and behavioral symptoms, as well as fewer hallucinations. Referral to a neurologist or geriatric psychiatrist is warranted if the disease is suspected.

Alzheimer disease (AD) is an irreversible, progressive disorder that proceeds in stages, gradually destroying memory, reason, judgment, language, and eventually the ability to carry out even the simplest of tasks. Alzheimer disease is the most common neurodegenerative disorder, affecting an estimated 4 million people in the United States. One recent study found that AD was present in 47.2% of people age 85 and older.

The emotional and financial burden of this disease on individuals and their families and the impact on society are difficult to measure, but currently, AD is estimated to cost the nation $80–$90 billion a year. Caring for a person with AD is estimated to cost $47,000 per year, whether the patient lives at home or is in a nursing home. It is clear that as life expectancy increases and the United States experiences the demographic impact of the baby boom generation, AD will have an even greater effect on society in coming years.

The pathological hallmarks of the disease are extraneuronal amyloid plaques (fragmented brain cells surrounded by amyloid-family proteins) and intraneuronal neurofibrillary tangles (tangles of filaments largely composed of protein associated with the cytoskeleton). These 2 findings are associated with neuronal death and decreased levels of the neurotransmitter acetylcholine, as well as abnormalities in other neurotransmitter systems. Signs of neuronal death first appear in the entorhinal cortex, with eventual extension into the hippocampus (an area essential for memory storage). As the disease progresses, the basal forebrain and eventually the cerebral cortex become involved.

Amyloid plaques and neurofibrillary tangles

Amyloid precursor protein (APP) appears to play a role in normal membrane growth and survival and protrudes through the neuronal membrane, with extensions inside and outside the cell. This protein is continually replaced by new APP molecules manufactured in the cell. Amyloid precursor protein is cleaved by enzymes known as secretases, with 1 such cleavage product being the highly amyloidogenic protein A-beta-42, which subsequently aggregates into plaques. Once plaque has formed, secondary cascades of inflammation, neuronal overactivity, and likely apoptosis (programmed cell death) result in progressive damage.

The other pathologic hallmark of AD is the presence of *neurofibrillary tangles (NFT)*. The tangles consist of a hyperphosphorylated form of the microtubule-associated protein, tau. Tau proteins are best known for their ability to bind and help stabilize microtubules, which are like long, parallel railroad tracks that carry nutrients from the body of the cells down to the ends of the axons. In AD, tau is changed chemically, altering its ability to hold microtubules together and causing them to twist into paired helical filaments, like 2 threads wound around each other. This collapse of the transport system may first result in malfunction in communication between nerve cells and may later lead to neuronal death. Formation of NFT seems to be secondary to amyloid deposition rather than vice versa.

The degree of cognitive decline in AD seems to correlate more closely with the NFT burden than with the amount of amyloid deposition. If the mechanism linking amyloid formation and NFT development can be identified, a significant breakthrough in terms of therapy might be possible. For instance, amyloid accumulation seems to activate a class of enzymes known as *caspases,* which in turn result in cleavage of tau proteins and then production of NFTs. It may be possible to control disease activity by interfering with APP cleavage to A-beta-42 and with tau cleavage by caspase.

Etiology

The exact etiology of AD is unknown, but both genetic and environmental factors play a role.

Genetic factors There are 2 types of AD: *familial AD,* which follows a certain inheritance pattern, and *sporadic AD,* in which no inheritance pattern is obvious. Alzheimer disease is further described as *early onset* (occurring in people younger than age 65) and *late onset* (occurring in those older than age 65). Early-onset AD is rare (10% of cases) and generally affects persons between 30 and 60 years of age. Some forms of early-onset AD are inherited and typically progress faster than the more common late-onset forms.

All known familial AD cases have been of early onset, and to date these hereditary forms of AD have mutations that accelerate the production of A-beta-42. This acceleration occurs either by abnormal APP-production or by excessive processing via mutations in the secretase enzymes. For instance, the *APP* gene is on chromosome 21, and patients with Down syndrome have trisomy of chromosome 21 and an excess of APP. As they grow older, such patients usually develop plaques and tangles like those found in AD. There is no evidence that any of these specific familial mutations play a role in the most common sporadic, or nonfamilial, form of late-onset AD.

Nevertheless, there does appear to be a genetic component in the more common form of late-onset AD. Patients who have a first-degree relative with dementia have a 10%–30% increased risk of developing the disorder. A possible marker for the development of AD is the presence of the epsilon 4 genotype of the protein apolipoprotein E. The apolipoprotein E protein has many functions, including participation in the transport of cholesterol throughout the body. There are 3 alleles of the gene: epsilon 2, epsilon 3, and epsilon 4. People who inherit two epsilon 4 genes are 8 times more likely to develop AD than those who inherit two of epsilon 3, the most common version. The least common allele, epsilon 2, seems to actually lower the risk for AD.

Nongenetic factors Numerous factors have been implicated as playing a role in contributing to the cascade of events that produce AD. Oxidative stress from free radicals may damage cells. Unique characteristics of the brain, including its high rate of metabolism and the long life span of its nondividing cells, may make it particularly vulnerable to oxidative stress. Inflammation is another important mechanism that is under intense investigation as a possible cause of AD. Inflammation in the brain increases with age but is more pronounced in patients with AD. Yet another area of interest involves cerebrovascular disease, including small infarcts in specific regions of the brain that accelerate the findings of AD.

Diagnosis
There is no definitive antemortem diagnostic test for AD other than a brain biopsy. Physicians rely on a variety of methods including history, physical examination, laboratory tests, brain scans, and assessments of memory, language skills, and other brain functions. Cerebrospinal fluid levels of tau and amyloid protein are under investigation as possible diagnostic markers. A few years ago, some investigators suggested that patients with AD had a more pronounced pupil dilation response to dilute tropicamide, presumably reflecting a generalized cholinergic deficit. Subsequent studies indicated that this was not useful as a diagnostic test, and it is no longer used.

Several imaging techniques are useful, and all may have specific utility in aiding the diagnosis of AD or at least eliminating other causes of dementia. Positron emission tomography detects changes in glucose metabolism in the parts of the brain most affected by AD. Single-photon emission computed tomography can be combined with genetic and psychological testing to predict which patients with memory loss will eventually develop AD. Magnetic resonance imaging can be particularly useful in measuring atrophy in the hippocampus, a sign of early AD in patients who demonstrate problems with memory. The precise clinical usefulness of these studies is not yet well defined; as better preventive therapies are developed, early recognition of disease will be more valuable.

Treatment
Given the tremendous toll the disease takes on the patient, caregivers, and society, there is great interest in identifying factors that may prevent onset of the disease. Some

epidemiologic studies suggested that NSAIDs may be useful in the prevention of AD. However, more recent studies indicate that there appears to be no significant benefit with these drugs and that they appear to put patients at increased risk for other problems, such as cardiovascular events. Until there is stronger clinical trial evidence of benefit, these drugs have no role in dementia prevention or treatment. The lipid-lowering HMG-CoA reductase inhibitors (statins) may also decrease the risk of developing AD, but definitive studies are pending. Other proposed interventions include exercise, cognitive activity, high n-3 fatty acid intake, consumption of vitamin E–rich foods, use of ginkgo biloba, and moderate alcohol intake, but none of these have been proven in a prospective trial.

Once the disease is diagnosed, the first steps involve addressing psychosocial issues. Patients and family members will need to deal with matters such as driving and cooking safety, emotional lability, wandering, and falls. There are a number of resources to assist with these issues, such as the Alzheimer's Association (http://www.alz.org). Pharmacologic treatment includes use of the cholinesterase inhibitors donepezil (Aricept), rivastigmine (Exelon), and galantamine (Reminyl). These drugs cannot stop or reverse progression of the disease, but they can decrease the rate of progression for some patients for a few months up to 2 years. They do not seem to alter significant endpoints, such as admission to a nursing home or progression to advanced dementia. Memantine (Namenda) is an N-methyl-D-aspartate (NMDA) receptor antagonist that has a neuroprotective effect and that appears to be effective in treating more advanced AD, although further studies are required to better define its role in treatment. High doses of memantine may also have a role in slowing progression. Use of antidepressants and antipsychotics may be necessary to treat specific behavioral symptoms.

Immunization with amyloid beta peptide has been attempted because it has been shown to reduce the amyloid plaque burden. However, phase 1 testing was suspended because in some of the human subjects there was brain inflammation that led to irreversible CNS damage. Interestingly, a follow-up report of patients without complications found that cognitive decline was significantly less in patients who had an increase in serum beta amyloid plaque–related antibodies. Perhaps other immunologic-based approaches will be safer and more successful. Efforts are also under way to develop drugs that modify secretase activity and thereby minimize plaque formation.

Ophthalmologic considerations
Patients with AD may present to the ophthalmologist with vague visual complaints such as poor vision and reading difficulties. In general, AD does not seem to have any direct pathologic effect on the optic nerve and retina, and these visual problems are caused by disruption of central pathways. Specific findings include spatial contrast sensitivity disturbance, fixation instability, saccadic latency prolongation with hypometric saccades, and saccadic intrusions during smooth-pursuit eye movements. Patients with AD can also manifest disorders of higher cortical function, such as visual agnosia and surface dyslexia. Defective motion perception (cerebral akinetopsia) has been described, as has Balint syndrome (simultanagnosia [an inability to recognize 2 or more things at the same time], acquired ocular apraxia, and optic ataxia).

Goetz CG, ed. *Textbook of Clinical Neurology*. 2nd ed. Philadelphia: WB Saunders; 2003.

Pelak VS, Hall DA. Neuro-ophthalmic manifestations of neurodegenerative disease. *Ophthalmol Clin North Am*. 2004;17(3):311–320.

UpToDate Web site. Available at http://www.uptodate.com.

The authors would like to thank Michael A. Keys, MD, and James Heckaman, MD, for their contributions to this chapter.

CHAPTER 13

Preventive Medicine

Recent Developments

- More than 95% of all cervical cancers are positive for human papillomavirus (HPV).
- Virtual colonoscopy with high-resolution computed tomography (CT) is currently being studied as a screening tool for colon cancer.
- Oseltamivir (Tamiflu) is effective for the treatment and prophylaxis of influenza types A and B.
- Diphtheria-tetanus-pertussis (DTP) vaccine has been replaced with the newer vaccine DTaP (diphtheria and tetanus toxoid with acellular pertussis vaccine).
- New childhood immunization recommendations now also include vaccines for hepatitis B, *Haemophilus influenzae* type B, *Pneumococcus, Varicella,* influenza, and hepatitis A.
- New vaccines are now available for meningococcus, Lyme disease, typhoid fever, anthrax, yellow fever, and Japanese encephalitis. Other new vaccines are being evaluated for HIV, cholera, respiratory syncytial virus, rabies, herpes simplex type 2, *Pseudomonas,* plague, rotavirus, malaria, tuberculosis, smallpox, and anthrax.

Screening Procedures

The goal of preventive medicine is not only the reduction of premature morbidity and mortality but also the preservation of function and quality of life.

Screening techniques can be used both for research and for practical disease prevention or treatment. Screening for nonresearch purposes is useful if the disease in question is

- detectable with some measurable degree of reliability
- treatable or preventable
- significant because of its impact (prevalence or severity)
- progressive
- generally asymptomatic (or has symptoms a patient might deny or might not recognize)

Screening techniques should not be applied to a certain population until the following concerns have been addressed:

- sensitivity and specificity of the test

- convenience and comfort of the test
- cost of finding a problem
- cost of not finding a problem

Cost can and should be measured in both economic and human terms, including the cost of suffering, losing function, or dying.

The term *sensitivity* describes how often a test result is positive among persons with a target disease. *Specificity* measures the test's ability to exclude truly negative results. *Relative risk* is the probability of a disease based on a specific finding divided by the probability of that disease in the absence of that specific finding.

Screening can be done as a 1-time venture or by the sequential application of screening tests. Initially, a more sensitive test is administered; when appropriate, it is followed by a more specific test (which is often more costly or difficult to use). In judging the predictive value of the screens for an individual patient, the physician should account for the patient's clinical history and current medications.

Cardiovascular Diseases

Hypertension

The consequences of uncontrolled hypertension include significantly increased risk of thrombotic and hemorrhagic stroke, atherosclerotic heart disease, atrial fibrillation, congestive heart failure, left ventricular hypertrophy, aortic aneurysm and dissection, peripheral vascular disease, and renal failure. Approximately 30% of end-stage renal disease is related to hypertension. There are more than 65 million cases of hypertension in the United States, about half of which have been diagnosed and a third of which are being treated in some way. Hypertension currently afflicts 1 billion people worldwide. The prevalence of hypertension in many developed countries is about 20% of the adult population, and it has reached as high as 28% in the United States. Hypertension in childhood is becoming a more widely recognized problem. Hypertension meets all 5 of the criteria mentioned previously for screening: it is detectable, treatable, highly prevalent, progressively damaging, and characteristically asymptomatic until late in its course.

Elevation in either systolic or diastolic blood pressure is associated with increased cardiovascular risk. *Hypertension* is defined as systolic blood pressure of 140 mm Hg or higher, diastolic blood pressure of 90 mm Hg or higher, or both. *Pre-hypertension* is defined as systolic blood pressure between 120 and 139 or diastolic blood pressure between 80 and 89 on multiple readings. The classification of hypertension is included in Chapter 2.

The primary screening method is blood pressure measurement, but several prospective studies have shown that ambulatory blood pressure monitoring provides a better prediction of major cardiovascular events. Abnormal measurements, unless urgently high, should be confirmed on 2 more occasions. Once hypertension is detected, the cause should be sought to allow appropriate treatment. Regular exercise, weight loss, and dietary modifications such as reduction of dietary salt intake and increased dietary potassium and folate intake may enhance blood pressure normalization. Chapter 2 discusses the pharmacologic treatment of hypertension.

Brown MJ, Haydock S. Pathoaetiology, epidemiology and diagnosis of hypertension. *Drugs.* 2000;59(suppl 2):1–12.

Krousel-Wood MA, Muntner P, He J, et al. Primary prevention of essential hypertension. *Med Clin North Am.* 2004;88:223–238.

Staessen JA, Wang J, Bianchi G, et al. Essential hypertension. *Lancet.* 2003;361:1629–1641.

Verdecchia P, Angeli F, Gattobigio R, et al. Ambulatory blood pressure monitoring and prognosis in the management of essential hypertension. *Expert Rev Cardiovasc Ther.* 2003;1:79–89.

Atherosclerotic cardiovascular disease

In the United States, atherosclerosis is responsible for approximately half of all deaths and for one third of deaths between ages 35 and 65. Three fourths of deaths related to atherosclerosis are from coronary artery disease (CAD). Atherosclerosis is the leading cause of permanent disability and accounts for more hospital days than any other illness.

The rationale for early screening emerged with the demonstration that reducing risk factors does reduce the incidence of coronary disease events. Epidemiologic studies demonstrate that each 1% of reduction in total cholesterol produces a 2% reduction in the risk of coronary disease events, including fatal and nonfatal myocardial infarctions. Several studies also confirm that reduction in cholesterol results in reduced cardiovascular morbidity and mortality in patients with previous coronary heart disease.

Established clinical risk factors for CAD include family history of early-onset coronary disease, increased age, male sex, hypertension, left ventricular hypertrophy, smoking, diabetes mellitus, physical inactivity, stress, and cocaine abuse. Laboratory risk factors are elevated plasma cholesterol level (also elevated low-density-lipoprotein [LDL] cholesterol and low high-density-lipoprotein [HDL] cholesterol levels), elevated plasma homocysteine level, and increased C-reactive protein. Patients in the top 20th percentile for risk factors experienced approximately 50% of the fatal and nonfatal atherosclerotic events. Counseling on smoking cessation, lifestyle modification, and diet should be an important element of all primary care and preventive care encounters.

Hypertriglyceridemia alone, without elevated cholesterol level, is not associated with a significant incidence of coronary disease; however, the combination of cholesterol and triglyceride elevation confers a greater risk of coronary disease than does cholesterol elevation alone.

Dyslipoproteinemia has become an important concept. We now recognize that excesses or deficiencies of specific lipoproteins and apolipoproteins are more significantly correlated with atherosclerosis than the more general category of lipids. Indeed, screening for cholesterol and triglycerides alone will miss 50% of cases of hyperlipoproteinemia. Therefore, it is valid and important to measure the LDL and HDL cholesterol every 5 years. Total, LDL, and HDL cholesterol screening is recommended for all persons aged 21 and older. If the level is normal (<200 mg/dL), the screen should be repeated every 5 years. If the level is abnormal, the screen should be repeated with a complete cholesterol profile. Hyperlipoproteinemias are discussed in greater detail in Chapter 5.

The presence of xanthelasma and corneal arcus, especially in young patients, increases the probability of concomitant dyslipoproteinemia. Although these signs are low in specificity, they are easily detected during a routine eye examination and should prompt a more specific lipid-lipoprotein screening.

Screening for significant coronary artery atherosclerosis is more expensive and time-consuming than screening for associated reversible risk factors. In general, it is reasonable to screen for a history of cardiovascular symptoms and events (chest pain, dyspnea, syncope, arrhythmias, claudication, stroke) and reserve more specific testing (eg, exercise stress testing, dobutamine stress echocardiography, or exercise myocardial scintigraphy) for those in increased risk categories. Single-photon emission computed tomography (SPECT) is a rapid, noninvasive, high-resolution imaging study that detects coronary artery calcium as a means of screening asymptomatic patients for coronary atherosclerosis. This technique can noninvasively detect and even quantitate the presence of coronary atherosclerosis.

> Cosson E, Paycha F, Paries J, et al. Detecting silent coronary stenoses and stratifying cardiac risk in patients with diabetes: ECG stress test or exercise myocardial scintigraphy? *Diabet Med*. 2004;21:342–348.
>
> Yokoshima T, Honma H, Kusama Y, et al. Improved stratification of perioperative cardiac risk in patients undergoing noncardiac surgery using new indices of dobutamine stress echocardiography. *J Cardiol*. 2004;44:101–111.

Cancer

In women, the most common cancers are lung, breast, and colorectal. In men, they are lung, prostate, and colorectal. The types of cancer most amenable to screening are cervical cancer, breast cancer, urologic cancer, lung cancer, colorectal cancer, and melanoma. Table 13-1 shows a set of recommendations for early cancer detection.

Cervical cancer

Cervical cancer is the most common gynecologic cancer in patients between the ages of 15 and 34. Overall, approximately 15,000 cases of invasive cancer of the cervix (about 5000 resulting in death) and 45,000 cases of carcinoma in situ occur each year in the United States. About 80% of the 470,000 cervical cancer cases diagnosed worldwide each year occur in developing countries. Despite advances in the treatment of cervical cancer, approximately half of the women with the disease will die. Cervical cancer is the eighth most common cause of cancer mortality in the United States.

The risk factors for cervical cancer are the number of lifetime sexual partners, the presence of high-risk serotypes of HPV, low socioeconomic status, positive smoking history, use of steroid contraceptive hormones, and a history of other sexually transmitted diseases. More than 95% of all cervical cancers are positive for HPV. Early detection and appropriate treatment markedly reduce the morbidity and mortality from invasive cancer of the cervix. Cervical cancer is asymptomatic when it occurs in situ, and the most effective screening technique remains the Papanicolaou test ("Pap smear"). HPV can be detected with PCR assay techniques, and high-risk patients should receive HPV testing at the time of the PAP smear examination. Vaccines to prevent HPV infection and its sequelae have recently become available.

Breast cancer

Though recently surpassed by lung cancer as the most common cause of death in women older than age 40, breast cancer remains the most common malignancy in women. The

Table 13-1 American Cancer Society Recommendations for Early Cancer Detection in Asymptomatic Patients

Test or Procedure	Sex	Population Age (Years)	Frequency
Sigmoidoscopy	M, F	>50	After 2 negative exams 1 year apart, perform every 3–5 years
Stool guaiac slide test	M, F	>50	Annual
Digital rectal examination	M, F	>40	Annual
Papanicolaou test	F	20–65; <20, if sexually active	After 2 negative exams 1 year apart, perform at least every 3 years
Pelvic examination	F	20–40	Every 3 years
		>40	Annual
Endometrial tissue sample	F	Women at high risk* and at menopause	At menopause
Breast self-examination	F	>20	Monthly
Breast physical examination	F	20–40	Every 3 years
		>40	Annual
Mammography	F	35–40	Baseline
		40–49	Annual
		>50	Annual
Chest x-ray			Not recommended
Sputum cytology			Not recommended
Health counseling and cancer checkup†	M, F	>20	Every 3 years
	M, F	>40	Annual

*History of infertility, obesity, failure to ovulate, abnormal uterine bleeding, or estrogen therapy.
†To include examination for cancers of the thyroid, testis, prostate, ovary, lymph nodes, oral region, and skin.

overall incidence of breast cancer in the United States is 10%–12%; 50% of these patients are curable. In 2004, approximately 215,990 new cases of breast cancer and more than 40,110 related deaths were reported in the United States alone. More than 75% of all breast cancers are cured with current therapy.

The importance of specific screening is increased by the presence of known risk factors, all of which are identifiable by history: (1) first-degree relative with breast cancer, (2) prior breast cancer, (3) nulliparity, (4) first pregnancy after age 30, and (5) early menarche or late menopause. Additional risk factors are elevated serum estrogen levels, elevated testosterone levels, high-fat diet, obesity, and sedentary lifestyle. Fibrocystic disease is not a risk factor unless there is demonstrated hyperplasia or atypia on biopsy.

Hormone replacement therapy (HRT) with estrogen and progesterone was associated with an increased risk of invasive breast cancer and abnormal mammograms in the Women's Health Initiative randomized trial. In the same trial, postmenopausal hormone therapy was also associated with an increased risk for venous thromboembolism, stroke, coronary heart disease, and breast cancer, and these risks have also been reported in other controlled trials. The beneficial effects that were noted in the Women's Health Initiative trial included reductions in the incidence of fractures and colorectal cancer.

Approximately 42% of breast cancers detectable by mammography are not detectable by physical examination alone, and one third of those found by mammographic screening are noninvasive or less than 1 cm in size if invasive. Because mammograms can yield false-negative results, the best detection strategy involves a physical examination plus mammography, with fine-needle aspiration or biopsy if either reveals an abnormality. Mammograms have been shown to be safe as well as effective, with current low-dose radiation not inducing added cancer risk. Mammographic screening should be performed yearly in women at or beyond age 40. A woman should undergo mammographic screening until at least age 70. Recently, new tools advocated for breast cancer screening have included ultrasound, digital mammography, magnetic resonance imaging, magnetic resonance spectroscopic imaging, and positron emission tomography.

Urologic cancer
The prostate, bladder, kidney, and testes yield approximately 16% of new cancer cases per year, with most of the common malignancies in middle-aged and older men. About 230,000 new cases of prostate cancer and nearly 40,000 related deaths occur each year in the United States. Screening remains controversial, but preliminary estimates suggest that screening can reduce mortality. Prostate and testicular cancer can be detected early by digital examination of the prostate, serum prostate-specific antigen (PSA) measurements, and physical examination of the testes. It is now generally accepted that PSA should be measured yearly in men older than age 45 with more than 10 years of life expectancy. For patients with a family history of prostate cancer, screening should begin at age 40 or earlier. PSA levels greater than 10 ng/mL strongly suggest metastatic disease; levels less than 4 ng/mL usually suggest benign hypertrophy or a normal prostate. A trend of increasing PSA levels is an even more sensitive indicator of prostate cancer than an individual elevated PSA level.

Although prostate cancer is a potentially lethal illness, there are many detectable prostate cancers that are of little threat to life. Some men with low-grade prostate cancer receive curative treatment, even though their disease may not require treatment. Some studies suggest that more than 75% of men with screen-detected localized disease may not even need treatment. More specific screening methods are needed to allow differentiation between lethal and nonlethal cancers.

Lung cancer
Lung cancer is the leading form of cancer in adults. Among male patients with lung cancer, 93% are smokers. The number and percentage of cases in women have risen with the increased incidence of smoking in women. In one study of lung cancer, 40% of cases were detected by chest radiography and 60% were detected by symptoms. The usefulness of radiographic and sputum cytologic screening is generally considered to be low, but some studies have suggested that annual chest radiography may reduce morbidity and mortality. Chest radiography can be improved with digital radiography, image processing, and computer-aided detection, as these methods have been shown to enhance lung nodule detection. In high-risk patient groups, screening protocols effect a higher yield and may include sputum cytology, low-dose helical chest CT (with possible fine-needle aspiration

for suspicious lesions), and bronchoscopy with possible endobronchial biopsy. Fluorescent bronchoscopy is a promising new tool in identifying early malignant changes in the central airways, because it is significantly more sensitive than white light bronchoscopy. Also, new molecular markers detected in sputum and serum show some promise in the future of lung cancer screening.

Gastrointestinal cancer

The primary risk factors for squamous cell carcinoma of the esophagus are tobacco use and alcohol consumption, accounting for 80%–90% of these neoplasms. The main risk factors for adenocarcinoma of the esophagus are gastroesophageal reflux disease, obesity, and history of Barrett esophagus. Treatment has poor results; thus, prevention or elimination of the risk factors is worthwhile. The incidence of adenocarcinoma of the esophagus is increasing in developed countries, but squamous cell carcinoma remains dominant in underdeveloped areas. Currently, no effective preventative screening programs are available, and most patients present with advanced or metastatic disease. Barrett esophagus is a complication of long-standing gastroesophageal reflux disease (GERD) and is the premalignant condition for the majority of esophageal adenocarcinomas. Although duration of gastroesophageal reflux (GER), male sex, and, possibly, a strong family history are directly related to risk of Barrett esophagus, the role of endoscopic screening in those with GERD and the role of endoscopic surveillance in those with confirmed Barrett syndrome remain controversial.

Gastric cancer appears to be associated with certain geographic areas (Japan, China, Central and South America, Eastern Europe, and parts of the Middle East), high ingestion of nitrates, loss of gastric acidity, lower socioeconomic status, and blood type A. It remains the second most frequent and lethal malignancy worldwide. Although routine endoscopic screening is not cost-effective, widespread screening for and treatment of *Helicobacter pylori* infection, in high-incidence populations, could be an effective strategy.

Pancreatic cancer is 2 to 3 times more common in heavy smokers than in nonsmokers, and it has also been associated with chronic pancreatitis, diabetes mellitus, and obesity. Familial pancreatic cancer is well documented, but the genes responsible for this condition have not yet been identified, and familial cases represent only about 5% of all pancreatic cancer cases. Hepatocellular cancer is more common in persons with preexisting liver disease, especially cirrhosis and hepatitis C.

Colorectal cancer

Colorectal cancer is a major killer in Western society, second only to lung cancer in incidence and mortality. The cumulative lifetime probability of developing colon cancer is roughly 6%, with 3% probability of dying from this disease. The chance for survival 5 years after diagnosis remains only 40%, despite the optimistic theory that early detection would lead to curative surgery. Potentially modifiable risk factors such as fiber and fat intake are important in primary prevention.

Most authorities accept the theory that colorectal cancer develops from an initially benign polyp in a mitotic process that occurs over 5–10 years. Supportive evidence shows that many operative specimens containing colon cancer have at least 1 adenoma and that invasive cancer frequently occurs near adenomatous tissue. Histologic studies have shown that growth of adenomas is associated with increasing cellular atypia. This theory is supported by the malignant potential of adenomas in familial polyposis; furthermore, patients who refuse removal of polyps frequently develop cancer at the same site and at other sites in their colon.

Studies to date lack the necessary longevity to prove definitively that polyp removal prevents carcinoma. Yet colonoscopic removal or ablation of all polyps has become the standard of care where facilities and trained personnel are available.

A national polyp study is under way to define the biology of these tumors, to identify factors that seem to promote invasive carcinoma, and to clarify whether early removal prevents invasive cancer. One study reported characteristics associated with high-grade dysplasia in colorectal adenomas. The major independent risk factors were adenoma size and extent of the villous component in the adenoma. Increasing age was associated with increased risk for high-grade dysplasia. Gender was not an independent factor.

Increased dietary fiber and reduced dietary fat intake have been associated with reduced risk of colorectal cancer. Some studies have suggested that regular use of nonsteroidal anti-inflammatory drugs is correlated with reduced risk of colorectal cancer. Also, calcium supplementation is associated with a moderate reduction in the risk of recurrent colorectal adenomas.

Detection must be improved with more widespread use of screening studies such as Hemoccult slides, flexible sigmoidoscopy, barium enema, and colonoscopy, with aggressive follow-up of positive cases. It is estimated that widespread adoption of these recommendations could reduce the mortality rate of colorectal cancer by more than 50%. Fecal DNA testing for molecular tumor markers is a new, investigational noninvasive method of colorectal cancer screening with high sensitivity and specificity. Because this testing is easier to use and more sensitive than fecal occult blood testing, patient compliance may be better. Although fecal DNA testing is expensive, initial studies suggest it is cost-effective.

Periodic sigmoidoscopy (every 3 years) and annual digital rectal examination with fecal occult blood testing have been recommended in asymptomatic adults older than 50 years. Recommendations remain controversial because of a lack of randomized trials. Sigmoidoscopy offers good specificity but misses proximal cancers. Nevertheless, several case-control studies have demonstrated a 50%–70% reduction in the risk of colorectal cancer in patients screened with sigmoidoscopy. Similarly, fecal occult blood testing every 2 years has been shown to decrease the mortality rate of colon cancer by up to 40%.

The sensitivity of the barium enema is the main disadvantage of this type of screening study. Historically, this test has been ineffective in examination of the rectum. Double-contrast, or air-contrast, barium enema is more sensitive but is still not the standard examination in many radiology departments.

Colonoscopy as a screening test for asymptomatic patients older than age 50 has been gaining popularity. When results are negative, the test is repeated every 10 years in low-risk patients. Colonoscopy is thought to be about twice as sensitive as barium enema for detection of colon cancers. Also, many of the lesions discovered with colonoscopy would not be detected with sigmoidoscopy. Yearly colonoscopy has been advocated in populations at very high risk, such as patients with familial polyposis and first-degree relatives of patients with colon cancer. The disadvantages of colonoscopy are the increased cost, the number of trained personnel required, and the risks of intravenous sedation and colonic perforation (approximately 0.2%). Virtual colonoscopy with high-resolution CT is currently being evaluated as a screening tool. It may offer the ability to screen out patients without neoplasia, thus allowing colonoscopy to be reserved for patients with significant lesions. Virtual colonoscopy has a high sensitivity for large adenomas and colorectal cancers.

Melanoma
Melanoma is the most deadly form of skin cancer, and its incidence is increasing faster than that of all other cancers. In the United States, about 1 in 75 persons will develop melanoma during his or her lifetime. More than 44,000 new cases and more than 7000 related deaths are reported per year in the United States.

Most melanomas probably arise from dysplastic nevi. Risk factors for melanoma include history of melanoma or atypical moles, presence of more than 75–100 moles, positive melanoma family history, history of previous nonmelanoma skin cancer, giant congenital nevus (greater than 20 cm), xeroderma pigmentosum, treatment with UV-A and psoralens, frequent tanning with UV-A light, and a history of 3 or more severe (blistering) sunburns. Other, less significant risk factors are light complexion of the hair and eyes, freckles, inability to tan, indoor occupation with outdoor hobbies, and proximity to the equator.

Ultraviolet damage probably causes most melanomas. Intense intermittent exposures are directly related to melanoma, whereas other skin cancers are more associated with cumulative exposure. Ultraviolet radiation causes DNA damage, which is usually corrected by DNA repair enzymes. These DNA repair processes decrease with increasing age.

A pigmented lesion with any of the following characteristics, easily remembered by the *ABCDE* mnemonic, is suggestive of melanoma: *a*symmetrical lesions, *b*order (irregular), *c*olor (variable), *d*iameter (greater than 6 mm), and *e*levation. Other characteristics suggestive of melanoma are pruritus, bleeding, changing morphology, and new lesions or scalp lesions. Everyone should perform self skin examinations every 1 or 2 months, and suspicious lesions require referral and possible biopsy. Sun avoidance and use of sunblock can reduce the risk of melanoma and other skin cancers. In addition to providing simple visualization, dermoscopy (epiluminescence microscopy) can increase the specificity of clinical examination for the detection of melanomas.

> Brawley OW. Prostate cancer screening: clinical applications and challenges. *Urol Oncol.* 2004;22:353–357.
>
> Carli P, Mannone F, De Giorgi V, et al. The problem of false-positive diagnosis in melanoma screening: the impact of dermoscopy. *Melanoma Res.* 2003;13(2):179–182.
>
> Chang JT, Katzka DA. Gastroesophageal reflux disease, Barrett esophagus, and esophageal adenocarcinoma. *Arch Intern Med.* 2004;164:1482–1488.
>
> Chlebowski RT, Hendrix SL, Langer RD, et al. Influence of estrogen plus progestin on breast cancer and mammography in healthy postmenopausal women: the Women's Health Initiative Randomized Trial. *JAMA.* 2003;289:3243–3253.
>
> Deenadayalu VP, Rex DK. Fecal-based DNA assays: a new, noninvasive approach to colorectal cancer screening. *Cleve Clin J Med.* 2004;71(6):497–503.

Diederich S, Wormanns D. Impact of low-dose CT on lung cancer screening. *Lung Cancer.* 2004;45(suppl 2):S13–S19.

Franco EL, Schlecht NF, Saslow D. The epidemiology of cervical cancer. *Cancer J.* 2003;9: 348–359.

Genta RM. Screening for gastric cancer: does it make sense? *Aliment Pharmacol Ther.* 2004;20(suppl 2):42–47.

Jansen KU. Toward vaccines against cervical cancer. *Curr Opin Drug Discov Devel.* 2004;7: 228–232.

Lieberman DA, Weiss DG, Bond JH, et al. Use of colonoscopy to screen asymptomatic adults for colorectal cancer. Veterans Affairs Cooperative Study Group 380. *N Engl J Med.* 2000;343:162–168.

Mak T, Lalloo F, Evans DG, et al. Molecular stool screening for colorectal cancer. *Br J Surg.* 2004;91:790–800.

Michaud DS. Epidemiology of pancreatic cancer. *Minerva Chir.* 2004;59(2):99–111.

Moodley M, Moodley J, Chetty R, et al. The role of steroid contraceptive hormones in the pathogenesis of invasive cervical cancer: a review. *Int J Gynecol Cancer.* 2003;13(2):103–110.

Nanda K, McCrory DC, Myers ER, et al. Accuracy of the Papanicolaou test in screening for and follow-up of cervical cytologic abnormalities: a systematic review. *Ann Intern Med.* 2000;132:810–819.

Newcomb PA, Storer BE, Morimoto LM, et al. Long-term efficacy of sigmoidoscopy in the reduction of colorectal cancer incidence. *J Natl Cancer Inst.* 2003;95:622–625.

Patel M, Ferry K, Franceschi D, et al. Esophageal carcinoma: current controversial topics. *Cancer Invest.* 2004;22:897–912.

Sharma P. Barrett esophagus: will effective treatment prevent the risk of progression to esophageal adenocarcinoma? *Am J Med.* 2004;117(suppl 5A):79S–85S.

Smith JA, Andreopoulou E. An overview of the status of imaging screening technology for breast cancer. *Ann Oncol.* 2004;15(suppl 1):I18–I26.

Stanzel F. Fluorescent bronchoscopy: contribution for lung cancer screening? *Lung Cancer.* 2004;45(suppl 2):S29–37.

Tjalma WA, Arbyn M, Paavonen J, et al. Prophylactic human papillomavirus vaccines: the beginning of the end of cervical cancer. *Int J Gynecol Cancer.* 2004;14:751–761.

Warren MP. A comparative review of the risks and benefits of hormone replacement therapy regimens. *Am J Obstet Gynecol.* 2004;190:1141–1167.

Wilkinson NW, Loewen GM, Klippenstein DL, et al. The evolution of lung cancer screening. *J Surg Oncol.* 2003;84:234–238.

Wilson SS, Crawford ED. Screening for prostate cancer: current recommendations. *Urol Clin North Am.* 2004;31:219–226.

Winawer SJ. Screening of colorectal cancer: progress and problems. *Recent Results Cancer Res.* 2005;166:231–244.

Winawer SJ, Stewart ET, Zauber AG, et al. A comparison of colonoscopy and double-contrast barium enema for surveillance after polypectomy. National Polyp Study Work Group. *N Engl J Med.* 2000;342:1766–1772.

Metabolic Diseases

Diabetes

The prevalence of diabetes mellitus (DM) is difficult to determine accurately because many cases remain undiagnosed until patients experience significant symptoms. Also, prevalence rates differ according to race, age, and sex. Prevalence in the United States is estimated to be 1%. (See Chapter 9 for a detailed discussion on the classification of DM.) Type 1 DM, previously called *insulin-dependent DM,* accounts for one fourth of cases. Blood glucose screening is recommended for anyone older than age 45. Persons at higher risk for type 2 DM should be screened earlier, including patients with symptoms suggestive of DM, obese patients, pregnant women, those with a positive family history of DM, long-term users of corticosteroids, blacks, and Native Americans.

A random fasting blood glucose test is very sensitive for detecting DM but not specific. A fasting glucose level of 126 mg/dL or higher on 2 separate occasions or a positive glucose tolerance test result is diagnostic of DM. Hemoglobin A_{1c} levels provide additional helpful screening information regarding a patient's long-term glycemic status.

Thyroid diseases

The prevalence of abnormal thyroid test results is high, particularly in older persons. Up to 15% of women older than age 60 have asymptomatic elevated thyroid-stimulating hormone levels or low thyroxine (T_4) levels. A low percentage of such persons progress to clinical hypothyroidism. Although no clinical trials justify widespread screening, it would be reasonable to test women older than age 60. The availability of the newer ultrasensitive thyroid-stimulating hormone tests has simplified screening for thyroid disease. To evaluate newborns for congenital hypothyroidism, clinicians should check the thyroid-stimulating hormone and T_4 levels of newborns. Thyroid peroxidase antibodies in pregnancy are useful as a marker for postpartum and long-term thyroid dysfunction.

> Premawardhana LD, Parkes AB, John R, et al. Thyroid peroxidase antibodies in early pregnancy: utility for prediction of postpartum thyroid dysfunction and implications for screening. *Thyroid.* 2004;14:610–615.
>
> Raikou M, McGuire A. The economics of screening and treatment in type 2 diabetes mellitus. *Pharmacoeconomics.* 2003;21:543–564.
>
> Zamboni G, Zaffanello M, Rigon F, et al. Diagnostic effectiveness of simultaneous thyroxine and thyroid-stimulating hormone screening measurements. Thirteen years' experience in the Northeast Italian Screening Programme. *J Med Screen.* 2004;11:8–10.

Infectious Diseases

The major public health screening efforts in the United States have been for tuberculosis and sexually transmitted diseases. Hepatitis screening is used primarily for blood donation, institutionalized populations, and health care workers rather than for general population screening.

Tuberculosis

The prevalence of tuberculosis (TB) has recently increased in the United States, reversing decades of steady decline. High-incidence clustering occurs in certain subgroups: HIV-infected patients; inner city, economically disadvantaged males; nursing home residents (3.5% incidence of skin test results converting to positive); health care workers, including physicians; people older than age 50; recent immigrant groups; drug-dependent and alcohol-dependent groups; and patients who have undergone gastrectomy or who have debilitating diseases. Tuberculosis skin testing should be performed in these high-risk groups. Such testing is sensitive, although interpretation of results may be complicated by coinfection with HIV. Positive results should prompt chest radiography and consideration of chemoprophylaxis. Some experts advocate routine skin testing of all people younger than 35 years at the time of routine health examination (for detection as well as for baseline data). The Occupational Safety and Health Administration requires annual TB skin testing of all health care workers.

A new PCR assay, the BDProbeTec ET System, is capable of rapidly detecting *Mycobacterium tuberculosis* DNA in respiratory specimens and compares favorably with microscopy of smear material using Ziehl-Neelsen stain and with TB cultures. In a recent study, the overall sensitivity and specificity for BDProbeTec ET compared with culture were 93.7% and 98.7%, respectively, while with smear-positive and smear-negative specimens, the sensitivities were 100% and 81.5%, respectively. BDProbeTec ET, in parallel with cultures, can be used to monitor the regression of TB DNA in treated patients. Also, it can be very useful for rapid detection of *M tuberculosis* complex, especially in smear-negative respiratory specimens.

Although the bacille Calmette-Guérin (BCG) vaccine seems to reduce the mortality of childhood TB in developing countries, the vaccine does not significantly affect the 90% of cases that occur in adults. Several candidate vaccines for TB are currently being developed, including subunit, DNA, microbial vector, and live attenuated vaccines.

Syphilis

Syphilis is almost always transmitted sexually; congenital disease transmitted in utero is now rare. In fact, the incidence of congenital syphilis has dropped 90% since the 1940s because of required premarital screening and pregnancy screening. Better prenatal care and increased syphilis screening during pregnancy improve the chances of detecting infants at risk for congenital syphilis, thus allowing early maternal treatment.

Latent, untreated cases of syphilis in which the primary or secondary mucocutaneous lesion is no longer present can be detected only by screening. It is important to detect early latent disease: in approximately 25% of cases, infectious mucocutaneous lesions reemerge spontaneously in the first 2 years. Late latent disease should be detected and treated because of the long-term destructive effects on the central nervous system, the aorta, and the skeletal system.

Screening is generally performed with the more sensitive, but less specific, nontreponemal antigen tests (VDRL, RPR). Positive results are then confirmed with treponemal antigen tests (FTA-ABS, MHA-TP, HATTS), which are more expensive.

Centers for Disease Control and Prevention (CDC). Congenital syphilis—United States, 2002. *MMWR Morb Mortal Wkly Rep.* 2004;53:716–719.

Jesus de la Calle I, Jesus de la Calle MA, Rodriguez-Iglesias M. Evaluation of the BDProbeTec ET system as screening tool in the direct detection of *Mycobacterium tuberculosis* complex in respiratory specimens. *Diagn Microbiol Infect Dis.* 2003;47:573–578.

Immunization

The development of immunization as a means of preventing the spread of infectious disease began in 1796, when Edward Jenner injected cowpox virus, which causes a mild disease, into a child to prevent smallpox, a severe, potentially fatal illness. Immunization today still relies on Jenner's inoculation methods in protecting against disease. There are 2 types: active and passive.

In *active immunization,* the recipient develops an acquired immune response to inactivated or killed viruses, viral subtractions, bacterial toxoids or antigens, or synthetic vaccines. Once the immune response to a particular pathogen has developed, it protects the host against infection. The persistence of acquired immunity depends on the perpetuation of cell strains responsive to the target antigenic stimulus, and booster inoculations may be required for certain immunogens.

In general, live inactivated vaccines produce longer-lasting immunity; however, they are contraindicated in immunocompromised persons or pregnant women because the pathogen can potentially replicate in the host. Ideally, active immunization should be completed before exposure; however, life-saving postexposure immunity can be developed through combining active and passive immunization.

The current Recommended Childhood Immunization Schedule for the year 2005, developed by the American Academy of Pediatrics Committee on Infectious Diseases, is summarized in Table 13-2. The new schedule includes "catch-up" protocols for children who have missed some of the recommended immunization doses.

Passive immunization depends on the transfer of immunoglobulin in serum from a host with active immunity to a susceptible host. Passive immunity does not result in active immunity and sometimes even blocks the development of active immunity. Passive immunity is short-lived and without immune memory; however, it confers immediate protection on the recipient who has been exposed to the pathogen. Pooled human globulin, antitoxins, or human globulin with high antibody titers for specific diseases are the usual products available for passive immunization.

Immunization should be avoided in persons who have allergic reactions to the vaccine or its components. Idiopathic autoantibody or cross-reacting antibody development may occur after vaccination, resulting in systemic disease such as Guillain-Barré syndrome, a rare but devastating complication of vaccination. Immunization should be avoided during a febrile illness. Multidose immunization schedules that are interrupted can be resumed; however, doses given outside the schedule should not be counted toward completion of the vaccination sequence.

Hepatitis B

Approximately 100,000 symptomatic cases of hepatitis B occur annually in the United States. Between 6% and 10% of adult patients with hepatitis B become carriers. Chronic active hepatitis occurs in 25% of carriers. Of those patients with chronic active disease, 20% will die of cirrhosis and 5% will die of hepatocellular carcinoma.

The available recombinant vaccines based on hepatitis B virus (HBV) surface antigen are Engerix-B, Recombivax HB, and Bio-Hep-B. In Europe, a new triple antigen vaccine, Hepacare, is indicated for vaccination of patients who did not respond to the current single antigen vaccines and for persons who require rapid protection against hepatitis B infection. HBV vaccine is usually administered in 3 sessions, with the second and third occurring 1 and 6 months after the initial injection in adults. On this regimen, 90% of

Table 13-2 Recommended Childhood Immunization Schedule

Age	Immunizations
Birth	HepB #1
2 mo	DTaP #1, Hib #1, IPV #1, PCV #1, HepB #2
4 mo	DTaP #2, Hib #2, IPV #2, PCV #2
6 mo	DTaP #3, Hib #3, IPV #3, PCV #3, HepB #3 (HepB #3 must be given at least 2 mo after HepB #2)
12–15 mo	HepB #3 (if not given at 6 mo) Hib #4 (booster) IPV (or OPV) #3 (if not given at 6 mo), MMR #1, PCV #4 Varivax (if no chickenpox by 12 mo of age)
15–18 mo	DTaP #4 HepB #3 (if not previously given) IPV (or OPV) #3 (if not given at 12–15 mo) PCV (if not previously given)
4–6 yr	DTaP #5, MMR #2, IPV (or OPV) #4
11–12 yr	Td MMR #2 (booster; if not given at age 4–6 yr) Varivax (if not previously immunized, and if no reliable history of chickenpox)
13–18 yr	Td (if not given at 11–12 yr) Check anti-HBV titers: consider HepB booster

DTaP = diphtheria/tetanus/acellular pertussis vaccine; HepB = hepatitis B virus vaccine; Hib = *Haemophilus influenzae* type B conjugate vaccine; IPV = inactivated polio vaccine; MMR = measles/mumps/rubella; OPV = oral polio vaccine; PCV = pneumococcal conjugated vaccine; Td = tetanus and diphtheria toxoid vaccine; Varivax = live attenuated *Varicella* vaccine

Additional recommendations:
PCV is also recommended for children with chronic illnesses between 2 and 5 yr of age. Influenza vaccine is recommended annually for children 6–59 months of age. Hepatitis A vaccine is recommended for children over 2 yr of age and adolescents living in endemic areas or in contact with infected patients. Give a Td booster every 10 yr, sooner if severe traumatic wound occurs. Oral live rotavirus vaccine is recommended at ages 2, 4, and 6 months. A second dose of *Varicella* vaccine is recommended at ages 4–6 years. Human papillomavirus vaccine is recommended for girls 11–12 years, with catch-up immunization of girls 13–18 years.

Adapted from Committee on Infectious Diseases. Recommended immunization schedules for children and adolescents—United States, 2007. *Pediatrics.* 2007;119:207–208. Updated from Centers for Disease Control and Prevention. Recommended childhood and adolescent immunization schedule—United States, 2005. *MMWR.* 2005;53(Nos. 51&52):Q1–Q3.

recipients develop protective antibody levels for at least 3 years. The recombinant vaccine can also be given on an accelerated dosing schedule, which requires vaccination at 0, 1, and 2 months followed by a booster dose at 12 months. Antibody levels that are greater than 10 milli-International Units (mIU) per milliliter are considered to be adequate protection. Booster injections are advised for persons whose antibody levels are less than 10 mIU/mL. Approximately 3%–4% of healthy persons lack the immune response gene needed to produce antibodies after receiving the vaccine. Repeat vaccination results in the development of protective antibodies in 50% of the nonresponders. Vaccines are also available for hepatitis A and are being developed for hepatitis C and E.

Vaccination before exposure is recommended and cost-effective for all infants and children and in certain high-risk groups: health care workers, hemodialysis patients, residents and staff of institutions for the retarded, household and sexual contacts of chronic carriers of hepatitis B, hemophiliacs, users of illicit injectable drugs, prison inmates, sexually active homosexual men, and HIV-positive patients. Vaccination can be combined with passive immunization for postexposure prophylaxis without affecting the development of active immunity. The incorporation of the vaccine into childhood immunization schedules has resulted in a decrease in the number of new hepatitis B cases reported annually, and there has also been a significant reduction in the number of hepatocellular carcinoma cases reported in children.

Twinrix is a new combination hepatitis A and hepatitis B vaccine, combining the antigenic components contained in Havrix (inactivated hepatitis A vaccine) and Engerix-B (recombinant hepatitis B vaccine). When administered in a standard 3-dose schedule at 0, 1, and 6 months, Twinrix provides immunity that is comparable to the monovalent vaccines.

Postexposure prophylaxis with hepatitis B immune globulin should be considered when there is perinatal exposure of an infant born to a carrier, accidental percutaneous or permucosal exposure to blood positive for HBV surface antigen, or sexual exposure (within 14 days) to a carrier of hepatitis B. Hepatitis B immune globulin should be given as soon as possible after exposure in a single intramuscular dose of 0.06 mL/kg body weight; the recombinant HBV vaccine should be concurrently administered in an accelerated dosing schedule.

Lamivudine (Epivir) is a nucleoside analogue inhibitor of reverse transcriptase and was initially developed for the treatment of HIV infection. Interferon-α and lamivudine have been found to be very effective against HBV and are considered to be the drugs of choice for the treatment of patients with chronic HBV infection. Promising new treatments for hepatitis B include adefovir, entecavir, telbivudine, and peginterferon alfa-2a.

Influenza

Although influenza is usually a self-limited disease with rare sequelae, it can be associated with severe morbidity and mortality in elderly persons or those with chronic diseases. Influenza vaccines produce long-lasting immunity. However, antigenic shifts, primarily in type A rather than type B influenza virus, necessitate yearly reformulation of the vaccine to contain the antigens of strains considered most likely to cause disease. Protection is correlated with the development of antihemagglutinin and antineuraminidase antibodies, which decrease the patient's susceptibility and the severity of the disease. The influenza vaccine is as effective in HIV-positive patients as it is in HIV-negative patients, regardless of CD4 T-cell counts. Annual vaccination is recommended for adults and children with chronic diseases requiring medical care, immunosuppressed patients (including HIV-infected patients), nursing home residents, children who require long-term aspirin therapy, healthy children younger than 5 years, persons older than age 65, and medical personnel with extensive contact with high-risk patients. The vaccine is well tolerated, and there has been no increased risk of neurological complications with the vaccines administered after 1991. Influenza vaccine should not be administered to persons with anaphylactic hypersensitivity to eggs or to pregnant women in their first trimester. A trivalent intranasal influenza vaccine (FluMist) is available and provides protection against type A and type B influenza virus. Newer antiviral agents, such as zanamivir (Relenza) and oseltamivir, are active against influenza types A and B. These drugs are effective for the treatment of influenza infection as well as the prophylactic treatment of the contacts of infected persons.

Varicella-Zoster

Varivax, the approved varicella-zoster vaccine, is recommended for immunocompetent patients older than 12 months with no history of previous varicella infection. For patients older than 12 years, 2 doses of vaccine are given 4–8 weeks apart. Also, health care workers who have not been exposed to chickenpox should be vaccinated. Varivax is safe and provides immunity for up to 20 years. Data from the Centers for Disease Control show that there was a dramatic decline in the incidence of varicella (up to 87%) from 1995 to 2000.

Measles

Vaccination has dramatically reduced the incidence of measles, along with associated encephalitis, mental retardation, and mortality. Introduced in 1963, the initial vaccine was an inactivated virus that did not provide a long duration of protection; therefore, many young adults are at risk for measles, which is more severe as an adult disease. Vaccination before age 1 with any form of vaccine is ineffective because maternal antibodies block the development of immunity. In 1967, a live attenuated vaccine that causes long-lasting immunity was introduced. Vaccination with the attenuated strain should be routine not only at age 15 months but also for persons born between 1957 and 1967 who were neither vaccinated nor infected and for persons who received the inactivated viral vaccine. Individuals born before 1957 are considered immune by virtue of natural infection. For persons who cannot have the vaccine (which should be given within 72 hours of exposure), postexposure prophylaxis with immune globulin should be considered within 6 days. The vaccine is contraindicated for persons with hypersensitivity to eggs. Measles-mumps-rubella (MMR) vaccination is recommended for all children and is usually given at about age 15 months and again between ages 4 and 6. Past concerns about the adverse effects of thimerosal-containing MMR vaccines are no longer an issue, as this preservative is no longer used in this vaccine. In addition, several studies have refuted previous fears of an association between MMR vaccines and autism.

Mumps

The number of reported cases of mumps in the United States has decreased steadily since the introduction of a live mumps vaccine in 1967. Although mumps is generally self-limited, meningeal signs may appear in up to 15% of cases and orchitis in up to 20% of clinical cases in postpubertal males. Other possible complications include permanent deafness and pancreatitis. Mumps vaccination is indicated in all children and all susceptible adults, particularly postpubertal males.

Rubella

Rubella immunization is intended to prevent fetal infection and consequent congenital rubella syndrome, which can occur in up to 80% of fetuses of mothers infected during the first trimester of pregnancy. The number of reported cases of rubella in the United States has decreased steadily from more than 56,000 in 1969, the year rubella vaccine was licensed, to 954 cases in 1983. A single subcutaneously administered dose of live, attenuated rubella vaccine provides long-term (probably lifetime) immunity in approximately 95% of persons vaccinated.

Rubella vaccine is recommended for adults, particularly women, unless proof of immunity is available (documented rubella vaccination on or after the first birthday or a positive serologic test result) or the vaccine is specifically contraindicated. Rubella vaccine should be given at least 14 days before administration of immune globulin or deferred for 3 months after administration. Because of the theoretical risk to the fetus, women of childbearing age should receive the vaccine only if they are not pregnant. A new nonreplicating rubella virus DNA vaccine is being evaluated and may offer a safer alternative for pregnant patients.

Polio

Before the introduction of the first polio vaccine in 1955, polio caused thousands of cases of paralysis. Despite widespread immunization with oral vaccine in 1962, there has been a steady decline in polio immunization and a growing number of susceptible persons. Although the incidence of polio is low, the possibility of large-scale outbreaks increases as the number of susceptible persons increases. There are 2 forms of the vaccine: an oral form that is a live attenuated virus (OPV, Sabin vaccine) and a subcutaneous injectable form of killed virus (IPV, Salk vaccine). Vaccine-associated paralytic poliomyelitis has been associated more with the OPV than with the IPV. Therefore, the American Academy of Pediatrics has recommended that the IPV be administered for all 4 vaccinations in the series, or for the first 2 of the series. Either IPV or OPV can be used for the last 2 vaccinations of the series. OPV is contraindicated in pregnant women, who should receive only the killed virus vaccine.

Tetanus and Diphtheria

The combined tetanus and diphtheria toxoid vaccine (Td) is highly effective. It is used for both primary and booster immunization of adults. The pediatric vaccine, diphtheria-tetanus-pertussis (DTP), has been the standard vaccine for years but has been replaced recently with the newer vaccine DTaP (diphtheria and tetanus toxoids with acellular pertussis vaccine). Now, DTaP is the preferred vaccine formulation for all doses in the immunization series. These vaccines should not be given to adults because of the risk of adverse neurological reactions among adults to the pertussis component. All young adults should have completed a primary series of tetanus and diphtheria toxoids. Persons who have completed a primary series of tetanus and diphtheria immunization should receive a booster dose every 10 years. If serious doubt exists about the completion of a primary series of immunization, 2 doses of 0.5 mL of the combined toxoids should be given intramuscularly at monthly intervals, followed by a third dose 6–10 months later. Thereafter, a booster dose of 0.5 mL should be given at 10-year intervals.

In wound management of tetanus, previously immunized persons with severe wounds should receive a booster if more than 5 years have elapsed since the last injection. The management of previously unimmunized patients with severe wounds should include tetanus immune globulin as well as Td. Although tetanus is uncommon, more than 60% of cases occur in persons older than 60 years. Therefore, older adults should be given a single booster at age 65.

Pneumococcal Pneumonia

Pneumococcal pneumonia is the most serious and prevalent of the community-acquired respiratory infections. Although pneumococcal disease affects children and adults, the incidence of pneumococcal pneumonia increases in persons older than 40 years. Pneumococci that are resistant to penicillin have emerged since 1974. The mortality rate from bacteremic pneumococcal infection exceeds 25% despite treatment with antibiotics.

The current unconjugated pneumococcal vaccine contains polysaccharide antigens from 23 of the types of pneumococci most commonly found in bacteremic pneumococcal disease. The 23-valent vaccine has been designed to induce a protective level of serum antibodies in immunocompetent adults. The vaccine is highly effective in healthy young adults, but its effectiveness in elderly persons and those in poor health has not been precisely determined. However, the vaccine is well tolerated and is recommended for the elderly, for patients who have cardiac or respiratory disease, and for other patients who are at high risk for pneumococcal infection, including those with sickle cell disease, splenic dysfunction, renal and hepatic disease, or immunodeficiency. The pneumococcal vaccine is given subcutaneously or intramuscularly as a 0.5-mL dose. In most circumstances, persons who have previously received the 14-valent vaccine should not be revaccinated with the 23-valent vaccine because doing so may be associated with increased local and systemic reactions. The duration of protection afforded by primary vaccination with pneumococcal vaccine seems to be 9 years or more. Persons who received pneumococcal vaccine before age 65 should be reimmunized at 65 if more than 6 years have passed since the initial vaccination.

A new conjugated heptavalent pneumococcal vaccine (Prevnar, PCV7) is now approved and recommended for all children younger than age 5. It is administered in 4 intramuscular doses at 2, 4, 6, and 12–15 months of age. The vaccine provides coverage for approximately 80% of the invasive pneumococcal diseases in children in the United States. The conjugated pneumococcal vaccine is recommended for all infants and toddlers younger than age 2 and for all children with chronic cardiopulmonary disorders or immune suppression between ages 2 and 5. A recent epidemiologic study revealed that the addition of pneumococcal vaccine to the childhood immunization schedule was associated with a 10-fold greater reduction in pneumonia and a 100-fold greater reduction in otitis media when compared with a previously reported reduction in culture-confirmed invasive pneumococcal infections.

Haemophilus influenzae

A vaccine against *H influenzae* type B (Hib vaccine) has been endorsed by the American Academy of Pediatrics and the Immunization Practices Advisory Committee. They have recommended that the vaccine be given to all children before age 24 months. The vaccine has significantly reduced the number of infections caused by encapsulated *H influenzae* type B, which previously affected 1 in every 200 children in the United States during the first 5 years of life. Approximately 60% of these infections were meningitis, amounting to about 10,000 cases each year. The type B capsule enhances the invasive potential of *H influenzae*. These encapsulated strains may result in life-threatening bacteremic infections. A critical factor that determines an individual's susceptibility to systemic *H influenzae* type B infection is the presence or absence of serum antibodies to capsule antigens. Thus, the induction of serum antibodies by immunization with Hib vaccine is a reasonable strategy.

The vaccine significantly reduces the risk of contracting systemic *H influenzae* type B infection and is protective in reducing the incidence of epiglottitis, meningitis, and orbital cellulitis. The majority of children who develop these *H influenzae* type B infections are older than 2 years. The vaccine is estimated to be 90% effective when given before age 24 months. Hib is one of the safest vaccine products approved for use in children. A newer combination vaccine (Hib-DTaP), which includes Hib conjugate vaccine and DTaP, is available and is effective and safe, offering the increased convenience of fewer injections for pediatric immunization. Other combined vaccines include the tetravalent acellular pertussis combined vaccine (DTacP-IPV; Tetravac) and the pentavalent 2-component acellular pertussis combined vaccine (DTacP-IPV-Hib; Pentavac). The hexavalent vaccine, DTPa-HBV-IPV/Hib, provides immunization for 6 diseases in a series of 3 single injections at 3, 4, and 5 months of age. In trials, the vaccine was shown to be safe, well tolerated, and immunologically equivalent to primary immunization with separately administered vaccines.

Meningococcus

A polysaccharide vaccine for the prevention of meningococcal meningitis is available and is recommended for use in military personnel, college students living in dormitories, travelers to endemic areas, close contacts of infected patients, new outbreaks, and high-risk patients, especially splenectomized and complement-deficient patients. The vaccine is approximately 85% effective in preventing the spread of group C meningococcal infections. The vaccine is used primarily in controlling spread of the disease and is generally not given as a routine immunization.

Travel Immunizations

Precise travel vaccination recommendations depend on the geographic regions planned as travel destinations, the duration of travel, consumption of local food and untreated water, and likelihood of close contact with local populations. Routine childhood vaccinations should be reviewed in all travelers and updated as needed. Yellow fever vaccination may be required for those who plan to enter a country located within a yellow fever endemic area or for travelers returning from an endemic area in order to prevent introduction of the disease. Immunization against HBV should be considered in travelers who expect to have close contact with local populations known to have high rates of hepatitis B transmission. Japanese encephalitis vaccine should be offered to those whose travel plans include prolonged trips to rural areas in Southeast Asia or the Indian subcontinent during the endemic season. Typhoid fever and hepatitis A immunizations are recommended for travelers who may be exposed to potentially contaminated food and water sources. Preexposure rabies vaccination should be considered in travelers whose plans include a prolonged visit in a remote area or in those who engage in activities that might involve working near animals.

New and Future Vaccines

New vaccines are now available for typhoid fever *(Salmonella typhi)*, anthrax, yellow fever, and Japanese encephalitis. Additional vaccines are currently undergoing clinical trials for HIV, hepatitis C, cholera, dysentery, *Campylobacter*, rotavirus, *Clostridium difficile*, respiratory syncytial virus, Ebola virus, malaria, cytomegalovirus, rabies, viral encephalitis, herpes simplex type 2, Epstein-Barr virus, TB, *Pseudomonas aeruginosa, Helicobacter pylori, Staphylococcus, Streptococcus,* HPV, parainfluenza virus, leishmaniasis, plague, smallpox, and anthrax.

Passive immunization with human hyperimmune globulin is currently available to treat or prevent rabies, tetanus, respiratory syncytial virus, cytomegalovirus, hepatitis A, hepatitis B, hepatitis C, herpes virus, and varicella-zoster infections.

Considering the worldwide impact of many other infectious diseases, there is considerable interest in developing new vaccines for the organisms that cause TB, AIDS, malaria, gonorrhea, syphilis, toxigenic *Escherichia coli* infection, leprosy, trachoma, and others. It is hoped that ongoing research will lead to safe and effective vaccines for many or all of these illnesses.

American Academy of Pediatrics. Prevention of influenza: recommendations for influenza immunization of children, 2006–2007. *Pediatrics.* 2007;119:846–851.

Centers for Disease Control and Prevention. Recommended childhood and adolescent immunization schedule—United States, 2005. *MMWR Morb Mortal Wkly Rep.* 2005;53(Nos. 51&52):Q1–Q3.

Chartrand SA. Varicella vaccine. *Pediatr Clin North Am.* 2000;47:373–394.

Committee on Infectious Diseases. Recommended immunization schedules for children and adolescents—United States, 2007. *Pediatrics.* 2007;119:207–208.

Glezen WP. New vaccines for old diseases: trivalent cold-adapted influenza vaccine. *Pediatr Ann.* 2004;33:545–50.

Hinman AR, Orenstein WA, Papania MJ. Evolution of measles elimination strategies in the United States. *J Infect Dis.* 2004;189(suppl 1):S17–S22.

Lavanchy D. Hepatitis B virus epidemiology, disease burden, treatment, and current and emerging prevention and control measures. *J Viral Hepat.* 2004;11:97–107.

Lo Re V 3rd, Gluckman SJ. Travel immunizations. *Am Fam Physician.* 2004;70:89–99.

Poehling KA, Lafleur BJ, Szilagyi PG, et al. Population-based impact of pneumococcal conjugate vaccine in young children. *Pediatrics.* 2004;114:755–761.

Pollard AJ, Levin M. Vaccines for prevention of meningococcal disease. *Pediatr Infect Dis J.* 2000;19:333–344.

Vazquez M. Varicella zoster virus infections in children after the introduction of live attenuated varicella vaccine. *Curr Opin Pediatr.* 2004;16:80–84.

Venters C, Graham W, Cassidy W. Recombivax-HB: perspectives past, present and future. *Expert Rev Vaccines.* 2004;3:119–129.

Welliver R, Monto AS, Carewicz O, et al. Effectiveness of oseltamivir in preventing influenza in household contacts. A randomized controlled trial. *JAMA*. 2001;285:748–754.

Zepp F, Knuf M, Heininger U, et al. Safety, reactogenicity and immunogenicity of a combined hexavalent tetanus, diphtheria, acellular pertussis, hepatitis B, inactivated poliovirus vaccine and *Haemophilus influenzae* type b conjugate vaccine, for primary immunization of infants. *Vaccine*. 2004;22:2226–2233.

Zuckerman JN, Zuckerman AJ. Recombinant hepatitis B triple antigen vaccine: Hepacare. *Expert Rev Vaccines*. 2002;1:141–144.

CHAPTER **14**

Medical Emergencies

Recent Developments

- Adult basic life-support rescuers should "phone first" for unresponsive adults. *Exceptions:* "phone fast" (provide cardiopulmonary resuscitation first) for adult victims of submersion, trauma, and drug intoxication.
- The availability of portable defibrillators in ambulances, public places, and airline jets increases the probability of survival for victims of out-of-hospital ventricular fibrillation.
- Victims of suspected ischemic stroke should be transported to a facility capable of initiating fibrinolytic therapy within 1 hour of arrival unless that facility is more than 30 minutes away by ground ambulance.

Introduction

Although only occasionally called upon to manage a patient in acute distress, the ophthalmologist must be aware of the diagnostic and therapeutic steps necessary for proper care of these emergencies. Infrequent use of these techniques makes periodic review of life-support techniques particularly important. Both the American Red Cross and the American Heart Association offer courses in, and periodic review of, basic life support and advanced cardiac life support (ACLS).

Cardiopulmonary Arrest

Cardiopulmonary resuscitation (CPR) is intended to rescue patients with acute circulatory failure, respiratory failure, or both. The most important determinant of short-term and long-term neurologically intact survival is the interval from the onset of the arrest to the restoration of effective spontaneous circulatory and respiratory function. Numerous studies have demonstrated that early defibrillation is the most important factor influencing survival and the minimization of sequelae. The sequences included here have been developed to optimize treatment. They are useful guidelines for most patients, but they do not preclude other measures that may be indicated for individual patients. The most crucial aspects of treatment are contained in the mnemonic *ABC—a*irway maintenance, *b*reathing, and *c*irculation.

Following are the steps to perform in an encounter with an unconscious patient:

1. Determine unresponsiveness. Attempt to arouse the patient by shaking the shoulders and saying, "Are you OK?" Do not shake the head or neck unless trauma to this area has been ruled out.
2. Activate the Emergency Medical Service (EMS) system if there is no response (911 where available). Rescuers should "phone first" for unresponsive adults. *Exceptions:* "phone fast" (provide CPR first) for adult victims of submersion, trauma, and drug intoxication. Be prepared to give the location and nature of the emergency and condition of the victim.
3. Position the victim supine on a firm, flat surface. Patients with suspected stroke should be rapidly transported to a hospital capable of initiating fibrinolytic therapy within 1 hour of arrival unless that facility is more than 30 minutes away by ground ambulance. These patients merit the same priorities for dispatch as patients with acute myocardial infarction or major trauma.
4. Open the airway. The head-tilt, chin-lift maneuver is preferred because it is most likely to provide a good airway opening; the jaw thrust and the neck lift are alternative maneuvers. The rescuer can use the chin lift to tilt the head backward by applying firm pressure to the forehead while placing the fingers of the other hand under the chin, supporting the mandible. The modified jaw thrust should be used if a neck injury is suspected.
5. Determine breathlessness. If spontaneous respiration is not present, gently pinch the nose closed with the index finger and thumb of the hand that is on the forehead. Make a tight seal over the patient's mouth and ventilate twice with slow, full breaths (1.5–2.0 seconds each). A 2-second pause should be observed between breaths. Slow breaths result in less gastric distension.

    Health care professionals should be proficient in the use of barrier devices for basic life support. A face shield can help prevent transmission of most infections and exposure to HIV in saliva. (One such device is the Microshield from Medical Devices International.) The mouth-to-nose technique is recommended when it is impossible to ventilate through the victim's mouth. Masks are more effective than face shields in delivering adequate ventilation. Features can include a non-rebreathing (1-way) valve, an extension tube to eliminate close proximity, low resistance, a bacterial filter, transparency, and ease in maintaining a seal over the mouth (eg, the Seal Easy Mask from Respironics). Alternative airway devices (eg, laryngeal mask airway and the esophageal-tracheal Combitube) may be acceptable when rescuers are trained in their use.
6. Determine presence or absence of pulse. Palpate the carotid pulse for at least 5 seconds to ensure that a pulse is not missed because of bradycardia.
7. Call for help again. If a carotid pulse is present, rescue breathing should be continued at a rate of 10–12 ventilations per minute. If there is no pulse, begin chest compressions.
8. To ensure good hand placement for chest compressions, place the heel of 1 hand at the midsternal region, with the bottom of the hand 1–2 fingerbreadths above the xiphoid process.

9. The recommended cardiac compression rate is 100 per minute. Cardiac output varies, but on average, 30% of normal cardiac output can be expected with CPR. The depth of chest compression is critical; optimal compressions are 1.0–1.5 inches for children and 1.5–2.0 inches for adults. Duration of chest compression should be at least 50% of the total duration of the cycle.
10. For 1- and 2-rescuer CPR: when the victim's airway is unprotected, 15 compressions should be performed before the victim is ventilated twice. About 3–5 seconds should be taken for 2 ventilations, and there should be a pause between each ventilation.
11. The rescuer responsible for airway management should assess the adequacy of compressions by periodically palpating for the carotid pulse. Once the patient is intubated, ventilations are continued at a rate of 12–15 per minute, without pausing for compressions. The rescuer should stop and check for return of pulse and spontaneous breathing every few minutes.
12. CPR is most effective when started immediately after cardiac arrest. If cardiac arrest has persisted for more than 10 minutes, CPR is unlikely to restore the patient's central nervous system (CNS) to prearrest status. If there is any question about the exact duration of cardiac arrest, the patient should be given the benefit of the doubt, and resuscitation should be started. In sharp contrast with cardiac arrest in adults, most causes of cardiopulmonary arrest in infants and children (younger than 8 years) are related to airway or ventilation problems rather than sudden cardiac arrest. In these patients, rescue support (especially rescue breathing) is essential and should be attempted first before activation of the EMS system (if the rescuer is trained).

The following adjuncts are helpful in CPR and are suggested components for a medical emergency tray, crash cart, or tackle box:

- oxygen, to enhance tissue oxygenation and to prevent or ameliorate a hypoxic state
- airways, adult and child, oral and nasal, to be used on unconscious or sedated patients
- a barrier device, such as a face shield or mask-to-mouth unit, to prevent disease transmission. Both can be used with supplemental oxygen and are especially useful if the rescuer is inexperienced in using a standard bag-valve device (eg, Ambu Bag), which should also be included as standard equipment to help secure the airway. Alternative airway devices may also be acceptable when appropriate (see No. 5 in the preceding list).
- intravenous drugs (Table 14-1)
- intravenous solutions: 5% dextrose and water, D5 lactated Ringer's, normal saline
- syringes (1, 5, and 10 mL), hypodermic needles (20, 22, and 25 gauge), and venous catheters
- a suction apparatus, tourniquet, taped tongue blade, and tape
- laryngoscope and endotracheal tubes (adult and child)

If there is no 911 community emergency phone system, it is essential to have the phone number of the local paramedic emergency squad posted near all office telephones.

Table 14-1 Medications Used in Acute Medical Emergencies

Drugs	Indications	Adult Dose	Adverse Effects
Epinephrine (1:1000)	Anaphylaxis	0.3–0.5 mg subcutaneously every 5 minutes	Tachycardia, hypertension
Epinephrine (1:10,000)	Asystole, ventricular fibrillation, EMD	Bolus 0.5–1.0 mg every 5 minutes	Hypertension in excess doses
Lidocaine	PVCs, ventricular tachycardia, ventricular fibrillation	Bolus 1.0 mg/kg with subsequent doses of 0.5 mg/kg to a maximum total dose of 3.0 mg/kg	Focal and grand mal seizures in excess doses
Atropine	Bradycardia, EMD, asystole	Bolus 0.5–1.0 mg every 5 minutes	Induced ventricular fibrillation, ventricular tachycardia, or supraventricular tachycardia
Diphenhydramine HCl (Benadryl)	Anaphylaxis and anaphylactoid reactions	12.5–25 mg (IV)	Drowsiness
Diazepam (Valium)	Seizures	5–10 mg	Sedation
Hydrocortisone sodium succinate (Solu-Cortef)	Anaphylaxis and anaphylactoid reactions	500 mg every 6 hours	Adrenal-pituitary axis suppression
Sodium bicarbonate	Severe metabolic acidosis	Bolus 1 mEq/kg	Hypernatremia, hypocalcemia, and metabolic alkalosis
Calcium chloride (ampule of 10% solution)	Acute hyperkalemia and hypocalcemia, calcium-channel blocker toxicity	2–4 mg/kg	Bradycardia
Aminophylline	Bronchospasm	6 mg/kg (loading dose)	Tachycardia
Glucose (D 50)	Profound hypoglycemia	Bolus 10 mL	Hyperglycemia

EMD = electro-mechanical dissociation
PVCs = premature ventricular contractions

Basic life support also outlines methods for aiding persons who are choking, including the Heimlich maneuver and appropriate manual techniques for removing foreign bodies from the oral pharynx. Epigastric thrusts should be attempted; up to 10–12 thrusts may be necessary. Thereafter, ventilation should be attempted. If these efforts are unsuccessful, the mouth should be cleared with a finger sweep and ventilation attempted again. Transtracheal ventilation by means of cricothyrotomy may be necessary. The increasing availability of portable defibrillators in ambulances, public places, and airline jets improves the probability of survival for victims of out-of-hospital ventricular fibrillation. Recent clinical trials showed that induced hypothermia after cardiac arrest could improve neurological outcome as well as reduce overall mortality.

In addition to providing guidelines for basic CPR, the American Heart Association has established guidelines and procedures for ACLS. ACLS includes intubations, defibrillation, cardioversion, pacemaker placement, administration of drugs and fluids, and communication with ambulance and hospital systems. Protocols and algorithms have been established in critical cardiac care for ventricular fibrillation, ventricular tachycardia, asystole, electro-mechanical dissociation, premature ventricular contractions, atrial tachycardia, and bradycardia. The provider of ACLS must precisely understand the actions, indications, doses, and adverse effects of the cardiac drugs used in the specific protocols. Except in dire emergencies, these drugs should be administered to treat cardiac arrhythmias *only* by physicians who use them routinely. Because of the comprehensive and changing nature of ACLS algorithms, these procedures are beyond the scope of this chapter.

Competency in pediatric emergency care may be enhanced with training in PLS (pediatric life support). In addition, ophthalmologists should be familiar with the ophthalmic manifestations of child abuse and shaken baby syndrome. These are discussed in BCSC Section 6, *Pediatric Ophthalmology and Strabismus*.

Shock

Shock is a state of generalized inadequacy of tissue perfusion that leads to impaired cellular metabolism and—if uncorrected—progresses to multiple organ failure and death.

Classification

Shock is classified according to the 4 primary pathophysiologic mechanisms involved:

- oligemic or hypovolemic (eg, hemorrhage, diabetic ketoacidosis, burns, or sequestration)
- cardiogenic (eg, myocardial infarction or arrhythmia)
- obstructive (eg, pericardial tamponade, pulmonary embolus, or tension pneumothorax)
- distributive, characterized by maldistribution of the vascular volume secondary to altered vasomotor tone (eg, sepsis, anaphylaxis, spinal cord insult, beriberi, or an arteriovenous fistula)

The type of shock can often be determined by history, physical examination, and appropriate diagnostic tests. Regardless of the event that precipitated the state of shock, microcirculatory failure is the common factor that eventually leads to death in advanced shock. Ventilatory failure appears to be the most significant factor in the morbidity and mortality of shock, with subsequent hypoxemia and metabolic acidosis leading to many complications.

If one rules out vasovagal syncope (by virtue of its short duration and because of knowledge of the situations that produce this condition), the basic life-support measures for the initial emergency care of the unconscious patient are similar. The most important aspects of treatment are the ABCs, the same principles used in CPR.

Failure of respiratory gas exchange is the most frequent single cause of death in patients with shock. One must first rule out respiratory obstruction. Oxygen is then given by mask, and if respiratory movements are shallow, mechanical ventilation is necessary. If laryngeal edema is present, as with anaphylaxis, endotracheal intubation (if possible), tracheotomy, or cricothyrotomy is indicated. Respiratory obstruction can be assumed if there is stridor with respiratory movements or if cyanosis persists even when adequate ventilatory techniques have been applied. A conscious patient in distress who cannot speak but is developing cyanosis may be choking on food or a foreign body; the Heimlich maneuver has been shown to be an effective means of treatment.

Assessment

The vital signs must be monitored. The clinical syndrome is usually characterized by an altered sensorium, relative hypotension, tachycardia, tachypnea, oliguria, metabolic acidosis, weak or absent pulse, pallor, diaphoresis, and cool skin (however, the skin may be warm in septic shock). Decreased pulse pressure is often an early sign of shock, and systolic pressures of less than 90 mm Hg are often associated with vital organ hypoperfusion. Blood pressure, however, is not always a reliable indicator of tissue perfusion. The following tests and procedures are useful for assessment:

- arterial blood gases
- electrocardiogram (ECG)
- pulmonary artery (Swan-Ganz) catheter monitoring
- complete blood count: a low hematocrit may indicate blood loss; a high hematocrit may indicate intravascular volume depletion
- serum electrolytes and creatinine
- renal function: oliguria, increased urinary osmolarity, and decreased urinary sodium are signs of tissue hypoperfusion

Treatment

Treatment of shock is often complex; specific guidelines are beyond the scope of this text. General guidelines for the treatment of shock are as follows:

- The patient should be positioned with the legs elevated.
- Supplemental oxygen should be administered to enhance tissue oxygenation. Mechanical ventilation may be necessary to maintain the Po_2 and to prevent respiratory acidosis.
- Volume expansion with an IV infusion is of primary importance in maintaining circulation. Initially, a crystalloid solution (ie, normal saline or Ringer's lactate) should be administered rapidly.
- Sodium bicarbonate, given intravenously over 5–10 minutes, is indicated for correction of severe metabolic acidosis. The dosage should be titrated according to arterial blood gas results.
- Vasopressor drugs (norepinephrine bitartrate or dopamine) may be needed for augmentation of cardiac output and perfusion of vital organs after an adequate circulating volume is established.

- Antibiotic therapy should be initiated promptly if sepsis is suspected.
- Low-dose corticosteroids have recently been recommended in the treatment of cases of septic shock.

Anaphylaxis

One specific cause of shock that requires immediate and specific therapy is anaphylaxis. *Anaphylaxis* is an acute allergic reaction following antigen exposure in a previously sensitized person. It is usually mediated by immunoglobulin E antibodies and involves release of chemical mediators from mast cells and basophils. *Anaphylactoid reactions,* which are more common yet less severe, are the result of direct release of these chemical mediators triggered by nonantigenic agents. Anaphylaxis or anaphylactoid reactions may occur after exposure to pollen, drugs, foreign serum, insect stings, diagnostic agents such as iodinated contrast materials or fluorescein, vaccines, local anesthetics, and food products. The most important parameter for prediction of such an attack is a history of a previous allergic reaction to any other drug or possible antigen. Unfortunately, a history of known sensitivity may not always be elicited.

Anaphylaxis is particularly important to the ophthalmologist, in view of the increasing number of surgical procedures and fluorescein angiograms being performed in the office setting. It is estimated that allergic reactions to fluorescein (including urticaria) occur in up to 1% of all angiograms. In one survey, the overall risk of a severe reaction was 1 in 1900 patients, including a risk of respiratory compromise in 1 in 3800 subjects. Any patient developing diaphoresis, apprehension, pallor, a rapid and weak pulse, or any combination thereof after administration of a drug should be considered to have an allergic reaction until proven otherwise. The diagnosis is certain if there is associated generalized itching, urticaria, angioedema of the skin, dyspnea, wheezing, or arrhythmia. This process may lead rapidly to loss of consciousness, shock, cardiac arrest, coma, or death.

Once an acute allergic reaction is suspected, prompt treatment is indicated:

- Epinephrine (0.3–0.5 mL of 1:1000) injected subcutaneously or intramuscularly in a limb opposite to the antigenic agent exposure site is usually effective to maintain circulation and blood pressure.
- Intravenous volume expansion may be needed to restore and maintain tissue perfusion.
- Oxygen should be administered to all patients in respiratory distress.
- Tracheotomy or cricothyrotomy is indicated when laryngeal edema is unresponsive to the previous methods or when oral intubation cannot be performed.
- Hydrocortisone should be administered for serious or prolonged reactions. When given early, corticosteroids help control possible long-term sequelae.
- Antihistamines are also helpful in slowing or halting the ongoing allergic response but are of limited value in acute anaphylaxis.
- All patients with anaphylaxis or anaphylactoid reactions should be observed for at least 6 hours.

In cases of mild allergic reactions, the physician can give 25–50 mg of diphenhydramine (Benadryl) orally or intramuscularly and observe the patient closely to determine whether further treatment is necessary. Pretreating high-risk patients with an antihistamine, corticosteroids, or both prior to a fluorescein angiogram may reduce the risk of an allergic reaction. In all cases of anaphylaxis, supportive treatment should be maintained until the emergency medical team arrives.

For patients with a known history of anaphylaxis, personal emergency kits containing epinephrine are available and can be used until medical help arrives. The kits are designed to allow self-treatment by the patient or administration by a family member or an informed bystander. The Ana-Kit contains a syringe and needle preloaded with 0.6 mL of 1:1000 epinephrine. The physician who prescribes this kit must give detailed instructions concerning the use of the device. The EpiPen or EpiPen Jr contains a spring-loaded automatic injector, which does not permit graduated doses to be given but automatically injects 0.3 mg of epinephrine (0.15 mg in the junior version) when the device is triggered by pressure on the thigh. The epinephrine ampules contained in these self-treatment kits have a limited shelf life and should be replaced when the expiration date is reached or if the solution becomes discolored.

> Annane D, Bellissant E, Cavaillon JM. Septic shock. *Lancet.* 2005;365:63–78.
> Cummins RO, ed. *Advanced Cardiac Life Support Provider Manual.* Dallas: American Heart Association; 2003.
> Graham CA, Parke TR. Critical care in the emergency department: shock and circulatory support. *Emerg Med J.* 2005;22:17–21.
> Guidelines 2000 for Cardiopulmonary Resuscitation and Emergency Cardiovascular Care. The American Heart Association in collaboration with the International Liaison Committee on Resuscitation. *Circulation.* 2000;102(8 suppl):I129–135.
> Holzer M, Sterz F; Hypothermia After Cardiac Arrest Study Group. Therapeutic hypothermia after cardiopulmonary resuscitation. *Expert Rev Cardiovasc Ther.* 2003;1:317–325.
> Keh D, Sprung CL. Use of corticosteroid therapy in patients with sepsis and septic shock: an evidence-based review. *Crit Care Med.* 2004;32(11 suppl):S527–S533.
> Noone MC, Osguthorpe JD. Anaphylaxis. *Otolaryngol Clin North Am.* 2003;36:1009–1020.
> Roth CS, Weaver DT, eds. *Pocket Manual of Emergency Medical Therapy.* 4th ed. Toronto: Decker; 1987.

Seizures and Status Epilepticus

A *seizure* is a paroxysmal episode of abnormal electrical activity in the brain resulting in involuntary transient neurological, motor activity, behavioral, or autonomic dysfunction. Seizures can present with many different clinical manifestations, but most fit into the categories of simple partial, complex partial, or generalized tonic-clonic. See also Chapter 12, Behavioral and Neurologic Disorders, for further discussion.

As in the treatment of all medical emergencies, the first consideration is airway maintenance. This becomes particularly important if the seizure progresses to *status epilepticus,* which is defined as a prolonged seizure or as multiple seizures without intervening periods of normal consciousness. Status epilepticus, like seizures, may have a local onset with secondary generalization or may be generalized from onset. A seizure is considered status epilepticus when it lasts for 30 minutes or longer. Status epilepticus is often found concomitantly with hyperthermia, acidosis, hypoxia, tachycardia, hypercapnia, and mydriasis and, if persistent, may be associated with irreversible brain injury. Status epilepticus that is completely stopped within 2 hours usually has relatively minor morbidity compared with episodes lasting longer than 2 hours.

Major causes of seizures and status epilepticus include

- drug withdrawal, such as from anticonvulsants, benzodiazepines, barbiturates, or alcohol
- metabolic abnormalities, such as hypoglycemia, hyponatremia, hypocalcemia, or hypomagnesemia
- conditions that affect the CNS, such as infection, trauma, stroke, hypoxia, ischemia, or sleep deprivation
- toxic levels of various drugs

In management, it is important not only to stop the seizure activity but also to identify and treat the underlying cause. Following is a general treatment protocol:

1. Note time of seizure onset. Monitor airway, vital signs, and ECG.
2. Establish IV line. Position patient on side to allow gravity drainage of saliva. Insert oral airway if possible. Some experts advocate using a washcloth or taped tongue blade as a bite block.
3. Draw blood immediately; check level of glucose, electrolytes, calcium, and magnesium; and check toxicology screen.
4. Give 50 mL of 50% dextrose IV push (or 1 mL/kg).
5. Administer a benzodiazepine such as diazepam (Valium) or lorazepam (Ativan) slowly by IV line, titrated to an effective dose, usually 5.0 mg/min to a total dose of 0.5 mg/kg.
6. Proceed immediately to administer phenytoin (or fosphenytoin) intravenously. Monitor pulse rate, blood pressure, and ECG. Watch especially for hypotension.
7. If seizures continue for 20 minutes, administer a loading dose of phenobarbital.
8. Emergency medical management of seizures is best left to physicians who perform this routinely. Activation of the emergency response (911) team is indicated in all cases of acute seizure onset.

Gaitanis JN, Drislane FW. Status epilepticus: a review of different syndromes, their current evaluation, and treatment. *Neurologist.* 2003;9:61–76.

Toxic Reactions to Local Anesthetics and Other Agents

Toxic overdose is an additional cause of unconsciousness or of acute distress in a conscious patient, and it must be considered whenever the patient is undergoing a procedure that requires local anesthesia. Table 14-2 lists commonly used local anesthetics with their maximum safe dose.

Reactions following the administration of local anesthetics are almost always toxic and only rarely allergic. A high blood level of local anesthetic can be produced by the following: too large a dose, unusually rapid absorption (including inadvertent IV administration), and unusually slow detoxification or elimination (especially in liver disease). Hypersensitivity (ie, decreased patient tolerance) and idiosyncratic reactions are rare, but

Table 14-2 Maximum Recommended Local Anesthetic Doses

Agent	Commercially Available Concentrations (%) 1% = 10 mg/cc	Plain Solutions, mg	Epinephrine-Containing Solutions, mg
Chloroprocaine	1.0, 2.0, 3.0	800	1000
Lidocaine	0.5, 1.0, 1.5, 2.0, 4.0, 5.0	300	500
Mepivacaine (Carbocaine)	1.0, 1.5, 2.0	300	225
Bupivacaine	0.25, 0.5, 0.75	175	225
Tetracaine	1.0	100	100

they may occur with local anesthetic agents, as with any drug. Although true allergic or anaphylactic reactions are also rare, they may occur, particularly with agents belonging to the aminoester class.

Toxic reactions cause overstimulation of the CNS, which may lead to excitement, restlessness, apprehension, disorientation, tremors, and convulsions (cerebral cortex effects), as well as nausea and vomiting (medulla effects). Cardiac effects initially include tachycardia and hypertension. Ultimately, however, depression of the CNS and the cardiovascular system occurs, which may result in sleepiness and coma (cerebral cortex effects) as well as in irregular respirations, sighing, dyspnea, and respiratory arrest (medulla effects). Cardiac effects of CNS depression are bradycardia and hypotension.

Injected local anesthetic agents can also produce a direct toxic effect on muscle tissue. In the case of retrobulbar injections, this can result initially in muscle weakness, which in some patients is followed by muscle contracture. Extraocular motility can be affected, resulting in diplopia (usually hypertropia) that may require surgical revision. Hyaluronidase may be partially protective by allowing more rapid diffusion of the anesthetic agent following injection.

Signs of cortical stimulation require immediate treatment, before progressive changes to cortical and medullary function and cardiac depression occur. Increased metabolic activity of the CNS and poor ventilatory exchange lead to cerebral hypoxia. Treatment consists of oxygenation, supportive airway care, and titrated IV administration of midazolam, which is used to suppress cortical stimulation. Respiratory stimulants are to be avoided because the medullary respiratory center has already been stimulated by the local anesthetic, and these drugs lead to eventual respiratory depression.

In cases of toxic overdose, other emergency procedures include suctioning if vomiting occurs and using a taped tongue blade if convulsions develop. If shock develops, the appropriate drugs can be administered by IV infusion.

The addition of *epinephrine* to the local anesthetic can also cause adverse reactions. Epinephrine can produce symptoms similar to early CNS stimulation by local anesthetic, such as anxiety, restlessness, tremor, hypertension, and tachycardia. Unlike local anesthetics, however, epinephrine does not produce convulsions or bradycardia as the toxic reaction proceeds. Oxygen is useful in the treatment of epinephrine overdoses.

One study looked at the effect of intraocular epinephrine irrigation at a concentration that maintained pupillary dilation during routine extracapsular cataract surgery. The study found no additional risk of significant interval changes in either arterial blood pressure or heart rate in patients with or without preexisting hypertension.

The administration of retrobulbar *bupivacaine* has been associated with respiratory arrest. This reaction may be caused by intra-arterial injection of the local anesthetic, with retrograde flow to the cerebral circulation. It could also result from puncture of the dural sheath of the optic nerve during retrobulbar block, with diffusion of the local anesthetic along the subdural space in the midbrain. A large prospective study comparing retrobulbar injection of 0.75% bupivacaine plus 2.0% lidocaine to 0.75% bupivacaine plus 4.0% lidocaine found that those patients receiving 4.0% lidocaine mixed with bupivacaine had an almost 9 times greater risk of respiratory arrest than the patients receiving 2.0% lidocaine mixed with bupivacaine. (See also Chapter 15, Perioperative Management in Ocular Surgery, for further discussion of reactions to local anesthetics.)

The use of *edrophonium chloride* (Tensilon) in the diagnosis of myasthenia gravis can have toxic side effects. The signs and symptoms result from cholinergic stimulation and may include nausea, vomiting, diarrhea, sweating, increased bronchial and salivary secretions, muscle fasciculations and weakness, and bradycardia. Some of these signs may be transient and self-limited because of the very short half-life of IV edrophonium. Whenever a Tensilon test is to be performed, a syringe containing 0.5 mg of atropine sulfate must be immediately available. (Some physicians routinely pretreat, with atropine, all patients undergoing Tensilon testing.)

If signs of excess cholinergic stimulation occur, 0.4–0.5 mg of atropine sulfate should be administered intravenously. This dose may be repeated every 3–10 minutes if necessary. The total dose of atropine necessary to counteract the toxic effects is seldom more than 2 mg. If toxic signs progress, the treatment described earlier for toxic overdose may be necessary.

> Brown SM, Brooks SE, Mazow ML, et al. Cluster of diplopia cases after periocular anesthesia without hyaluronidase. *J Cataract Refract Surg.* 1999;25:1245–1249.
> Capo H, Guyton DL. Ipsilateral hypertropia after cataract surgery. *Ophthalmology.* 1996;103:721–730.
> Wittpenn JR, Rapoza P, Sternberg P, et al. Respiratory arrest following retrobulbar anesthesia. *Ophthalmology.* 1986;93:867–870.
> Yamaguchi H, Matsumoto Y. Stability of blood pressure and heart rate during intraocular epinephrine irrigation. *Ann Ophthalmol.* 1988;20:58–60.

Ocular Side Effects of Systemic Medications

Because of the development of compartmentalized medical specialties and the proliferation of specific therapeutic agents, patients frequently have multiple simultaneous drug regimens. Often, no single physician (among the several to whom a patient may relate) is aware of all the drugs the patient is taking. The clinical problem is compounded by several factors. For example, the physician is often not aware of what other drugs a patient uses or might not be familiar with agents used outside of his or her specialty. In addition, the patient may have a drug interaction that affects a bodily system not usually monitored by a given specialist. Finally, the patient might not associate a symptom with a particular drug that has been used, if that symptom is not related to the system for which the drug was given. For example, the association between ophthalmic epinephrine therapy and cardiac arrhythmia might not be readily apparent to the patient. Conversely, the commonly prescribed erectile dysfunction agent sildenafil (Viagra) has been noted to block photoreceptor signals, causing electroretinographic changes, visual disturbances, and increased light sensitivity. The spectrum of systemic side effects with commonly used ophthalmic drugs is covered extensively elsewhere in this series (see BCSC Section 9, *Intraocular Inflammation and Uveitis*, and Section 10, *Glaucoma*). The ocular side effects of several commonly prescribed systemic medications are presented in Table 14-3. Drug interactions must always be suspected in patients on multiple topical and systemic agents.

Table 14-3 Potential Ocular Effects of Popular Drugs*

Drug (Trade Name)	Side Effects
Antibiotics	
Cefaclor (Ceclor)	Mild inflammation of ocular surface (rare); eyelid problems; nystagmus; visual hallucinations
Cefuroxime axetil (Ceftin)	Mild inflammation of ocular surface (rare)
Ciprofloxacin (Cipro)	Eyelid problems; exacerbation of myasthenia; visual sensations
Tetracycline, doxycycline, minocycline (Dynacin, Minocin)	Papilledema secondary to pseudotumor cerebri; transient myopia; blue-gray, dark blue, or brownish pigmentation of the sclera; hyperpigmentation of eyelids or conjunctiva; diplopia
Rifampin (Rifadin and others)	Conjunctival hyperemia; exudative conjunctivitis; increased lacrimation
Antidepressants/anxiolytics	
Alprazolam (Xanax)	Diplopia; decreased or blurred vision; decreased accommodation; abnormal extraocular muscle movements; allergic conjunctivitis
Fluoxetine (Prozac)	Blurred vision; photophobia; mydriasis; dry eye; conjunctivitis; diplopia
Imipramine (Tofranil)	Decreased vision; decreased accommodation; slight mydriasis; photosensitivity
Antiepileptics	
Topiramate (Topamax)	Conjunctivitis, abnormal accommodation, photophobia, strabismus, mydriasis, iritis, acute myopia, secondary angle-closure glaucoma
Analgesics, anti-inflammatory agents	
Aspirin	Transient blurred vision; transient myopia; hypersensitivity reactions
Ibuprofen (Advil)	Blurred vision; decreased vision; diplopia; photosensitivity; dry eyes; decrease in color vision; optic or retrobulbar neuritis
Naproxen (Anaprox, Aleve)	Decreased vision; changes in color vision; optic or retrobulbar neuritis; papilledema secondary to pseudotumor cerebri; photosensitivity; corneal opacities
Piroxicam (Feldene)	Decreased vision; photosensitivity
Hydroxychloroquine (Plaquenil)	Maculopathy with decreased vision and color perception
Disease-modifying agents	
Isotretinoin (Accutane)	Corneal opacities, decreased night vision
Interferon	Cotton-wool spots

(Continued)

Table 14-3 *(continued)*

Drug (Trade Name)	Side Effects
Asthma, allergy drugs	
Corticosteroids (general)	Decreased vision; posterior subcapsular cataracts; increased IOP
Antihistamines (general)	Decreased vision; may induce or aggravate dry eye; pupillary changes; decreased accommodation; blurred vision; decreased mucoid or lacrimal secretions; diplopia
Cardiovascular drugs	
Amiodarone (Cordarone, Pacerone)	Photophobia; blurred vision; corneal opacities; subcapsular lens opacities; optic neuropathy
β-Blockers (general)	Decreased vision; visual hallucinations; decreased IOP; decreased lacrimation
Alpha-1a selective antagonists, tamsulosin (Flomax)	Intraoperative floppy iris syndrome (IFIS), with a sluggish hypotonic iris, miosis, iris prolapse
Calcium channel blockers	Decreased or blurred vision; periorbital edema; ocular irritation (general)
Captopril/enalapril (Vaseretic)	Angioedema of the eye and orbit; conjunctivitis; decreased vision
Digitalis glycosides	Decreased vision; color vision defects; glare phenomenon; flickering vision
Diuretics (thiazide-type)	Decreased vision; myopia; color vision abnormalities; retinal edema
Flecainide (Tambocor)	Blurred vision; decreased vision; decreased accommodation; abnormal visual sensations; decreased depth perception; nystagmus
Warfarin (Coumadin)	Retinal hemorrhages in susceptible persons; hyphema; allergic reactions; conjunctivitis; lacrimation; decreased vision
Drugs used in the treatment of impotence	
Cialis (Tadalafil)	Sudden loss of vision, retinal vascular occlusions, decreased color perception, conjunctivitis, photophobia
Sildenafil (Viagra)	
Hormones, hormone-related drugs	
Clomiphene (Clomid and others)	Visual sensations; decreased vision; mydriasis; visual field constriction; photophobia; diplopia
Danazol (Danocrine)	Decreased vision; diplopia; papilledema secondary to pseudotumor cerebri; visual field defects
Estradiol (general)	Decreased vision; retinal vascular disorders; papilledema secondary to pseudotumor cerebri; fluctuations of corneal curvature and corneal steepening; color vision abnormalities
Leuprolide (Lupron)	Blurred vision; papilledema secondary to pseudotumor cerebri; retinal hemorrhage and branch vein occlusion; eye pain; lid edema
Oral contraceptives (general)	Decreased vision; retinal vascular disorders; papilledema secondary to pseudotumor cerebri; color vision abnormalities
Tamoxifen (Nolvadex)	Decreased vision; corneal opacities; retinal edema or hemorrhage; optic disc swelling; retinopathy; decreased color vision; possible optic neuritis or neuropathy

*For ocular side effects of cancer chemotherapy agents, see Chapter 11, Table 11-1.

Modified with permission from Doran M. When good drugs go bad. *EyeNet.* 2001;5:43–48. Chart updated 2005.

The ophthalmologist can minimize adverse effects from multiple drug therapy by doing the following:

- Maintain a high level of suspicion for drug interactions.
- Question the patient closely about other drug therapy and general symptoms.
- Encourage all patients to carry a card listing the drugs they use.
- Keep in close communication with the patient's primary care physician.
- Consult with a clinical pharmacologist or internist whenever a question of drug interaction arises.

Unrecognized adverse effects of topical or systemic medications should be reported to the National Registry of Drug-Induced Ocular Side Effects:

Frederick Fraunfelder, MD
Casey Eye Institute
Oregon Health Sciences University
3375 SW Terwilliger Blvd.
Portland, OR 97201-4197
Phone: 503-494-5686
Fax: 503-494-6864

Doran M. When good drugs go bad. *EyeNet*. 2001;5:43–48.

Fraunfelder FT, Fraunfelder FW. *Drug-Induced Ocular Side Effects*. 5th ed. Boston: Butterworth-Heinemann; 2001.

Parssinen O, Leppänen E, Keski-Rahkonen P, Mauriala T, Duqué B, Lehtonen M. Influence of tamsulosin on the iris and its implications for cataract surgery. *Invest Ophthalmol Vis Sci.* 2006;47:3766–3771.

CHAPTER **15**

Perioperative Management in Ocular Surgery

Ocular surgery is generally associated with low morbidity and mortality, as it is usually (though not always) of short duration and, in general, there is not much blood loss. Still, the perioperative management of eye patients can be challenging. Patients are frequently elderly and have numerous medical conditions. Sometimes the surgery may be directly related to a systemic disease such as diabetes mellitus or thyroid disease. Ophthalmic surgery is also very delicate and may have specific requirements about the patient's level of alertness during the procedure. The level of sedation is particularly important during topical cataract surgery.

This chapter divides the discussion of perioperative management into preoperative medical assessment, intraoperative complications, and postoperative care.

Preoperative Assessment

Adult Patients

All patients require a history and physical examination (Table 15-1). The goals of the preoperative assessment are to review any known medical problems that might have some impact on the patient's surgical course (eg, the patient has a chronic cough that might make surgery difficult). The history or physical should identify any unknown medical conditions that may affect the patient's course, such as recent angina or stroke symptoms that have not been evaluated. The history and physical should ensure that the patient is in the best condition possible for the procedure (eg, the patient's diabetes should be under control). Adjustments in the patient's therapy, such as stopping aspirin or other anticoagulants, may be necessary so that the chances for a successful procedure are optimized. Furthermore, according to the American Academy of Ophthalmology ethics policy statement regarding pretreatment assessment, the responsibilities of the ophthalmologist include medical diagnosis and preoperative treatment of the patient. The ophthalmologist may delegate the acquisition of the data required for the preoperative history and physical examination. However, the synthesis of that data and the preoperative planning must be done by the operating ophthalmologist.

It is accepted that all patients should have a history and physical examination prior to surgery. There is not, however, universal agreement about the extent of the preoperative

Table 15-1 Suggested Elements of an Admission History and Physical

History
Presenting diagnosis/condition
History of present illness
Past medical history
Allergies
Current medications
Family history
Social history
Review of systems

Physical Examination
Vital signs
General appearance
Eyes, ears, nose, and throat
Head and neck
Cardiovascular system
Abdomen
Respiratory tract
Genitourinary tract
Musculoskeletal system
Skin
Neurological system

testing that should be performed in asymptomatic patients. A study by Schein and co-workers has questioned the value of routine preoperative medical testing before cataract surgery. The direct cost to Medicare for such testing prior to cataract surgery is estimated at $150 million each year. Routine medical tests before cataract surgery may be unnecessary for asymptomatic patients because these tests do not increase the safety of the procedure. Preoperative medical tests can be ordered when a finding on a history or physical examination indicates a need.

Pediatric Patients

There is no evidence that abnormalities in a complete blood count affect the choice of anesthetic management for asymptomatic children. In general, if the child is healthy and there is no long-term use of prescribed medications, then laboratory tests are unnecessary even for general anesthesia. African American patients, if they have not been tested previously, should be screened for sickle cell disease or trait because some aspects of anesthetic management will change in patients with hemoglobinopathy. Routine pregnancy testing of female patients of childbearing age, prior to anesthesia, is a complex issue—even more so in minors because individual states may have statutes concerning parental notification of test results. The anesthesiologist will likely discuss the need for preoperative pregnancy testing; however, pregnancy testing without consent is neither legal nor ethical.

The issue of elective eye surgery in children with an upper respiratory tract infection is controversial. A child who is already ill will feel even worse after surgery, and the significance of a postoperative fever may be difficult to interpret. Furthermore, contaminated nasal discharge could possibly enter the ocular area during surgery. If a child has a fever above 101°F, has purulent nasal discharge, or appears systemically ill, a bacterial lower respiratory tract infection should be considered. This circumstance argues for a delay so that the increased risk of laryngospasm and bronchospasm associated with general anesthesia can be avoided. However, in the absence of such findings—such as a child who appears well except for a runny nose—many anesthesiologists elect to proceed.

Specific Preoperative Concerns

Obstructive pulmonary disease

Chronic obstructive pulmonary disease (COPD) can pose a distinct problem in ophthalmic surgery. Cessation of smoking is extremely helpful in reducing intraoperative and postoperative coughing. Preoperative bronchopulmonary care with chest physiotherapy can decrease a patient's susceptibility to infection and improve air exchange. General anesthesia may be preferred over local anesthesia because the anesthesiologist may have better control over tracheal bronchial secretions and the cough reflex. (See also Chapter 6.)

Beta-blockers

Preoperative use of beta-blockers has been shown to reduce mortality in patients undergoing noncardiac surgery. The surgeries that carry the highest cardiac risk and the most benefit from preoperative use of beta-blockers are major operations on elderly patients. Some ophthalmic surgeries, such as orbital surgery or facial surgery, may benefit from preoperative use of beta-blockers in selected patients. Patients who should receive beta-blockers before surgery include patients with previous myocardial infarction, those with a positive stress test, or patients with 2 or more risk factors for coronary artery disease. This protocol is based on American Heart Association/American College of Cardiology guidelines, available on the Internet at http://www.acc.org/clinical/guidelines/perio/update/pdf/perio_update.pdf.

Malignant hyperthermia

Malignant hyperthermia (MH), which is discussed at greater length later in this chapter, is a serious intraoperative complication triggered by certain anesthetic agents. Potentially fatal if diagnosis and treatment are delayed, MH can occur as an isolated case or as a dominantly inherited disorder with incomplete penetrance. Physical disorders associated with MH include strabismus, muscular dystrophy, and congenital ptosis. The incidence is reported variously as between 1:6000 and 1:30,000 and is generally thought to be higher in children. Malignant hyperthermia can occur in all age groups, however.

The preoperative personal and family history is helpful in determining whether the patient is at risk for MH. Patients with a history of masseter muscle rigidity after the administration of succinylcholine may be at risk for MH. The diagnosis of MH should be considered if the patient or other family members have a history of any of the following during anesthesia:

- sudden onset of tachycardia

- breathing problems
- high fever
- ventricular arrhythmias
- cardiac failure

Muscle biopsy with in vitro halothane and caffeine contraction testing is the most specific test to confirm the clinical diagnosis. Patients who have a relative with MH or a history that is unconfirmed for but suggestive of MH should undergo testing to detect susceptibility. Creatine kinase measurement is not reliable. Although levels are elevated in up to two thirds of patients with MH, normal results have no predictive value.

Malignant hyperthermia occurs most commonly with the use of succinylcholine, often combined with an inhalation anesthetic such as halothane. Safer agents include nitrous oxide, barbiturates, narcoleptics, antipyretics, nondepolarizing muscle relaxants, propofol, and droperidol. However, even the stress of having surgery itself can trigger this complication.

Latex allergy

Latex allergy is a condition that has caused growing concern in the last few years. The overall prevalence of latex allergy has not been determined, but certain populations appear to be at particular risk for reactions. Health care workers and hospital employees can experience progressive sensitization to latex because of repeated occupational exposure. This sensitivity is accentuated if the health care worker has a history of atopy. Certain patient populations also are at significant risk for latex allergy and anaphylaxis, including patients with myelodysplasia or spina bifida and those who have undergone repeated urinary catheterization or frequent surgical procedures. A cross-reactivity with bananas, avocados, mangoes, and chestnuts has been demonstrated, and allergies to these foods have also been associated with latex allergy. Other implicated foods include apricots, celery, figs, grapes, papayas, passion fruit, peaches, and pineapples. A history of reactivity to balloons also suggests a latex allergy.

Any patient suspected of having latex allergy should be referred to an allergist, and the surgery should be delayed until this concern can be evaluated. The entire operating room environment must be changed to care for the patient allergic to latex. Furthermore, the allergic patient should be the first case of the day in that particular operating room.

Local anesthetic allergies

A patient reporting an allergy to local anesthetics should be quizzed about the nature of the "allergic" reaction. Occasionally, the patient may have experienced an intravascular injection of epinephrine, a vasovagal attack, or even a panic attack rather than a true allergic reaction. A true allergic reaction to a "-caine" medication includes wheezing, urticaria, and respiratory distress. A history of sweating, tachycardia, headache, or hypertension suggests intravascular injection of epinephrine. An overdose of local anesthetic produces tinnitus, a bad taste in the mouth, or central nervous system (CNS) changes such as confusion, slurred speech, or respiratory arrest. An overdose is unlikely in ophthalmic anesthesia, given the relatively small volumes that are used.

A true allergy to local anesthetics is more likely with the ester derivatives such as procaine, tetracaine, chloroprocaine, and benzocaine. An allergy can even occur to the preservative Paraben, which is widely used in multidose vials of local anesthetics, as well as in other medicines, cosmetics, and foods.

If a patient is suspected of having a true allergy to local anesthetics, preoperative skin testing by appropriate personnel with adequate monitoring and resuscitation equipment nearby is recommended. If the patient proves to have true ester allergy, *amides* (lidocaine, bupivacaine, or mepivacaine) can be used as an alternative. Conversely, if the patient has a true allergy to amides, an ester-type of anesthetic such as chloroprocaine or tetracaine can be used. Preservative-free agents are also available. (Allergic or toxic reactions to local anesthetics are discussed more fully later in this chapter, as well as in Chapter 14, Medical Emergencies.)

Preoperative Fasting

Questions often arise as to how long the patient must be kept on NPO status before surgery. A pediatric patient who is kept on NPO status for 10–12 hours preoperatively may become hypotensive as a result of dehydration. It has been shown that use of clear liquids orally up to 2 hours prior to surgery does not lead to any higher incidence of aspiration or other gastrointestinal complications of general anesthesia or local anesthesia.

The purpose of preoperative fasting is to reduce the particulate matter in the stomach and to lower the gastric fluid volume and acidity in case aspiration of stomach contents occurs. Patients with diabetes, particularly those with autonomic neuropathy, are at risk for gastroparesis. Pregnant patients have a higher-than-normal risk of aspiration. In addition, patients with known gastroesophageal reflux disease and those with peptic ulcer disease may also have some increased risk of aspiration.

Oral administration of an H_2 blocker such as *ranitidine* or *famotidine* 2–4 hours before surgery reduces the percentage of patients with low gastric pH or high gastric volume. *Metoclopramide* or *cisapride* (restricted access for cisapride in the United States) also promotes intestinal motility and decreases reflux; these drugs are especially useful in a nonfasting patient who requires urgent surgery. (See Table 15-2 for selected perioperative medications.)

Management of Medications

Anticoagulants

Drugs that interfere with platelet function should be discontinued before eyelid, orbit, or retinal surgery. Most surgeons do not routinely stop antiplatelet drugs or anticoagulants prior to topical cataract surgery (no retrobulbar or peribulbar injection). Aspirin irreversibly acetylates platelet cyclooxygenase. Because cyclooxygenase is not regenerated in the circulation within the life span of the platelet, and because this enzyme is essential for the aggregation of platelets, a single aspirin may affect platelet function for a week. All other drugs that inhibit platelet function (eg, vitamin E, indomethacin, sulfinpyrazone, dipyridamole, tricyclic antidepressants, phenothiazines, furosemide, steroids) do not inhibit cyclooxygenase function irreversibly; these drugs disturb platelet function for only

Table 15-2 **Selected Perioperative Medications**

Name (Generic and Brand)	Uses
Metoclopramide (Reglan)	Relief of gastric paresis, reduction of gastroesophageal reflux, perioperative antiemetic
Cisapride (Propulsid)	Reduction of gastroesophageal reflux
Midazolam (Versed)	Preoperative sedation
Propofol (Diprivan)	Preoperative sedation/general anesthesia
Diazepam (Valium)	Preoperative sedation
Alfentanil (Alfenta)	Analgesic/anesthetic
Fentanyl citrate (Sublimaze)	Analgesic/anesthetic
Methohexital (Brevital Sodium)	Analgesic/anesthetic
Sufentanil (Sufenta)	Analgesic/anesthetic
Ondansetron (Zofran)	Postoperative antiemetic
Ketorolac (Toradol)	Postoperative analgesic

24–48 hours. Usually it takes approximately 8 days for platelet function to return entirely to normal after aspirin administration; however, platelet function may become adequate 1–2 days earlier. If emergency surgery is needed before the 8-day aspirin waiting period, or the 2-day period for other drugs, has elapsed, consultation with an internist or hematologist, platelet transfusions, or both may be advisable. Patients who need retrobulbar injection or surgery for which anticoagulation is contraindicated may stop anticoagulation or aspirin with minimal risk.

The management of anticoagulation in the perioperative setting must be individualized because the risk of thrombosis and the strength of the indication for anticoagulation vary greatly. As no single regimen satisfies all patient needs, consultation with an internist, family practitioner, or hematologist is advisable. Anticoagulation with warfarin may be continued in patients undergoing routine topical cataract or glaucoma surgery. In most patients undergoing other types of ophthalmic surgeries, warfarin should be stopped 3–5 days before surgery, and the prothrombin time should be checked. As the international normalized ratio level drops below 2.0, heparin therapy with either IV unfractionated heparin or subcutaneous low-molecular-weight heparin should be started and dosed to maintain adequate anticoagulation. Intravenous heparin is discontinued approximately 12 hours before surgery and restarted 24 hours after surgery. Low-molecular-weight heparin can be discontinued 12–24 hours prior to surgery and restarted on the first postoperative day. If gastrointestinal function is normal, warfarin may be restarted on the day of surgery. Heparin may be discontinued once therapeutic warfarin levels have been reached.

Medications for diabetes mellitus

Oral hypoglycemic medications are usually withheld the day of surgery. These medications have a relatively long duration of action, which could lead to hypoglycemia late in the day if the patient's oral caloric intake is inadequate.

As discussed in Chapter 9, *management of blood glucose* is important so that CNS dysfunction can be avoided. Whenever possible, insulin-dependent patients should undergo surgery early in the day to allow for postoperative insulin management. Successful perioperative glucose management depends on careful monitoring, and no single regimen works for all patients. Perioperative management of blood glucose during a brief surgical procedure in the *diet-controlled diabetic patient* generally involves only monitoring of blood glucose levels immediately perioperatively and every 3 hours until oral intake is resumed.

For cases of relatively well-controlled insulin-requiring diabetes with reasonable glucose control (<250 mg/dL), one option is to hold all short-acting insulin and give half the intermediate-acting or long-acting insulin the morning of the surgery. It is imperative to provide close preoperative, intraoperative, and postoperative glucose and electrolyte monitoring. In addition, careful titration of a dextrose 5% in water drip with an initial intravenous rate of 75 mL/hour should prevent hypoglycemia or hyperglycemia. Blood glucose levels should be monitored hourly and the infusion rate adjusted to maintain the glucose level at 120–200 mg/dL. Alternatively, for patients who are on insulin and who are undergoing procedures lasting less than 2 hours, the "no insulin, no glucose" regimen works well preoperatively on the morning of surgery. Monitoring blood glucose before, during, and after surgery is important. The availability of 1-touch monitoring makes such measurements very easy, even in the operating room. During the procedure, intravenous solutions without dextrose (lactated Ringer's or saline) are given. After the surgical procedure, the patient should receive a portion (usually one half or one third) of the usual insulin dose, once oral intake is established. If a procedure lasts more than 2 hours, insulin may have to be given as an infusion of at least 4 units per hour, with monitoring of the blood glucose level every 30–60 minutes. The anesthesiologist and primary care physician should be involved in managing the blood glucose level in such patients.

The patient who uses an insulin pump can be easily managed perioperatively: the pump is left on the basal rate, and because the patient is not taking meals before surgery, the dosing used for meals is not given.

Other medications

In general, medication regimens should not be interrupted if possible. Treatments for hypertension, asthma, angina, and congestive heart failure should be continued throughout the day of surgery. The following are guidelines, although individual practice can vary from locality to locality.

Patients should continue use of *antihypertensive medications* until the time of surgery to avoid rebound hypertensive crises and the risk of end-organ damage associated with uncontrolled hypertension (specifically myocardial ischemic diseases). Such medications include clonidine (both dermal patch and orally administered), beta-blockers, and angiotensin-converting enzyme inhibitors. Oral antihypertensive medications can be taken with a sip of water the day of surgery whether or not the patient is on NPO status.

Digoxin can be withheld the day of surgery for many patients, given its long half-life. However, if a patient is receiving digoxin to control the ventricular response to atrial fibrillation, it is important to be sure that the resting heart rate is appropriate on the morning of surgery; digoxin should be given if the resting heart rate is more than 90 beats per minute.

Anticonvulsant medications should be administered (with sips of water) on the patient's usual schedule because stress and particularly general anesthesia can lower the seizure threshold.

Thyroid medications can be held the day of surgery, given their long half-life.

The patient who has taken *systemic corticosteroids* for more than 1 month within the previous 6 months before surgery is customarily "covered" with the equivalent of 300 mg/day of hydrocortisone perioperatively. At the start of the procedure, 100 mg is given intravenously, an additional 100 mg is given at the end of the procedure, and the last 100 mg is administered 6 hours after the end of surgery. Lower doses can be administered for procedures associated with minimal physiologic stress, in the range of 25–30 mg of hydrocortisone intravenously in the first 24 hours after surgery.

In general, *antimicrobial prophylaxis* of bacterial endocarditis is not necessary in patients with cardiac valvular disease prior to ocular surgery. An exception to this guideline is when there is a chance of exposure to pathogens in the upper respiratory system, such as during dacryocystorhinostomy, orbital surgery, or incision and drainage of infected tissue. Prophylaxis is not recommended for elective oral endotracheal intubation. Mitral valve prolapse without valvular regurgitation is not an indication for prophylaxis. Guidelines from the American Heart Association (AHA) for antibiotic prophylaxis are available on the AHA Web site at http://www.americanheart.org/presenter.jhtml?identifier=9459.

It may be desirable to discontinue diuretics on the day of surgery. A patient under local anesthesia may become uncomfortable from a full bladder caused by a preoperative dose of diuretic. A patient undergoing general anesthesia who continues diuretic use on the morning of surgery may become hypotensive because of intravascular volume depletion prior to surgery.

Nicotinic acid should be discontinued before general anesthesia because it can cause an exaggerated hypotensive response from vasodilation. It is generally taught that *monoamine oxidase (MAO) inhibitors* should be discontinued 2–3 weeks before elective surgery because these medications are associated with an exaggerated hypertensive response to systemically released vasopressors during general anesthesia. In addition, the ephedrine or dopamine that is sometimes needed to increase blood pressure intraoperatively can cause marked elevation in blood pressure in patients who are on MAO inhibitors. The administration of meperidine to patients who are taking MAO inhibitors can result in hyperpyrexia, muscle rigidity, seizures, coma, hypotension, and respiratory depression, probably in response to an increase in cerebral serotonin occurring secondary to MAO inhibition. Nevertheless, there is some debate as to whether MAO inhibitors need to be discontinued in that anesthesiologists can use anesthetic techniques with vasoactive medications other than ephedrine and dopamine to avoid the risk of hypertension or sympathetic stimulation in the patient. This is an issue that is best discussed with the anesthesiologist.

Although echothiophate iodide eyedrops are rarely used today, their use affects the choice of muscle relaxant prior to endotracheal intubations. Ideally, the drops should be stopped 3 weeks before the elective surgery so that the cholinesterase enzyme system can recover. However, if echothiophate iodide must be continued, succinylcholine cannot be used during intubations. Alternative medications are available in such cases.

Preoperative Sedation

Preoperative sedation is an important part of comfortable regional or general anesthesia in a patient undergoing elective surgery. Anxiolytics such as midazolam can be given intramuscularly (1–4 mg) 30–60 minutes before the procedure or intravenously (0.5–2.0 mg) 2–3 minutes before the stimulus of the anesthetic block (see Table 15-2). For outpatient surgery, midazolam is a more appropriate sedative than diazepam, because its elimination half-life is 2–4 hours; diazepam's half-life is 20–40 hours. The effects of midazolam can also be reversed with administration of flumazenil. Careful IV titration of sedatives and narcotics is important, particularly in the elderly, so that oversedation and respiratory depression can be avoided.

Alfentanil can be given intravenously in titrated doses with appropriate anesthesia monitoring. Its peak effect occurs in 1–2 minutes and lasts 10–20 minutes. *Fentanyl citrate,* which has a peak effect in 3–5 minutes and lasts about 30 minutes, is also given in titrated doses for ophthalmic monitored anesthesia. The effects of narcotics can be reversed with administration of the antagonist *naloxone,* which is given intravenously. The duration of naloxone reversal is 1 hour or less.

Propofol is a drug with unique properties of rapid hypnosis and a tendency to produce bradycardia, but it has rapid clearance with very little hangover. It must be given through a large-bore vein or administered after a lidocaine flush of the IV line so that significant burning on administration can be minimized. Propofol is a lipid-based medication that supports rapid bacterial growth at room temperature. Indeed, extrinsically contaminated propofol has been associated with postoperative infections, including endogenous endophthalmitis. Hospital personnel involved in the preparation, handling, and administration of this drug must therefore adhere to strict aseptic technique during its use.

Preoperative sedation for children can include midazolam or methohexital.

Intraoperative Complications

Adverse Reactions to Local Anesthesia

Screening for possible allergies to local anesthetic agents was discussed previously. Following is a discussion of other types of adverse reactions.

Local anesthetic injection into the retrobulbar space can lead to apnea, respiratory arrest, and cranial nerve palsies on the side being injected or even on the opposite side. Anatomic studies of the position of the retrobulbar needle in relation to the optic nerve when the adducted or supraducted position of the eye is used during injection show that it is possible to inadvertently inject anesthetic into the subdural space with a standard Atkinson-type needle. Cases of cranial nerve palsies in association with respiratory difficulties represent actual brain stem anesthesia from injection of the anesthetic agent into the subdural space, with subsequent diffusion into the circulating cerebrospinal fluid.

Several suggestions have been made so that such complications of retrobulbar injection can be avoided, including changing the traditional positioning of the eye during the retrobulbar anesthetic injection so that the nerve is rotated away from the track of the needle—for example, by having the patient look straight ahead. Using less sharp, nondisposable retrobulbar needles less than 1¼ inch long also reduces the chance of perforating the optic nerve sheath. Although one series implicated the concentration of anesthetic as the cause of respiratory arrest, it is more likely that a larger volume and, therefore, a larger total dose of anesthetic was delivered to the brain stem through an inadvertent subdural injection. The peribulbar technique was devised, in part, to avoid such complications. If apnea, respiratory arrest, or cranial neuropathies occur after a retrobulbar injection, the patient's airway must be supported with mask ventilation. Intubation and mechanical ventilation may be necessary. Apnea seldom lasts more than 30–50 minutes, but it is important that experienced medical personnel stabilize the patient's condition during this time.

Respiratory distress and dysphagia can result from the Nadbath block, an injection into the stylomastoid foramen that is used to provide facial akinesia. These complications occur when the anesthetic agent is injected deeply into the area of the facial nerve as it exits the stylomastoid foramen, and the anesthetic bathes cranial nerves IX, X, and XI as they exit the jugular foramen. This leads to paralysis of these nerves, and the patient becomes dysphagic, begins to cough or has a hoarse voice, and may develop stridor or severe respiratory insufficiency. These complications tend to occur in thin persons, in whom it is easier to bury the needle deeply. Management of the respiratory distress requires suctioning the pharynx, positioning the patient on his or her side, and supplementing the patient's inspired gases with oxygen or even intubation. This complication can be avoided if a short hypodermic needle is used and advanced only part way into the area to be injected, injecting a small volume (<3 mL).

Anesthetic toxicity can occur when high concentrations of anesthetic agent are given. For example, if 4% lidocaine is used for a peribulbar injection, the total volume that can be safely given to a 70-kg patient is limited to 8 mL. A smaller patient would be able to tolerate no more than 5 mL of 4% lidocaine without risking complications of systemic toxicity, including confusion, cardiac arrhythmias, and respiratory depression.

Seizures have occurred because of the intra-arterial injection of local anesthetic agent into the ophthalmic artery. Such seizures are instantaneous with injection and short in duration. Supportive measures should include airway maintenance and blood pressure support.

Malignant Hyperthermia

As discussed earlier in this chapter, preoperative evaluation can help to identify some patients who are at risk for MH. Nevertheless, such preoperative screening is not infallible, and the surgeon should be prepared to respond to this complication.

Malignant hyperthermia is a disorder of calcium binding by the sarcoplasmic reticulum of skeletal muscles. In the presence of an anesthetic triggering agent, unbound intracellular calcium increases, stimulating muscle contracture. This increased metabolism outstrips oxygen delivery, and anaerobic metabolism develops, with the production of lactate and subsequent massive acidosis. Hyperthermia thus results from the hypermetabolic state.

The earliest signs of MH include tachycardia that is greater than expected for the patient's anesthetic and surgical status, and an elevated end-tidal carbon dioxide level

Table 15-3 Malignant Hyperthermia Protocol

1. Stop the triggering agents immediately, and conclude surgery as soon as possible.
2. Hyperventilate with 100% oxygen at high flow rates.
3. Administer:
   a. Dantrolene: 2–3 mg/kg initial bolus with increments up to 10 mg/kg total. Continue to administer dantrolene until symptoms are controlled. Occasionally, a dose greater than 10 mg/kg may be needed.
   b. Sodium bicarbonate: 1–2 mEq/kg increments guided by arterial pH and pCO_2. Bicarbonate will combat hyperkalemia by driving potassium into cells.
4. Actively cool patient:
   a. If needed, IV iced saline (not Ringer's lactate) 15 mL/kg q 10 minutes × 3. Monitor closely.
   b. Lavage stomach, bladder, rectum, and peritoneal and thoracic cavities with iced saline.
   c. Surface cool with ice and hypothermia blanket.
5. Maintain urine output. If needed, administer mannitol 0.25 g/kg IV, furosemide 1 mg/kg IV (up to 4 doses each). Urine output greater than 2 mL/kg/hr may help prevent subsequent renal failure.
6. Calcium channel blockers *should not* be given when dantrolene is administered, as hyperkalemia and myocardial depression may occur.
7. Insulin for hyperkalemia: Add 10 units of regular insulin to 50 mL of 50% glucose and titrate to control hyperkalemia. Monitor blood glucose and potassium levels.
8. Postoperatively: Continue dantrolene 1 mg/kg IV q 6 hours × 72 hours to prevent recurrence. Lethal recurrences of MH may occur. Observe in an intensive care unit.
9. For expert medical advice and further medical evaluation, call the MHaus MH hotline consultant at (800) 644–9737. For nonemergency professional or patient information, call (800) 986–4287.

---

when the patient is monitored by capnography. Labile blood pressure, tachypnea, sweating, muscle rigidity, blotchy discoloration of skin, cyanosis, and dark urine all signal progression of the disorder. Temperature elevation, which can reach extremely high levels, is a relatively late sign. Ultimately, respiratory and metabolic acidosis, hyperkalemia, hypercalcemia, myoglobinuria, and renal failure can occur, as can disseminated intravascular coagulation and death.

Although volatile anesthetics such as halothane, enflurane, isoflurane, and intravenous succinylcholine are all known to trigger MH, haloperidol, trimeprazine, and promethazine also can cause MH.

If a surgeon wishes to avoid the use of succinylcholine, a laryngeal mask airway can be considered for strabismus surgery in adults if muscle relaxation is not otherwise required. Use of the laryngeal mask airway reduces the soreness and irritation of the throat that occurs after oral endotracheal intubation.

Malignant hyperthermia is treated as a medical emergency (Table 15-3 shows the treatment protocol). The Malignant Hyperthermia Association of the United States staffs a 24-hour hotline to advise medical personnel on the diagnosis and treatment of MH at (800) 644-9737.

Postoperative Care

The use of balanced general anesthesia—in which small amounts of several different types of medications are titrated so that the side effects of a large dose of any one type can be avoided—has been effective in reducing prolonged anesthesia and prolonged recovery time. Neuromuscular blocking agents of short duration (12 minutes for mivacurium and 30 minutes for atracurium and vecuronium) administered with an infusion pump allow the anesthesiologist to fine-tune the degree of neuromuscular blockade during balanced anesthesia.

The shorter-acting narcotics such as sufentanil have potencies up to 1000 times that of morphine. These agents help provide short-term stability of hemodynamics during intensive stimulation without the cost of prolonged excessive sedation postoperatively. Using such agents immediately before intubation as part of an anesthetic induction has become nearly universal.

Management of postoperative nausea and vomiting after general anesthesia has become easier with more powerful antinausea medications such as ondansetron and metoclopramide. Ondansetron and metoclopramide do not cause sedation as droperidol does, thus speeding recovery of the patient in same-day surgery settings.

Postoperative pain can be prophylactically treated during the procedure with IV ketorolac in a 30–60 mg dose or with small titrated doses of IV fentanyl in the range of 50–100 μg. Because of the reported gastrointestinal complications with higher doses of ketorolac, patients older than age 60 should receive no more than 30 mg of IV ketorolac, total. Longer-acting narcotics, such as morphine or meperidine, can delay the patient's discharge because of excessive sedation. Also, there is evidence that IV ketorolac, because of its pain-reducing qualities, can reduce the amount of postoperative nausea and vomiting in patients undergoing strabismus surgery and other procedures requiring general anesthetic. There is no evidence that this particular nonsteroidal anti-inflammatory drug increases postoperative bleeding following ophthalmic surgery.

> Bennett SN, McNeil MM, Bland LA, et al. Postoperative infections traced to contamination of an intravenous anesthetic, propofol. *N Engl J Med.* 1995;333(3):147–154.
>
> Everett LL, Kallar SK. Current status of treatment to prevent aspiration in outpatients. *Anesthesiol Clin North America.* 1996;14:679–693.
>
> Kallio H, Rosenberg PH. Advances in ophthalmic regional anesthesia. *Best Pract Res Clin Anaesthesiol.* 2005;19(2):215–227.
>
> Miller RD, ed. *Miller's Anesthesia.* 6th ed. New York: Elsevier/Churchill Livingstone; 2005.
>
> Van Norman G. Preoperative management of common minor medical issues in the outpatient setting. *Anesthesiol Clin North America.* 1996;14:655–677.

CHAPTER 16

Using Statistics in Practice and Work

The role of clinical research is vital in establishing a standard of care for patients. Such research is best performed using an interdisciplinary approach that combines the efforts of the clinician, statistician, and epidemiologist from the conception of the study through data analyses and interpretation. The choice of study design depends on the research questions to be answered, the population available, and the resources and effort to be expended. If a study finds a statistical association, that association may be considered valid after alternative explanations—such as chance, bias, and confounding—have been ruled out. Furthermore, the association may be more credible if it is a consistent finding in other studies. This chapter is intended to encourage the clinician to critically review the results of clinical research and to apply the results to the clinical practice of ophthalmology.

Obtaining Useful Information From Published Studies

In trying to obtain useful information from studies for resolving either diagnostic or management issues, first assess the question to be answered. If the data exist, numerous tools are available to obtain information from the literature for answers to questions requiring specific factual information—questions such as the following: What is the prevalence of glaucoma in African Americans? Are African Americans and Mexican Americans at greater risk of having open-angle glaucoma than Caucasians are? It can also be relatively straightforward to obtain information on the outcome of specific surgical procedures. For example, a question such as the following is easy to obtain the answer to: What is the expected survival of a corneal graft in a person with Fuchs dystrophy? However, responses to other questions may not be available. For example, how soon can a person go swimming in the ocean after cataract extraction? The response to this type of question is unlikely to be found in any database, existing instead primarily in the experience of experts in the field. Therefore, before attempting to access medical literature, stop a moment to ascertain whether the type of information sought is likely to be available in the literature.

Once it is determined that such information is likely to be found in the literature, there are various sources from which to choose. These include general textbooks of ophthalmology such as *Duane's Ophthalmology*. More detailed information on specific subjects is available in review articles (eg, as can be found in the *Survey of Ophthalmology* [www.ophsource.org/periodicals/sop]; American Academy of Ophthalmology [AAO] *Preferred Practice Patterns* [PPP]; and AAO *Focal Points* [www.aao.org/aao/education/]). In addition, high-quality meta-analyses of specific management issues (eg, surgery for nonarteritic ischemic optic neuropathy, intervention for involutional lower lid ectropion) can be obtained from the Cochrane Library (www.cochraneeyes.org). For more specific, primary sources of information, use Medline/PubMed (www.ncbi.nlm.nih.gov/entrez) to perform a search for original articles. Yet other sources include the references cited in review articles or other papers of interest, and back issues of various journals, such as the following:

- *American Journal of Ophthalmology* (www.ophsource.org/periodicals/ajopht)
- *Archives of Ophthalmology* (archopht.ama-assn.org/)
- *Ophthalmology* (www.ophsource.org/periodicals/ophtha)

When performing online searches, refine the search question and use specific keywords. A more detailed description of how to perform such a search with the use of appropriate keywords can be found on the PubMed Web site. Such searches usually reveal various types of primary sources, from laboratory basic science studies (cell culture, molecular biology) to animal studies (testing new drugs or specific surgical techniques); and from clinical case reports or case series to randomized clinical trials. Based on the question of interest, the search can be narrowed or widened.

This type of search often retrieves articles that may suggest different answers to the question of interest. At this stage, it is important to consider some critical issues with regard to each specific study. A careful consideration of these issues can provide the clinician with the confidence needed to translate the findings into clinical practice.

In an evaluation of a published study, the first and foremost issue to consider before committing time to a critical reading is whether the question that is being posed in the study aims or introduction is the question of interest. For example, if the clinician is interested in determining whether use of a prostaglandin is beneficial in patients with open-angle glaucoma (OAG), then examining data from the Early Manifest Glaucoma Trial (EMGT) would not be useful (prostaglandins were not used in EMGT), whereas data from specific drug trials would be important to consider. The key issue here is that the intervention in the 2 studies was different, even though the effect of both interventions was to lower intraocular pressure (IOP). On the other hand, if the question of interest is whether lowering IOP is beneficial in patients with OAG, then both types of studies might be useful. Thus, it is critical to carefully evaluate the question being asked in the aims or introduction of the study and determine its relevance to the question of interest.

Next, determine whether the conclusions of the study are believable. There are 2 specific questions to consider:

- Are the results valid, reliable, and reproducible?
- Are the results generalizable, or are they applicable to particular patients?

A consideration of these 2 critical questions entails examining several additional factors: specific issues related to the participants/patients, sample size, intervention, outcomes, and the statistical methodology and inferences.

Participants and Setting

Is there a clear description of the selection of the study participants (which patients were included and excluded)? This description lays the groundwork for understanding the setting of the study. Was it a clinic-based study, was it multicentered, or was it a community-based trial? For therapeutic trials, the patient inclusion and exclusion criteria identify the characteristics of those who were or were not treated with an intervention. There may be specific patient groups that were excluded because they were considered a vulnerable population. For example, because most ocular hypotensive drug trials exclude children and pregnant women, there is minimal data on the safety and efficacy of most ocular hypotensive agents in these 2 groups. Thus, if a decision needs to be made on whether to use a specific ocular hypotensive agent in a pregnant woman or in a child, most of the evidence can be found only in individual case reports or retrospective case series.

The next consideration is determining whether the results of a specific study can be directly applied to particular patients, the first step of which is finding out if there was any *selection bias* in assigning an intervention to certain participants. The questions to be considered here are, Was the intervention randomly assigned? Was the treated group comparable to the control group? The purpose of randomly assigning an intervention to a specific participant is that randomization helps minimize bias. If only those participants with particular characteristics are assigned a particular intervention, and the control group is not, then an underestimate or an overestimate of the effect of the intervention is likely, making it difficult to know the true treatment effect of the intervention. This selection bias can be found when well-meaning clinicians assign a more invasive intervention to those patients with more advanced disease. Such a selection bias would make it likely that the more invasive treatment would have poorer outcomes. When an intervention is allocated randomly, the participant has an equal chance of being assigned to either treatment group, thereby reducing the likelihood of selection bias. However, randomization does not always ensure that the participants assigned to each of the intervention groups are similar. To determine whether the groups were similar, study the baseline participant characteristics that may impact the outcome. For example, in a study assessing the effect of lasers for treatment of diabetic retinopathy, the diabetic control, the blood pressure, and the types of medications should be similar in the 2 groups, because these factors are likely to have an effect on progression and regression of retinopathy.

Another consideration in evaluating the generalizability and applicability of a study's results is the severity of disease in the participants included in the study. Was only 1 disease severity group studied, or were the participants representative of different stages of disease, such as mild, moderate, and severe disease? Clinical trials usually study a selected disease severity, making the results applicable and generalizable only to patients with similar disease severity. One common error is extrapolating the data from patients with a specific disease severity to all patients and their varying severity of disease. For example, if a particular treatment effect size was noted in patients with mild glaucomatous damage who underwent trabeculectomy but not in those with advanced glaucomatous damage, the application of this study's results should be limited to patients with early glaucoma damage, not generalized to those with advanced glaucomatous damage. Thus, the generalizability of a study's results is guided by the characteristics of the participants included in the study, and any application of the results should be limited to patients with similar characteristics.

Sample Size Determination

Was the sample size (the number of participants in the study) determined before the initiation of the trial and if so, what criteria were used to determine the sample size? Any clinical trial is aimed at disproving the *null hypothesis,* which states that the impact of the intervention in terms of the primary outcomes is no different from outcomes without the intervention. The sample size is calculated to maximize the likelihood of disproving this null hypothesis. The estimate of sample size is usually based on the expected size of the treatment effect on the primary outcome (eg, improvement in visual acuity, reduction of IOP, proportion of participants with resolution of macular edema). In general, if a large treatment effect is expected, then the sample size needed in a particular study is smaller than that which would be needed if a small treatment effect is expected. The estimated effect size is usually based on the available literature. The sample size must be determined carefully. It is not appropriate to change the sample size midway in a study when the initial results do not bear out the prior assumptions of the effect size.

Issues Related to Intervention

Was the intervention clearly described, and is it reproducible? In most drug studies, the concentration of the drug is provided in the report, but the details of the other components in the medication may not always be clearly stated. Similarly, in surgical studies, a clear description of the procedure is needed to assess whether and how well other surgeons can perform the procedure. In addition, it is useful to know whether the intervention is reproducible, a critical aspect often not addressed. In studies assessing the benefits of drugs, standardization of concentration and content of the drugs is rigorous, as manufacturers have to comply with strict federal guidelines for the preparation of medications. The concentration and content of the medications can be tested during the course of the trial. This testing ensures that the medications have been formulated in a consistent manner. In contrast with drug studies, similar rigor in ensuring consistency is not generally exercised or reported in surgical studies. The surgical procedure should be such that different surgeons can perform it in the same manner in each case. In studies comparing different surgical methods or use of medications versus surgery, the surgical method must be performed in a reproducible manner across all participants who received that intervention. Although surgical standardization cannot be perfect, training all participating surgeons before starting the study, monitoring specific aspects of the surgical procedure during the study, and standardizing postoperative care would go a long way in ensuring such uniformity.

Issues Related to Outcome

Were the outcome measures clearly defined, and were they measured in a reliable/objective manner? The outcome measures are usually specific for the disease under study.

However, most ocular studies include a measure of visual acuity. In addition, ocular studies may include other clinical measurements, for example, an assessment of visual fields, color vision, IOP, or change in a structural abnormality such as macular edema or leakage of fluid in the retina. At the outset of the study, the primary and secondary outcomes of the study should be clearly stated. These outcomes are then used to determine whether the study was able to prove or disprove the null hypothesis. In most studies, not only the outcome measure must be mentioned, but also the magnitude of the outcome measure. For example, if the primary outcome measure is improvement in visual acuity, it is essential to state whether it is a 2-line (or 10-letter) or a 3-line (15-letter) improvement. Similarly, the magnitude of the outcome measure can be stated clearly for other measures such as IOP, intraocular inflammation, and pain relief.

Many of the outcomes in vision research are subject to measurement error (eg, vision; IOP; macular thickness, measured with optical coherence tomography [OCT]). Assessment of these outcomes needs to be standardized across different observers and at different centers. For example, for the assessment of change in the lens, a specific description of the appearance of the lens, as well as comparisons of the lens to a photographic standard similar to that currently used to assess lens opacification, would be useful. Also, it is desirable for assessment of the outcome measures to be performed by individuals who are masked to the intervention, because this reduces the likelihood of measurement bias in the observations. *Measurement bias* is present when an observer assesses a particular outcome variable as either higher or lower than its true value based on the type of intervention. Such an underestimation or overestimation is likely to affect the outcome of the trial.

Validity

The validity of a study is anchored on (1) adequate duration of follow-up, and (2) follow-up of all participants. Thus, in evaluating a study, ask, Was there adequate follow-up of the participants after the intervention? Was the outcome in all participants reported at the conclusion of the study? The duration of follow-up of study participants can determine whether or not a specific outcome is realized. For example, for an evaluation of the value of atropine eyedrops versus patching for the treatment of amblyopia, a follow-up of 3–6 months may be adequate; similar follow-up periods may be adequate and appropriate for the evaluation of macular edema resolution after laser or drug therapy, or improvement of visual acuity after cataract extraction. On the other hand, because of glaucoma's slow progression rates, trials assessing visual field loss in glaucoma would require many years of follow-up. Thus, the typical rate of progression of disease is an important guide to the duration of follow-up required.

Follow-up of all participants in terms of the primary outcome is also critical to the validity of a study. This may not be practical or feasible in all cases, because of dropout from a study (eg, due to death during follow-up). For cases of dropout not due to death during the follow-up period, the reasons for loss to follow-up are essential to ascertain, as they may suggest certain problems with the treatments given to those participants. For example, participants in a drug trial may drop out if they frequently get untoward ocular side effects such as burning or stinging from the drug.

Clinical Relevance Issues

- Is the intervention clinically applicable in the current practice environment?
- Are the outcomes clinically important?
- Are all clinically important outcomes evaluated?
- Is the effect of the treatment both statistically and clinically significant?

Issues related to clinical relevance are central to the decision of whether a study's results can be applied to the management of patients. The first issue to consider is if the intervention being studied is likely to be used in practice. If the intervention is too expensive, if it can be performed by only a few physicians, or if it is no longer in general use, then there is little benefit in evaluating such a study.

Next, attention should be directed at the outcomes being evaluated. Usually, the statistical tests used to determine the difference between 2 groups depend on the nature of the data. If the data are *normally distributed* (ie, conform more or less to a bell-shaped curve) and are of a continuous nature (eg, macular thickness in a trial determining the value of intravitreal steroids for treatment of diabetic macular edema), then a Student t test comparing the treated and control groups can be performed. For normally distributed data that are expressed as categories (present or absent; small, medium, or large), a chi-square test is used. For data that are not normally distributed, nonparametric tests such as the Wilcoxon rank sum test can be used. All of these tests provide a P value that states the likelihood with which a difference between the 2 groups may be from chance alone. Thus, a P value of $<.05$ means that the likelihood that the difference between the 2 groups is due to random chance alone is less than 5%. The lower the P value, the lower the likelihood that the difference is by chance and the more likely it is that the difference is a true difference.

Statistical differences are not the only important factor. *Clinically meaningful* differences must also be present. In vision research, visual acuity is often a primary outcome variable. However, if the magnitude of the difference being evaluated is an improvement of 3–5 letters, or 1 line or less, on the visual acuity chart, then this difference is within the margin of measurement error and likely does not provide clinically meaningful results. A change of more than 10 letters of acuity or 2 lines on the visual acuity chart is clinically meaningful. Similarly, in an ocular hypotensive drug trial, an IOP difference of 1 mm Hg is within the measurement error and is likely to not be clinically meaningful, whereas a difference of 3 mm Hg or more may be. Thus, even though a statistical test may suggest a statistically significant difference, the magnitude and nature of the difference are critical to determining whether there is a clinically meaningful difference between 2 interventions. This point needs to be highlighted because it is useful to consider implementing only those interventions that are both statistically and clinically significant. In addition to evaluating these primary outcome variables, the study should also evaluate secondary clinically important variables related to the safety of the intervention. These variables include dropout rates, pain, allergic reactions, systemic reactions, and death.

Clinical Study Designs

Information about a disease process and its appropriate management can be gained from a wide array of study designs. In *observational studies,* also known as *nonexperimental studies,* people are assessed with respect to their personal characteristics, behaviors, and exposures in relation to their having a particular disease or condition or having a particular complication of the disease. The investigator notes only what has happened and does not directly manipulate the behavior (eg, cigarette smoking) or exposures (eg, use of a medication or treatment with laser) of the patient. In *experimental studies,* typically clinical trials, subjects are assigned a particular treatment, where *treatment* is used broadly to describe a prescribed behavior (eg, eat a diet high in antioxidant foods) or a therapeutic or preventive intervention (eg, oral neuroprotective agent for patients with glaucoma or antioxidant vitamin supplement for patients with early age-related maculopathy [ARM] at risk of vision loss from the development of late ARM).

When well conducted and appropriately interpreted, each study design yields valuable information. Observational studies are best used for describing the presentation and progression of disease, generating hypotheses, and efficiently assessing data that may already exist for consistency with a hypothesis about an intervention. However, the best evidence on the effects of an intervention is obtained through randomized clinical trials and, when multiple clinical trials have been conducted to address the same or a very similar question, meta-analyses (Fig 16-1).

Case Reports

A report on a single patient can provide valuable information by demonstrating that something unusual can happen under particular circumstances. Reporting unusual presentations of a serious disease may aid others in recognizing the condition. For example, Friedman reported on a patient who presented with retinal vasculitis and who was apparently healthy and free of conditions typically associated with retinal vasculitis, such as toxoplasmosis, syphilis, Behçet syndrome, sarcoidosis, lupus, and herpes. A magnetic resonance image of the brain revealed findings typical of multiple sclerosis (MS). Although patients with an established history of MS are known to develop retinal vasculitis, this was the first patient reported with retinal vasculitis as the initial presentation of MS. The

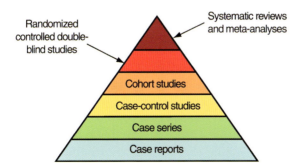

Figure 16-1 The pyramid of evidence from different study designs. *(Adapted from Medical Research Library of Brooklyn. Available at http://library.downstate.edu/ebm/2100.htm.)*

author advised evaluating a patient for MS when the etiology of retinal vasculitis remains unclear after testing for the more common causes.

Case reports cannot provide information on treatment efficacy or on causal mechanisms. At most, they can suggest that a previously unsuspected effect or mechanism might exist. Other study designs, as described below, can be used to address efficacy and mechanisms.

Case Series

Case series are investigations of the presentation, history, and/or follow-up of patients that can provide valuable information on the natural history of a disease or on the prognosis for groups of patients managed in the same way. The methods for subject selection, the assessment of patient characteristics, and the length and completeness of follow-up determine the quality of a case series, and clinicians must consider all of these in deciding whether the results of a case series pertain to their particular patients.

Case selection factors

Often, case series are based on patients seen in university-based clinical practices that may serve as tertiary referral centers. These settings may serve patients with particularly severe disease or may have a higher proportion of patients with features that make the disease not amenable to widely available treatments. Characteristics of the presentation and prognosis of patients in the case series may differ dramatically from those of patients seen by a community ophthalmologist. A case series by Margherio and coworkers provided the characteristics of consecutive patients with choroidal neovascularization secondary to age-related macular degeneration seen in a large practice of retina specialists. The location and composition of neovascular lesions that determined a patient's suitability for either thermal laser treatment or photodynamic therapy with verteporfin may not have been representative of all neovascular lesions that can be seen, because the ophthalmologists whom patients saw for routine care might not have referred all cases, some because they could be treated easily with a thermal laser and some because they were already too large for any treatment. The time period of the collection of the case series may also have a major effect on the prognosis of patients, because of changes in medical management of diseases. A striking example of this is how the prognosis of HIV patients with cytomegalovirus retinitis changed after the introduction of highly active antiretroviral therapy (HAART).

Assessment of patient characteristics

The methods for measurements, tests, and other evaluations in case series are typically not standardized and may be subject to a high degree of variability. Often, case series are prepared from a review of existing medical records provided by a number of ophthalmologists. Such retrospective collection of data suffers from differing levels of degree of detail across patients and from missing or incomplete information. For example, the technicians, examination rooms, lighting, and/or charts used for the measurement of visual acuity may differ among ophthalmological offices. In addition to the variability introduced by nonstandardized testing conditions, the acuity may be recorded only to the nearest whole line in some charts (20/25) but recorded to the letter (20/25 + 2) in other charts.

Length and completeness of follow-up
Case series that report on the course of patients need to appropriately accommodate the differing lengths of follow-up for patients. Often, cases are collected over a long period, as for example, 1996–2000, so that at the time of chart review in 2005, patients would be expected to have between 5 and 9 years of follow-up. Particularly for characteristics that are likely to change progressively over time (eg, mean deviation in patients with glaucoma), reporting on the average change observed among all patients does not provide an adequate description of the course of disease. When the length of follow-up varies, the data should be reported at specific follow-up times, such as at 1, 2, and 3 years after the initiation of treatment. When the outcome measure is an event, such as corneal graft failure, survival analysis can account appropriately for the varying lengths of follow-up. If not all patients are followed up for the full length of the possible follow-up period, the reported outlook for the case series may be biased because of losses to follow-up. Especially when the case series is based on review of medical charts, losses to follow-up may be related strongly to how the patient fares over time. For example, in a case series of patients with macular edema from branch vein occlusion, some patients may have chosen not to return because their macular edema resolved and their vision improved; some patients may have suffered further loss of vision and sought care from another ophthalmologist; and some patients may have had no major change in vision and moved to another location. When a large percentage of patients have not returned for complete follow-up, the generalizability of the description of the course of patients becomes limited, because the returning patients may have had an unusually good or unusually bad course.

Case-Control Studies
Case-control studies are observational study designs used to investigate the association between exposures, or potential risk factors (eg, smoking, medical conditions, therapies), and outcomes (eg, loss of visual acuity, development of glaucoma, corneal graft failure, cataract surgery). In case-control studies, one group of participants is selected because these individuals have the disease of interest (cases), and another group of comparable individuals who are free of disease (controls) is selected. The past exposures and characteristics of the cases and controls are compared. If an exposure is more (or less) common in the cases than in the controls, the exposure is considered associated with the disease (Fig 16-2).

Case-control studies are often performed as a first approach to investigating a hypothesis, generated from laboratory findings or from case reports and series, that a factor is associated with a disease. Typically, though not always, the cases and controls are selected from currently available groups, and the history of exposures is obtained through patient interview and/or review of medical records. Thus, compared with cohort studies (discussed later) that often require extended periods of subsequent follow-up, case-control studies can be performed relatively quickly and inexpensively. In addition, many

Case-control study

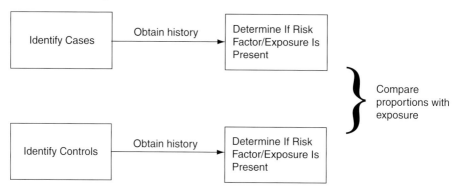

Cohort study

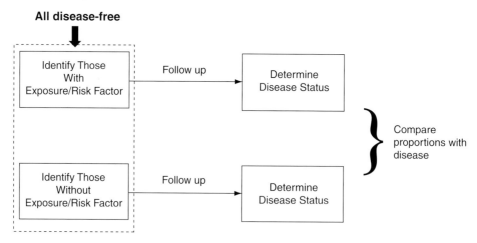

Figure 16-2 Simplified schematics of observational study designs.

potential risk factors can be evaluated simultaneously if the history on many factors is gathered while records are reviewed or the patient is questioned.

However, these advantages are often overshadowed by the inaccuracies introduced because of gathering the exposure data from records and patient recall. In addition to the problems described previously for case series, case-control studies may suffer from many types of bias that may distort the true association between the exposure and the disease. For example, patients with retinal vein occlusion (cases) may be much more likely to recall taking medications of any type (eg, aspirin) because of efforts to figure out what caused the occlusion, whereas controls might be less likely to remember taking medications because they have not been motivated to scrutinize their past behavior. Therefore, a higher proportion of cases than controls might report use of aspirin in the last 6 months, even if in truth the proportion of aspirin users was the same in both cases and controls. The apparent increased exposure to aspirin in cases would be attributable solely to *recall bias*.

Another common challenge in case-control studies is selection of an appropriate control group. For example, if controls for cases with retinal vein occlusion are chosen from a general ophthalmology practice, the proportion of cases with myopia might be much lower than the proportion of controls because a high proportion of some general ophthalmology practices may be devoted to providing refractive correction for myopes. Comparing the proportion of myopes in the case and control groups would show an apparent protective effect of myopia. However, the apparent association could be attributable totally to selection bias. A full discussion of the many potential sources of bias is beyond the scope of this chapter; however, a full discussion can be found in most textbooks in epidemiology.

The association between statin use and ARM was investigated by McGwin and colleagues through a database compiled as part of a major study on atherosclerosis. Study participants had fundus photographs taken at 1 of the required visits; subjects were classified as cases if macular drusen and/or pigmentary changes were present. Electronic records from previous visits were assessed for statin use. Among 871 cases of ARM, 11% had a history of statin use; of 11,717 controls, 12.3% had used statins. After consideration of additional factors known to be associated with ARM, the authors found that the slightly higher proportion of statin users in the control group was statistically significant and concluded that the data support statin use as a protective factor. In this study, the authors collected data prospectively using standard methods because the patients were involved in an atherosclerosis study. The data were complete and relatively free of bias because of the use of standardized questionnaires that asked about current, rather than past, use of medications. However, in this instance, it is not possible to know whether the drusen and pigmentary changes were present before the drugs were used or if they developed afterward. As patients with early ARM are usually asymptomatic, these subjects may have had the macular changes for a long time before they were photographed.

Cross-sectional Studies

Cross-sectional studies also relate exposures and risk factors to the presence or absence of a disease or condition; however, the timing or sequencing of exposure and development of disease is not known. A study in which an ophthalmologist notes the lens status (phakic, pseudophakic, or aphakic) for all scheduled patients arriving for their appointments and in which each of the patients provides a blood sample would be an example of a cross-sectional study. Patients could be classified with respect to whether they have had cataract surgery (case status) and with respect to their cholesterol level and gender (potential risk factors). We might find that the mean cholesterol level in the patients with cataract surgery was much higher than the mean for those without cataract surgery, a finding that would be consistent with the association between high cholesterol level and increased risk of cataract surgery. However, it would not be known whether the cholesterol level was elevated before the onset of lens opacification and the cataract surgery. In addition, as with both case-control and cohort studies (discussed next), there is the concern that the apparent association is attributable to confounding factors. For this study, age could be acting as a *confounding factor,* because cholesterol levels are known to increase with age, and the likelihood of cataract surgery also increases with age. Researchers could use stratification and/or regression analyses to adjust for age and to see if the cholesterol–cataract surgery association persisted.

Cohort Studies

Cohort studies are another observational study design used to investigate the association between exposures, or potential risk factors, and patient outcomes. In *cohort,* or *follow-up, studies,* individuals who are free of the disease of interest are identified and classified by the presence or absence of potential risk factors, and their subsequent development of the disease is assessed (see Fig 16-2).

The Beaver Dam Eye Study has yielded many cohort studies examining several ocular conditions and many different potential risk factors. Approximately 5000 residents of Beaver Dam, Wisconsin, were examined and interviewed and then followed up for 10 years for the incidence of ocular disease. Researchers explored potential risk factors for diseases such as ARM, diabetic retinopathy, glaucoma, and cataract using the residents' exposures at the beginning of the study and the incidence of the diseases 5 and 10 years later. For example, the investigators classified participants without late ARM at the initial examination according to a number of potential risk factors (age, gender, presence of pigmentary changes, drusen characteristics) for progression to late ARM. The incidence of late ARM was 15% among eyes with pigmentary changes, 0.4% among eyes without pigmentary changes; the incidence for eyes with soft, indistinct drusen was 20%, compared with 0.8% for eyes without such drusen.

The Beaver Dam Eye Study is an example of a population-based cohort study with prospective data collection. However, the groups with and without the potential risk factors may be clinic-based, and the data collection may be retrospective. For example, Strahlman and colleagues were interested in the development of choroidal neovascularization in the second eye of patients who already had neovascularization in the first eye. At the clinical center, retinal photography was available for the fellow eye at the time the patient presented with neovascularization in the first eye. Patients were recalled and examined for the development of neovascularization in the second eye. Patients with large, confluent drusen present at the time of the diagnosis of neovascularization in the first eye were found to have a higher risk of developing neovascularization in the second eye. Because the retinal photographs were retrieved from the patients' medical records for past visits, the data collection is considered retrospective. But because patients were classified based on their earlier fellow-eye drusen status, and because the incidence of neovascularization was compared between the groups with and without confluent drusen, the study is considered a cohort study.

Cohort studies can provide apparently strong links between risk factors and disease; however, the primary weakness of this study design is that the participants with the risk factor of interest may differ in many ways from those without the risk factor. If those with the risk factor differ from those without it on other factors that affect the incidence of the disease, then the apparent association may have been induced by those other differences.

An example of this is the use of interrupted sutures, rather than running sutures, in corneal transplantation. If researchers follow up patients for incidence of graft failure, they find a much higher proportion of graft failure among patients with interrupted sutures. However, concluding that use of interrupted sutures increases the risk of graft failure would be wrong. Interrupted sutures are often used on patients at high risk of graft failure because of such conditions as stromal vascularization, which increases the risk of immunologic rejection. These eyes are much more likely to have an established, strong risk factor for graft failure; hence, the apparent higher risk of graft failure in the eyes with interrupted sutures. In this example, stromal vascularization is a confounding factor. Statistical analysis techniques, such as stratified analysis and regression analysis, can adjust for the effect of known confounding factors. However, most often, not all of the factors that affect the incidence of disease are known or measured, and confounding factors may be hidden from view. For this reason, cohort studies may identify strong associations between risk factors and disease incidence, but these associations are not considered clear evidence of a causal role.

Clinical Trials

Clinical trials are similar to cohort studies (see Fig 16-2) in concept, with 1 major difference: in clinical trials, patients are assigned to treatment groups (exposure groups) *randomly* (Fig 16-3). Randomized treatment assignment generally yields treatment groups that are similar on all known and unknown risk factors for developing the disease or condition of interest. Randomized treatment assignment is the only way to substantially reduce the effect of confounding variables that bedevil other study designs. Its importance cannot be overstated.

However, randomization alone does not ensure that the information generated from clinical trials on the effects of interventions is valid. All of the features mentioned previously as improving the quality of observational studies should be applied to randomized clinical trials:

- well-defined trial objective
- explicit inclusion and exclusion criteria
- adequate sample size
- standardized procedures

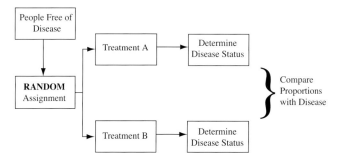

Figure 16-3 Simplified schematic of a clinical trial.

- predefined and objective primary and secondary outcome measures
- patients, treaters, and evaluators who are masked to the assigned treatment
- complete follow-up of all patients

The CONSORT (Consolidated Standards of Reporting Trials) guidelines, which have been adopted by most medical journals, provide a comprehensive listing of the features that should be considered when designing trials and that should be included in reports of clinical trials.

Although the results of a properly designed, well-executed, randomized clinical trial should be easy to interpret, 2 issues often arise in interpreting the results of clinical trials. The first is excluding patients from data analysis for any of the following reasons: they did not meet all of the eligibility criteria; they had side effects and stopped treatment; or they were noncompliant with the treatment regimen. Exclusion of patients can strongly bias the apparent results of a clinical trial, because the reasons for exclusion are nearly always related in some way to the trial outcome measure. An *intention-to-treat analysis* includes the data from all patients assigned treatment in a clinical trial and should be the primary analysis.

The second issue is the interpretation of results from subgroups of patients (eg, young versus old; hypertensive or not). Even if there is no benefit of treatment overall, when researchers look at many subgroups, they can almost always identify a subgroup of patients that have a statistically significant benefit of treatment. Minor differences in treatment effect across subgroups are expected because of random variation. Conclusions that a particular subgroup benefits more from treatment than do others are strongest when the subgroup is identified *before* the trial data were examined; when there is statistical evidence of treatment variability across the subgroups; and when there is a biologically plausible explanation for the finding.

Systematic Reviews and Meta-analyses of Clinical Trials

The strongest evidence for assessing interventions comes from systematic reviews and meta-analyses that combine the evidence from 2 or more clinical trials studying the intervention for a particular condition. Although there have been few instances in ophthalmology of more than 1 high-quality randomized clinical trial of any 1 treatment, the Cochrane Eyes and Vision Group publishes these types of analyses. For example, Leyland and Zinicola reviewed the results of 3 multicenter and 5 single-center randomized clinical trials of multifocal versus monofocal intraocular lenses after cataract extraction. Using special statistical methods for combining data from multiple trials, they found no statistically significant difference between the 2 lens types in unaided and aided distance visual acuity; statistically significant better near vision and less need for glasses with multifocal lenses; and significantly more patients experiencing glare, haloes, and reduced contrast sensitivity with multifocal lenses.

> Friedman SM. Retinal vasculitis as the initial presentation of multiple sclerosis. *Retina.* 2005;25:218–219.
> Klein R, Klein BEK, Tomany SC, et al. Ten-year incidence and progression of age-related maculopathy. The Beaver Dam Eye Study. *Ophthalmology.* 2002;109:1767–1779.

Leyland M, Zinicola E. Multifocal versus monofocal intraocular lenses after cataract extraction (Cochrane Review). From *The Cochrane Library, Issue 3, 2005*. Chichester, UK: John Wiley & Sons, Ltd.

Margherio RR, Margherio AR, DeSantis ME. Laser treatments with verteporfin therapy and its potential impact on retinal practices. *Retina*. 2000;20:325–330.

McGwin G Jr, Xie A, Owsley C. The use of cholesterol-lowering medications and age-related macular degeneration. *Ophthalmology*. 2005;112:488–494.

Moher D, Schutz KF, Altman DG, for the CONSORT Group. The CONSORT statement: revised recommendations for improving the quality of reports of parallel-group randomised clinical trials. *Lancet*. 2001;357:1191–1194.

Rothman KJ, Greenland S. *Modern Epidemiology*. 2nd ed. Philadelphia: Lippincott-Raven Publishers; 1998.

Strahlman ER, Fine SL, Hillis A. The second eye of patients with senile macular degeneration. *Arch Ophthalmol*. 1983;101:1191–1193.

Interpreting Diagnostic or Screening Tests

The best way to learn how to interpret diagnostic or screening tests is to start with the simplest, most straightforward clinical situation: a screening test with a binary (yes/no) outcome that has been well studied by multiple investigators and that has been used in a wide variety of populations; a disease that the patient definitely either has or does not have; and a patient about whom nothing is known at the time of screening. Gradually, complicating features are inserted, those that often appear in routine ophthalmic practice and in research concerning testing for screening and diagnostic tests. In reporting such research, the investigators should have considered these complicating features; in reading these papers, the discriminating reader should ask whether these complicating features were addressed.

The Straightforward Case

Consider a hypothetical screening test for childhood strabismus in 100 children. A thorough examination of this clinic population reveals that 30 children have strabismus and 70 do not. The screening test identifies 60 children with abnormal results and 40 with normal results. Twenty of those failing the screening truly have strabismus; 40 failing the screening do not. Ten strabismic patients pass the screening test. Table 16-1 shows the results.

The data are presented in the *2 × 2 table*. From this table, much can be learned about the screening test. Note that the "truth" is expressed along the horizontal title

Table 16-1 Screening Test for Strabismus in Clinic

Screening Test Result	Strabismus	No Strabismus	Totals
Abnormal	Truly abnormal (20)	Falsely abnormal (40)	60
Normal	Falsely normal (10)	Truly normal (30)	40
Totals	30	70	100

row, and the screening test verdict down the vertical row. *Accuracy* is found by adding "truly normal" and "truly abnormal." The screening test performance is described as follows:

- *Sensitivity:* The test correctly identifies 20 of every 30 children with strabismus (67%).
- *Specificity:* The test correctly passes 30 of every 70 children who do not have strabismus (42%).
- *Positive predictive value (PPV):* If a child has abnormal test results, there is only a 1 in 3 chance (20/60) that the child actually has strabismus (33%).
- *Negative predictive value (NPV):* If a child passes the screening test, the child has a 3 in 4 chance (30/40) of actually being disease-free (75%).
- *Accuracy:* The screening test is correct in 50 of 100 cases (50%).

Sensitivity and specificity are attractive measures because they are intuitively obvious. *Sensitivity* is the percentage of those who have the disease of interest and fail the test, and *specificity* is the percentage of disease-free persons who pass the test. Confidence limits can be stated for both sensitivity and specificity, based in large part on the sample size used. However, an important caveat is that neither sensitivity nor specificity takes into account the relative frequency of healthy and unhealthy persons in a population. For example, if the hypothetical strabismus test was taken to a shopping center and used to screen children, Table 16-2 might result.

The sensitivity is still 67%, and the specificity is about the same at 41%. But because of screening failure, 58 disease-free persons and only 2 truly strabismic children would be referred for complete examinations. The PPV and the NPV alert us to the problem. For this shopping center population, the PPV (if a person has positive test results, what is the probability that the disease is present?) is 2/(2 + 58), or only 3%. The NPV (if a person has negative test results, what is the probability that the disease is absent?) is 39/(1 + 39), or 98%. But the point of screening is not to reassure disease-free persons, but to detect treatable disease. Clearly, this test, which found 67% of the patients with strabismus and which had a 33% PPV in a clinic population, failed miserably when used in a wider population. PPV and NPV, then, are better parameters to employ in an assessment of a screening test that is to be used in a wider population, because these values take into account the prevalence of disease in the population. Of course, the PPV and NPV are much more relevant when calculated on the basis of disease prevalence in the wider population, and not on a disease-rich clinic population.

Table 16-2 Screening Test for Strabismus in Shopping Center

Screening Test Result	Strabismus	No Strabismus	Totals
Abnormal	Truly abnormal (2)	Falsely abnormal (58)	60
Normal	Falsely normal (1)	Truly normal (39)	40
Totals	3	97	100

Complicating Features

Number 1: a screening test with a continuous outcome

Now consider the situation in which the screening test has a continuous value, as opposed to a binary outcome. Intraocular pressure (IOP) is such a variable. Assume for the moment that people are able to be definitively classified, on the basis of a thorough examination, into those with glaucoma and those without glaucoma. For each value of IOP in mm Hg, persons above that value of IOP could be classified as having failed the screening, and those below it, as having passed the screening, thus converting the result into a yes/no format at that value of IOP. Percentages for sensitivity and for specificity can be derived for each value of IOP and graphically displayed (Fig 16-4).

Thus, there is a series of paired sensitivity/specificity values, 1 for each level of IOP. This series can be plotted graphically: sensitivity, by convention, is on the ordinate (y-axis); and (1 – specificity) is on the abscissa (x-axis). In this form, it is known as a *Receiver Operating Characteristics (ROC)* curve. (The ROC curve was originally designed to evaluate early radio sets on their ability to separate signal from noise.) The ability of IOP to discriminate glaucoma from non-glaucoma is shown in Figure 16-5; data are from the population-based Baltimore Eye Survey. (The data points are actually connected by steps, but the continuous line graph is easier to view.)

It is obvious that IOP is not a very good screening tool for glaucoma, because the graph does not curve strongly toward the upper left of the ROC plot, where good sensitivity is paired with good specificity. The diamond-shaped symbols represent a hypothetical optimal screening test; the triangular symbols represent a test with a 50:50 sensitivity and specificity, nothing better than chance alone. The usual cutoff for "normal" IOP, 21 mm Hg, gives a sensitivity of 91% with a specificity of only 47%. The optimal mix of sensitivity and specificity is at 18 mm Hg, where sensitivity is 65%; specificity, 66%. Despite the inadequate performance of IOP as a screening methodology, it can be seen that for a continuous variable test like IOP, there is a trade-off between sensitivity and specificity. The more specific we want a test result (left side of x-axis), the less sensitive it becomes, and vice versa. An ROC curve can help in the choice of an optimal cutoff point in that the curve selects a sensitivity–specificity pair located toward the upper left of the ROC plot.

Other significant factors in choosing a cutoff point are the population to be screened and the fact that sensitivity and specificity may not be equally important. If the consequence of missing a diagnosis is blindness, and the price of a false-positive test is negligible, then a high sensitivity with a poorer specificity would be an appropriate choice. An example of this might be a cutoff value for an erythrocyte sedimentation rate in a person who has fugitive visual loss and who is suspected of having giant cell arteritis.

Number 2: the diagnosis is not yes/no, but has arbitrary, consistent criteria

Of course, the presence or absence of glaucoma is dependent on how glaucoma is defined. No test or examination is capable of detecting the first optic nerve axon that is damaged in glaucoma. Therefore, in research, a consistent and verifiable, though arbitrary, criterion for a glaucoma diagnosis must be used. If this criterion is applied, there is a risk of misclassifying an early glaucoma patient as disease-free. A test that correctly identifies

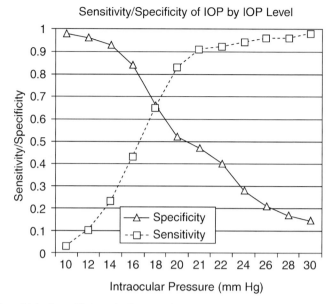

Figure 16-4 Sensitivity/specificity of IOP by IOP level. For each level of IOP along the abscissa, the values for sensitivity and specificity are plotted. *(Data from Tielsch JM, Sommer A, Witt K, et al. Blindness and visual impairment in an American urban population: the Baltimore Eye Survey. Arch Ophthalmol. 1990;108:286.)*

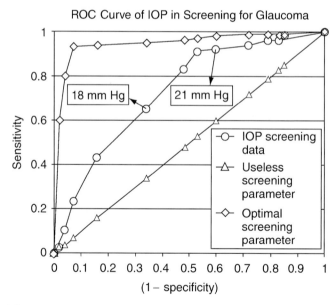

Figure 16-5 ROC curve of IOP in screening for glaucoma. In this ROC curve, the data from Figure 16-4 are replotted, with sensitivity on the ordinate and (1 − specificity) on the abscissa. The middle line shows these pairs. Two of these plotted points are identified with the IOP cutoff represented. *(Data from Tielsch JM, Sommer A, Witt K, et al. Blindness and visual impairment in an American urban population: the Baltimore Eye Survey. Arch Ophthalmol. 1990;108:286.)*

such a patient as having glaucoma is misclassified as a false-positive. Therefore, evaluation of new diagnostic modalities that may detect glaucoma earlier than do current tests is challenging. The problem is that there is no gold standard against which to compare a new diagnostic test. But even without the benefit of longitudinal follow-up to see who later develops glaucoma, a new test can still be evaluated if it is compared with others. ROC curves are useful as a means of comparing the relative efficacy of different screening methods or of different diagnostic tests. A good example from the recent literature is shown in Figure 16-6. In this study, 3 devices that image the optic disc and nerve fiber layer were compared on their ability to discriminate between healthy eyes and eyes with glaucomatous visual field loss.

Using ROC curves to compare tests is especially useful when the tests express results in different units or on completely different scales. The area under the ROC curve (AUC) is a summary measure of the relative efficacy of competing tests. The AUC must be better than 0.5, which a useless test can achieve (see Fig 16-5).

Number 3: pretest probability of disease

Now consider the case in which something relevant is known about the patient before the screening or diagnostic test is performed. In the case of glaucoma, perhaps it is known that the patient has a first-degree relative with glaucoma and has a thinner-than-average central corneal thickness (both risk factors for glaucoma). This information lets us know

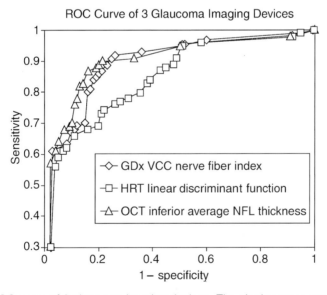

Figure 16-6 ROC curve of 3 glaucoma imaging devices. The single parameter chosen for display for each instrument was the one that performed the best in the authors' study. The HRT linear discriminant function is from a paper by Bathija et al, referenced by Medeiros et al; the OCT and GDx parameters are standard test outputs provided by the manufacturers. No statistically significant difference in the area under the ROC curves for these 3 parameters was present. *(Graph redrawn with data from Medeiros FA, Zangwill LM, Bowd C, et al. Comparison of the GDx VCC scanning laser polarimeter, HRT II confocal scanning laser ophthalmoscope, and Stratus OCT optical coherence tomograph for the detection of glaucoma. Arch Ophthalmol. 2004;122:827–837.)*

that the patient has a pretest probability of glaucoma 3 times that of a person picked at random from the general population. How much does a diagnostic test improve the ability to diagnose glaucoma in this patient? How much does the relative risk of glaucoma increase as a result of a positive test?

For this problem, apply *Bayes' theorem*, which allows the combination of a pretest probability of disease with test results, producing a posttest probability. Among the statistical applications of this theorem, one of the most useful is the *likelihood ratio* and its derived positive and negative predictive values. Although the likelihood ratio sounds complicated, it is simple to understand, because it is calculated using sensitivity and specificity. First, the likelihood ratio of a positive test is the sensitivity divided by (1 – specificity), numbers that can be found in the 2 × 2 table or the ROC curve. For a test with 80% sensitivity and 90% specificity (0.8/1 – 0.9), the positive likelihood ratio is 8. Second, the likelihood ratio of a negative test is (1 – sensitivity) divided by specificity. For the same 80%/90% test, the negative likelihood ratio is (1 – 0.8)/0.9, or 0.22. Positive likelihood ratios start at 1 and continue to infinity—the bigger, the better. Negative likelihood ratios vary from 0 to 1; the smaller, the better. If the interest is in diagnosing disease, the test with the larger positive likelihood ratio is the better test; conversely, if the goal is ruling out disease, the test with the smaller negative likelihood ratio is better.

If the positive likelihood ratio is multiplied by the pretest odds of disease, the result is the posttest odds of disease. Thus, for the example patient with the positive family history, thin cornea, and pretest odds of 3—if there is a positive test with a positive likelihood ratio of 8, then the posttest odds of glaucoma are 24 times that of a person drawn at random from the population.

Now consider the case of a 65-year-old woman with no risk factors for glaucoma and a pretest probability of disease of 1% (Table 16-3). A positive test result for glaucoma would raise her probability of disease to 7.5%. However, an 85-year-old man with a strong positive family history, thin central corneal thickness, and an IOP of 30 might have a pretest probability of disease of 50%. If his test result were negative, he would still have a posttest probability of 18.2%, greater than that of the 65-year-old woman. This example illustrates how important the pretest probability of disease becomes in deciding whether to employ a diagnostic test.

Often in clinical practice there is an intermediate diagnostic category, such as "glaucoma suspect," between the diseased and the normal condition. Successful statistical treatment of such a category is another advantage that likelihood ratios have and that sensitivity/specificity and ROC curves do not. Sensitivity/specificity and ROC curves require

Table 16-3 Example of a Test With 80% Sensitivity/90% Specificity and Changes in PPV and NPV Depending on Pretest Probability

Pretest Probability	Predictive Value of a Positive Test	Predictive Value of a Negative Test
1%	7.5%	99.8%
10%	47.1%	97.6%
50%	88.9%	81.8%
90%	98.6%	33.3%

that borderline subjects be placed in 1 of 2 categories: "those with disease" (eg, glaucoma) or "those without disease" (eg, no glaucoma). But a separate likelihood ratio for the borderline category can be constructed, thereby reflecting the risk of patients exhibiting that characteristic (eg, a "glaucoma suspect").

Number 4: combining tests

Sometimes clinicians may make a diagnosis by using 2 tests, the second employed if the first is positive. Likelihood ratios for each test may be known, because of clinical research done independently for each test. It is tempting to use the product of the 2 likelihood ratios and the pretest probability to calculate a posttest probability, but this is unwise because the test results are usually not completely independent of each other.

Consider the following case: the Stratus OCT is used as a diagnostic test, and if the result is positive, the GDx is employed. Reference to Medeiros et al provides likelihood ratios for each test. But both tests measure nerve fiber layer thickness, albeit using different technologies, and are highly correlated. Because the 2 tests are not independent, the actual performance of the 2-test strategy is likely to be disappointing in comparison with the posttest probability calculated from the product of the pretest probability and the 2 likelihood ratios.

Another test combination strategy is performing 2 tests and considering the result positive if either test result is positive. This strategy works best when tests have good specificity (because combining tests this way makes overall specificity deteriorate) and when the 2 tests address different aspects of a disease (such as a functional test and a structural test for glaucoma). A clinical example would be combining an optic nerve imaging test with a visual field test to determine whether glaucoma is present.

Number 5: clinical acceptance

So far, it has been assumed that the clinical test under consideration is not burdensome, either physically or financially, on the patient. The test's performance characteristics have been evaluated in a vacuum. But all tests carry some burden, including the potential for side effects or the need to repeat them and/or order additional tests if they are failed. A test that produces a small increment in likelihood ratio of detecting disease, but that is expensive or painful, is not likely to achieve clinical acceptance.

Number 6: generalizability

Most investigations of new screening or diagnostic tests are performed on patients presenting to a clinic. Only after these tests have passed the test of usefulness in that setting are they investigated in a population-based sample (largely because of the high cost of performing population-based research). Because the data for new tests are based on clinic patients, not populations, the generalizability of the results for a screening application is questionable. Even when new tests are being evaluated for diagnostic usefulness, the mix of patients tested may not reflect the usual mix of patients in an office practice. For example, only those patients who clearly have glaucoma and those who are young and disease-free may be studied. This leads to excellent sensitivity and specificity, which would not be replicated in a sample of patients who have borderline glaucoma and those who are older.

Summary

A variety of measures are available for evaluating the efficacy of screening and diagnostic tests. Sensitivity and specificity are the simplest and easiest to understand, but they suffer from the disadvantage of not considering the prevalence of disease in the target population. PPV and NPV are more useful in that regard. ROC curves can make more comprehensible the relationship of sensitivity and specificity in tests with a continuously variable result; they can also be used for comparing diagnostic tests with one another. Likelihood ratios, and their effect on pretest probability of disease, provide help in critically evaluating screening and diagnostic tests in the context of the clinical setting to which they are to be applied.

> Medeiros FA, Zangwill LM, Bowd C, et al. Comparison of the GDx VCC scanning laser polarimeter, HRT II confocal scanning laser ophthalmoscope, and Stratus OCT optical coherence tomograph for the detection of glaucoma. *Arch Ophthalmol.* 2004;122:827–837.
>
> Riegelman RK. *Studying a Study and Testing a Test: How to Read the Medical Evidence.* 5th ed. Baltimore: Lippincott Williams & Wilkins; 2005.
>
> Tielsch JM, Sommer A, Witt K, et al. Blindness and visual impairment in an American urban population: the Baltimore Eye Survey. *Arch Ophthalmol.* 1990;108:286–290.

Discussing Benefits, Risks, Probabilities, and Expected Outcomes With Patients

Interpreting results of scientific studies for patients is one of the most important duties of a physician. The origin of the word *physician* in Greek is *to educate*. Physicians should always remember that one of their main responsibilities is to educate the patient regarding his or her disease, as well as the potential treatments, preventions, and outcomes. Although increasingly complex scientific analyses have made the interpretation of findings challenging at times, even for the most knowledgeable, if those scientific findings cannot be interpreted for patients, then physicians have failed an important duty.

Most clinical studies present research findings as a percentage or as an absolute change in a disease status (eg, presence of ARM) or in a continuous outcome (eg, IOP). Concrete findings such as these can be straightforward to discuss with patients. However, it is more difficult to discuss odds ratios and concepts such as absolute and relative risk. *Risk* is defined as an expected loss within a distribution of possible outcomes, as when homeowners buy insurance to guard against the risk of a flood. But in the context of clinical research, risk can often be characterized as a conditional probability of an event, usually an adverse event. The condition might be as basic as survival to a particular point or exposure to some phenomenon, for example, persons "at risk" for disease or "in the risk set."

There are 2 potential summaries for comparing risk between groups of individuals. *Risk difference* is the absolute difference in the risk measured between groups. *Relative risk* is the ratio of 2 risk measures. The risk difference depends on the unit of measurement, whereas relative risk is dimensionless because it involves division of 2 risk measurements. In the Ocular Hypertension Treatment Study (OHTS), the absolute risk difference of developing glaucoma for subjects who were not treated compared with those who were treated was 5% (9.5% − 4.5%) across 5 years. The relative risk of not being treated compared with treatment was 211% (9.5/4.5).

Both of these summaries are consistent with the data, but the interpretation of these 2 estimates of the risk in the untreated compared with the treated can be vastly different. Numerically, a 5% increased risk of glaucoma if ocular hypertension is not treated might seem small to a patient, and a 211% increased risk of glaucoma with untreated ocular hypertension might seem large. A key piece of information that may assist in the interpretation is the *baseline probability of the outcome*. In everyday life, people may be willing to board an airplane, doubling their relative risk of accidental death, because the baseline probability of an adverse outcome is so low. In this context, if there is a choice between 2 airlines, for which the risk difference is 5% per million miles flown, the risk difference would not seem small. Thus, it is important to give patients the baseline probabilities or expected outcomes being used for comparison, as these can be interpreted more easily by patients. This is especially true when the risk ratio is less than 100% and may be wrongly interpreted as a risk difference. For example, a difference in adverse outcome rates of between 10% and 13% could be described as involving a relative risk of approximately 30%, but to those unfamiliar with the baseline probabilities, this 30% figure may sound as though the comparison were between 10% and 40%, when it is not.

In observational studies, investigators may present their results as odds ratios. In an *odds ratio*, the odds of a subject with a disease (case) having an exposure (eg, smoking) are compared with the odds of a subject without the disease (control) having the exposure. When the disease is rare, the odds ratio approximates the relative risk of that exposure, because the denominators for both of the odds being compared are close to 1 for rare events. For example, in the meta-analyses on the potential risk factors for late ARM, which occurs relatively infrequently, the odds ratio for smoking is 2.35. This can be interpreted that smokers have 235% of the risk of developing late ARM, compared with nonsmokers.

A *risk factor* is a factor to which patients are exposed either voluntarily or not and with which an increased or decreased likelihood of a disease is associated. Thus, risk factors influence the occurrence of a disease. Exposures to specific factors may or may not be clinically significant. For example, use of seat belts may not be a clinically significant exposure for ARM, whereas smoking is. One of the subsets of risk factors is *causal risk factors*, which are root causes of the disease. Because it is difficult to distinguish causal risk factors from noncausal risk factors in observational studies, researchers often use inductively oriented causal criteria to determine which risk factors are causal and which are not. The Surgeon General's 1964 report on smoking and health broke new ground by describing criteria for evaluating causal relationships in observational data.

When research findings from clinical trials or observational studies are being interpreted, the generalizability of the findings to individual patients must be considered. Questions to raise are, Do the study inclusion criteria include factors that would be applicable to the patient? Or can the findings be extrapolated to the patient? One concept that is essential to understand is the distinction between an *individual effect* and an *average effect*. For example, in the OHTS, the investigators reported that a 1 mm Hg increase in IOP was associated with approximately a 10% increase in the risk of developing glaucoma. Does this necessarily mean that lowering the IOP 1 mm Hg in all ocular hypertensive patients would decrease the overall risk of glaucoma in each patient by 10%, or does it mean that some patients would have more than a 10% risk reduction, and others less? The correct answer is that this statement is referring to an *average effect* in the overall population of ocular hypertensive patients and not to an individual patient. It is important to understand that this concept is population-based and analogous to the health advantages of lower cholesterol levels. In medicine, there is a history of finding an average effect from a treatment in a study and then administering that treatment to everyone who has the disease or condition being studied, with the hope that this helps. Thus, in general, lowering IOP is useful as an overall goal for ocular hypertensive patients, but its benefits may differ from one patient to another.

The literature on causal inference makes clear that it is impossible to draw inferences about individual effects unless an assumption is made that individual effects are the same in a subgroup of patients as in the population studied. A goal of research should be to continue refining estimates of individual effects so that they are tailored as closely as possible to individual characteristics. A goal of patient care should be that treatment decisions are made so that both patient and physician have a clear understanding of the risks involved.

> Kass MA, Heuer DK, Higginbotham EJ, et al. The Ocular Hypertension Treatment Study: a randomized trial determines that topical ocular hypotensive medication delays or prevents the onset of primary open-angle glaucoma. *Arch Ophthalmol.* 2002;120:701–713.
>
> Rubin DB. Bayesian inference for causal effects: the role of randomization. *Ann. Statist.* 1978;6:34–58.
>
> *Smoking and Health: Report of the Advisory Committee to the Surgeon General of the Public Health Service.* Washington, DC: US Dept of Health, Education, and Welfare, Public Health Service; 1964. Public Health Service Publication No. 1103.
>
> Tomany SC, Wang JJ, Van Leeuwen R, et al. Risk factors for incident age-related macular degeneration: pooled findings from 3 continents. *Ophthalmology.* 2004;111:1280–1287.

Applying Statistics to Measure and Improve Clinical Practice

As awareness of the variation in the content and quality of eye care increases, insurers, professional organizations, physician practices, hospitals, and patients will need to understand and use systems that both measure and seek to improve care. Donabedian's organization of quality into 3 distinct elements—structure, process, and outcomes—provides an organizational framework within which eye care can be monitored. *Structure* refers to how the care system is designed, such as whom the patient sees initially, what pathways exist for obtaining various diagnostic tests, and what the financial arrangements are for care reimbursement. *Process* is the content of care, what the provider does or does not do. The principle that drives process quality is "doing the right thing at the right time," to which structure adds "by the right person at the right place." *Outcomes* are the results of care, or the completion of the principle " … so that the right results occur."

Several important statistical principles and techniques are applied in the creation and use of a system that enhances care. At the outset, when the system is being planned or designed, issues of validity, reliability, and population bias are essential considerations. If the system is not designed to measure every occurrence, sampling concerns and nonresponse and missing data issues will need to be addressed when the system is implemented. Analysis of results, particularly comparisons across different providers, can raise important questions about statistical and clinical significance, confounders and adjustments, use of appropriate comparisons, and the extent to which the observed variability of the results is explained through the analyses being used. The final component needed to improve the system is methods of data presentation that facilitate a continual feedback process whereby performances can be tracked and then improved over time. Issues related to comparisons over time thus become important to understand.

Issues in Designing a Measurement System

The first requirement of a useful system is that proposed indicators actually reflect the quality or characteristic to be assessed. This is referred to as *validity*. One question commonly faced by ophthalmologists is whether a patient's eye was dilated during an eye examination, as several national assessments of quality of care measure whether a retinal examination is performed on a patient with diabetes at least every year or two. What might indicate that a dilated exam was done? The single best way, also referred to as the *gold standard,* is to have every ophthalmic examination videotaped, so that a reviewer, through observing the use of an indirect ophthalmoscope or a mirrored contact lens after dilating drops had been placed, could note that a dilated exam was indeed done. An alternative gold standard, according to practice guidelines, is to see that photographs of the retina, including the periphery, had been obtained. The following also could lead to the conclusion that a dilated exam was performed: (1) documentation indicating that dilating drops were placed in the eye; (2) chart notations indicating that a peripheral dilated exam was performed, such as "P" or "periphery," noted as being "normal" or "abnormal"; (3) a diagram or drawing of the retina, on which the periphery or peripheral findings are indicated. All of these would be considered "valid" measures in that their presence in the chart would most likely indicate that a dilated exam had been done; their absence, that it had not. The use of proxies for a gold standard is referred to as *construct validity*.

Once there is a valid measure, *reliability* needs to be determined, that is, whether that measure gives the same answer when it is repeated under a different set of assessment conditions but without a change in the underlying document or service being assessed. How exactly might conditions change? First, a clinician may review a medical chart and may be distracted or tired. When the test or review is repeated by the same clinician at a different time, does the analysis show the same results? Measures that are designed to minimize errors when repeated are noted to have good *test–retest* reliability or reproducibility. Are the same results obtained when the measure is made with the same instrument the second time and the third? Second, if the person doing the measurement gets the same results on the same subject, with multiple attempts, then there is good *intrarater* reliability. Third, measures should be designed (as should the training system and support system that capture and analyze the data) so that many different people can use the measure and obtain the same results. Measures that have this characteristic are said to have good *interrater* reliability.

Two common statistical techniques are used to determine whether there is "good" agreement. One method is to simply tally the number of identical answers between 2 different tests and then divide that number by the total number of items being assessed, thereby yielding a "percent agreement." A second method is to use the *κ (kappa) statistic*, a measure of agreement between 2 or more persons or entities which takes into account that sometimes observers agree through chance alone. Kappas greater than 0.70 are thought to denote good agreement; those of 0.50 or more are thought to have only moderate agreement; less than 0.30, not in agreement.

Once there is a valid and reliable measure, the *population* must be considered, specifically, the population in which the measure is to be used. First, *inclusion criteria* and *exclusion criteria* (who is in and who is out of the population to be measured) need to be carefully defined. For example, a study of the quality of care provided by ophthalmologists might exclude retina specialists (exclusion criterion) and include only comprehensive ophthalmologists who see patients at least 50% of the time (inclusion criterion).

Second, it needs to be ascertained whether the population is one in which there is sufficient frequency of occurrences for meaningful differences to be found. Or are the events so rare ("floor effect") or so common ("ceiling effect") that there is little value to be gained in using such a measurement system? Often, such issues do not become apparent until after at least a pilot analysis is done; but more often, these issues are overlooked when the system is designed. However, even rare events (eg, endophthalmitis or appropriate workups obtained in patients with third nerve palsies) can be meaningful clinically, as can common events (eg, patients surviving surgery or having their vision checked postoperatively). Both, therefore, should be measured on that basis. Such decisions should be made with an understanding of the number of observations (sample size) needed to find statistically and clinically significant differences.

Third, the measures should be easily obtained in the population of interest (including validity and reliability). Systems that do not require much additional work are more practical for the purpose of monitoring practices. Thus, billing files may provide sufficient information on the likelihood of specific process quality steps, such as the performance of regular visual field testing in patients with glaucoma; or of outcomes, such as suprachoroidal hemorrhage after intraocular surgery.

Implementing a Monitoring System

An ideal monitoring system would capture every patient of interest for a given practitioner. Doing so gives the maximum number of cases for statistical analyses and thus provides maximum statistical power while allowing for more reliable estimates of uncommon or rare events. In addition, a 100% analysis minimizes bias that is due to missing patients. For administrative data, 100% review is made feasible by the presence of data in accessible electronic formats. For example, every patient who had intraocular surgery in a practice (defined by specific CPT codes) can be identified during a specified period, and then subsequent surgeries (again defined by CPT codes) within the next 30 or 90 days can be determined, as can a subsequent diagnosis of a specific complication (by ICD codes) such as retinal detachment or endophthalmitis.

In contrast, questions about process quality—such as whether a target pressure range was set for every patient with glaucoma—are not amenable to a 100% review because that type of data (target pressure ranges) is not captured in current administrative databases (but registration and billing data are). Also, a trained reviewer is required to abstract that type of information from charts. Other process quality measures that are separately billed services, such as gonioscopy, are identifiable by analyses of billing databases.

Thus, to the extent that many structure, process, and outcomes quality indicators are not included in electronic databases, they may be feasible to use only when the care of a limited number of patients is reviewed. As electronic medical records become more popular, such reviews will become more feasible, since specific process steps would then become electronically accessible.

The review of a smaller population of interest thus requires *sampling* of the larger pool of patients. First, the universe of patients of interest is clearly defined, with explicit inclusion and exclusion criteria. Second, a list of eligible patients (as complete as possible) is compiled. Third, ideally, the sample for review is drawn in a random fashion by a disinterested party or method. Allowing providers to select charts for review creates substantial selection bias, because the providers are likely to pick those charts that are likely to have the most complete data. Using a convenient sample of the last 20 or so consecutive patients also raises the concern that the sample is not truly representative of the provider's care over the entire period of interest (eg, the clinic may sometimes have been overbooked, causing the provider to defer certain steps of the examination).

Once the sample is drawn, the records are then reviewed. What are the standards that should be used for a review? What criteria should be used? Evidence clearly suggests that having explicit criteria with yes/no or limited categories (eg, having options for optic nerve documentation such as a statement that nerve normal/vertical cup to disc ratio/drawing/photograph) is more reliable than having implicit criteria (the reviewer's judgment that overall quality was good or not good), particularly for interrater reliability. For ophthalmology, the American Academy of Ophthalmology (AAO) has *Preferred Practice Patterns,* as well as Benchmarks, both of which can be easily used as explicit criteria. Similarly, the American Board of Ophthalmology (ABO) has explicit criteria in the Office Record Review Module for board maintenance of certification. These are available at http://www.aao.org/aao/education/library/benchmarks and at http://www.abop.org/recert/recertorl.html.

In many reviews, charts may not be available, or they are incomplete, with missing data or visits. Efforts should be made to obtain unavailable charts. If, after reasonable effort, these charts remain unavailable, the number of unavailable charts are recorded, and replacement charts from the randomization should be reviewed. If the missing-chart rate exceeds a specific rate (eg, the typical rate for missing charts in a particular clinic for patient visits), then issues of bias (perhaps intentional) are more likely to be present. For charts with missing visits, there may be specific review criteria that can be answered completely from available visits. For those review criteria that require every visit to be checked, the options are to (1) exclude that patient; (2) exclude that patient only for those analyses needing that missing visit data; (3) impute the missing values by statistical modeling of available data; or (4) treat the missing visit as either meeting or not meeting the criteria (generally the latter). The key steps are to make a decision on what to do and then apply that decision consistently over time (and report the decision with the data and results). Finally, patients with missing data from a specific visit are typically treated as having not met the review criteria—which is in essence, determining if something is or is not documented in the chart.

One concern is the number of charts that should be reviewed. The sample size required depends on the underlying rates of performance and the amount of difference sought. In general, rates at either extreme (very rare or very common) require a greater sample size. The smaller a difference (eg, in how one provider performs compared with the group average) the researcher wishes to determine to be statistically significant, the greater the sample size required. An important element of establishing a monitoring system for quality of care is performing power calculations to determine sample sizes, as these calculations provide confidence that a nonsignificant difference is truly that (and not due to having insufficient sample size).

A related concern is the route of administering the measure, as the route or method used can have significant effects on the results. The dilated eye examination quality indicator in patients with diabetes can be used as an example. McGlynn et al (2004) noted that use of a chart review format (as described previously) yielded an annual dilated eye examination rate of only 19% among patients with diabetes. Yet a rate of approximately 50% resulted when billing levels were used, specifically, when an appropriate eye examination was imputed to those who had had any eye visit with an eye care professional at a billing level sufficient to support that a dilation could have been done. Clearly, there are significant validity issues with the measure that uses claims data.

Regardless of the method used, systematic errors may occur. First, the data may have been recorded incorrectly, on the part of either the observer or the person abstracting the data from the data source. Errors related to administrative databases include coding issues, data entry problems, and incorrect diagnoses. Errors for chart review approaches, in addition to the above-mentioned, include those made by the abstractor and those made later in the calculation of quality scores. These errors can be minimized by (1) upfront training of all personnel; (2) review of cases with values outside the expected range; and (3) duplicate review of a 5%–10% sample of cases.

Analyzing the Results

Once the results have been compiled, they have to be understood and used appropriately. For projects designed to detect important deviations from expected performance, it is vital to use appropriate statistical tests developed to determine if any differences are statistically significant. For many measures, comparisons of mean performance are satisfactory—as in the percentage of AAO benchmark process indicators for cataract met across 25 patients for every provider. However, for others, the best way to compare performance may be to use the number of persons whose care meets a given threshold. For example, investigators may want to know the percentage of patients who have at least a 90% quality score. Once they have obtained that measure, they can then compare it among providers.

Even if differences are found to be statistically significant, they still may not be clinically meaningful. The greater the sample size, the more likely it is that a statistically significant difference can be found. But it is a separate question whether such differences are truly meaningful. For example, one provider may document the optic nerve 78% of the time; another provider, 81% of the time. With a large enough sample size, this difference can be statistically significant. However, most would be hard-pressed to state that this is clinically meaningful, and most would deny that this difference finds one doctor to be technically of higher quality than the other. Indeed, an appreciation of clinically significant differences is very useful for calculating the sample sizes in the first place.

There may be factors beyond the provider's control that may have resulted in a certain finding. Thus, even if investigators find a difference that means something clinically, they also need to take into account these other factors. For technical performance of process steps such as taking a history or performing a dilated exam, the only likely confounders are the patient's refusal or inability to allow that process step to be performed and the patient's inability to afford any additional tests. For outcomes of chronic diseases, however, the weight of confounders and other factors may often overwhelm the provider's ability to influence the results by doing the right thing, especially over a longer period. For example, the rate of blindness from glaucoma over 20 years is subject to the physiological severity (on presentation) and the risk for progression of the pool of patients. Even beyond this concern for "case-mix" of severity, however, there are many other issues at play, such as the ability of patients to return for regular care and to use their recommended treatments regularly, and the impact of their socioeconomic and cultural states. Thus, measuring whether the provider performs specific examination steps, such as examining the optic nerve (process) is appropriate, whereas looking at rates of blindness over 20 years (outcomes) may not be appropriate.

In other words, even if adjustments are made for case-mix and other confounders, caution still needs to be exercised so that appropriate comparisons are used. The fundamental question is whether it is fair to hold the provider accountable for the indicator in question. Where the criterion is wholly or even largely within the control of the provider, it certainly is. Where the criterion is within the control of an agent or factor independent of the provider, it most likely is not. If providers are held accountable, they are, in essence, being made responsible for the behaviors of their patients and the patients' families. Under such a circumstance, providers would most likely find a strong disincentive to accept poorer, less compliant patients, instead focusing on only those with the attitudes, skills, and resources to follow recommended care. For example, a provider caring for indigent patients in an inner-city neighborhood may be penalized relative to a lower-quality provider in a wealthy suburb, unless such adjustments and appropriate comparisons are made.

In making statistical comparisons *and* including confounding factors, investigators specify a defined set of factors and conditions that may be helpful in understanding the results of the analyses. A key step, often overlooked, is to see how important these indicators are to the overall quality of care and thence to how the patient fares (the AAO *Preferred Practice Patterns* grade each process indicator as to the "importance to care"). If a step is not truly crucial to either defining a condition, in relating to overall quality, or assessing how a patient does over time, then its nonperformance may be less of a problem.

One technique commonly used to perform this key analysis is looking at how much of the *variance* in the dependent variable of interest is accounted for by all of the independent variables in the analysis. This is often stated as the percent of variance that is "explained" by the variables included in the analysis. Where the proportion of variability explained is high, we would expect that paying greater attention to the specific criteria in the analysis would be important; where the proportion of variability explained is low, less weight would be given to the criteria. From a statistical perspective, one shorthand method of expressing variance explained is assessing the R^2 of the variables in the analysis. The fundamental question is, How much do the statistically (and clinically) meaningful variables explain the dependent variable of interest?

Methods of Data Presentation to Facilitate Continuous Improvement of Practices

Once the initial system has been designed, implemented, and analyzed, the quality monitoring and improvement system can enhance care only if the results from the analyses are disseminated and used to improve care processes and structures. Just measuring and feeding back results have been shown to improve subsequent care by between 3% and 6% in the performance indicators. Those delivery systems that make a dedicated effort to implementing continual quality improvement are able to demonstrate significantly greater performance gains. A discussion of the methods of continuous quality improvement (CQI) and total quality management (TQM) is beyond the scope of this chapter; however, there are several useful tools for data analysis and presentation that have broader use.

First, plotting the data on a frequency distribution, or *histogram* (Fig 16-7), or using a *scatter diagram* (Fig 16-8) to show the distribution along 2 or more variables is vital to understanding the nature of the data. Are the data "normally distributed" in a bell-shaped curve, or are they skewed? The answer to this question affects the choice of statistical tools and analyses, and it can also provide important insights into potential underlying factors. Or, 2 distinct subgroups may be found in the data, thereby calling for additional insights as to defining those subgroups. For example, care in solo practices is likely to differ significantly from large single-specialty groups for a particular disease area.

Second, use of a *pareto chart* (Fig 16-9) provides insights into a cumulative distribution of key factors of interest. The chart combines a histogram with a cumulative frequency line, making it possible to assess performance across the range of values for the variable of interest.

Third, the rates of events, especially uncommon ones, can fluctuate over time. Are the fluctuations significant, both statistically and clinically, compared with those of prior periods and other institutions or practices? The use of *run diagrams,* or *control charts* (Fig 16-10), in which event rates are plotted over time with both SD (standard deviation) and benchmark lines, enables reviewers to determine (1) if an aberrant data point is really a meaningful finding or one due to random error and (2) how the organization is faring compared with peer comparisons.

The purpose of these data analyses is to identify variation in the factor of interest. Those factors that are due to the way the system is established and that are inherent in its current state of operations are referred to as *common cause* factors. To improve per-

CHAPTER 16: Using Statistics in Practice and Work • 369

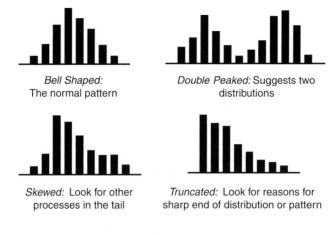

Bell Shaped:
The normal pattern

Double Peaked: Suggests two
distributions

Skewed: Look for other
processes in the tail

Truncated: Look for reasons for
sharp end of distribution or pattern

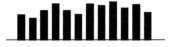

Ragged Plateau: No single clear
process or pattern

Figure 16-7 Types of histograms. *(Reproduced from the Quality Assurance Project. Available at http://qaproject.org/methods/reshistorgram.html.)*

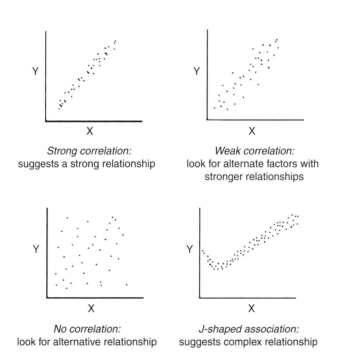

Strong correlation:
suggests a strong relationship

Weak correlation:
look for alternate factors with
stronger relationships

No correlation:
look for alternative relationship

J-shaped association:
suggests complex relationship

Figure 16-8 Scatter diagram interpretation. *(Reproduced from the Quality Assurance Project. Available at http://qaproject.org/methods/resscatter.html.)*

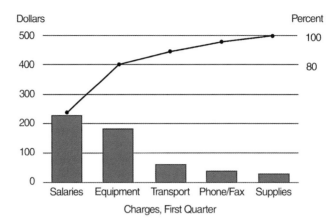

Figure 16-9 Pareto chart. *(Reproduced from the Quality Assurance Project. Available at http://qaproject.org/methods/resparetochart.html.)*

formance in this area, the system will have to be redesigned and reengineered. For example, there may be a known rate of "unreliable" visual fields in glaucoma, despite the best training of technicians and screening of patients. In contrast, there are "special causes" of variation that are due to a specific, identifiable factor, often a specific provider or person. Rapid identification of "special cause" variance allows for quick correction of variation that exceeds normal rates. However, it is improving the performance of the overall system and reducing "common cause" variation that provide the opportunity to improve care and impact the most patients. It is by "shifting the curve" that care for every patient may be improved, as opposed to just identifying the outlier providers and assisting in their rehabilitation.

Other Features of Continuous Quality Improvement

Use of continuous quality improvement tools also requires significant thought on how to then improve care structures and processes. An essential step in consciously trying to improve care processes, before or after initial analyses, is developing a *checklist* of the steps and parties involved and then creating a *flowchart* (Fig 16-11) of the system of care involved. By looking at the overall process for a specific outcome (eg, making sure a patient with diabetes gets an annual eye examination), researchers can identify opportunities for streamlining the process.

An additional tool is the *fishbone,* or *cause and effect* diagram (Fig 16-12), which provides detailed information on the different factors, including personnel, that are significant inputs to each step of the process of care. Mapping each of these important steps can help clarify where problems may occur and where work may be improved. Changes in those steps can then be measured and the results monitored. Those interested in improving the quality of care are, in this way, provided with continuous feedback.

Summary

Efforts to improve the quality of care—and ensuring that fair and meaningful quality measures are part of this endeavor—bring key statistical concepts to the forefront. Par-

CHAPTER 16: Using Statistics in Practice and Work • 371

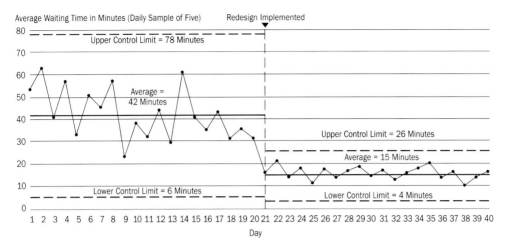

Figure 16-10 Control chart of average wait time before and after a redesign. *(Reproduced from the Quality Assurance Project. Available at http://qaproject.org/methods/resstattools2.html.)*

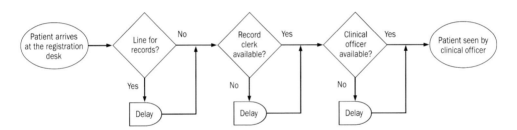

Figure 16-11 Flowchart of patient registration. *(Reproduced from the Quality Assurance Project. Available at http://qaproject.org/methods/resflowchart.html.)*

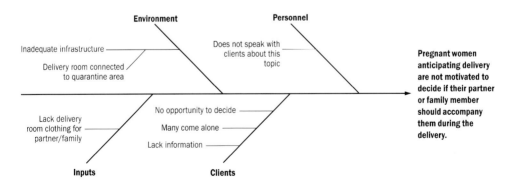

Figure 16-12 Fishbone diagram used at a hospital. *(Reproduced from the Quality Assurance Project. Available at http://qaproject.org/methods/resc&e.html.)*

ticularly since *quality* is likely to become an important component of reimbursement for federal government programs as well as private managed-care companies ("pay for performance"), creation and maintenance of an appropriate system are essential. Indeed, to the extent quality measures are also used to select providers for participation in provider panels of insurance companies, having meaningful systems that entail appropriate statistical approaches in their design and implementation is even more important. Thus, statistics is useful not only for understanding the scientific literature and providing care for patients, but also for influencing the practices and livelihoods of providers, including ophthalmologists.

> Abrams LS, Scott IU, Spaeth GL, et al. Agreement among optometrists, ophthalmologists, and residents in evaluating the optic disc for glaucoma. *Ophthalmology*. 1994;101(10): 1662–1667.
>
> Committee on Quality of Health Care in America, Institute of Medicine. *Crossing the Quality Chasm: A New Health System for the 21st Century.* Washington, DC: National Academy Press; 2001.
>
> Donabedian A. Evaluating the quality of medical care. *Milbank Mem Fund Q*. 1966;44(3): suppl:166–206.
>
> Ferguson TB Jr, Peterson ED, Coombs LP, et al. Use of continuous quality improvement to increase use of process measures in patients undergoing coronary artery bypass graft surgery: a randomized controlled trial. *JAMA*. 2003;290(1):49–56.
>
> Fong DS, Sharza M, Chen W, et al. Vision loss among diabetics in a group model Health Maintenance Organization (HMO). *Am J Ophthalmol*. 2002;133(2):236–241.
>
> Fremont AM, Lee PP, Mangione CM, et al. Patterns of care for open-angle glaucoma in managed care. *Arch Ophthalmol*. 2003;121(6):777–783.
>
> McGlynn EA, Asch SM, Adams J, et al. The quality of health care delivered to adults in the United States. *N Engl J Med*. 2003;348(26):2635–2645.
>
> Oliver JE, Hattenhauer MG, Herman D, et al. Blindness and glaucoma: a comparison of patients progressing to blindness from glaucoma with patients maintaining vision. *Am J Ophthalmol*. 2002;133(6):764–772.
>
> Schuster MA, McGlynn EA, Brook RH. How good is the quality of health care in the United States? *Milbank Q*. 1998;76(4):517–563.
>
> Sloan FA, Brown DS, Carlisle ES, et al. Monitoring visual status: why patients do or do not comply with practice guidelines. *Health Serv Res*. 2004;39(5):1429–1448.

The BCSC faculty wishes to acknowledge the following individuals for their contributions to this chapter: Paul P. Lee, MD, JD; Maureen Maguire, MD; and Richard P. Mills, MD, MPH.

Dr. Lee states that he receives financial compensation from Pfizer and from Allergan, Inc. Dr. Mills states that he has an affiliation with Pfizer and with Allergan, Inc.

Basic Texts

General Medicine

Beers MH, Berkow R, eds. *The Merck Manual of Diagnosis and Therapy.* 17th ed. Rahway, NJ: Merck Research Laboratories; 1999.

Braunwald E, Zipes DP, Libby P, eds. *Heart Disease: A Textbook of Cardiovascular Medicine.* 6th ed. Philadelphia: Saunders; 2001.

Cancer: Rates and Risks. 4th ed. Bethesda, MD: National Institutes of Health; 1996.

Cummins RO, ed. *Advanced Cardiac Life Support Provider Manual.* Dallas: American Heart Association; 2003.

Cush JJ, Kavanaugh A, Stein CM. *Rheumatology: Diagnosis and Therapeutics.* 2nd ed. Philadelphia: Lippincott Williams & Wilkins; 2005.

DeVita VT Jr, Hellman S, Rosenberg SA, eds. *Cancer: Principles and Practice of Oncology.* 7th ed. Philadelphia: Lippincott Williams & Wilkins; 2005.

Diabetes in America. 2nd ed. Bethesda, MD: National Institutes of Health; 1995.

Fraunfelder FT, Fraunfelder FW. *Drug-Induced Ocular Side Effects.* 5th ed. Boston: Butterworth-Heinemann; 2001.

Goetz CG, ed. *Textbook of Clinical Neurology.* 2nd ed. St Louis: Elsevier; 2003.

Goldman L, Ausiello D, eds. *Cecil Textbook of Medicine.* 22nd ed. Philadelphia: Saunders; 2004.

Harris ED Jr, Budd RC, Firestein GS, et al, eds. *Kelley's Textbook of Rheumatology.* 7th ed. Philadelphia: Saunders; 2005.

Henderson KE, Baranski TJ, Bickel PE, eds. *The Washington Manual Endocrinology Subspecialty Consult.* Philadelphia: Lippincott Williams & Wilkins; 2005.

Kasper DL, Braunwald E, Fauci A, eds. *Harrison's Principles of Internal Medicine.* 16th ed. New York: McGraw-Hill; 2004.

Larsen PR, Kronenberg H, Melmed S, et al, eds. *Williams Textbook of Endocrinology.* 10th ed. Philadelphia: Saunders; 2003.

Mandell GL, Bennett JE, Dolin R, eds. *Mandell, Douglas, and Bennett's Principles and Practice of Infectious Diseases.* 6th ed. New York: Churchill Livingstone; 2004.

Moore DP, Jefferson JW. *Handbook of Medical Psychiatry.* 2nd ed. St Louis: Mosby; 2004.

Ropper AH, Brown RJ, eds. *Adams and Victor's Principles of Neurology.* 8th ed. New York: McGraw-Hill, 2005.

Credit Reporting Form

Basic and Clinical Science Course, 2009–2010
Section 1

The American Academy of Ophthalmology is accredited by the Accreditation Council for Continuing Medical Education to provide continuing medical education for physicians.

The American Academy of Ophthalmology designates this educational activity for a maximum of 30 *AMA PRA Category 1 Credits*™. Physicians should only claim credit commensurate with the extent of their participation in the activity.

If you wish to claim continuing medical education credit for your study of this Section, you may claim your credit online or fill in the required forms and mail or fax them to the Academy.

To use the forms:

1. Complete the study questions and mark your answers on the Section Completion Form.
2. Complete the Section Evaluation.
3. Fill in and sign the statement below.
4. Return this page and the required forms by mail or fax to the CME Registrar (see below).

To claim credit online:

1. Log on to the Academy website (www.aao.org/cme).
2. Select Review/Claim CME.
3. Follow the instructions.

Important: These completed forms or the online claim must be received at the Academy by June 2012.

I hereby certify that I have spent _____ (up to 30) hours of study on the curriculum of this Section and that I have completed the study questions.

Signature: _____
                                                                                        Date
Name: _____

Address: _____

City and State: _____   Zip: _____

Telephone: (_____) _____   Academy Member ID# _____
                 area code

Please return completed forms to: **Or you may fax them to:** 415-561-8575
American Academy of Ophthalmology
P.O. Box 7424
San Francisco, CA 94120-7424
Attn: CME Registrar, Customer Service

2009–2010
Section Completion Form

Basic and Clinical Science Course

Answer Sheet for Section 1

Question	Answer	Question	Answer	Question	Answer
1	a b c d	20	a b c d	39	a b c d
2	a b c d	21	a b c d	40	a b c d
3	a b c d	22	a b c d	41	a b c d
4	a b c d	23	a b c d	42	a b c d
5	a b c d	24	a b c d	43	a b c d
6	a b c d	25	a b c d	44	a b c d
7	a b c d	26	a b c d	45	a b c d
8	a b c d	27	a b c d	46	a b c d
9	a b c d	28	a b c d	47	a b c d
10	a b c d	29	a b c d	48	a b c d
11	a b c d	30	a b c d	49	a b c d
12	a b c d	31	a b c d	50	a b c d
13	a b c d	32	a b c d	51	a b c d
14	a b c d	33	a b c d	52	a b c d
15	a b c d	34	a b c d	53	a b c d
16	a b c d	35	a b c d	54	a b c d
17	a b c d	36	a b c d	55	a b c d
18	a b c d	37	a b c d		
19	a b c d	38	a b c d		

Section Evaluation

Please complete this CME questionnaire.

1. To what degree will you use knowledge from BCSC Section 1 in your practice?

    ☐ Regularly

    ☐ Sometimes

    ☐ Rarely

2. Please review the stated objectives for BCSC Section 1. How effective was the material at meeting those objectives?

    ☐ All objectives were met.

    ☐ Most objectives were met.

    ☐ Some objectives were met.

    ☐ Few or no objectives were met.

3. To what degree is BCSC Section 1 likely to have a positive impact on health outcomes of your patients?

    ☐ Extremely likely

    ☐ Highly likely

    ☐ Somewhat likely

    ☐ Not at all likely

4. After you review the stated objectives for BCSC Section 1, please let us know of any additional knowledge, skills, or information useful to your practice that were acquired but were not included in the objectives. [Optional]

5. Was BCSC Section 1 free of commercial bias?

    ☐ Yes

    ☐ No

6. If you selected "No" in the previous question, please comment. [Optional]

7. Please tell us what might improve the applicability of BCSC to your practice. [Optional]

Study Questions

Although a concerted effort has been made to avoid ambiguity and redundancy in these questions, the authors recognize that differences of opinion may occur regarding the "best" answer. The discussions are provided to demonstrate the rationale used to derive the answer. They may also be helpful in confirming that your approach to the problem was correct or, if necessary, in fixing the principle in your memory. The authors wish to acknowledge Edward J. Rockwell, MD, for his contributions.

1. Which of the following statements about vancomycin is incorrect?
    a. Vancomycin-resistant staphylococcal infections have not yet been reported in the medical literature.
    b. Vancomycin-resistant enterococcal infections have been reported in the medical literature.
    c. Vancomycin is a member of the glycopeptide antibiotic family.
    d. Teicoplanin is effective against some vancomycin-resistant bacterial strains.

2. PCR (polymerase chain reaction) DNA assays are now available for the rapid and highly sensitive detection of which of the following organisms?
    a. *Clostridium difficile*
    b. *Chlamydia trachomatis*
    c. cytomegalovirus
    d. all of the above

3. Which of the following is not a type of viral hepatitis?
    a. hepatitis C
    b. chronic delta hepatitis
    c. hepatitis K
    d. TTV-associated (transfusion-transmitted virus) hepatitis

4. All of the following statements are true regarding HAART (highly active antiretroviral therapy) *except*
    a. Since the advent of HAART, a smaller percentage of HIV-infected patients are developing AIDS.
    b. In HAART, multiple antiretroviral drugs are given sequentially, rather than simultaneously.
    c. HAART often results in dramatic reduction of HIV viral load and increased CD4 lymphocyte levels.
    d. Some studies have shown more than an 80% reduction in the number of opportunistic infections in patients on HAART.

5. Newer antibiotic agents currently available to treat serious bacterial infections include all of the following *except*
   a. trovafloxacin, a fluoroquinolone
   b. quinupristin/dalfopristin, a streptogramin
   c. cefzolapine, a cephalosporin
   d. linezolid, an oxazolidinone

6. Blood pressure monitoring should begin
   a. in childhood
   b. after age 18
   c. after age 35
   d. depending on symptoms

7. Which one of the following statements is incorrect?
   a. The risk of cardiovascular disease, beginning at 115/75 mm Hg, doubles with every 20/10 mm Hg rise in blood pressure.
   b. Systolic blood pressure is a more important risk factor for cardiovascular disease than is diastolic blood pressure.
   c. Hypertension, generally, is symptomatic above 160/90 mm Hg.
   d. Cardiovascular complication rates differ according to ethnic group and socioeconomic status.

8. Lifestyle modifications to manage hypertension include all of the following *except*
   a. weight reduction
   b. dietary sodium reduction
   c. exercise
   d. abstinence from alcohol

9. Ocular conditions associated with hypertension include which of the following?
   a. retinal vein occlusion
   b. ischemic optic neuropathy
   c. glaucoma
   d. all of the above

10. Carotid endarterectomy has been proven to be of benefit in reducing stroke in patients with symptoms and
    a. 70%–99% carotid artery stenosis
    b. 40%–69% carotid artery stenosis
    c. 20%–39% carotid artery stenosis
    d. 100% carotid artery stenosis

11. Statin use reduces the risk of
    a. coronary events in patients with hyperlipidemia
    b. stroke in patients with coronary artery disease
    c. stroke in patients with previous stroke of atherosclerotic origin
    d. all of the above

12. Magnetic resonance imaging is more sensitive than computed tomography in the diagnosis of which one of the following?
    a. intracranial hemorrhage
    b. early cerebral infarction
    c. ischemic stroke
    d. none of the above

13. Which of the following is the number one killer of women in the United States?
    a. breast cancer
    b. lung cancer
    c. ovarian cancer
    d. atherosclerotic heart disease

14. Which one of the following does not increase serum high-density-lipoprotein cholesterol (HDL-C)?
    a. aerobic exercise
    b. moderate alcohol consumption
    c. gemfibrozil (Lopid)
    d. lovastatin (Mevacor)

15. Hypercholesterolemia is a risk factor for all but which one of the following?
    a. arteritic ischemic optic neuropathy
    b. ischemic heart disease
    c. cerebrovascular disease
    d. peripheral vascular disease

16. The first line of treatment in reducing serum cholesterol should be
    a. dietary therapy
    b. aerobic exercise
    c. weight loss
    d. drug therapy

17. Therapeutic lifestyle changes (TLC) alone should be considered if the patient has
    a. coronary heart disease and a low-density-lipoprotein cholesterol (LDL-C) level of >90 mg/dL
    b. coronary heart disease risk equivalents and an LDL-C level of ≥100 mg/dL
    c. 2 risk factors for coronary heart disease and an LDL-C level of >120 mg/dL
    d. 1 risk factor for coronary heart disease and an LDL-C level of >150 mg/dL

18. Which one of the following is true?
    a. Statin use reduces the risk of age-related macular degeneration (AMD).
    b. Hormone replacement therapy can be used as an alternative to cholesterol-lowering therapy in postmenopausal women with elevated cholesterol levels.
    c. For every 30-mg/dL change in LDL-C, the risk of coronary heart disease (CHD) is changed by 30%.
    d. Use of statins in acute coronary syndromes does not reduce the risk of recurrent coronary events.

19. Which one of the following is most indicative of restrictive pulmonary disease?
    a. abnormal-appearing chest radiograph
    b. FEV_1 less than 80% predicted
    c. low Po_2 in arterial blood gas
    d. total lung capacity less than 70% predicted

20. Which of the following may be used as therapy for chronic obstructive pulmonary disease?
    a. adrenergic agonists
    b. anticholinergic drugs
    c. anti-inflammatory drugs
    d. all of the above

21. Which of the following is the best test to monitor heparin therapy?
    a. prothrombin time (PT)
    b. partial thromboplastin time (PTT)
    c. bleeding time
    d. platelet count

22. Adverse ocular reactions seen with use of digoxin include which one of the following?
    a. glare phenomenon and disturbances with color vision
    b. corneal microdeposits
    c. keratoconjunctivitis sicca
    d. bull's-eye maculopathy

23. All of the following statements about iron deficiency anemia are correct *except*
    a. This is the most common type of anemia worldwide.
    b. In iron deficiency anemia, the serum ferritin level is low.
    c. It is safe to give iron supplements to patients with iron deficiency anemia and to repeat the blood count in 1 year.
    d. Severe iron deficiency can cause mucosal changes, such as a smooth tongue, brittle nails, and cheilosis.

24. All of the following can interfere with platelet function and increase bleeding time *except*
    a. aspirin
    b. nonsteroidal anti-inflammatory drugs
    c. severe renal disease
    d. vitamin K

25. Which one of the following statements is not correct about rheumatoid arthritis?
    a. It tends to affect the large joints.
    b. Approximately 80% of patients are positive for rheumatoid factor.
    c. Stiffness at rest often improves with use.
    d. Extra-articular disease may be found.

26. A 50-year-old white male presents with acute nongranulomatous anterior uveitis. He has had chronic back pain for years. Which one of the following does not fit with his clinical syndrome?
    a. sacroiliitis on radiography
    b. spinal ankylosis on radiography
    c. positive HLA-DR4
    d. restrictive lung disease

27. Which one of the following is the most common ophthalmic manifestation of systemic lupus erythematosus?
    a. cranial nerve palsies
    b. retinal vascular disease
    c. cortical blindness
    d. Sjögren syndrome

28. Which one of the following is most effective for treating Wegener granulomatosis?
    a. aspirin
    b. nonsteroidal anti-inflammatory agents
    c. cyclophosphamide
    d. methotrexate

29. The definitive test for giant cell arteritis is which one of the following?
    a. Wintrobe sedimentation rate
    b. Westergren sedimentation rate
    c. C-reactive protein
    d. temporal artery biopsy

30. In addition to uveitis, with or without hypopyon, which one of the following is the most common ophthalmic manifestation of Behçet syndrome?
    a. glaucoma
    b. retinal vasculitis
    c. corneal disease
    d. eyelid ulcers

31. Which one of the following is a potential adverse effect of newer anticytokine drugs such as etanercept (Enbrel) and infliximab (Remicade)?
    a. disc edema
    b. angle-closure glaucoma
    c. demyelinating disease, including optic neuritis
    d. increased risk of diabetes

32. The preferred test for diagnosing type 2 diabetes is
    a. hemoglobin A_{1c}
    b. fasting plasma glucose
    c. oral glucose tolerance test
    d. urine glucose and ketones

33. Which one of the following is correct as a significant side effect associated with the class of oral hypoglycemic agents given?
    a. sulfonylureas—nausea and vomiting
    b. α-glucosidase inhibitors—thrombocytopenia
    c. biguanides—hypertension
    d. thiazolidinediones—fluid retention and heart failure

34. Ophthalmic findings that can be diagnostic for multiple endocrine neoplasia type IIB are
    a. subconjunctival neuromas
    b. asymmetric bitemporal visual field defects
    c. prominent corneal nerves
    d. diplopia and visual field loss associated with a severe headache

35. Type 2 diabetes is characterized by all of the following *except*
    a. genetic predisposition
    b. low basal insulin secretion early in the disease
    c. later age of onset than with type 1 diabetes
    d. increased visceral fat

36. Which one of the following is the leading cause of death in the United States?
    a. coronary artery disease
    b. stroke
    c. cancer
    d. accidents

37. Which one of the following is the most sensitive and specific test(s) for screening for thyroid disease?
    a. T_3 level
    b. free T_4 and sensitive TSH levels
    c. radioactive iodine uptake
    d. thyroid-binding globulin level

38. Cancer is predominantly a genetic disease. Which one of the following cancers may have a viral cause?
    a. breast
    b. colon
    c. lung
    d. cervical

39. Lung cancer is
    a. occurring in an increasing percentage of patients
    b. more common in women than in men
    c. not associated with smoking
    d. all of the above

40. Viruses
    a. do not cause cancer in animal models
    b. that contain RNA are most likely to cause cancer
    c. that contain single-stranded DNA are most likely to cause cancer
    d. have been implicated in nasopharyngeal carcinoma

41. Which one of the following statements is not correct about bipolar disorder (formerly known as manic depression)?
    a. It is the most common form of depression.
    b. There may be alternating periods of depression and elevated mood.
    c. It is treated with psychotherapy.
    d. It is treated with lithium.

42. Fetal alcohol syndrome includes all but which one of the following?
    a. blepharophimosis
    b. cataract
    c. telecanthus
    d. optic nerve hypoplasia

43. Antidepressants include all of the following *except*
    a. lithium
    b. monoamine oxidase inhibitors
    c. fluoxetine (Prozac)
    d. haloperidol (Haldol)

44. Parkinson disease is characterized by all but which one of the following?
    a. increased rigidity
    b. excess dopamine production
    c. potential worsening of symptoms with neuroleptic drugs
    d. loss of neurons in the substantia nigra

45. Alzheimer disease is characterized by all of the following *except*
    a. neurofibrillary tangles
    b. progressive dementia in later life
    c. a toxic cause in most cases
    d. extraneuronal amyloid plaques

46. Which one of the following would argue against widespread screening for a disease?
    a. It is treatable or preventable.
    b. It has a low prevalence.
    c. It is generally asymptomatic.
    d. The cost of the disease and its complications is high.

47. Which one of the following is *not* a risk factor for breast cancer?
    a. fibrocystic disease
    b. first-degree relative with breast cancer
    c. early menarche
    d. nulliparity

48. Which of the following is *not* true regarding cervical cancer?
    a. More than 95% of cervical cancers are positive for human papillomavirus.
    b. Cervical cancer is the most common gynecologic cancer in women between the ages of 15 and 34.
    c. Number of sexual partners is a risk factor for cervical cancer.
    d. The Papanicolaou test ("Pap smear") is now considered obsolete and is no longer used to diagnose cervical cancer.

49. Which statement is true regarding the American Cancer Society's recommendations for cancer screening?
    a. Mammography should begin with a baseline examination at age 45.
    b. Chest x-ray is an effective screening test for lung cancer.
    c. Sigmoidoscopy is recommended for patients older than 50 years of age, every 3 to 5 years, after 2 negative annual examinations.
    d. Pelvic examination is recommended every 5 years for women between the ages of 20 and 40 years.

50. Which one of the following is not a routine childhood immunization?
    a. hepatitis B
    b. varicella
    c. cytomegalovirus
    d. polio virus

51. Which one of the following is not a component of the management of anaphylaxis?
    a. epinephrine (0.3–0.5 mL of 1:1000 subcutaneous or intramuscular injection)
    b. terbutaline 10 mg intravenous injection
    c. intravenous volume expansion
    d. hydrocortisone for serious or prolonged reactions

52. An anesthesiologist would avoid which one of the following in a patient with a history of malignant hyperthermia?
    a. thiopental sodium
    b. nitrous oxide
    c. midazolam (Versed)
    d. succinylcholine

53. Routine preoperative testing
    a. should be performed before all cataract surgery
    b. effectively reduces malpractice liability
    c. is not necessary for many patients
    d. is an effective public health measure

54. Which one of the following would be the most important for a preoperative patient to take the morning of surgery?
    a. antihypertensive agent
    b. digoxin
    c. thyroid medication
    d. estrogen supplements

55. Which one of the following studies would best demonstrate the incidence of a disease?
    a. case series
    b. case-control study
    c. cohort study
    d. randomized, prospective, controlled clinical trial

Answers

1. **a.** In fact, the first case of vancomycin-resistant *Staphylococcus aureus* was reported in the literature in July 2002. The other statements are true. Teicoplanin is a newer member of the glycopeptide class of antibiotics.
2. **d.** PCR testing is now available for detection of all of these organisms and many more.
3. **c.** Hepatitis A, B, C, D, E, and G, as well as TTV-associated hepatitis, are documented in the medical literature, but thus far, there is no hepatitis K.
4. **b.** The multiple antiretroviral agents used in HAART are given simultaneously, not sequentially, to prevent early drug resistance.
5. **c.** Cefzolapine does not exist. The others are antibiotics, including 2 new classes of antibiotics—the streptogramins and the oxazolidinones.
6. **a.** Evidence suggests that hypertension in the young is more common than previously recognized and has substantial long-term health consequences. It is recommended that children older than 3 years of age who are seen in a medical setting should have their blood pressure measured.
7. **c.** Individuals with hypertension are often asymptomatic. Most patients with hypertension either do not know that they have it or are inadequately treated, and symptoms are not a reliable indicator of the severity of hypertension. Significant racial and ethnic disparities in awareness, treatment, and control of hypertension exist in the United States, and socioeconomic and lifestyle factors continue to be barriers to treatment in many minority patients.
8. **d.** Maintenance of normal body weight, reduced dietary sodium intake, and regular aerobic physical activity are all beneficial for controlling blood pressure. Although moderation of alcohol consumption is advised, abstinence is not required.
9. **d.** Retinal vascular complications (including hypertensive retinopathy and retinal vein occlusions), glaucoma, and ischemic optic neuropathy are commonly associated with hypertension.
10. **a.** Carotid endarterectomy is beneficial for symptomatic patients with recent nondisabling carotid artery ischemic events and ipsilateral 70%–99% carotid artery stenosis. Carotid endarterectomy is not beneficial for symptomatic patients with 0%–29% or 100% stenosis. The potential benefit of carotid endarterectomy for symptomatic patients with 30%–69% stenosis is uncertain.
11. **d.** Statin use reduces the risk of stroke and other coronary events in patients with coronary artery disease or in those who have had an ischemic stroke of atherosclerotic origin. Statin use also reduces the risk of coronary events in patients with hyperlipidemia.
12. **b.** All suspected cases of stroke and threatened stroke should prompt *computed tomography (CT)* of the brain. Computed tomography is very sensitive to the presence of intracranial hemorrhage. *Magnetic resonance imaging (MRI)* is often more sensitive than CT in detecting an evolving stroke within hours of its onset and an early cerebral infarction, whereas CT results may be negative for up to several days after an acute cerebral infarct.

13. **d.** Atherosclerotic coronary artery disease is by far the number one killer not only in the United States, but also in the world. It is estimated that every minute, 1 person dies in the United States because of coronary artery disease. The number of women who die from cardiovascular disease is 10 times that of breast cancer.

14. **d.** Aerobic exercise, moderate alcohol consumption, and gemfibrozil have all been demonstrated to increase serum high-density-lipoprotein cholesterol (HDL-C), which may have a beneficial effect against atherogenesis. High levels of low-density-lipoprotein cholesterol (LDL-C) and low levels of HDL-C have been shown to increase the risk of coronary artery disease. Lovastatin reduces serum LDL-C but does not increase HDL-C.

15. **a.** Hypercholesterolemia is a risk factor for ischemic heart disease, cerebrovascular disease, peripheral vascular disease, and nonarteritic ischemic optic neuropathy. Arteritic ischemic optic neuropathy is seen in giant cell arteritis, a vascular inflammatory condition, associated with polymyalgia rheumatica.

16. **a.** Dietary therapy should be the first line of treatment in reducing serum cholesterol. Regular aerobic exercise and limited alcohol intake have a beneficial effect on serum cholesterol by increasing HDL cholesterol. Medications are used after other modalities such as diet and exercise have not lowered cholesterol adequately. Weight loss can be associated with a lowering of cholesterol; however, in and of itself, it is not the first line of treatment for reducing serum cholesterol.

17. **b.** Therapeutic lifestyle changes alone should be considered if the patient has coronary heart disease (CHD) or CHD risk equivalents and an LDL-C level of 100 mg/dL or higher; 2 or more risk factors and an LDL-C level of 130 mg/dL or higher; or 1 risk factor and an LDL-C level of 160 mg/dL or higher.

18. **c.** Numerous clinical trials have demonstrated that effective LDL-C reduction substantially reduces the risk of coronary heart disease. For every 30-mg/dL change in LDL-C, the risk of CHD is changed by 30%. Physicians should advise against the use of hormone replacement therapy as an alternative to cholesterol-lowering drugs. Use of statins in acute coronary syndromes reduces the risk of recurrent coronary events. There is no definitive evidence that statin use reduces the risk of age-related macular degeneration.

19. **d.** Low arterial Po_2 can have a number of causes and is not specific for the type of pulmonary disease. An abnormal-appearing chest radiograph may show severe kyphosis, one cause of restrictive lung disease, but is not usually diagnostic of restrictive lung disease. An FEV_1 less than 80% of predicted suggests obstructive pulmonary disease. A total lung capacity less than 70% predicted suggests restrictive pulmonary disease, such as pulmonary fibrosis.

20. **d.** All of these drug classes may be used as therapy for chronic obstructive pulmonary disease.

21. **b.** Heparin therapy is monitored by the partial thromboplastin time (PTT). Prothrombin time or the international normalized ratio (INR) is used to monitor oral warfarin therapy. Bleeding time reflects platelet count and function. Platelet abnormalities do not affect the PTT.

22. **a.** The glare phenomenon and disturbances with color vision are the most striking and the most common adverse ocular reactions seen with use of digoxin. Corneal microdeposits occur with use of chloroquine and amiodarone. Keratoconjunctivitis sicca is not a specific side effect of digoxin but may be observed in patients using beta-blockers. Bull's-eye maculopathy may be a side effect of chloroquine.

23. **c.** By far the most common type of anemia worldwide, iron deficiency anemia is diagnosed when serum ferritin is less than 30 µg/L. Every adult with iron deficiency anemia is suspected to be bleeding until proven otherwise. Menstrual blood loss in women plays a major role, as does gastrointestinal bleeding in both men and women. For many patients today, treatment of various conditions includes aspirin, which can cause gastrointestinal bleeding. The signs and symptoms of iron deficiency anemia are the same as those of the other anemias (pallor, cool skin, exercise intolerance or fatigue at rest, and so forth), but severe iron deficiency can cause mucosal changes, such as a smooth tongue, brittle nails, and cheilosis.

24. **d.** Vitamin K affects the coagulation factors but not platelet function. A single aspirin tablet taken orally irreversibly inhibits platelet aggregation for the life span of the circulating platelets present, causing a modest prolongation of the bleeding time for at least 48–72 hours following ingestion. This reaction has remarkably little effect in normal persons, although intraoperative blood loss may be slightly increased. Nonsteroidal anti-inflammatory drugs cause reversible inhibition of platelet function in the presence of the drug; the effect disappears as the drug is cleared from the blood. Uremia caused by renal failure may interfere with platelet function.

25. **a.** Patients with rheumatoid arthritis (RA) often have stiffness at rest that improves with activity (morning stiffness), and extra-articular disease (lungs, skin, cardiac, ocular) may be seen. RA tends to involve the small joints of the fingers and feet, but all joints may be affected.

26. **c.** Patients with ankylosing spondylitis may have anterior nongranulomatous uveitis and axial skeletal disease manifested as sacroiliitis as well as bony fusion (ankylosis), which may cause restrictive lung disease. Men are more often affected than women. HLA-B27 is associated with ankylosing spondylitis; HLA-DR4 with rheumatoid arthritis.

27. **b.** Sjögren syndrome, cranial nerve palsies, and cortical blindness may be seen in systemic lupus erythematosus. However, retinal vascular disease is the most common ophthalmic manifestation of systemic lupus erythematosus.

28. **c.** Aspirin and nonsteroidal anti-inflammatory agents may be helpful in the management of many forms of arthritis and other inflammatory disorders. Methotrexate is beneficial for some patients with severe rheumatoid arthritis. Wegener granulomatosis is a potentially fatal systemic disease. Cyclophosphamide and prednisone are usually used in the management of Wegener granulomatosis.

29. **d.** C-reactive protein, the Westergren sedimentation rate, and the Wintrobe sedimentation rate may each be elevated in giant cell arteritis. However, temporal artery biopsy is the definitive test for giant cell arteritis.

30. **b.** In addition to uveitis, with or without hypopyon, retinal vasculitis is the most common ophthalmic manifestation of Behçet syndrome. Corneal disease and glaucoma may result from chronic intraocular inflammation. Oral and genital ulcers, not eyelid ulcers, are common in Behçet syndrome.

31. **c.** Etanercept and infliximab have been associated with demyelinating disease and optic neuritis. The antiepileptic medication topiramate (Topamax) has been associated with acute angle-closure glaucoma. The newer atypical antipsychotic agents, such as olanzapine (Zyprexa) and clozapine (Clozaril), may be associated with initiating or worsening diabetes. Cyclosporine (Neoral, Sandimmune) has been associated with disc edema.

32. **b.** The fasting plasma glucose (FPG) is the preferred test. The oral glucose tolerance test may be more sensitive than the FPG, but it is not routinely used because it is more costly, inconvenient, and difficult to reproduce. The hemoglobin A_{1c} measurement is not currently recommended for diagnosing diabetes, although this may change when the test is more standardized. Although measuring urine glucose is much easier than measuring blood glucose, it is not sensitive, because blood glucose levels need to be quite elevated before glucose appears in urine. Measurement of urinary ketones is useful during periods of illness or stress, because any positive value suggests the presence of ketonemia; however, measurement of urinary ketones is not used for the diagnosis of diabetes.

33. **d.** Fluid retention that can lead to heart failure is a side effect of the thiazolidinediones (rosiglitazone [Avandia] and pioglitazone [Actos]). Flatulence may be a limiting side effect of the α-glucosidase inhibitors (acarbose [Precose] and miglitol [Glyset]). First-generation sulfonylureas compete for carrier protein-binding sites with many other drugs. Because the pharmacologic effect of the sulfonylureas may be increased when they are displaced from their albumin-combining sites, combination drug therapy may have unforeseen toxic consequences. Second-generation sulfonylureas are less likely to cause such problems. The only available biguanide is metformin (Glucophage), and it has the potential to cause severe lactic acidosis in the setting of renal insufficiency.

34. **c.** Prominent corneal nerves are reported to occur in 100% of patients with multiple endocrine neoplasia type IIB (MEN IIB). Subconjunctival neuromas may also occur but may not be as obvious or diagnostic. Early recognition of this syndrome may be lifesaving because of the high risk of associated thyroid cancer. Ophthalmologists, therefore, have a critical role in diagnosing MEN IIB. Bitemporal visual field defects are associated with pituitary tumors, which can be seen in MEN type I (in addition to parathyroid and enteropancreatic tumors). The acute onset of diplopia, visual field loss, and a severe headache suggests pituitary apoplexy.

35. **b.** Type 2 diabetes is characterized by later age of onset than type 1 (formerly referred to as *juvenile*) diabetes and increased visceral fat. Both type 1 and type 2 diabetes have a genetic predisposition. Type 1 diabetes is characterized by reduced insulin production, usually with destruction of insulin-producing beta cells in the pancreas. Early in the course of type 2 diabetes, basal insulin secretion is usually normal or increased.

36. **a.** Coronary artery disease is the leading cause of death in the United States; cancer, the second; and cerebrovascular disease, the third.

37. **b.** Radioactive iodine uptake measures the thyroid gland's ability to concentrate a dose of radioactive iodine. It is not a good measure of thyroid metabolic status. Thyroid-binding globulin and T_3 levels vary in many other disease states, but the free T_4 level may be normal. Free T_4 and sensitive TSH have a sensitivity of 99.5% and a specificity of 98% in screening for thyroid disease and are better measures for thyroid disease.

38. **d.** Breast and colon cancer have a genetic basis in many patients. The incidence of colon cancer may also be affected by diet. Lung cancer, especially squamous cell carcinoma, is associated with cigarette smoking. Carcinoma of the cervix may be associated with herpes infection.

39. **b.** The incidence of lung cancer has been on the rise in women, in whom the mortality rate is increasing approximately 6% per year. Even though breast cancer remains more prevalent, lung cancer kills more women than does breast cancer. Lung cancer deaths among men dropped nearly 7% between 1991 and 1995.

40. **d.** Several human cancers (Burkitt lymphoma, nasopharyngeal carcinoma, carcinoma of the cervix, and hepatocellular carcinoma) show a definite correlation with viral infection, as well as reveal the presence and retention of specific virus nucleic acid sequences and virus proteins in the tumor cells.

41. **a.** In bipolar disorder (formerly known as manic depression) periods of depression often alternate with elevated mood, although this pattern varies. Lithium is the cornerstone of therapy, and psychotherapy is used as an adjunct. Major depression is far more common than bipolar disorder.

42. **b.** Fetal alcohol syndrome may include blepharophimosis, telecanthus, ptosis, optic nerve hypoplasia or atrophy, and tortuosity of the retinal arteries and veins. Cataract is not a part of fetal alcohol syndrome.

43. **d.** Monoamine oxidase inhibitors, fluoxetine, and lithium are used to treat depression. Haloperidol is a major tranquilizer.

44. **b.** Parkinson disease is characterized by tremor, bradykinesia, akinesia, rigidity, and a shuffling and stooped gait. Neuroleptic drugs may cause Parkinson disease. Parkinson disease leads to a loss of neurons in the substantia nigra with decreased, not increased, production of dopamine. Levodopa (L-dopa) is commonly used to treat Parkinson disease.

45. **c.** Alzheimer disease (AD) is characterized by progressive dementia, usually in patients older than 65 years. Extraneuronal amyloid plaques and neurofibrillary tangles are seen histopathologically. AD has genetic factors that follow either a familial autosomal dominant or sporadic autosomal dominant inheritance pattern. Toxins and free radicals may also play a role in the pathogenesis of AD.

46. **b.** Ideal diseases to screen for are the ones that are reliably detectable, treatable or preventable, progressive (especially if untreated), and generally asymptomatic. A high, rather than low, prevalence argues in favor of screening. For a rare disease, screening may not prove cost-effective.

47. **a.** Nulliparity, early menarche, and history of a first-degree relative with breast cancer are all risk factors for breast cancer. Fibrocystic disease is not a risk factor for breast cancer.

48. **d.** The "Pap smear" is indeed still the primary screening tool for detecting cervical cancer. The other statements are true.

49. **c.** Mammography should begin with a baseline examination for women between the ages of 35 and 40. Chest x-ray is not considered to be an effective screening test for lung cancer. Pelvic examination is recommended every 3 years for women between the ages of 20 and 40 years.

50. **c.** Although cytomegalovirus vaccination is now available, it has not yet become a routine childhood immunization. The others are routine childhood immunizations.

51. **b.** Terbutaline is not typically used for the treatment of anaphylaxis, but the others are.

52. **d.** An anesthesiologist would avoid succinylcholine in a patient with a history of malignant hyperthermia. There would be no contraindication to the use of the other agents. The inhaled agents halothane, enflurane, and isoflurane also may trigger malignant hyperthermia.

53. **c.** A study by Schein and coworkers has questioned the value of routine preoperative medical testing before cataract surgery. Routine medical tests before cataract surgery may be unnecessary for asymptomatic patients because these tests do not increase the safety of the procedure.

54. **a.** Of the listed medications, antihypertensive agents are the most important to take the morning of surgery. Rebound hypertensive crises can be precipitated by abrupt withdrawal of beta-blockers, clonidine, or angiotensin-converting enzyme inhibitors. However, diuretics can usually be withheld the morning of surgery. Digoxin and thyroid or estrogen supplements have a long half-life and can be resumed after surgery.

55. **c.** A cohort study would be the best study to demonstrate the incidence of a disease. In a cohort study, persons who are initially free of the disease are followed over time, during which time some subjects develop the disease. A case series or case-control study would not be capable of determining the incidence of a disease. A randomized, prospective, controlled clinical trial is the best way to compare different treatments or treatment versus no treatment, but such a trial is not good for establishing the incidence of a disease.

Index

i = image; *t* = table
Drugs are listed under generic names; when a drug trade name is listed, the reader is referred to the generic name.

A-beta-42, in Alzheimer disease, 286
Abacavir, 41
   for postexposure HIV prophylaxis, 46–47*t*
Abciximab, 111, 115, 123
Absence epilepsy, 282
Absorptiometry, dual-photon x-ray, 243
Abstinence (withdrawal) syndrome, 267. *See also specific drug*
   hypertension and, 97–98
ABT-773. *See* Cethromycin
Abuse, elder, 236–237
Acarbose, 212*t*, 213
Accolate. *See* Zafirlukast
Accupril. *See* Quinapril
Accuracy, of screening/diagnostic test, 354
Accuretic. *See* Quinapril
Accutane. *See* Isotretinoin
ACE inhibitors. *See* Angiotensin-converting enzyme (ACE) inhibitors
Acebutolol, 88*t*
Acenorm. *See* Captopril
Aceon. *See* Perindopril
Acetohexamide, 212*t*
Acetylsalicylic acid. *See* Aspirin
ACLS. *See* Advanced cardiac life support
Acquired immunodeficiency syndrome (AIDS), 36–53
   atypical mycobacterial infections and, 23, 49–50
   CDC definition of, 37, 40*t*
   classification of, 40*t*
   clinical syndrome of, 37–39, 40*t*
   cytomegalovirus infections and, 29, 47–48
   diagnosis of, 39
   encephalopathy in, 37
   etiology of, 36–37
   immunization against, development of vaccine for, 44–45
   incidence of, 36
   influenza vaccine in patients with, 305
   lymphoma in, 50–51
   malignancies associated with, 50–51
   management of, 40–45
      chemoprophylaxis and, 45, 46–47*t*
      drug resistance and, 41, 43, 44
      HAART in, 43–44
      immune reconstitution syndromes and, 51
      recent developments in, 3, 42, 44
   nephropathy associated with, 37–38
   occupational exposure to, 39
      precautions in health care setting and, 51–52
      prophylaxis for, 45, 46–47*t*
   ocular infection/manifestations and, 51–52
   opportunistic infections associated with, 45–51
   pathogenesis of, 36–37
   Pneumocystis carinii (Pneumocystis jiroveci) infections and, 45–47
   primary (retroviral syndrome), 38
   prognosis of, 40–45
   seroepidemiology of, 39
   spore-forming intestinal protozoa and, 48–49
   superinfection and, 40
   syphilis/syphilitic chorioretinitis in, 18
   transmission of, 39–40
   transplacental transmission of, chemoprophylaxis for, 45
   tuberculosis and, 24, 49–50, 301, 302
Acrodermatitis chronica atrophicans, in Lyme disease, 19
Acromegaly, 228
ACS. *See* Acute coronary syndrome
ACTH (adrenocorticotropic hormone), pituitary adenoma producing, 228–229
Actinomycin-D (dactinomycin), 257, 259*t*
Activase. *See* Alteplase
Activated protein C, 164, 165
   deficiency of, 170
Activated protein C resistance, 170
Active immunization, 303
Activities of daily living (ADL), assessment of, 233, 234
Actos. *See* Pioglitazone
Acular. *See* Ketorolac tromethamine
Acute coronary syndrome, 113–115
   hypercholesterolemia and, 143
   management of, 111, 122–125
Acyclovir, 65*t*, 76–77
   for herpes simplex virus infections, 28, 76
   for herpes zoster infections, 28, 76–77
Acylureidopenicillins, 67
AD. *See* Alzheimer disease
Adalat. *See* Nifedipine
Adalimumab, 199
Adefovir, 41, 77
Adenoma, pituitary, 228–229
Adenosine
   in atrial flutter diagnosis, 138
   for atrial tachycardia, 136–137
Adnexa. *See* Ocular adnexa
Adolescents, hypertension in, 81, 91
Adrenergic agents
   centrally acting, for hypertension, 89*t*, 93–94
   for heart failure, 130
   inhibitors. *See* Alpha-blockers; Beta-blockers
Adrenocorticotropic hormone (ACTH), pituitary adenoma producing, 228–229
Adriamycin. *See* Doxorubicin
Adult-onset diabetes. *See* Diabetes mellitus, type 2
Adult Treatment Panel (ATP) reports, 144, 144*t*
Advance directives, surgery in elderly patients and, 238
Advanced cardiac life support (ACLS), 317
Advanced glycosylation end products, diabetes complications and, 217
Advil. *See* Ibuprofen
AeroBid. *See* Flunisolide

396 • Index

Aerolate. *See* Theophylline
Affective disorders (mood disorders), 265–266
    drugs for treatment of, 277
Afterload, 129
    reduction of for heart failure, 130
Age/aging, 233–249
    elder abuse and, 236–237
    falls and, 247, 248*t*
    hypertension and, 96
    medication use and, 235–236
    osteoporosis and, 240–247, 242*t*, 243*t*, 245*t*
    outpatient visits and, 236
    physiologic/pathologic eye changes and, 235
    psychology/psychopathology of, 238–240, 265
        normal changes and, 238–239
    surgical considerations and, 237–238
    systemic disease incidence and, 247–249
Age-related macular degeneration/maculopathy (senile macular degeneration), statin drugs and, 143, 150–151, 349
Agenerase. *See* Amprenavir
Aggrastat. *See* Tirofiban
Aging. *See* Age/aging
Agnosia, visual, in Alzheimer disease, 288
Agranulocytosis, clozapine causing, 271
AIDS. *See* Acquired immunodeficiency syndrome
AIDS-dementia complex (HIV encephalopathy), 37. *See also* HIV infection/AIDS
AIDS-related virus (ARV), 36–37. *See also* Human immunodeficiency virus
Airway management, in CPR, 314
Akinetopsia, cerebral, in Alzheimer disease, 288
Albaconazole, 76
Albuterol, 157, 157*t*
    with ipratropium, 157*t*
Alcohol (ethanol)
    hypertension affected by, 85, 87*t*
    malformations associated with maternal use of, 270
    use/abuse of, 268*t*, 269–270
Alcohol abstinence syndrome, 269–270
Aldactazide. *See* Spironolactone
Aldactone. *See* Spironolactone
Aldochlor. *See* Methyldopa
Aldomet. *See* Methyldopa
Aldoril. *See* Methyldopa
Aldose reductase inhibitors, for diabetes mellitus, 217, 218
Aldosterone-receptor blockers, for hypertension, 88*t*
Alendronate, for osteoporosis, 245*t*
Aleve. *See* Naproxen
Alfenta. *See* Alfentanil
Alfentanil, perioperative, 332*t*, 335
Alkeran. *See* Melphalan
Alkylating agents, for cancer chemotherapy, 258*t*
Allergic granulomatosis and angiitis (Churg-Strauss syndrome), 189*t*, 193
Allergic reactions
    anaphylaxis as, 319–320
    to drugs, 319–320
    drugs for, 319
        ocular effects of, 325*t*
    immunization and, 303, 305
    to insulin, 211
    to latex, in ocular surgery candidate, 330
    to local anesthetics, 330–331
    to penicillin, 67–68
Allylamines, 64*t*, 76
Alpha-blockers
    for heart failure, 130
    for hypertension, 89*t*, 93
        with beta-blockers, 89*t*, 93
Alpha-glucosidase inhibitors, 212*t*, 213
Alpha (α)-hemolytic bacteria, endocarditis prophylaxis and, 7, 8–11*t*
Alpha (α)-interferon, 261
    for Behçet syndrome, 193
    in cancer therapy, 260*t*, 261
    for hepatitis C, 31
Alpha (α)-thalassemia, 161
Alprazolam, ocular effects of, 324*t*
Altace. *See* Ramipril
Alteplase, for ST-segment elevation acute coronary syndrome, 124
Alzheimer disease, 240, 284, 285–289
    recent developments in, 263
Amantadine, 65*t*, 77
    for Parkinson disease, 280
Amaryl. *See* Glimepiride
Amaurosis fugax, carotid artery disease and, 107
Ambien. *See* Zolpidem
AmBisome. *See* Amphotericin B
Ambulatory blood pressure monitoring, 92, 292
AMD-3100, 42
Amdoxovir (DADP), 41
Amikacin, 62*t*, 70
Amikin. *See* Amikacin
Amiloride, 88*t*, 90*t*
Aminocyclitols. *See* Aminoglycosides
Aminoglycosides, 61–62*t*, 70–71. *See also specific agent*
Aminopenicillins, 67
Aminophylline, for medical emergencies, 316*t*
Amiodarone
    for heart failure, 131
    ocular effects of, 141, 325*t*
Amlodipine
    for angina, 120
    for heart failure, 130
    for hypertension, 89*t*, 90*t*
Amoxicillin, 56*t*, 67
    with clavulanic acid, 56*t*, 69
    for endocarditis prophylaxis, 10*t*, 11*t*
Amoxil. *See* Amoxicillin
Amphetamine abuse, 268*t*, 270
Amphotec. *See* Amphotericin B
Amphotericin B, 25, 64*t*, 76
Ampicillin, 56*t*, 67
    for endocarditis prophylaxis, 10*t*, 11*t*
    Haemophilus influenzae resistance and, 12
    with sulbactam, 56*t*, 69–70
Amprenavir, 42
    for postexposure HIV prophylaxis, 46–47*t*
Amyloid beta peptide immunization, for Alzheimer disease, 288
Amyloid plaques, in Alzheimer disease, 285, 286
Amyloid precursor protein (APP), 286
Amyloidosis/amyloid deposits, 166
ANA. *See* Antinuclear (antineutrophil) antibodies
Ana-Kit, 320

Anabolism, glucose, 202
Anakinra, 199
Analgesics, ocular effects of, 324t
Anaphylactoid reactions, 319
Anaphylaxis, 319–320
  penicillin allergy causing, 68
Anaplasma phagocytophilum, 19
Anaplastic carcinoma, of thyroid gland, 227
Anaprox. *See* Naproxen
Ancef. *See* Cefazolin
Ancobon. *See* 5-Fluorocytosine
Ancotil. *See* 5-Fluorocytosine
Ancrod, for stroke, 105
Anemia, 160–163
  aplastic, chloramphenicol causing, 74
  of chronic disease, 161
    iron deficiency differentiated from, 159
  in elderly, 247
  hemolytic, 162–163
    autoimmune, 163
  iron deficiency, 159, 161
  pernicious, 162
  sickle cell. *See* Sickle cell disease
  sideroblastic, 162
Anesthesia (anesthetics)
  in elderly patients, 238
  local (topical/regional)
    adverse reactions to, 321–323, 330–331, 335–336
      allergic, 330–331
      toxic overdose, 321–323, 331, 336
    maximum safe dose of, 322t
  malignant hyperthermia caused by, 329–330, 336–337, 337t
  retrobulbar, adverse reactions to, 322, 323, 335–336
Aneurysms
  berry (saccular), 105–106
  cerebral, ruptured, intracranial hemorrhage caused by, 105, 106
Angiitis
  in Churg-Strauss syndrome, 193
  cutaneous leukocytoclastic, 189t
Angina pectoris, 113. *See also* Ischemic heart disease
  ECG changes in, 113, 116
  stable, 113
    management of, 120–122
    risk stratification for, 121t
  unstable, 114
  variant (Prinzmetal), 113
Angiogenesis inhibitors, in cancer therapy, 251, 257
Angiography
  cerebral
    in cerebrovascular ischemia, 104
    in subarachnoid hemorrhage, 106
  coronary, 115, 119–120, 123–124
  magnetic resonance, in cerebral ischemia/stroke, 103–104
Angioplasty, percutaneous transluminal coronary (PTCA/balloon angioplasty)
  for angina, 121
  for ST-segment elevation acute coronary syndrome, 125
  troponin levels in determining need for, 117
Angiotensin-converting enzyme (ACE) inhibitors
  for heart failure, 130

  for hypertension, 88t, 90t, 92
  for non-ST-segment elevation acute coronary syndrome, 123
  ocular effects of, 142
  in perioperative setting, 333
Angiotensin II receptor blockers
  for heart failure, 130
  for hypertension, 88t, 90t, 93
Anhedonia, 265
Anidulafungin, 76
Anisoylated plasminogen streptokinase activator complex (APSAC), for ST-segment elevation acute coronary syndrome, 124
Ankylosing spondylitis, 175–176
  juvenile, 178
Ansaid. *See* Flurbiprofen
Anspor. *See* Cephradine
Anterior uveitis
  HLA association and, 175, 176
  in spondyloarthropathies, 175, 178
Anthracyclines, in cancer chemotherapy, 257
Antianxiety drugs, 273–277, 274t
  ocular effects of, 324t
  preoperative, 335
Antibacterial agents, 54–72, 55–63t. *See also specific agent and* Antibiotics
Antibiotic-associated colitis, *Clostridium difficile* causing, 8
Antibiotics, 53–78, 55–65t. *See also specific agent and* Antimicrobial therapy
  beta (β)-lactam, 54–66, 67–70
  in cancer chemotherapy, 257, 259t
  new classes of, 63–65t, 74–75
  ocular effects of, 324t
  prophylactic
    for endocarditis, 10t
      ocular surgery and, 334
    for tuberculosis reactivation, 24
  resistance to, 3, 66. *See also specific agent and specific organism*
    new drug classes and, 74–75
  for septic shock, 319
Anticardiolipin antibodies, in antiphospholipid antibody syndrome, 182, 183
Anti-CCP antibodies. *See* Anti-citrulline–containing peptide antibodies
Anticholinergic agents
  for Parkinson disease, 279–280
  for pulmonary diseases, 157–158, 157t
Anti-citrulline–containing peptide antibodies, in rheumatoid arthritis, 174
Anticoagulant therapy, 171–172. *See also specific agent*
  for antiphospholipid antibody syndrome, 184
  for cerebral ischemia/stroke, 104
  for non-ST-segment elevation acute coronary syndrome, 123
  in perioperative setting, 331–332
  after PTCA with stenting, 121
  tailoring dosages and, 165
Anticonvulsant drugs, 282–283, 283t
  as mood stabilizers, 277
  ophthalmic side effects of, 263, 284, 324t
  in perioperative setting, 334
Anticytokine therapy, 199–200

Antidepressants, 274–276, 275t
    ocular effects of, 324t
Antidiabetic agents. *See* Insulin therapy; Oral hypoglycemic agents
Anti-double-stranded DNA (dsDNA) antibodies, in systemic lupus erythematosus, 181, 181t
Antiepileptic drugs, 282–283, 283t
    as mood stabilizers, 277
    ophthalmic side effects of, 263, 284, 324t
    in perioperative setting, 334
Antifungal agents, 64–65t, 75–76. *See also specific type*
Antigenic surface variation, as microbial virulence factor, 4
Antihistamines, 319
    ocular effects of, 325t
Anti-HIV antibody tests, 39
Antihypertensive drugs, 86, 87–94, 88–89t, 90t, 91i, 91t. *See also specific agent*
    for children and adolescents, 97
    combination, 90t
    high-risk conditions affecting selection of, 86, 91t
    new developments and, 81
    in older patients, 96
    parenteral, 94
    in perioperative setting, 333
    during pregnancy, 96–97
    withdrawal from, rebound hypertension and, 97–98
Anti-infective agents, 53–78, 55–65t. *See also specific type*
Anti-inflammatory agents. *See also specific type and* Corticosteroids; Nonsteroidal anti-inflammatory drugs
    ocular effects of, 324t
    for pulmonary diseases, 157t, 158
Anti-La (SSB) autoantibodies, in Sjögren syndrome, 186, 187t
Antimetabolites
    in cancer chemotherapy, 258t
    for rheumatic disorders, 200
Antimicrobial prophylaxis, for endocarditis, 7, 8–11t
    ocular surgery and, 334
Antimicrobial susceptibility testing, 66–67
Antimicrobial therapy, 53–78, 55–65t. *See also specific agent*
Antineoplastic drugs. *See* Chemotherapy
Antinuclear (antineutrophil) antibodies
    in juvenile idiopathic arthritis, 178
    in scleroderma, 185
    in systemic lupus erythematosus, 180–182, 181t
    in Wegener granulomatosis, 192
Antiphospholipid antibody syndrome (phospholipid antibody syndrome), 171, 182–184
Antiplatelet therapy. *See also* Aspirin
    for carotid disease, 107
    for cerebral ischemia/stroke, 104
    in perioperative setting, 331
    after PTCA with stenting, 121
Antipsychotic drugs, 271–273, 272t
    atypical, 263, 271–272, 272t
    ocular side effects of, 272–273
Antipyrimidines
    in cancer chemotherapy, 258t
    for rheumatic disorders, 199
Antiretroviral therapy, 40–45
    drug resistance and, 41, 43, 44
    HAART, 43–44
    prophylactic, 45, 46–47t
    recent developments in, 3, 42, 44
Anti-Ro (SSA) autoantibodies, in Sjögren syndrome, 186, 187t
Anti-Smith (anti-Sm) antibodies, in systemic lupus erythematosus, 181, 181t
Antithrombin III, 164, 165
    deficiency of, 170
Antithrombin therapy, for non-ST-segment elevation acute coronary syndrome, 123
Antithyroid antibodies, testing for, 223
Antitumor antibiotics, 257, 259t
Anti-VEGF agents, for diabetes mellitus, 217
Antiviral agents, 65t, 76–77
    for HIV infection/AIDS, 40–45. *See also* Antiretroviral therapy
Anxiety, 266–267
    drugs for management of (antianxiety drugs/anxiolytics), 273–277, 274t
    ocular effects of, 324t
    preoperative, 335
Anxiolytics. *See* Antianxiety drugs
Aortic arch (Takayasu) arteritis, 189t, 191
Aortic coarctation, hypertension in, 83, 84t
Aortic dissection, cerebral ischemia/stroke and, 102
Aortitis syndrome (Takayasu arteritis), 189t, 191
APC. *See* Activated protein C
Apidra. *See* Glulisine insulin
Aplastic anemia, chloramphenicol causing, 74
Apolipoprotein E epsilon 3 and epsilon 4 (ε3 and ε4) genes, in Alzheimer disease, 287
Apoplexy, pituitary, 229–230
APP. *See* Amyloid precursor protein
APP gene, in Alzheimer disease, 286–287
Apresazide. *See* Hydralazine
Apresoline. *See* Hydralazine
APS. *See* Antiphospholipid antibody syndrome
APSAC. *See* Anisoylated plasminogen streptokinase activator complex
Aptamers, in cancer chemotherapy, 257
Aqueous penicillin, 55t
Ara-C. *See* Cytarabine
Aralen. *See* Chloroquine
Arava. *See* Leflunomide
ARBs. *See* Angiotensin II receptor blockers
ARC. *See* Lymphadenopathy syndrome
Arcus (corneal), in dyslipoproteinemia/hyperlipoproteinemia, 151, 293
Argon laser therapy, for coronary revascularization, 122
Aricept. *See* Donepezil
Arrhythmias, 132–141. *See also specific type*
    heart failure and, 131–132
    sudden cardiac death and, 115
Artane. *See* Trihexyphenidyl
Arteriography. *See* Angiography
Arteriovenous anastomoses, retinal, in Takayasu arteritis, 191
Arteriovenous malformations, intracranial hemorrhage caused by, 105, 106
Arteritis
    cerebral ischemia/stroke and, 102
    giant cell (temporal), 188–190, 189t
    Takayasu (aortic arch arteritis/aortitis syndrome/pulseless disease), 189t, 191

Arthritis
  in Behçet syndrome, 193
  enteropathic, 177
  juvenile idiopathic, 178–179
  Lyme, 19
  mutilans, 178
  psoriatic, 178
  reactive (Reiter syndrome), 176–177
  rheumatoid, 173–174
  in systemic lupus erythematosus, 179, 181t
Arthrotec. See Diclofenac, with misoprostol
ARV. See AIDS-related virus
AS. See Ankylosing spondylitis
Ascorbic acid (vitamin C), deficiency of (scurvy), 166
Asparaginase, 260t
Aspart insulin, 209, 209t
Aspiration (respiratory), during surgery, prevention of, 331
Aspirin, 197t
  for carotid artery disease, 107
  for cerebral ischemia/stroke, 101, 104
  discontinuing before surgery, 331–332
  for non-ST-segment elevation acute coronary syndrome, 122
  ocular effects of, 324t
  platelet function affected by, 167–168, 331–332
Asthma, 153–154
  drug treatment for, 158
  ocular effects of, 325t
AT III. See Antithrombin III
Atacand. See Candesartan
Atazanavir, 42
Atenolol, 88t, 90t
Atevirdine, 41
Atheroma-cutting blades, for coronary revascularization, 122
Atherosclerosis, coronary artery (coronary heart disease), 111. See also Ischemic heart disease
  in diabetes, 218
  hypercholesterolemia and, 143, 143–144
  risk factors for, 112–113
  screening for, 293–294
Atorvastatin, for hypercholesterolemia, 149t, 150t
  heart disease prevention and, 148
Atovaquone, for *Pneumocystis carinii* (*Pneumocystis jiroveci*) pneumonia, 45
ATP reports. See Adult Treatment Panel (ATP) reports
Atrial complexes, premature (PACs), 135
Atrial fibrillation, 138
  heart failure and, 131, 132
  stroke and, 102
Atrial flutter, 137–138
Atrial tachycardia, paroxysmal, 136–137
Atrioventricular block, 134
Atrioventricular (AV) junction, 133
Atrioventricular junctional rhythm, 133
Atropine
  for cholinergic stimulation in toxic overdose, 323
  for medical emergencies, 316t
Atrovent. See Ipratropium
Attachment, as microbial virulence factor, 4
Atypical antipsychotic agents, 263, 271–272, 272t
Atypical mycobacteria, 23
  in HIV infection/AIDS, 23, 49–50

Augmentin. See Amoxicillin, with clavulanic acid
Aura (seizure), 281
Auricular chondritis, in relapsing polychondritis, 187
Autism, MMR vaccine and, 306
Autoantibodies. See also specific type
  in diabetes mellitus, 203
  in Sjögren syndrome, 186, 187t
  in systemic lupus erythematosus, 180–182, 181t
  in Wegener granulomatosis, 192
Autoimmune diseases
  Graves hyperthyroidism as, 224
  systemic lupus erythematosus as, 179
Autoimmune hemolytic anemia, 163
Automatisms, 281
AV block. See Atrioventricular block
AV junction. See Atrioventricular junction
Avalide. See Irbesartan
Avandamet. See Rosiglitazone, with metformin
Avandia. See Rosiglitazone
Avapro. See Irbesartan
Avelox. See Moxifloxacin
Average versus individual effect, 361–362
Avilamycin, 63t, 75
AVM. See Arteriovenous malformations
Azactam. See Aztreonam
Azalides, 60t, 71. See also specific agent
Azathioprine, 200
  for Behçet syndrome, 194
AZD2563, 75
Azidothymidine. See Zidovudine
Azithromycin, 60t, 71
  for endocarditis prophylaxis, 10t
Azlocillin, 67
Azmacort. See Triamcinolone
AZT (azidothymidine). See Zidovudine
AZTEC. See Zidovudine
Aztreonam, 59t, 70
Azulfidine. See Sulfasalazine

B-cell lymphomas, in HIV infection/AIDS, 50
B cells (B lymphocytes), in HIV infection/AIDS, 37
Babesiosis, 19
Bacille Calmette-Guérin (BCG) vaccination, 302
  PPD test affected by, 24
Bacteria, treatment of infection caused by. See Antibiotics
Bactericidal drugs, 54
Bacteriostatic drugs, 54
Bactrim. See Trimethoprim-sulfamethoxazole
BAL9141, 68
Balint syndrome, in Alzheimer disease, 288
Balloon angioplasty. See Percutaneous transluminal coronary angioplasty
Bamboo spine, in ankylosing spondylitis, 176
Barbiturates, 274t
  abuse of, 268t, 269
Bariatric surgery, for obesity in type 2 diabetes, 208–209
Barium enema, in cancer screening, 298
Barrett esophagus, 297
Barrier devices, for basic life support, 314, 315
Basal ganglia, in Parkinson disease, 278
Baseline probability of outcome, 361
Basic life support, 313–317
  medications used in, 316t

for ventricular fibrillation, 140
Bayes' theorem, 358
BB isoenzyme, in myocardial infarction, 117
BCG (Bacille Calmette-Guérin) vaccination, 302
  PPD test affected by, 24
Beaver Dam Eye Study, 360
Beclomethasone, for pulmonary diseases, 157t
Beclovent. See Beclomethasone
Behavioral/psychiatric disorders, 264–277. See also specific type
  aging and, 239–240
  anxiety disorders, 266–267
  mental disorders due to general medical condition, 264
  mood (affective) disorders, 265–266
  noncompliance and, 277
  ophthalmic considerations and, 277
  pharmacologic treatment of, 271–277, 272t, 274t, 275t
    ocular side effects and, 277
    recent developments and, 263
  schizophrenia, 264–265
  somatoform disorders, 266
  substance abuse disorders, 267–271, 268t
Behçet syndrome, 193–194
Benadryl. See Diphenhydramine
Benazepril, 88t, 90t
Benicar. See Olmesartan
Benzathine penicillin, 55t
Benzodiazepines, 273–274, 274t
  abuse of, 269, 273
  for seizures, 283t
Benztropine, for Parkinson disease, 279
Benzylamines, 65t, 76
Berry (saccular) aneurysm, 105–106
Beta-adrenergic agonists, for pulmonary diseases, 157, 157t
Beta-blockers
  for angina, 120–121
  cholesterol levels affected by, 150
  for heart failure, 131
  for hypertension, 88t, 90t, 92
    with alpha-blockers, 89t, 93
  for hyperthyroidism, 225
  for non-ST-segment elevation acute coronary syndrome, 122
  ocular effects of, 141–142, 325t
  in perioperative setting, 329, 333
Beta (β) cells, pancreatic, in diabetes mellitus, 202
  genetic defects and, 204t
Beta (β)-hemolytic group A streptococci (Streptococcus pyogenes), 6
Beta (β)-interferon, 261
Beta (β)-lactam antibiotics, 54–66, 67–70. See also specific agent
Beta (β)-lactam ring, 54, 67
Beta (β)-lactamase inhibitors, 69–70. See also specific antibiotic combination
Beta (β)-thalassemia, 161
  bone marrow transplantation for, 159, 161
Betaxolol, 88t
Bextra. See Valdecoxib
BFU-E. See Burst-forming unit-erythroid
Biapenem, 69

Bias (statistical)
  measurement, 343
  recall, 349
  selection, 341
    in case-control studies, 349
    in case series, 346
Biaxin. See Clarithromycin
Bicarbonate
  for malignant hyperthermia, 337t
  for medical emergencies, 316t
  for shock, 318
Bicillin. See Benzathine penicillin
BiCNU. See Carmustine
Bifonazole, 76
Biguanides, 212t, 213
Bile acid sequestrants, for hypercholesterolemia, 149t
Bio-Hep-B. See Hepatitis B vaccine
Biofilms, microbial virulence and, 4
Biologic response modifiers. See also Immunotherapy
  in cancer chemotherapy, 257–262, 260t
Biotherapy. See Biologic response modifiers; Immunotherapy
Bipolar disorder, 265
  lithium for, 277
Bisoprolol
  for heart failure, 131
  for hypertension, 88t, 90t
Bisphosphonates, for osteoporosis, 246
Bitolterol, 157t
Bleeding/blood loss. See Hemorrhages
Bleeding time, 165
  aspirin affecting, 167–168
Bleomycin, 257, 259t
Blindness
  diabetic retinopathy causing, 201
  "hysterical." See Functional visual loss
Blocadren. See Timolol
Blood
  clotting pathways of, 164, 164i. See also Coagulation
  composition of, 159
Blood cells, 159
  development of, 160
Blood clotting/coagulation. See Coagulation
Blood glucose
  in diabetes
    in diagnosis/screening, 301
    self-monitoring of, 215–216
    surgery and, 220, 332–333
    surveillance of (glycemic control), 215–216
  normal, 203t
Blood-pool isotope scans, 119
Blood pressure. See also Hypertension
  ambulatory monitoring of, 92, 292
  classification of, 81, 82, 82t
  normal, 81, 82, 82t
  screening, 292
    oral contraceptives/pregnancy and, 96
  in shock, 318
Blue bloaters, 154
Blurred vision/blurring, SSRIs causing, 276
Body dysmorphic disorder, 266
Bone
  cortical and trabecular, 241
  physiology of, 241

Bone density, measurement of, 242–243
Bone marrow transplantation, for thalassemia, 159, 169
Borrelia burgdorferi, 18–21
Bradyarrhythmias, 133–135
Bradykinetic movement disorders, 278. *See also*
    Parkinson disease/parkinsonism
Breast cancer, 252
    eye involvement and, 262
    screening for, 294–296, 295*t*
Breast examination, for cancer screening, 295*t*, 296
Breathing exercises, 156
Brethaire. *See* Terbutaline
Brethine. *See* Terbutaline
Brevibloc. *See* Esmolol
Brevital. *See* Methohexital
Bricanyl. *See* Terbutaline
Brief psychotic disorder, 265
Brivudine, 77
Bromfenac, 197
Bromides, abuse of, 268*t*
Bromocriptine, for Parkinson disease, 279
Bronchial lavage, 155
Bronchiectasis, 154
Bronchitis, 154
Bronchodilators, 156–157, 157*t*
Bronchoscopy, 155
    in cancer screening, 297
Bronchospasm, in asthma, 153–154
Bruits, carotid, 107. *See also* Carotid occlusive disease
Budesonide, for pulmonary diseases, 157*t*
Bull's-eye maculopathy, hydroxychloroquine causing, 198
Bumetanide
    for diastolic dysfunction, 131
    for hypertension, 88*t*
Bumex. *See* Bumetanide
Bundle branch block, left or right, 134–135
Bundle of His, 133, 134
Bupivacaine
    maximum safe dose of, 322
    toxic reaction to, 323
Bupropion, 276
Burkitt lymphoma, Epstein-Barr virus associated with, 30, 254
Burst-forming unit–erythroid, 160
Butazolidin. *See* Phenylbutazone
Butenafine, 65*t*, 76
Byetta. *See* Exenatide
Bypass grafting, coronary artery, 121–122
    troponin levels in determining need for, 117

C (parafollicular) cells, 221
C-reactive protein
    in coronary artery disease, 111
    in giant cell arteritis, 190
CABG. *See* Coronary artery bypass graft
Calan. *See* Verapamil
Calanolide, 42
Calcinosis, in scleroderma, 185
Calcitonin/calcitonin nasal spray, for osteoporosis, 245*t*, 246
Calcium, for osteoporosis, 244
Calcium channel blockers
    for angina, 120–121
    for heart failure, 130
    for hypertension, 89*t*, 90*t*, 93
    for non-ST-segment elevation acute coronary syndrome, 122–123
    ocular effects of, 325*t*
Calcium chloride, for medical emergencies, 316*t*
Cancer, 251–262. *See also specific type or organ or structure affected*
    carcinogenesis and, 253
    chemicals causing, 252–253
    chemotherapy for, 256–262, 258–260*t*
    etiology of, 252–255
    genetic and familial factors in, 254–255
    in HIV infection/AIDS, 50–51
    hypercoagulability and, 171
    incidence of, 251
    ophthalmic considerations and, 262
    radiation causing, 253
    radiation therapy for, 255–256
    recent developments in, 251
    screening for, 294–300, 295*t*
    therapy of, 255–262
        recent developments in, 251
    vaccines against, 262
    viruses causing, 254
Cancer checkup, 295*t*
Cancer chemotherapy. *See* Chemotherapy
Cancer-cluster families, 254
Cancer vaccines, 262
Candesartan, 88*t*, 90*t*
Candida albicans, 25
Cannabis use/abuse, 268*t*
Capillary telangiectasias, 106
Capoten. *See* Captopril
Capozide. *See* Captopril
Capravirine, 42
Captopril
    for heart failure, 130
    for hypertension, 88*t*, 90*t*
    for non-ST-segment elevation acute coronary syndrome, 123
    ocular effects of, 325*t*
Carbacephems, 59*t*, 69
Carbamazepine, 283*t*
    as mood stabilizer, 277
Carbapenems, 59–60*t*, 69–70. *See also specific agent*
Carbatrol. *See* Carbamazepine
Carbenicillin, 67
Carbidopa, for Parkinson disease, 279
Carbocaine. *See* Mepivacaine
Carboxypenicillins, 67
Carcinogenesis, 253
    chemical, 252–253
    genetic and familial factors in, 254–255
    radiation in, 253
    viral, 254
Cardene. *See* Nicardipine
Cardiac arrest. *See* Cardiopulmonary arrest
Cardiac disease. *See* Heart disease
Cardiac enzymes, in ischemic heart disease, 116–117
Cardiac failure. *See* Congestive heart failure
Cardiac glycosides. *See* Digitalis/digitoxin/digoxin
Cardiac rhythm, disorders of, 132–141. *See also* Arrhythmias

Cardiac-specific troponins (troponins T and I), in myocardial infarction, 117, 118i
Cardiac transplantation, for heart failure, 132
Cardiogenic shock, 317. *See also* Shock
Cardiolite scintigraphy. *See* Technetium-99m Sestamibi scintigraphy
Cardiopulmonary arrest, 313–317
Cardiopulmonary resuscitation, 313–317
  medications used in, 316t
  for ventricular fibrillation, 140
Cardioselective beta-blockers, 92
Cardiovascular disorders. *See also specific type*
  diabetes and, 216–217, 218
  hypertension and risk of, 81, 84, 86t
  in Lyme disease, 19
  screening for, 293–294
Cardioversion
  for atrial fibrillation, 138
  for atrial flutter, 137–138
  for atrial tachycardia, 137
  for torsades de pointes, 140
  for ventricular fibrillation, 140
  for ventricular tachycardia, 139
Cardizem. *See* Diltiazem
Cardura. *See* Doxazosin
Carmustine, 260t
Carotid arteries, disorders of, 107–109
Carotid bruits, 107. *See also* Carotid occlusive disease
Carotid endarterectomy, for carotid stenosis, 101, 107–108, 109
Carotid occlusive disease, 101, 107–109
Carotid siphon, cerebral ischemia/stroke and, 102
Carotid stenosis, 101, 107
Carrier (infection), in HIV infection/AIDS, 38–39
Carteolol, cholesterol levels affected by, 150
Cartrol. *See* Carteolol
Carvedilol
  for heart failure, 131
  for hypertension, 89t
Case-control studies, 345i, 347–349, 348i
Case reports, 345–346, 345i
Case series, 345i, 346–347
Caspases, in Alzheimer disease, 286
Caspofungin, 76
Catabolism, glucose, 202
Cataflam. *See* Diclofenac
Catapres. *See* Clonidine
Cataract
  quetiapine use and, 272
  radiation-induced, 256
Catastrophic antiphospholipid antibody syndrome, 183
Catheter-based reperfusion. *See* Percutaneous transluminal coronary angioplasty
Causal risk factors, 361, 362. *See also* Risk factor
Cause and effect diagram, 370, 371i
CCR5/CCR5 receptor, in HIV infection/AIDS, 44
CCR5 receptor antagonists, for HIV infection/AIDS, 42
CD4/CD8 ratio, in HIV infection/AIDS, 37
CD4 T cells
  in HIV infection/AIDS, 37, 40
  in SARS, 34
CD8 T cells, in SARS, 34
CDKs. *See* Cyclin-dependent kinases
CEA. *See* Carotid endarterectomy
Ceclor. *See* Cefaclor

Cedax. *See* Ceftibuten
CeeNU. *See* Lomustine
Cefaclor, 57t
  ocular effects of, 324t
Cefadroxil, 57t
  for endocarditis prophylaxis, 10t
Cefamandole, 57t
Cefazolin, 57t
  for endocarditis prophylaxis, 10t
Cefdinir, 59t
Cefditoren, 59t
Cefepime, 59t, 68
Cefixime, 58t
Cefizox. *See* Ceftizoxime
Cefmetazole, 59t
Cefobid. *See* Cefoperazone
Cefonicid, 57t
Cefoperazone, 58t
Cefotan. *See* Cefotetan
Cefotaxime, 58t
Cefotetan, 58t
Cefoxitin, 57t, 69
Cefozopran, 68
Cefpirome, 59t, 68
Cefpodoxime, 58t
Cefprozil, 58t
Ceftazidime, 58t
Ceftibuten, 59t
Ceftin. *See* Cefuroxime
Ceftizoxime, 58t
Ceftriaxone, 58t
Cefuroxime, 58t
  ocular effects of, 324t
Cefzil. *See* Cefprozil
"Ceiling effect," 364
Celebrex. *See* Celecoxib
Celecoxib, 173, 196, 197t
CellCept. *See* Mycophenolate mofetil
Cellular immunity (cell-mediated immunity), 4
  deficient, in HIV infection/AIDS, 37
Central nervous system
  disorders of. *See* Neurologic disorders
  systemic lupus erythematosus affecting, 180, 181t, 182
Cephalexin, 57t
  for endocarditis prophylaxis, 10t
Cephalosporins, 57–59t, 68–69. *See also specific agent*
Cephamycins, 59t
Cephradine, 57t
Cerebral akinetopsia, in Alzheimer disease, 288
Cerebral aneurysm, ruptured, intracranial hemorrhage caused by, 105, 106
Cerebral (intracerebral) angiography/arteriography. *See* Angiography
Cerebral ischemia, 101–105. *See also* Stroke
Cerebrovascular accident. *See* Stroke
Cerebrovascular disease, 101–109. *See also specific type and* Stroke
  in diabetes, 218
  hypertension management and, 91t, 95
Cerebyx. *See* Fosphenytoin
Cervical cancer
  screening for, 294
  viral carcinogenesis and, 254, 291
Cethromycin (ABT-773), 75

Chancre, syphilitic, 16
Chart review, monitoring systems and, 365–366
Checklist (system of care), 370, 371*i*
Chemical carcinogenesis, 252–253
Chemotherapy (cancer), 256–262, 258–260*t*. See also *specific agent*
    recent developments in, 251
Chest compressions, in CPR, 314–315
Chest pain, in angina pectoris, 113
Chest physiotherapy, postoperative, 156
Chest x-ray
    in cancer screening, 295*t*, 296
    in congestive heart failure, 127
    in pulmonary diseases, 155
CHF. *See* Congestive heart failure
Chi-square tests, 344
Chickenpox. *See* Varicella
Children
    cancer in, 251
    hypertension in, 81
    immunization schedule for, 303, 304*t*
    mydriasis in epilepsy and, 283–284
    preoperative assessment in, 328–329
    preoperative sedation for, 335
Chlamydia
    psittaci, 22
    trachomatis, 21–22
        gonococcal coinfection and, 13, 14, 22
Chlorambucil, 200, 258*t*
    for Behçet syndrome, 194
    in cancer chemotherapy, 258*t*
Chloramphenicol, 62*t*, 74
Chloromycetin. *See* Chloramphenicol
Chloroprocaine, maximum safe dose of, 322*t*
Chloroquine, 198
Chlorothiazide, 88*t*, 90*t*
Chlorpromazine, 271
Chlorpropamide, 212*t*
Chlorthalidone, 88*t*, 90*t*
Cholesterol levels
    classification of, 144, 144*t*
    drugs for modification of. *See* Lipid-lowering therapy
    elevated. *See* Hypercholesterolemia
    goals for, hypercholesterolemia management and, 145, 146, 147*t*
    risk assessment and, 144, 144*t*, 145, 145*t*, 146*i*, 147*t*
    screening, 293
Cholestyramine, for hypercholesterolemia, 149*t*
Choline magnesium trisalicylate, 197*t*
Chondritis, auricular or nasal, in relapsing polychondritis, 187
Chorioretinitis, toxoplasmic, 26
Chronic bronchitis, 154
Chronic disease, anemia of, 161
    iron deficiency differentiated from, 159
Chronic obstructive pulmonary disease, 154
    ocular surgery in patient with, 329
    recent developments in, 153
Churg-Strauss syndrome, 189*t*, 193
Cialis. *See* Tadalafil
Cidofovir, 48, 65*t*, 77
    for cytomegalovirus retinitis, 29, 48
    for herpes simplex virus infection, 28

Cigarette smoking
    cancer and, 252, 296, 297
    cessation of, 155–156
    heart disease and, 111
    hypertension and, 85
    thyroid disease and, 201, 225
Cilastin, with imipenem, 59*t*, 69
Cipro. *See* Ciprofloxacin
Ciprofloxacin, 62*t*, 73
    ocular effects of, 324*t*
Circulatory failure, 126
Cirrhosis, from hepatitis C, 31
Cisapride, perioperative, 331, 332*t*
Cisplatin, 260*t*
CK. *See* Creatine kinase
CK-MB, in myocardial infarction, 117
Claforan. *See* Cefotaxime
Clarithromycin, 49, 60*t*, 71
    for endocarditis prophylaxis, 10*t*
Clavulanic acid, 69–70. *See also specific antibiotic combination*
Cleocin. *See* Clindamycin
Clinafloxacin, 62*t*
Clindamycin, 60*t*, 71
    for endocarditis prophylaxis, 10*t*
    for *Pneumocystis carinii (Pneumocystis jiroveci)* pneumonia, 45
Clinical research/studies
    application to clinical practice and, 362–370
        data presentation and, 368–370, 369*i*, 370*i*, 371*i*
        measurement system design and, 363–364
        monitoring system implementation and, 364–366
        quality improvement and, 370, 371*i*
        results analysis and, 366–368
    designs for, 345–360, 345*i*
    evaluation of, 339–344
        clinical relevance and, 344
        intervention issues and, 342
        outcome issues and, 342–343
        participants and setting and, 341
        sample size and, 342
        validity and, 343, 363
    interpreting results for patients and, 360–362
Clinical trials (experimental/interventional studies), 345, 351–352, 351*i*. *See also* Clinical research
    systematic reviews/meta-analyses of, 352
Clinoril. *See* Sulindac
Clofazamine, 49
Clofibrate, for hypercholesterolemia, 149*t*
Clomid. *See* Clomiphene
Clomiphene, ocular effects of, 325*t*
Clonidine
    for heart failure, 130
    for hypertension, 89*t*
    in perioperative setting, 333
Clopidogrel
    for carotid disease, 107
    for cerebral ischemia/stroke, 104
Clostridium difficile, 8–10
Clotrimazole, 64*t*
Clotting. *See* Coagulation
Cloxacillin, 55*t*, 67
Clozapine, 271, 272

Clozaril. *See* Clozapine
Clusters A, B, and C personality disorders, 166
CMV. *See* Cytomegalovirus
Coactinon. *See* Emivirine
Coagulation. *See also* Hemostasis
  disorders of, 168–172
    acquired, 168–170
    hereditary, 168
  laboratory evaluation of, 165
  pathways of, 164, 164*i*
Coagulation factors, 164, 164*i*
  abnormalities/deficiencies of, 168
  vitamin K and, 168
Cocaine abuse, 270–271
Cocaine abstinence syndrome, 270
Cogan syndrome, 192
Cogentin. *See* Benztropine
Cohort studies (follow-up studies), 345*i*, 348*i*, 350–351
Colesevelam, for hypercholesterolemia, 149*t*
Colestipol, for hypercholesterolemia, 149*t*
Colistin, 54
Colitis
  granulomatous (Crohn disease), 177
  ulcerative, 177
Colon cancer. *See* Colorectal cancer
Colonoscopy, in cancer screening, 298–299
  virtual, 291, 299
Colony-forming unit–culture, 160
Colony-forming unit–erythroid, 160
Colony-forming unit–spleen, 160
Colony-stimulating factors, in cancer therapy, 261
Color flow Doppler imaging, in ischemic heart disease, 118
Colorectal cancer, 252, 297–299
  incidence of, 297
  screening for, 298–299
Coma
  myxedema, 226
  nonketotic hyperglycemic-hyperosmolar, 216
Combipres. *See* Clonidine
Combivent. *See* Albuterol, with ipratropium
Combivir. *See* Lamivudine (3TC), with zidovudine
Common cause factors, 368–370
Complete (third-degree) atrioventricular block, 134
Completed stroke, 102
Complex partial seizures, 281, 320
Compromised host. *See* Immunocompromised host
Computed tomography (CT scan)
  in cerebral ischemia/stroke, 103
  dual-energy quantitative, in osteoporosis, 243
  in intracranial hemorrhage, 106
  in pulmonary diseases, 155
Comtan. *See* Entacapone
Confounding factor, 350, 367
Confusion, 284
  in elderly patients, 237–238
Congenital syphilis, 15, 302
Congestive heart failure, 111, 125–132
  atrial fibrillation and, 131, 132
  classification of, 126, 126*t*
  clinical course of, 128–129
  clinical signs of, 126
  compensated, 126
  decompensated, 126
  diagnosis of, 127

  epidemiology of, 127
  etiology of, 128
  high-output, 128
  hypertension management and, 91*t*, 95, 130
  ischemic heart disease causing, 127, 128
  management of
    invasive or surgical, 132
    medical and nonsurgical, 130–132
    after myocardial infarction, 128
  pathophysiology of, 128–129
  refractory, 126
  symptoms of, 126
Conjunctivitis, in reactive arthritis/Reiter syndrome, 177
Connective tissue disorders, mixed, 185
CONSORT (Consolidated Standards of Reporting Trials) guidelines, 352
Construct validity, 363
Contact lenses, for trial fitting, disinfection of, 51
Continuous outcome, in screening/diagnostic test, 355
Continuous positive airway pressure (CPAP), 156
Continuous subcutaneous insulin infusion (CSII), 210–211
Contraceptives, oral
  hypercoagulability associated with, 171
  hypertension and, 96
  ocular effects of, 325*t*
Contractility, myocardial, 129
  enhancement of in heart failure management, 130–131
  reduction of in angina management, 120–121
Control charts, 368, 371*i*
Conversion disorders, 266
COPD. *See* Chronic obstructive pulmonary disease
Cor pulmonale, 154
Cordarone. *See* Amiodarone
Coreg. *See* Carvedilol
Corgard. *See* Nadolol
Corneal disorders/perforation, NSAID use and, 197–198
Corneal arcus, in dyslipoproteinemia/hyperlipoproteinemia, 151, 293
Corneal nerves, enlarged, in multiple endocrine neoplasia, 230–231, 231*i*
Coronary angiography/arteriography, 115, 119–120, 123–124
Coronary angioplasty, percutaneous transluminal (PTCA/balloon angioplasty)
  for angina, 121
  for ST-segment elevation acute coronary syndrome, 125
  troponin levels in determining need for, 117
Coronary artery bypass graft (CABG), 121–122
  troponin levels in determining need for, 117
Coronary artery stenosis, hemodynamically significant, 120
Coronary heart disease (coronary artery atherosclerosis), 111. *See also* Ischemic heart disease
  in diabetes, 218
  hypercholesterolemia and, 143, 143–144
  hypertension management and, 91*t*, 94
  risk factors for, 112–113
  screening for, 293–294
Coronary syndrome, acute. *See* Acute coronary syndrome
Coronary vasospasm, angina pectoris caused by, 113

Coronavirus, SARS caused by, 33
Cortical bone, 241
Corticosteroids (steroids), 194–196
    for anaphylaxis, 319
    for Behçet syndrome, 193–194
    for giant cell arteritis, 190
    ocular side effects of, 325t
    in perioperative setting, 334
    for pulmonary diseases, 157t, 158
    for rheumatic disorders, 194–196
    for shock, 319
    withdrawal from, 195
Corticotroph adenomas, 228
Corvert. See Ibutilide
Corzide. See Nadolol
Cotton-wool spots
    in radiation retinopathy, 256
    in systemic lupus erythematosus, 182
Cough, 153
Coumadin. See Warfarin
Covera. See Verapamil
COX-1/COX-2 (cyclooxygenase), 196
    aspirin affecting, 331
COX-2 inhibitors, 173, 196, 197t
Cozaar. See Losartan
CPAP. See Continuous positive airway pressure
CPK. See Creatine kinase
CPR. See Cardiopulmonary resuscitation
"Crack babies," 271
Creatine kinase (CK)/creatine kinase isoenzymes, in myocardial infarction, 117
CREST syndrome, 185
Cretinism, 221
Cricothyrotomy, 316
    for anaphylaxis, 319
Crixivan. See Indinavir
Croconazole, 64t, 76
Crohn disease (granulomatous ileocolitis), 177
Cromolyn, for pulmonary diseases, 157t, 158
Cross-sectional studies, 349–350
Cryoglobulinemic vasculitis, essential, 189t
Cryptosporidium parvum (cryptosporidiosis), in HIV infection/AIDS, 48
Crystalloids, for shock, 318
CSII. See Continuous subcutaneous insulin infusion
CSS. See Churg-Strauss syndrome
CT. See Computed tomography
Cushing syndrome
    corticotroph adenoma causing, 228–229
    hypertension in, 83, 84t
Cutaneous leukocytoclastic angiitis, 189t
CXCR4 receptor antagonists, for HIV infection/AIDS, 42
Cyclin-dependent kinases, in carcinogenesis, 253
Cyclooxygenase (COX-1/COX-2), 196
    aspirin affecting, 331
Cyclooxygenase-2 (COX-2) inhibitors, 173, 196, 197t
Cyclophosphamide, 200, 258t
    for Behçet syndrome, 194
    in cancer chemotherapy, 258t
    for rheumatoid arthritis, 174
    for Wegener granulomatosis, 192
Cyclospora cayatanensis (cyclosporiasis), in HIV infection/AIDS, 48, 49

Cyclosporine
    for Behçet syndrome, 194
    for rheumatoid arthritis, 174
Cyclothymic disorder, 265
Cymbalta. See Duloxetine
Cystic fibrosis, 154
Cytarabine, 258t
Cytokines
    in cancer therapy, 261
    in inflammation/rheumatic disorders, 199
Cytomegaloviruses, 29–30
    cancer association and, 254
    congenital infection caused by, 29
    in HIV infection/AIDS, 3, 29
        treatment of, 47–48
    retinitis caused by, 3, 29
        cidofovir for, 29, 48
        fomivirsen for, 48
        foscarnet for, 29, 48
        ganciclovir for, 29
        in HIV infection/AIDS, 3, 29, 47–48
Cytotoxic drugs, for Wegener granulomatosis, 192
Cytovene. See Ganciclovir
Cytoxan. See Cyclophosphamide

d4T. See Stavudine
Dactinomycin, 257, 259t
DADP. See Amdoxovir
Dalfopristin/quinupristin, 63t, 74
Danazol, ocular effects of, 325t
Danocrine. See Danazol
Dantrolene, for malignant hyperthermia, 337t
Dapsone, for *Pneumocystis carinii (Pneumocystis jiroveci)* pneumonia, 45
Daptomycin, 63t, 75
Data presentation, 368–370, 369i, 370i, 371i
Database, monitoring systems and, 364–365
Dawn phenomenon, 210
Daypro. See Oxaprozin
DCCT (Diabetes Control and Complications Trial), 210, 214–215
ddC. See Zalcitabine
ddI. See Didanosine
Death, sudden, 115–116
Deep brain stimulation, for Parkinson disease, 280
Defibrillator-cardioverters, implantable (ICDs), 111, 139–140
    for heart failure, 131
    for tachyarrhythmias, 139–140
Defibrillators, portable, public availability of, 313, 316
Dehydration, preoperative fasting and, 331
Delavirdine, 41
    for postexposure HIV prophylaxis, 46–47t
Delirium, 284
Delta hepatitis, 31–32
Delusions, 264
Demadex. See Torsemide
Dementia, 284–289
    AIDS-associated (HIV encephalopathy), 37
    Alzheimer, 240, 284–289
    in elderly, 240, 284
    hypertension and, 96
    Lewy body, 285
    mixed, 285

multi-infarct, 284
toxic, 285
vascular, 285
Demi-Regroton. *See* Reserpine
Depacon. *See* Valproate/valproic acid
Depakote. *See* Valproate/valproic acid
Dependence (drug), 267
Deprenyl. *See* Selegiline
Depression (mood disorder), 265
  drugs for (antidepressants), 274–276, 275*t*
    ocular effects of, 324*t*
  in elderly, 239, 265
    pseudodementia and, 240
Dermatographism, in Behçet syndrome, 193
Dermatomyositis, 186–187, 188*i*
Dermopathy, infiltrative, in hyperthyroidism, 224
Desyrel. *See* Trazodone
Detemir insulin, 209*t*, 210
Deviations, seizures causing, 284
DHPG. *See* Ganciclovir
DiaBeta. *See* Glyburide
Diabetes Control and Complications Trial (DCCT), 210, 214–215
Diabetes mellitus, 201–221
  classification of, 203–206, 204–205*t*
  clinical presentations of, 206–207
  complications of
    acute, 216
    long-term, 216–218
    ocular, 218–219
    tight glucose control affecting, 215
  definition of, 202, 203*t*
  diagnosis of, 203*t*, 207, 208*t*
  diet in management of, 207–209
  dyslipidemia and, 150
  exercise in management of, 207–209
  gestational, 203*t*, 205*t*, 206
  glucose metabolism and, 202
  glucose surveillance (glycemic control) and, 215–216
    importance of glucose control and, 214–215, 215*i*
    retinopathy incidence and progression affected by, 215, 215*i*
  hypertension management and, 91*t*, 95
  insulin therapy for, 208–211, 209*t*
  latent, in adults (LADA), 206
  management of, 207–216
    recent developments in, 201
  metabolic syndrome and, 206
  ophthalmologic considerations and, 218–220
  oral agents for, 211–214, 212*t*
  prediabetic disorders and, 206
  prevention of, 207, 208*t*
  screening for, 207, 208*t*, 300–301
  surgical considerations in patients with, 220–221, 332–333
  type 1 (insulin-dependent/IDDM/juvenile-onset), 203–205, 204*t*
  type 2 (non–insulin-dependent/NIDDM/adult-onset), 204*t*, 205–206
    approach to treatment of, 214
Diabetic ketoacidosis, 216
Diabetic nephropathy, 217–218
Diabetic neuropathy, 218
Diabetic retinopathy, 215
  glycemic control affecting, 215, 215*i*

Diabinese. *See* Chlorpropamide
Diagnostic tests. *See* Screening/diagnostic tests
Diarrhea, in HIV infection/AIDS, 48–49
Diastole (diastolic phase), 128
Diastolic dysfunction, 129
  causes of, 128
  management of, 131
Diazepam, 273
  for medical emergencies, 316*t*
  perioperative, 332*t*, 335
Diazoxide, for hypertensive emergency, 94
DIC. *See* Disseminated intravascular coagulation
Diclofenac, 196, 197*t*
  corneal problems associated with, 197–198
  with misoprostol, 197*t*
Dicloxacillin, 55*t*
Didanosine, 41
  for postexposure HIV prophylaxis, 46–47*t*
Diet/diet therapy
  cancer and, 252
  coronary artery disease and, 111
  in diabetes management/prevention, 207, 207–209
    surgery and, 220, 333
  in hypercholesterolemia, 146, 148*t*
Diffuse toxic goiter, 224. *See also* Graves hyperthyroidism
Diffusion-weighted magnetic resonance imaging (DWI), in cerebral ischemia/stroke, 104
Diflucan. *See* Fluconazole
Diflunisal, 197*t*
Digital rectal exam, in cancer screening, 295*t*
Digitalis/digitoxin/digoxin
  for heart failure, 130
  ocular effects of, 142, 325*t*
  in perioperative setting, 333
Dihydropyridines
  contraindications to in non-ST-segment elevation acute coronary syndrome, 122–123
  for hypertension, 89*t*, 93
Dihydroxy propoxymethyl guanine. *See* Ganciclovir
Dilacor. *See* Diltiazem
Dilantin. *See* Phenytoin
Diltiazem
  for angina, 120
  for heart failure, mortality increases and, 130
  for hypertension, 89*t*
  for non-ST-segment elevation acute coronary syndrome, 122
Diovan. *See* Valsartan
Diphenhydramine, for allergic reactions/medical emergencies, 316*t*, 319
Diphtheria, immunization against, 307–308
Diphtheria-tetanus-pertussis vaccine (DTP), 291, 307
Diphtheria and tetanus toxoid with acellular pertussis vaccine (DTaP), 291, 304*t*, 307
  in combination vaccines, 309
Diprivan. *See* Propofol
Dirithromycin, 60*t*, 71
Disalcid. *See* Salsalate
Discoid rash, in systemic lupus erythematosus, 179, 181*t*, 182
Disease-modifying (slow-acting) antirheumatic drugs, 174
Disseminated intravascular coagulation, 169–170
Distaclor. *See* Cefaclor

Distribution, normal, clinical relevance of research and, 344
Distributive shock, 317. *See also* Shock
Diupres. *See* Reserpine
Diuretics
    for diastolic dysfunction, 131
    for hypertension, 81, 86, 87–92, 88*t*, 90*t*
    ocular effects of, 325*t*
    in perioperative setting, 334
Diuril. *See* Chlorothiazide
DKA. *See* Diabetic ketoacidosis
DM. *See* Diabetes mellitus
DMARDs. *See* Disease-modifying (slow-acting) antirheumatic drugs
DNA, fecal, testing in cancer screening, 298
DNA probes, in infection diagnosis, 3
DNA viruses, cancer association of, 254
Do not resuscitate orders, surgery in elderly patients and, 238
Dobutamine, for heart failure, 130–131
Dobutrex. *See* Dobutamine
Dolobid. *See* Diflunisal
Donepezil, for Alzheimer disease, 288
Donor cornea, screening for HIV antibodies and, 51
L-Dopa, for Parkinson disease, 279
Dopamine
    antipsychotic mechanism of action and, 271
    for heart failure, 130–131
    in Parkinson disease, 278
Doppler imaging
    in amaurosis fugax, 107
    in cerebral ischemia/stroke, 103
    in ischemic heart disease, 118
Doripenem, 69
"Dowager's hump," 242
Doxazosin
    for heart failure, 130
    for hypertension, 89*t*
Doxorubicin, 257, 259*t*
Doxycycline, 61*t*
    ocular effects of, 324*t*
Dressler syndrome, 115
Drug dependence, 267
Drug resistance. *See also specific agent and specific organism*
    antibiotic, 3, 66
        new drug classes and, 74–75
    antiretroviral, 41, 43, 44
Drug tolerance, 267
Drugs
    allergic reaction to, 319–320
        penicillins, 67–68
    antibiotic, 53–78, 55–65*t*
    cytotoxic, for Wegener granulomatosis, 192
    diabetes mellitus associated with, 204*t*
    medication use by elderly and, 235–236
    ocular, age/aging and, 235–236
    ocular toxicity and, 323–326, 324–325*t*
    platelet dysfunction caused by, 167–168, 331–332
    thrombocytopenia caused by, 167
Dry eye
    radiation causing, 256
    in Sjögren syndrome, 186, 187*t*
DTacP-IPV-Hib vaccine, 309

DTacP-IPV vaccine, 309
DTaP (diphtheria and tetanus toxoid with acellular pertussis vaccine), 291, 304*t*, 307
    in combination vaccines, 309
DTP (diphtheria-tetanus-pertussis) vaccine, 291, 307
DTPa-HBV-IPV/Hib vaccine, 309
Dual-energy quantitative computed tomography, for bone density measurement, 243
Dual-photon x-ray absorptiometry, for bone density measurement, 243
Duloxetine, 276
Duplex ultrasonography, in cerebral ischemia/stroke, 103
Duracef. *See* Cefadroxil
DXA. *See* Dual-photon x-ray absorptiometry
Dyazide. *See* Triamterene
Dynabac. *See* Dirithromycin
Dynacin. *See* Minocycline
DynaCirc. *See* Isradipine
Dynapen. *See* Dicloxacillin
Dyrenium. *See* Triamterene
Dyslexia, surface, in Alzheimer disease, 288
Dyslipoproteinemia/dyslipidemia, 150
    diabetic, 150
    screening for, 293
Dyspnea, 153
Dysthymic disorder, 265

Early-onset Alzheimer disease, 286
Eberconazole, 76
Ebola virus/Ebola hemorrhagic fever, 35
EBV. *See* Epstein-Barr virus
EBV-associated hemophagocytic lymphohistiocytosis/syndrome (EBV-HLH), 30
Ecchymoses, 166. *See also* Purpura
ECG. *See* Electrocardiography
Echinocandins, 76
    for *Pneumocystis carinii* (*Pneumocystis jiroveci*) pneumonia, 45
Echocardiography
    in cerebral ischemia/stroke, 103
    in congestive heart failure, 127
    exercise (stress), 118
    in ischemic heart disease, 118
    transesophageal Doppler
        in amaurosis fugax, 107
        in cerebral ischemia/stroke, 103
Echothiophate, succinylcholine and, 334
Eclampsia, 96
Ecstasy (MDMA/3,4-methylenedioxymethamphetamine), 270
Edema, in hypothyroidism, 225
Edrophonium, toxic reaction to, 323
EEG. *See* Electroencephalography
EF. *See* Ejection fraction
Efavirenz, 41–42
    for postexposure HIV prophylaxis, 46–47*t*
Effexor. *See* Venlafaxine
Ehlers-Danlos syndrome, 166
Ehrlichiosis, human granulocytic, 19
Ejection fraction, in congestive heart failure, 127
Eldepryl. *See* Selegiline
Elder abuse, 236–237
Elderly patients. *See* Age/aging; Geriatrics

Electrocardiography (ECG)
  in atrial flutter, 137
  in atrial tachycardia, 136
  in congestive heart failure, 127
  exercise, 119
  in ischemic heart disease, 114, 116, 119
  in junctional tachycardia, 137
  in sinus tachycardia, 136
  in stroke evaluation, 103
  in torsades de pointes, 140
  in ventricular fibrillation, 140
  in ventricular tachycardia, 138
Electroencephalography (EEG), in epilepsy diagnosis, 282
ELISA. See Enzyme-linked immunosorbent assay
Elspar. See Asparaginase
Emboli, stroke caused by, 102
Emergencies, 313–326. See also specific type
  cardiopulmonary arrest, 313–317
  medications used in, 316t
  ocular side effects of systemic medications, 323–326, 324–325t
  recent developments and, 313
  seizures, 320–321
  shock, 317–320
  status epilepticus, 320–321
  toxic overdose, 321–323, 322t
Emivirine, 42
Emphysema, 154
Emtricitabine, 41
Emtriva. See Emtricitabine
Enalapril/enalaprilat
  for heart failure, 130
  for hypertension, 88t, 90t, 94
  ocular effects of, 325t
Enbrel. See Etanercept
Encapsulation, polysaccharide, as microbial virulence factor, 4
Encephalitis, herpes, 27
Encephalopathy, HIV, 37
Endarterectomy, carotid, for carotid stenosis, 101, 107–108, 109
Endarteritis, in syphilis, 16
Endocarditis prophylaxis, 7, 8–11t
  ocular surgery and, 334
Endocrine disorders, 201–231. See also specific type
  diabetes mellitus, 201–221
  hypothalamic-pituitary axis and, 227–230
  multiple endocrine neoplasia syndromes, 230–231
  recent developments in, 201
  thyroid disease, 221–227
Endocrinopathies. See Endocrine disorders
Endometrial tissue sampling, for cancer screening, 295t
Endotoxins, microbial, virulence and, 4
Energix-B. See Hepatitis B vaccine
Enfuvirtide, 42
Engerix-B. See Hepatitis B vaccine
Enoxacin, 62t, 73
Enoxaparin, for non-ST-segment elevation acute coronary syndrome, 123
Entacapone, for Parkinson disease, 279
Enteritis, regional (Crohn disease), 177
Enterococcus
  endocarditis caused by, 7
  vancomycin-resistant, 3, 5, 71, 72

Enterocolitis, pseudomembranous, *Clostridium difficile* causing, 8
Enteropathic arthritis, 177
Enthesitis, 175
Enzyme-linked immunosorbent assay (ELISA)
  in HIV infection/AIDS, 39
  in Lyme disease, 20
Eperezolid, 63t, 75
Epilepsy, 280–284. See also Seizures
Epinephrine
  for anaphylaxis, 319, 320
  with local anesthetic
    maximum safe dosage and, 322t
    toxic reaction to, 322
  for medical emergencies, 316t
  in personal emergency kits, 320
  for pulmonary diseases, 157
EpiPen/EpiPen Jr, 320
Epivir. See Lamivudine
Eplerenone, 88t
Eprosartan, 88t, 90t
Epstein-Barr virus, 30, 254
Eptifibatide, for non-ST-segment elevation acute coronary syndrome, 123
Ertapenem, 60t, 69
Erythema, chronicum migrans, in Lyme disease, 19
Erythrocyte sedimentation rate, in giant cell arteritis, 190
Erythrocytes, 159
  development of, 160
Erythromycin, 60t, 70
Erythropoiesis, 160
Erythropoietin, 160
  for HIV infection/AIDS, 44
Escape rhythm, idioventricular, 134
Eskalith. See Lithium
Esmolol, for hypertensive emergency, 94
Esophageal cancer, screening for, 297
Esophageal dysmotility, in scleroderma, 185
Essential cryoglobulinemic vasculitis, 189t
Essential hypertension, 82–83, 83i
Estazolam, 273
Estradiol, ocular effects of, 325t
Estrogen/estrogen replacement therapy
  breast cancer risk and, 295
  cholesterol levels and, 143
  osteoporosis and, 241, 245t, 246
Etanercept, 173, 199
Ethambutol, 24, 49
Ethnic differences
  cancer and, 252, 253, 254
  hypertension and, 97
Ethosuximide, 283t
Etodolac, 197t
Etoposide, 257, 259t
Etravirine, 42
Eulexin. See Flutamide
European Carotid Surgery Trial, 108
Euthyroid Graves ophthalmopathy, 224–225
Evernimicin, 63t, 75
Everninomicins, 63t, 75
Evolving stroke, 102
Examination, ophthalmic, HIV infection precautions and, 51–52
Excimer laser, for coronary revascularization, 122

Exclusion criteria, 364
Executive function deficit, 264
Exelon. *See* Rivastigmine
Exenatide, for diabetes, 214
Exercise
    diabetes management/prevention and, 201, 207, 207–209
    hypertension management and, 87*t*
Exercise stress tests, in ischemic heart disease, 119
    echocardiography, 118
Exotoxins, microbial, virulence and, 4
Experimental (interventional) studies (clinical trials), 345, 351–352, 351*i*. *See also* Clinical research
    systematic reviews/meta-analyses of, 352
Eye
    aging affecting, 235
    antipsychotic drugs affecting, 272–273
    radiation affecting, 255–256
    systemic drugs affecting, 323–326, 324–325*t*
    in systemic malignancies, 262
Eye movements, disorders of, in Parkinson disease, 280
Eyelids
    aging affecting, 235
    disorders of, in Parkinson disease, 280
    retraction of, seizures causing, 284
    in scleroderma, 186
    in systemic lupus erythematosus, 182
    tumors of, in multiple endocrine neoplasia, 230, 230*i*

F (flutter) waves, 137
Factitious disorders, 266
Factive. *See* Gemifloxacin
Factor V Leiden, 170
Factor VIII deficiency (hemophilia A/classic hemophilia), 168
Factor VIII transfusions, 168
Falls, in elderly, 247, 248*t*
Famciclovir, 65*t*, 77
    for herpes simplex virus infections, 28, 77
    for herpes zoster, 28, 77
Familial Alzheimer disease, 286
Family history/familial factors, in human carcinogenesis, 254–255
Famotidine, preoperative, 331
Famvir. *See* Famciclovir
Faropenem, 60*t*, 69
Fascicular block (cardiology), 134
Fasting, preoperative, 331
Fasting glucose
    in diabetes diagnosis/screening, 301
    impaired, 203*t*, 206
Fasting plasma glucose test, 207
Fecal DNA testing, in cancer screening, 298
Fecal occult blood testing, in cancer screening, 295*t*, 298
Felbamate, 283*t*
Felbatol. *See* Felbamate
Feldene. *See* Piroxicam
Felodipine, 89*t*, 90*t*
Felty syndrome, 174
Fenofibrate, for hypercholesterolemia, 149*t*
Fenoprofen, 197*t*
Fenoterol, 157
    with ipratropium, 157*t*

Fentanyl, perioperative, 332*t*, 335, 338
Ferric gluconate, 159, 161
Ferritin levels, in iron deficiency anemia, 161
Ferrous sulfate, for iron deficiency anemia, 161
Fetal alcohol syndrome, 270
Fetal hydantoin syndrome, 284
Fetal radiation, effects/ocular manifestations of, 255
FEV_1 (forced expiratory volume in 1 second), 155
Fibric acid derivatives, for hypercholesterolemia, 149*t*
Fibrillation
    atrial, 138
        heart failure and, 131, 132
        stroke and, 102
    ventricular, 140
Fibrinolytic system, 164
Fibrotic pulmonary disease, 154
Fine-needle aspiration biopsy (FNAB), of thyroid gland, 223
Fishbone diagram, 370, 371*i*
Fitting (contact lens), trial, disinfection and, 51
Flagyl/Flagyl IV. *See* Metronidazole
Flecainide, ocular effects of, 325*t*
"Floor effect," 364
Flovent. *See* Fluticasone
Flow cytometry, in paroxysmal nocturnal hemoglobinuria screening, 159, 162
Flowchart (system of care), 370, 371*i*
Floxin. *See* Ofloxacin
Flu. *See* Influenza
Fluconazole, 64*t*, 75–76
Flumadine. *See* Rimantadine
Flumazenil, for benzodiazepine reversal, 335
FluMist. *See* Intranasal influenza vaccine
Flunisolide, for pulmonary diseases, 157*t*
Flunitrazepam (date rape drug), 269
Fluorescein, allergic reactions to, 319
Fluorescent treponemal antibody absorption (FTA-ABS) test, 17, 17*t*, 302
5-Fluorocytosine, 64*t*
Fluoroquinolones, 54, 73. *See also* Quinolones
Fluoroscopy, magnetic resonance, in ischemic heart disease, 119
Fluorouracil, 258*t*
Fluoxetine, ocular effects of, 324*t*
Fluphenazine, 271
Flurbiprofen, 196, 197*t*
Flutamide, 260*t*
Fluticasone, for pulmonary diseases, 157*t*
Flutrimazole, 76
Flutter, atrial, 137–138
Flutter (F) waves, 137
Fluvastatin, for hypercholesterolemia, 149*t*, 150*t*
FNAB. *See* Fine-needle aspiration biopsy
Folate/folic acid
    antagonists of, in cancer chemotherapy, 258*t*
    deficiency of, 162
    homocysteine levels and stroke and, 109
Follicle-stimulating hormone, pituitary adenoma producing, 229
Follicular carcinoma, of thyroid gland, 227
Follow-up studies (cohort studies), 345*i*, 348*i*, 350–351
Fomivirsen, 48
    for cytomegalovirus retinitis, 48
Foradil. *See* Formoterol
Forced expiratory volume in 1 second (FEV_1), 155

Forced vital capacity (FVC), 155
Formed elements, 159. *See also* Blood cells
Formoterol, 157, 157*t*
Fortaz. *See* Ceftazidime
Fortovase. *See* Saquinavir
Fosamprenavir, 42
Foscarnet, 48, 65*t*, 77
 for cytomegalovirus retinitis, 29
  in HIV infection/AIDS, 48
Foscavir. *See* Foscarnet
Fosinopril, 88*t*
Fosphenytoin, 283*t*
FPG. *See* Fasting plasma glucose test
Free radicals (oxygen radicals), in Alzheimer disease, 287
Free T_4, 222
FTA-ABS (fluorescent treponemal antibody absorption) test, 17, 17*t*, 302
FTC. *See* Emtricitabine
5FU. *See* 5-Fluorouracil
Functional disorders, in elderly, 239–240
Functional visual loss, 266
Fungi, 25–26. *See also specific type*
 disseminated infection caused by, in HIV infection/AIDS, 50
 drugs for infection caused by (antifungal agents), 64–65*t*, 75–76. *See also specific type*
 endocarditis caused by, 7
Fungizone. *See* Amphotericin B
Furazolidone, 75
Furosemide
 for diastolic dysfunction, 131
 for hypertension, 88*t*
Furoxone. *See* Furazolidone
Fusidic acid, for *C difficile* colitis, 8
Fusion inhibitors, for HIV infection/AIDS, 42
Fuzeon. *See* Enfuvirtide
FVC (forced vital capacity), 155

G6PD deficiency. *See* Glucose-6-phosphate dehydrogenase deficiency
Gabapentin, 283*t*
Gabitril. *See* Tiagabine
GAD. *See* Generalized anxiety disorder
Galantamine, for Alzheimer disease, 288
Gamma (γ)-interferon, 261
Ganciclovir, 47–48, 65*t*, 77
 for cytomegalovirus retinitis, 29
  in HIV infection/AIDS, 47–48
Ganglioneuromas, in multiple endocrine neoplasia, 230, 230*i*
Gantrisin. *See* Sulfisoxazole
Garamycin. *See* Gentamicin
Gastric cancer, 252, 297
Gastric surgery, for obesity in type 2 diabetes, 208–209
Gastroesophageal reflux disease (GERD), cancer and, 297
Gastrointestinal disease
 cancer screening and, 297
 in HIV infection/AIDS, 48–49
 in scleroderma, 185
Gatifloxacin, 62*t*, 73
Gaze deviation, seizure activity and, 284
GCA (giant cell arteritis). *See* Arteritis, giant cell
GDM. *See* Gestational diabetes mellitus

Gel phenomenon, in rheumatoid arthritis, 173–174
Gemfibrozil, for hypercholesterolemia, 149*t*
Gemifloxacin, 62*t*, 73
Generalizability
 of clinical research study, 361–362
 of screening/diagnostic test, 359
Generalized anxiety disorder (GAD), 266–267. *See also* Anxiety
Generalized seizures, 281, 282, 320
Genetic/hereditary factors
 in Alzheimer disease, 286–287
 in diabetes, 205, 205*t*
 in epilepsy, 281
 in human carcinogenesis, 252, 254–255
 in Parkinson disease, 278
Genetic profiling, of tumors, 251
Genetic testing/counseling, in sickle cell disease, 159, 163
Genital ulcers, in Behçet syndrome, 193
Gentamicin, 61*t*, 70
 for endocarditis prophylaxis, 11*t*
GERD. *See* Gastroesophageal reflux disease
Geriatrics, 233–249. *See also* Age/aging
 elder abuse and, 236–237
 falls and, 247, 248*t*
 medication use and, 235–236
 osteoporosis and, 240–247, 242*t*, 243*t*, 245*t*
 outpatient visits and, 236
 physiologic/pathologic eye changes and, 235
 psychology/psychopathology of aging and, 238–240
 surgical considerations and, 237–238
 systemic disease incidence and, 247–249
Gestational diabetes mellitus, 203*t*, 205*t*, 206
Giant cell (temporal) arteritis. *See* Arteritis, giant cell
Gigantism, 228
Glargine insulin, 201, 209*t*, 210
Glaucoma, evaluation of screening tests for, 355–359, 356*i*, 357*i*, 358*t*
Glimepiride, 212, 212*t*
Glipizide, 212, 212*t*
 with metformin, 213
Global Initiative for Chronic Obstructive Lung Disease (GOLD), 153
Glucagon-like peptide, for diabetes, 214
Glucocorticoids/glucocorticosteroids, 194–196. *See also* Corticosteroids
Glucophage. *See* Metformin
Glucose
 for medical emergencies, 316*t*
 metabolism of, 202
 plasma levels of
  in diabetes
   diagnosis/screening and, 301
   self-monitoring of, 215–216
   surgery and, 220, 332–333
   surveillance of (glycemic control), 215–216
  normal, 203*t*
Glucose-6-phosphate dehydrogenase deficiency, 163
Glucose tolerance/intolerance
 in gestational diabetes, 203*t*, 206
 impaired, 203*t*, 206
 screening for, 301
Glucose tolerance test, 206
Glucose toxicity, 205–206

α-Glucosidase inhibitors, 212t, 213
Glucotrol. See Glipizide
Glucovance. See Glyburide, with metformin
Glulisine insulin, 209, 209t
Glyburide, 212, 212t
    with metformin, 213
Glycemic control (glucose surveillance), 215–216
    retinopathy incidence and progression affected by, 215, 215i
Glycopeptide antibiotics, 60–61t, 71–72
Glycopeptide-intermediate S aureus, 5
Glycoprotein IIb/IIIa receptor, 123
Glycoprotein IIb/IIIa receptor antagonists, 123
    for myocardial infarction, 111, 115, 123
Glycosylated hemoglobin (HbA_{1c}), in glucose control/surveillance, 215, 215i, 216, 219
Glynase. See Glyburide
Glyset. See Miglitol
Goiter
    diffuse toxic, 224. See also Graves hyperthyroidism
    nodular toxic, 225
GOLD. See Global Initiative for Chronic Obstructive Lung Disease
Gold compounds/salts, 199
Gold standard, 363
Gonadotroph adenomas, 229
Gonadotropins, pituitary adenoma producing, 229
Gonococcus (Neisseria gonorrhoeae/gonorrhea), 13–14
Gottron sign, in dermatomyositis, 186
gp160 vaccine, 44
Grand mal seizures, 282
Granulomatosis
    allergic, and angiitis (Churg-Strauss syndrome), 189t, 193
    Wegener, 189t, 192
Granulomatous disease
    ileocolitis (Crohn disease), 177
    pulmonary, 154
    subacute thyroiditis, 226–227
Graves hyperthyroidism, 224–225. See also Thyroid ophthalmopathy
Gray (Gy), radiation dose measurement, 255
Group A β-hemolytic streptococci (Streptococcus pyogenes), 6
Growth hormone, pituitary adenoma producing, 228
Guaiac stool test, in cancer screening, 295t, 298
Guanfacine, 89t
Guillain-Barré syndrome, immunization and, 303
Gummas, syphilitic, 16
Gyne-Lotrimin. See Clotrimazole

H_2-receptor blockers, preoperative, 331
HAART. See Highly active antiretroviral therapy
Haemophilus/Haemophilus influenzae, 10–12
    endocarditis caused by, 7
    immunization against, 12, 291, 304t, 308–309
    resistant strains of, 12
Haemophilus influenzae type B (Hib) vaccine, 12, 291, 304t, 308–309
    in combination vaccines, 309
Halcion. See Triazolam
Haldol. See Haloperidol
Hallucinations, 264

Hallucinogenic drugs, abuse of, 268t
Haloperidol, 271
Hand washing, in infection control, HIV transmission prevention and, 51
Hantavirus/hantavirus pulmonary syndrome, 35
Hashimoto thyroiditis, 226–227
    hypothyroidism caused by, 225, 226, 227
HATTS (hemagglutination treponemal test for syphilis), 17, 302
Havrix. See Hepatitis A vaccine
HBA. See Hepatitis, type A
HbA_{1c}. See Hemoglobin A_{1c}
HCV. See Hepatitis, type C
HDL cholesterol. See High-density-lipoprotein cholesterol
Head-tilt, chin-lift maneuver, for opening airway, 314
Headache
    in hypertensive-arteriosclerotic intracerebral hemorrhages, 105
    in subarachnoid hemorrhage, 105
Health counseling, in cancer prevention, 295t
Heart block, 134–135
Heart disease, 111–142
    congestive failure, 125–132
    in diabetes, 218
    endocarditis prophylaxis recommendations and, 7, 8–11t
    hypertension management and, 91t, 94
    hypertension and risk of, 81, 84, 86t
    ischemic, 111–125
    in Lyme disease, 19
    ophthalmic considerations and, 141–142
    recent developments in, 111
    rhythm disturbances, 132–141
    in scleroderma, 185
    screening for, 293–294
    in systemic lupus erythematosus, 179
Heart failure. See Congestive heart failure
Heart rate, reduction of in angina management, 120
Heart transplantation, for heart failure, 132
Heimlich maneuver, 316
Heinz bodies, 163
Helicobacter pylori infection, screening for, cancer screening and, 297
Heliotrope rash, in dermatomyositis, 186, 187, 188i
Helper T cells, in HIV infection/AIDS, 37
Hemagglutination antibody test, indirect, for Lyme disease, 20
Hemagglutination treponemal test for syphilis (HATTS), 17, 302
Hematocrit, in anemia, 160
Hematologic disorders, 159–172. See also specific type
    in systemic lupus erythematosus, 180, 181t
Hematopoietic growth factors
    in cancer therapy, 261
    for HIV infection/AIDS, 44
Hematopoietic stem cells, 160
Hemoccult slides. See Stool guaiac slide test
Hemoglobin A_{1c}, diabetes control and, 215, 215i, 216, 219
Hemoglobin S, 163
Hemoglobinuria, paroxysmal nocturnal, 162
    hypercoagulability and, 171
    screening test for, 159, 162

Hemolytic anemia, 162–163
  autoimmune, 163
Hemophilia A (classic hemophilia/factor VIII deficiency), 168
Hemorrhages
  coagulation disorders and, 166
  in hemophilia, 168
  hemostatic derangement and, 166
  intracranial, 105–106
    hypertensive-arteriosclerotic, 105, 106
    ruptured aneurysm causing, 105, 106
  iron deficiency anemia and, 161
  platelet disorders and, 166, 166–168
  subarachnoid, 105, 106
  vascular disorders and, 166
Hemorrhagic disease of newborn, 169
Hemorrhagic fever, Ebola, 35
Hemorrhagic telangiectasia, hereditary (Osler-Weber-Rendu disease), 166
Hemostasis, 164–165, 164i
  disorders of, 163–172
    clinical manifestations of, 166
    coagulation disorders and, 168–172
    hemorrhage and, 166
    hypercoagulable states and, 170–172
    platelet disorders and, 166–168
    vascular disorders and, 166
  laboratory evaluation of, 165
Henoch-Schönlein purpura, 189t
Hepacare. *See* Hepatitis B vaccine
Heparin therapy, 171
  for antiphospholipid antibody syndrome, 184
  for deep venous thrombosis prophylaxis in stroke patients, 101, 104
  for non-ST-segment elevation acute coronary syndrome, 123
  in perioperative setting, 332
Hepatitis, 31–32
  delta, 31–32
  HIV coinfection and, 50
  transfusion-transmitted virus causing, 32
  type A, 31
    immunization against, 31, 291, 305
    travel and, 309–310
  type B, 303–305
    cancer and, 254
    immunization against, 291, 303–305, 304t
    travel and, 309
  type C, 31–32
  type E, 32
Hepatitis A vaccine, 31, 291, 305
  travel and, 309–310
Hepatitis B immune globulin, 305
Hepatitis B vaccine, 291, 303–305, 304t
  in combination vaccines, 305, 309
  travel and, 309
Hepatitis D virus, 31–32
Hepatitis E virus, 32
Hepatitis G virus, 32
Hepatocellular carcinoma, 297
  viral carcinogenesis and, 254
HepB. *See* Hepatitis B vaccine
Hereditary hemorrhagic telangiectasia (Osler-Weber-Rendu disease), 166

Hereditary spherocytosis, 162
Heroin abuse, 269
Herpes simplex virus, 27–28
  acyclovir for infection caused by, 28, 76
  cancer association and, 254
  famciclovir for infection caused by, 28, 77
  perinatal infection caused by, 28
  type 1, 27
  type 2, 27
  valacyclovir for infection caused by, 28, 77
Herpes zoster, 28–29
  acyclovir for, 28, 76–77
  in elderly, 248–249
  famciclovir for, 28, 77
  valacyclovir for, 28, 77
Herpes zoster ophthalmicus
  acyclovir for, 76
  in elderly, 248–249
Herpesviruses, 27–30. *See also specific type*
  cancer association and, 254
Heterocyclic antidepressants, 275t
Hib (*Haemophilus influenzae* type B) vaccine, 12, 291, 304t, 308–309
  in combination vaccines, 309
Hib-DTaP vaccine, 309
High-density-lipoprotein cholesterol, 144, 144t. *See also* Cholesterol
  beta-blockers affecting, 150
  low levels of, 144t, 150
  risk assessment and, 144, 144t
  screening, 293
High-output failure, causes of, 128
High-speed rotary devices, for coronary revascularization, 122
Highly active antiretroviral therapy (HAART), 43–44
  CMV retinitis incidence and, 3, 48
  immune reconstitution syndromes and, 51
His bundle, 133, 134
Histogram, 368, 369i
History, preoperative assessment and, 327, 328t
HIV (human immunodeficiency virus), 36–37
  drug resistance and, 41, 43, 44
  superinfection and, 40
  testing for antibody to, 39
  vaccine development and, 44–45
HIV-1, 36–37. *See also* HIV infection/AIDS
  superinfection and, 40
HIV-1 delta 4 vaccine, 44
HIV-2, 37. *See also* HIV infection/AIDS
HIV infection/AIDS, 36–53
  atypical mycobacterial infections and, 23, 49–50
  CDC definition of, 37, 40t
  classification of, 40t
  clinical syndrome of, 37–39, 40t
  cytomegalovirus infections and, 29, 47–48
  diagnosis of, 39
  encephalopathy in, 37
  etiology of, 36–37
  immunization against, development of vaccine for, 44–45
  incidence of, 36
  influenza vaccine in patients with, 305
  lymphoma in, 50–51

malignancies associated with, 50–51
management of, 40–45
  chemoprophylaxis and, 45, 46–47*t*
  drug resistance and, 41, 43, 44
  HAART in, 43–44
  immune reconstitution syndromes and, 51
  recent developments in, 3, 42, 44
nephropathy associated with, 37–38
occupational exposure to, 39
  precautions in health care setting and, 51–52
  prophylaxis for, 45, 46–47*t*
ocular infection/manifestations and, 51–52
opportunistic infections associated with, 45–51
pathogenesis of, 36–37
Pneumocystis carinii (*Pneumocystis jiroveci*) infections and, 45–47
primary (retroviral syndrome), 38
prognosis of, 40–45
seroepidemiology of, 39
spore-forming intestinal protozoa and, 48–49
superinfection and, 40
syphilis/syphilitic chorioretinitis in, 18
transmission of, 39–40
transplacental transmission of, chemoprophylaxis for, 45
tuberculosis and, 24, 49–50, 301, 302
HIV p24 antigen testing, 39
HIV RNA
as predictor of response to therapy, 40, 43
testing for, 39
HIV vaccine, development of, 44–45
Hivid. *See* Zalcitabine
HLA antigens. *See* Human leukocyte (HLA) antigens
HMG-CoA (3-hydroxy-3-methyl glutaryl coenzyme-A) reductase inhibitors. *See also* Statins
cataracts and, 151
for hypercholesterolemia, 149*t*
Hodgkin disease, in HIV infection/AIDS, 50–51
Homocysteine
carotid artery disease and, 109
hypercoagulability and, 171
Hormone replacement therapy. *See also* Estrogen/estrogen replacement therapy
breast cancer risk and, 295
Hormones
in cancer chemotherapy, 260*t*
ocular effects of, 325*t*
osteoporosis and, 241, 245*t*, 246
pituitary adenoma producing, 228–229
Hospital-acquired infections, treatment of, 77–78
Host susceptibility, in carcinogenesis, 254
HPV. *See* Human papillomaviruses
HSV. *See* Herpes simplex virus
HTLV-I. *See* Human T-cell lymphotropic retrovirus type I
HTLV-III. *See* Human T-cell lymphotropic virus type III
Humalog. *See* Lispro insulin
Human granulocytic ehrlichiosis, 19
Human immunodeficiency virus (HIV), 36–37. *See also* HIV infection/AIDS
drug resistance and, 41, 43, 44
superinfection and, 40
testing for antibody to, 39
vaccine development and, 44–45

Human leukocyte (HLA) antigens
in ankylosing spondylitis, 175, 176
in anterior uveitis, 175, 176, 178
in Behçet syndrome, 193
in diabetes mellitus, 203–205
in enteropathic arthritis, 177
in psoriatic arthritis, 178
in reactive arthritis/Reiter syndrome, 176
in rheumatoid arthritis, 174
in spondyloarthropathies, 175, 178
in systemic lupus erythematosus, 179
Human papillomaviruses, 33
cancer association of, 33, 254, 291, 294
Human T-cell lymphotropic retrovirus type I (HTLV-I), 37
Human T-cell lymphotropic retrovirus type II (HTLV-II), 37
Human T-cell lymphotropic virus type III (HTLV-III), 37. *See also* Human immunodeficiency virus
Humira. *See* Adalimumab
Humoral immunity, 4
Hybridomas, 261
Hydralazine
for heart failure, 130
for hypertension, 89*t*, 94
Hydrochlorothiazide, 88*t*, 90*t*
Hydrocortisone
for anaphylaxis, 319
for medical emergencies, 316*t*
perioperative, 334
Hydrocortisone sodium succinate, for medical emergencies, 316*t*
HydroDIURIL. *See* Hydrochlorothiazide
Hydropres. *See* Reserpine
Hydroton. *See* Chlorthalidone
3-Hydroxy-3-methyl glutaryl coenzyme-A (HMG-CoA) reductase inhibitors. *See also* Statins
cataracts and, 151
for hypercholesterolemia, 149*t*
Hydroxyapatite, 241
Hydroxychloroquine, 174, 198
ocular effects of, 324*t*
Hyperaldosteronism, hypertension in, 83, 84*t*
Hypercholesterolemia, 143–152
classification of, 144, 144*t*
management of, 145–147, 146*i*, 147*t*, 148*t*, 149*t*, 150*t*, 151*t*. *See also* Lipid-lowering therapy
metabolic syndrome and, 146, 148, 152*t*
ophthalmologic considerations and, 150–151
recent developments in, 143
risk assessment and, 144, 144*t*, 145, 145*t*, 146*i*
screening for, 293
specific dyslipidemias and, 150
Hypercoagulable states (hypercoagulability), 170–172. *See also* Thrombophilia
fetal loss/preeclampsia and, 159
primary, 170–171
secondary, 171–172
Hyperglycemia. *See also* Diabetes mellitus
diabetic retinopathy incidence and progression and, 215, 215*i*
obesity and, 202
rebound, 210
Hyperhomocysteinemia, 171
carotid artery disease and, 109

Hypermetabolism, in hyperthyroidism, 223
Hyperparathyroidism, in multiple endocrine neoplasia, 230
Hyperstat. *See* Diazoxide
Hypertension, 81–99
   cardiovascular risk and, 81, 84, 86*t*
   in children and adolescents, 81, 97
   in diabetes, 218
   diagnosis/definition of, 82, 82*t*, 292
   etiology and pathogenesis of, 82–84, 83*i*, 84*t*
   evaluation of, 84
   incidence and prevalence of, 81–82
   intracranial hemorrhage and, 105, 106
   left ventricular hypertrophy and, 95
   MAO inhibitor interactions and, 97, 276
   metabolic syndrome and, 95
   minority populations and, 97
   obesity and, 85, 95
   in older patients, 96
   ophthalmic considerations and, 98–99, 98*t*
   orthostatic, 96
   peripheral arterial disease and, 96
   during pregnancy, 96–97
   primary (essential), 82–83, 83*i*
   rebound, 97–98
   resistant, 83, 85*t*
   retinal disease associated with, 98–99, 98*t*
   screening for, 292–293
   secondary, 83, 84*t*
   sleep disorders and, 95
   treatment of, 84–94, 91*i*
      cerebrovascular disease and, 95
      chronic renal disease and, 91*t*, 95
      diabetes and, 91*t*, 95
      heart failure and, 91*t*, 95, 130
      ischemic heart disease and, 91*t*, 94
      lifestyle modifications and, 85–86, 87*t*
      pharmacologic, 86, 87–94, 88–89*t*, 90*t*, 91*i*, 91*t*. *See also* Antihypertensive drugs
   white coat, 82
   withdrawal syndromes and, 97–98
   in women, 96–97
Hypertensive-arteriosclerotic intracerebral hemorrhages, 105, 106
Hypertensive crisis, 98
   MAO inhibitor interactions and, 276
   parenteral antihypertensive agents for, 94
Hypertensive retinopathy, 98–99, 98*t*
Hyperthermia, malignant, 336–337, 337*t*
   preoperative assessment of risk for, 329–330
Hyperthyroidism, 223–225
   in elderly, 249
   Graves, 224–225
   toxic nodular goiter, 225
Hypertriglyceridemia, screening for, 293
Hypnotic drugs, 273–277, 274*t*
   abuse of, 269
Hypochondriasis, 266
   in elderly, 240
Hypoglycemia
   insulin therapy causing, 211
   sulfonylurea-induced, 212
Hypoglycemia unawareness, 211
Hypoglycemic agents. *See* Insulin therapy; Oral hypoglycemic agents

Hypomania, 265
Hypometabolism, in hypothyroidism, 226
Hypopyon, in Behçet syndrome, 193, 194
Hypothalamic-pituitary axis, disorders of, 227–230, 229*i*
Hypothalamus, 227
Hypothyroidism, 225–226
Hypovolemic shock, 317. *See also* Shock
"Hysterical blindness." *See* Functional visual loss
Hytrin. *See* Terazosin
Hyzaar. *See* Losartan

Ibuprofen, 197*t*
   ocular effects of, 324*t*
Ibutilide, for atrial flutter, 137–138
ICDs. *See* Implantable cardioverter-defibrillators
Iclaprim, 75
IDDM. *See* Diabetes mellitus, type 1
Idiopathic thrombocytopenic purpura, 167
Idioventricular escape rhythm, 134
Ifex. *See* Ifosfamide
IFG. *See* Impaired fasting glucose
IFNs. *See* Interferons
Ifosfamide, 258*t*
Ig. *See under* Immunoglobulin
IGT. *See* Impaired glucose tolerance
IHD. *See* Ischemic heart disease
IL. *See under* Interleukin
Ileocolitis, granulomatous (Crohn disease), 177
Imidazoles, 64*t*, 75–76
Imipenem-cilastin, 59*t*, 69
Imipramine, ocular effects of, 324*t*
Immune reconstitution syndromes (IRS), 51
Immune response (immunity)
   cellular, 4
   humoral, 4
Immunization, 302–311. *See also specific disease*
   active, 303
   childhood, recommendations for, 303, 304*t*
   in immunocompromised host/HIV infection/AIDS, 41, 303, 305
   new developments in, 291, 310
   passive, 303
   for travel, 309–310
Immunocompromised host
   immunization in, 303, 305
   ocular infection in, cytomegalovirus retinitis, 29
Immunodot assay, for Lyme disease, 20
Immunofluorescence assay
   in HIV infection/AIDS, 39
   in Lyme disease, 20
Immunoglobulin A (IgA) protease, as microbial virulence factor, 4
Immunoglobulin E (IgE), in type I hypersensitivity/anaphylactic reactions, 319
Immunotherapy/immunosuppression, 199–200
   for Behçet syndrome, 193–194
   for cancer, 251, 257–262, 260*t*
   diabetes affected by, 203
   for HIV infection/AIDS, 44
   for pulmonary diseases, 158
   for rheumatic disorders, 199–200
   for rheumatoid arthritis, 174–175
Impaired fasting glucose, 203*t*, 206

Impaired glucose tolerance, 203*t*, 206
Implantable cardioverter-defibrillators (ICDs), 111,
    139–140
  for heart failure, 131
  for tachyarrhythmias, 139–140
Imuran. *See* Azathioprine
Inclusion criteria, 364
Incretins, for diabetes, 214
Indapamide, 88*t*
Inderal/Inderal LA. *See* Propranolol
Inderide. *See* Propranolol
Indinavir, 42
  for postexposure HIV prophylaxis, 46–47*t*
Indirect hemagglutination antibody test, for Lyme
    disease, 20
Individual versus average effect, 361–362
Indocin. *See* Indomethacin
Indomethacin, 197*t*
Infectious disease, 3–79. *See also specific organism and
    specific disorder*
  antimicrobial treatment for, 53–78, 55–65*t*
  diabetes mellitus and, 204*t*
  microbiologic principles and, 3–4
  recent developments in, 3
  screening for, 301–302
Infectious mononucleosis, Epstein-Barr virus
    causing, 30
Infiltrative dermopathy, in hyperthyroidism, 224
Inflammation (ocular), nonsteroidal anti-inflammatory
    agents for, 196–198
Inflammatory bowel disease, 177
Infliximab, 173, 199
  for Behçet syndrome, 194
Influenza virus
  antiviral agents for infection caused by, 77, 291
  vaccination against, 291, 305–306
Inhaled steroids, for pulmonary diseases, 158
Inhalers, metered-dose, β$_2$-adrenergics for pulmonary
    disease and, 157
Inotropic agents, for heart failure, 130–131
INR. *See* International normalized ratio
Inspra. *See* Eplerenone
Insulin. *See also* Insulin therapy
  in glucose metabolism/diabetes, 202
    genetic defects and, 204*t*
Insulin-dependent diabetes mellitus. *See* Diabetes
    mellitus, type 1
Insulin-neutralizing antibodies, 211
Insulin pump, 210–211
Insulin resistance
  immunologic, insulin therapy and, 211
  metabolic syndrome and, 148, 206
Insulin therapy, 208–211, 209*t*
  complications of, 211
  inhaled, 214
  intensive (tight control), 214–215
  recent developments in, 201
  surgery in diabetic patient and, 220–221, 333
  types of insulin for, 209–210, 209*t*
Intal. *See* Cromolyn
Integrase inhibitors, for HIV infection/AIDS, 42
Integrilin. *See* Eptifibatide
Intention-to-treat analysis, 352

Interferons (IFNs), 261
  α, 261
    for Behçet syndrome, 193
    in cancer therapy, 260*t*, 261
    for hepatitis B, 305
    for hepatitis C, 31
  β, 261
  γ, 261
  ocular effects of, 324*t*
Interleukin-2, in cancer therapy, 261
Interleukins
  in cancer therapy, 261
  for HIV infection/AIDS, 44
International normalized ratio (INR), 165
Interrater reliability, 363
Intervention, in clinical research, 342
Interventional (experimental) studies (clinical trials),
    345, 351–352, 351*i*. *See also* Clinical research
  systematic reviews/meta-analyses of, 352
Intracranial hemorrhage, 105–106
Intranasal influenza vaccine, 305
Intraocular pressure, measurement of, as screening tool,
    355, 356*i*
Intraocular tumors, 262
Intrarater reliability, 363
Intravascular ultrasound, in ischemic heart disease, 119
Intraventricular block (cardiology), 134
Intravitreal medications, for cytomegalovirus retinitis,
    29, 48
Intrinsic sympathomimetic activity, beta-blocker, 92
Intron-A. *See* Interferons (IFNs), α
Intropin. *See* Dopamine
Invirase. *See* Saquinavir
Iodine, radioactive
  for Graves hyperthyroidism, 225
  for thyroid scanning, 223
  thyroid uptake of, 223
Iodine-123, 223
Iodine-131, 225
Ionizing radiation. *See* Radiation
Ipratropium, 157–158, 157*t*
  in combination agents, 157*t*
IPV (Salk vaccine), 304*t*, 307
  in combination vaccines, 309
Irbesartan, 88*t*, 90*t*
Iridocyclitis
  in ankylosing spondylitis, 176
  in Behçet syndrome, 194
  HLA-associated diseases and, 177
Iron deficiency anemia, 161
  anemia of chronic disease differentiated from, 159
  treatment of, 159, 161
Iron dextran, 159, 161
IRS. *See* Immune reconstitution syndromes
ISA. *See* Intrinsic sympathomimetic activity
Ischemia
  cardiac. *See* Ischemic heart disease
  cerebral, 101–105. *See also* Stroke
  ocular, carotid artery disease and, 107
Ischemic heart disease, 111–125. *See also* Acute
    coronary syndrome; Angina pectoris
  asymptomatic patients with, 116
  clinical syndromes in, 113–116

in diabetes, 218
diagnosis of
  invasive procedures for, 119–120
  noninvasive procedures for, 116–119
heart failure and, 127, 128
hypercholesterolemia and, 143, 143–144
hypertension management in, 91t, 94
management of, 120–125
pathophysiology of, 112
risk factors for, 112–113
screening for, 293–294
Ischemic optic neuropathy, in giant cell arteritis, 190
Islet cells, injection of, for diabetes, 214
Isoantibody production, posttransfusion, 167
Isoniazid, 24, 49
Isoptin. *See* Verapamil
Isospora belli (isosporiasis), in HIV infection/AIDS, 48, 49
Isotretinoin, ocular effects of, 324t
Isradipine, 89t
ITP. *See* Idiopathic thrombocytopenic purpura
Itraconazole, 25, 64t, 75–76
Ixodes ticks, Lyme disease transmitted by, 18–19

Januvia. *See* Sitagliptin
Japanese encephalitis vaccine, 309
Jarisch-Herxheimer reaction, in Lyme disease treatment, 21
Jaw thrust, modified, for opening airway, 314
JIA. *See* Juvenile idiopathic (chronic) arthritis
Josamycin, 60t, 71
Junctional complexes, premature (PJCs), 135
Junctional rhythm, atrioventricular, 133
Junctional tachycardia, 137
Juvenile ankylosing spondylitis, 178
Juvenile idiopathic (chronic) arthritis, 178–179
  systemic onset (Still's disease), 178–179
Juvenile-onset diabetes mellitus. *See* Diabetes mellitus, type 1
Juvenile rheumatoid arthritis. *See* Juvenile idiopathic (chronic) arthritis
Juvenile spondyloarthropathy, 178

Kaletra. *See* Lopinavir/ritonavir
Kanamycin, 70
Kaposi sarcoma
  treatment of, 50
  viral carcinogenesis and, 254
Kappa (κ) statistic, 364
Kawasaki syndrome (mucocutaneous lymph node syndrome), 189t
Keflex. *See* Cephalexin
Kefurox. *See* Cefuroxime
Kefzol. *See* Cefazolin
Keppra. *See* Levetiracetam
Keratitis
  NSAID use and, 197–198
  peripheral, in Wegener granulomatosis, 192
Kerlone. *See* Betaxolol
Ketek. *See* Telithromycin
Ketoacidosis, diabetic, 216
Ketoconazole, 64t
Ketolides, 60t, 71, 75

Ketoprofen, 197t
Ketorolac tromethamine, 196–197
  perioperative, 332t, 338
  for postoperative pain, 197, 338
Kidneys, scleroderma (scleroderma renal crisis), 185
Kineret. *See* Anakinra
KM-1, 42
Kyphosis, in osteoporosis, 242

L-Dopa, for Parkinson disease, 279
Labetalol, 89t
  for hypertensive emergency, 94
Lactate dehydrogenase analysis, in myocardial infarction, 118
Lactotroph adenomas (prolactinomas), 228
LADA. *See* Latent autoimmune diabetes in adults
Lamictal. *See* Lamotrigine
Lamisil. *See* Terbinafine
Lamivudine (3TC)
  for hepatitis B, 305
  for HIV infection/AIDS, 41
  for postexposure HIV prophylaxis, 45, 46–47t
  with zidovudine, 41, 45
Lamotrigine, 283t
Lanoconazole, 76
Lantus. *See* Glargine insulin
Laser therapy (laser surgery), for coronary revascularization, 122
Lasix. *See* Furosemide
Late-onset Alzheimer disease, 286
Latency (viral), herpesvirus infection and, 27, 28
Latent autoimmune diabetes in adults (LADA), 206
Latex allergy, in ocular surgery candidate, 330
LAV. *See* Lymphadenopathy-associated virus
Lavage, bronchial, 155
LBBB. *See* Left bundle branch block
LBD. *See* Lewy body dementia
LDL cholesterol. *See* Low-density-lipoprotein cholesterol
Leflunomide, 199–200
Left anterior hemiblock, 134
Left bundle branch block, 134–135
Left posterior hemiblock, 134
Left ventricular hypertrophy, hypertension and, 95
Lens (crystalline), radiation affecting, 255–256
Lente insulin, 209t
Lescol. *See* Fluvastatin
Lesionectomy, for seizures, 283
Leukemia, ocular involvement in, 262
Leukeran. *See* Chlorambucil
Leukocytes, 159
Leukotriene modifiers, for pulmonary diseases, 157t, 158
Leuprolide, ocular effects of, 325t
Levaquin. *See* Levofloxacin
Levatol. *See* Penbutolol
Levemir. *See* Detemir insulin
Levetiracetam, 283t
Levodopa (L-dopa), for Parkinson disease, 279
Levodopa/carbidopa, for Parkinson disease, 279
Levofloxacin, 62t, 73
Levothyroxine, for hypothyroidism, 226
Lewy bodies, in Parkinson disease, 278, 285

Lewy body dementia (LBD), 285
Lexiva. *See* Fosamprenavir
Lexxel. *See* Felodipine
Lidocaine
   maximum safe dose of, 322*t*
   for medical emergencies, 316*t*
   toxic reaction to, 323, 336
Lifestyle modification
   in hypercholesterolemia management, 143, 145–146, 148*t*
   in hypertension management, 85–86, 87*t*, 91*i*
Likelihood ratio, 358–359
   combining screening tests and, 359
Linezolid, 63*t*, 74–75
Lipid-lowering therapy, 145–147, 146*i*, 147*t*, 148*t*, 149*t*, 150*t*, 151*t*. *See also specific agent*
Lipitor. *See* Atorvastatin
Lipoatrophy, at insulin injection site, 211
Lipohypertrophy, at insulin injection site, 211
Lipopeptide antibiotics, 63–64*t*, 75
Lipoprotein analysis, 144, 144*t*
Liraglutide, for diabetes, 214
Lisinopril
   for heart failure, 130
   for hypertension, 88*t*, 90*t*
   for non-ST-segment elevation acute coronary syndrome, 123
Lispro insulin, 209, 209*t*
Lithium, 277
Lithonate. *See* Lithium
Liver disease
   cancer, viral carcinogenesis and, 254
   hemostatic abnormalities and, 169
   hepatitis C and, 31
Living will, surgery in elderly patients and, 238
LMWHs. *See* Low-molecular-weight heparins
Lobectomy, for seizures, 283
Local anesthesia. *See* Anesthesia (anesthetics), local
Lodine. *See* Etodolac
Lodosyn. *See* Carbidopa
Lomefloxacin, 62*t*, 73
Lomustine, 260*t*
Loniten. *See* Minoxidil
Loop diuretics
   for diastolic dysfunction, 131
   for hypertension, 87, 88*t*, 89–92
Lopinavir/ritonavir, 42
   for postexposure HIV prophylaxis, 46–47*t*
Lopressor. *See* Metoprolol
Lorabid. *See* Loracarbef
Loracarbef, 59*t*, 69
Losartan, 88*t*, 90*t*
Lotensin. *See* Benazepril
Lotrel. *See* Amlodipine
Lotrimin. *See* Clotrimazole
Lovastatin
   cataracts and, 151
   for hypercholesterolemia, 149*t*, 150*t*
Lovenox. *See* Enoxaparin
Low-density-lipoprotein cholesterol, 144, 144*t*. *See also* Cholesterol
   beta-blockers affecting, 150
   goals for, hypercholesterolemia management and, 145, 146, 147*t*
   reducing levels of, 143, 145–147, 146*i*, 147*t*, 148*t*, 149*t*, 150*t*, 151*t*
   risk assessment and, 144, 144*t*, 145*t*, 146*i*, 147*t*
   screening, 293
   very high levels of, 144*t*, 150
Low-molecular-weight heparins
   for acute coronary syndrome, 111, 123
   in perioperative setting, 332
Lozol. *See* Indapamide
Luliconazole, 76
Lumbar puncture
   in cerebral ischemia/stroke, 103
   in subarachnoid hemorrhage, 106
   in syphilis, 17–18
Lung cancer, 252, 296–297
   eye involvement and, 262
   screening for, 296–297
Lung diseases. *See* Pulmonary diseases
Lupron. *See* Leuprolide
Lupus anticoagulant, in antiphospholipid antibody syndrome, 183–184
Lupus erythematosus, systemic, 179–182, 180*i*, 181*t*
Lupus nephritis, 179
Luteinizing hormone, pituitary adenoma producing, 229
Lyme disease/Lyme borreliosis, 18–21
Lymecycline, 72
Lymphadenopathy-associated virus (LAV), 36. *See also* Human immunodeficiency virus
Lymphadenopathy syndrome (ARC), 38–39
Lymphocytic thyroiditis, subacute ("painless"), 226
Lymphohistiocytosis, EBV-associated hemophagocytic (EBV-HLH), 30
Lymphoid stem cells, 160
Lymphomas
   Burkitt, Epstein-Barr virus associated with, 30
   in HIV infection/AIDS, 50–51
   ocular involvement in, 262
Lysosomal fusion, blocking, as microbial virulence factor, 4

MAC (*Mycobacterium avium* complex) infections, in HIV infection/AIDS, 49
Macroadenoma, pituitary, 228
Macrolides, 60*t*, 71. *See also specific agent*
Maculopathies, bull's-eye, hydroxychloroquine causing, 198
Magnetic resonance angiography (MRA), in cerebral ischemia/stroke, 103–104
Magnetic resonance fluoroscopy, in ischemic heart disease, 119
Magnetic resonance imaging (MRI)
   cardiac, in ischemic heart disease, 119
   in cerebral ischemia/stroke, 103–104
Magnetic source imaging (MSI), in epilepsy diagnosis, 282
Magnetoencephalography (MEG), in epilepsy diagnosis, 282
Major depression, 265
   drugs for (antidepressants), 274–276, 275*t*
      ocular effects of, 324*t*
   in elderly, 239
Major tranquilizer. *See* Antipsychotic drugs
Malar rash, in systemic lupus erythematosus, 179, 181*t*

Malignancy. *See* Cancer
Malignant hyperthermia, 336–337, 337t
    preoperative assessment of risk for, 329–330
Malingering, 266
Mammography, for cancer screening, 295t, 296
Mandol. *See* Cefamandole
Mania, 265
Manic depression. *See* Bipolar disorder
MAO inhibitors. *See* Monoamine oxidase inhibitors
Marax. *See* Theophylline
Marfan syndrome, 166
Marijuana use/abuse, 268t, 271
Mast cell stabilizers, for pulmonary diseases, 157t, 158
Mavik. *See* Trandolapril
Maxair. *See* Pirbuterol
Maxaquin. *See* Lomefloxacin
Maxipime. *See* Cefepime
Maxzide. *See* Triamterene
Maze procedure, 138
MB isoenzyme, in myocardial infarction, 117
MCTD. *See* Mixed connective tissue disease
MDMA (3,4-methylenedioxymethamphetamine/ecstasy), 270
MDRTB. *See* Multidrug resistant infections, tuberculosis
Measles-mumps-rubella (MMR) vaccine, 304t, 306
Measles virus, immunization against, 304t, 306
Measurement bias, outcome measures in clinical research and, 343
Measurement system, designing, 363–364
Mechlorethamine (nitrogen mustard), 258t
Meclofenamate, 197t
Meclomen. *See* Meclofenamate
Medullary carcinoma of thyroid gland, 227
    in multiple endocrine neoplasia, 230
Mefenamic acid, 197t
Mefoxin. *See* Cefoxitin
MEG. *See* Magnetoencephalography
Megaloblastic anemia, 161
Meglitinides, 213
Melanomas, 299
Melphalan, 258t
Memantine, for Alzheimer disease, 288
MEN. *See* Multiple endocrine neoplasia
Meningitis
    Haemophilus influenzae causing, 11, 12, 309
    meningococcal, 13
        immunization against, 13, 309
Meningococcemia, 13
Meningococcus *(Neisseria meningitidis)*, 12–13
    immunization against, 13, 309
Mental disorders due to general medical condition (organic mental syndromes), 264. *See also* Alzheimer disease; Behavioral/psychiatric disorders
    in elderly, 240
Mentax. *See* Butenafine
Meperidine, for postoperative pain, 338
Mepivacaine, maximum safe dose of, 322t
Mepron. *See* Atovaquone
6-Mercaptopurine, 258t
Meropenem, 60t, 69
Merrem. *See* Meropenem
Messenger RNA (mRNA), in antibiotic mechanism of action, 54
Meta-analyses, of clinical trials, 352

Metabolic disorders, screening for, 300–301
Metabolic syndrome, 95, 146, 148, 152t, 206
Metaglip. *See* Glipizide, with metformin
Metered-dose inhalers, β_2-adrenergics for pulmonary disease and, 157
Metformin, 212t, 213
Methadone maintenance, for heroin dependence, 269
Methamphetamine, abuse of, 270
Methicillin, 67
Methicillin-resistant *S aureus*, 5, 67, 71, 72
Methimazole, for Graves hyperthyroidism, 225
Methohexital, perioperative, 332t, 335
Methotrexate, 198, 258t
    in cancer chemotherapy, 258t
    for rheumatoid arthritis, 174
    for Wegener granulomatosis, 192
Methyldopa, 89t, 90t
3,4-Methylenedioxymethamphetamine (MDMA/ecstasy), 270
Metoclopramide, perioperative, 331, 332t, 338
Metolazone, 88t
Metoprolol
    for heart failure, 131
    for hypertension, 88t, 90t
Metronidazole, 62t, 74
    for *C difficile* colitis, 8
Mevacor. *See* Lovastatin
Mezlin. *See* Mezlocillin
Mezlocillin, 56t, 67
MH. *See* Malignant hyperthermia
MHA-TP (microhemagglutination assay for *T pallidum*), 17, 302
MI. *See* Myocardial infarction
Miacalcin. *See* Calcitonin/calcitonin nasal spray
MIC. *See* Minimal inhibitory concentration
Micafungin, 76
Micardis. *See* Telmisartan
Micatin. *See* Miconazole
Miconazole, 64t
Microadenoma, pituitary, 228
Microbiology, principles of, 3–4
Microcirculatory failure, in shock, 317
Microcytic anemia, 161
Microhemagglutination assay for *T pallidum* (MHA-TP), 17, 302
Micronase. *See* Glyburide
Microscopic polyangiitis (microscopic polyarteritis), 189t, 192
Microsporida (microsporidiosis), in HIV infection/AIDS, 48, 49
Microzide. *See* Hydrochlorothiazide
Midamor. *See* Amiloride
Midazolam, 273
    perioperative, 332t, 335
Miglitol, 212t, 213
Milrinone, for heart failure, 130–131
Minimal inhibitory concentration (MIC), 66–67
Minimal lethal concentration (MLC), 67
Minipress. *See* Prazosin
Minizide. *See* Prazosin
Minocin. *See* Minocycline
Minocycline, 61t
    ocular effects of, 324t
Minoxidil, for hypertension, 89t

Mirapex. *See* Pramipexole
Mitomycin/mitomycin-C, 257, 259*t*
Mixed connective tissue disease, 185
Mixed dementia, 285
MLC. *See* Minimal lethal concentration
MM isoenzyme, in myocardial infarction, 117
MMR vaccine, 304*t*, 306
MOABs. *See* Monoclonal antibodies
Mobitz type II atrioventricular block, 134
Moduretic. *See* Amiloride
Moexipril, 88*t*, 90*t*
Monistat. *See* Miconazole
Monitoring system, 364–366
Monoamine oxidase inhibitors, 275*t*, 276
 discontinuing before surgery, 334
 drug interactions and, 276
 hypertension and, 97, 276
Monobactams, 59*t*, 70
Monocid. *See* Cefonicid
Monoclonal antibodies, in cancer therapy, 261
Monocular transient visual loss, carotid artery disease and, 107
Mononucleosis, infectious, Epstein-Barr virus causing, 30
Monopril. *See* Fosinopril
Montelukast, 157*t*
Mood disorders (affective disorders), 265–266
 drugs for treatment of, 277
Morphine
 for diastolic dysfunction, 131
 for non-ST-segment elevation acute coronary syndrome, 122
 for postoperative pain, 338
Motor system disorders. *See also* Parkinson disease
 in schizophrenia, 264–265
Motrin. *See* Ibuprofen
Mouth-to-mouth resuscitation, 314
Mouth-to-nose resuscitation, 314
Movement disorders
 bradykinetic, 278. *See also* Parkinson disease/parkinsonism
 in schizophrenia, 264–265
Moxifloxacin, 62*t*, 73
6-MP. *See* 6-Mercaptopurine
MRI. *See* Magnetic resonance imaging
mRNA. *See* Messenger RNA
MRSA. *See* Methicillin-resistant *S aureus*
MSI. *See* Magnetic source imaging
MTX. *See* Methotrexate
Multidrug-resistant infections, tuberculosis (MDRTB), 24, 49
Multi-infarct dementia, 284
Multiple endocrine neoplasia, 230–231
Mumps virus, immunization against, 306
Mutation, carcinogenesis and, 252, 253
Mycelex. *See* Clotrimazole
Mycobacterium, 23–25
 avium, 49
 in HIV infection/AIDS, 23, 49–50
 kansasii, 49
 nontuberculous (atypical) infection caused by, 23, 49–50
 tuberculosis, 23–25. *See also* Tuberculosis
 screening/testing for, 23–24, 301–302

Mycophenolate mofetil, 200
Mycoplasma pneumoniae, 22
Mycostatin. *See* Nystatin
Mydriasis, seizures and, 283–284
Myeloid stem cells, 160
Myeloproliferative disorders, hypercoagulability and, 171
Mykrox. *See* Metolazone
Myocardial contractility, 129
 enhancement of in heart failure management, 130–131
 reduction of in angina management, 120–121
Myocardial infarction, 113–115. *See also* Acute coronary syndrome; Ischemic heart disease
 ECG changes in, 116
 heart failure and, 128
 hypertension management and, 91*t*
 management of, 122–125
 cardiac-specific troponins and, 117, 118*i*
 percutaneous coronary intervention for, 111
 pericarditis after (post-MI/Dressler syndrome), 115
 stroke and, 102
Myocardial oxygen requirements, reducing
 for acute coronary syndrome, 122
 for angina, 121
Myocardial scintigraphy, thallium-201, 119
Myoglobin, serum, in myocardial infarction, 117–118
Mysoline, 283*t*
Myxedema, 225, 226
 pretibial. *See* Infiltrative dermopathy
Myxedema coma, 226
Myxedema madness, 226

NAAT (nucleic acid amplification test). *See* Polymerase chain reaction
Nabumetone, 197*t*
Nadbath block, adverse reactions to, 336
Nadolol, 88*t*, 90*t*
Nafcillin, 55*t*, 67
Nalfon. *See* Fenoprofen
Nalidixic acid, 72–73
Naloxone, for narcotic reversal, 335
Namenda. *See* Memantine
Naprosyn. *See* Naproxen
Naproxen, 197*t*
 ocular effects of, 324*t*
Narrow complex tachycardias, 136
Nasal chondritis, in relapsing polychondritis, 187
Nasal CPAP, 156
Nasopharyngeal carcinoma, Epstein-Barr virus associated with, 30, 254
Nateglinide, 212*t*, 213
Nausea and vomiting, postoperative, management of, 338
Nebcin. *See* Tobramycin
Nedocromil, 157*t*
Needle stick, HIV transmission by, 39
 chemoprophylaxis for, 45, 46–47*t*
Nefazodone, 276
Negative predictive value (NPV), of screening/diagnostic test, 354
Neglect, elder, 236–237
Neisseria, 12–14
 gonorrhoeae (gonococcus), 13–14
 meningitidis (meningococcus), 12–13
 immunization against, 13, 309

Nelfinavir, 42
    for postexposure HIV prophylaxis, 46–47t
Neonates
    hemorrhagic disease of newborn in, 169
    herpes simplex infection in, 27
Neoral. See Cyclosporine
Nepafenac, 197
Nephritis, lupus, 179
Nephropathy
    diabetic, 217–218
    HIV-associated, 37–38
Nephrotoxicity, of aminoglycosides, 70
NES. See Nonepileptic seizures
Netilmicin, 61t, 70
Netromycin. See Netilmicin
Neuralgia, postherpetic, 28
Neurofibrillary tangles, in Alzheimer disease, 285, 286
Neuroimaging
    in Alzheimer disease, 287
    in epilepsy, 282
Neuroleptic malignant syndrome (NMS), 272
Neuroleptics. See Antipsychotic drugs
Neurologic disorders, 278–289. See also specific type
    Alzheimer disease/dementia, 284–289
    cerebrovascular disease, 101–109
    epilepsy, 280–284, 283t
    in Lyme disease, 19
    Parkinson disease, 278–280
    recent developments in, 263
    in systemic lupus erythematosus, 180, 181t, 182
Neurontin. See Gabapentin
Neuropathy
    diabetic, 218
    optic. See Optic neuropathy
Neurosyphilis
    treatment of, 18
    VDRL tests in, 16, 17t
Nevanac. See Nepafenac
Nevirapine, 41
    for HIV chemoprophylaxis during pregnancy, 45
Newborn, hemorrhagic disease of, 169
NFT. See Neurofibrillary tangles
Niacin (nicotinic acid)
    discontinuing before surgery, 334
    for hypercholesterolemia, 149t
Niaspan. See Nicotinic acid
Nicardipine
    for angina, 120
    for hypertension, 89t, 94
Nicotinic acid (niacin)
    discontinuing before surgery, 334
    for hypercholesterolemia, 149t
NIDDM. See Diabetes mellitus, type 2
Nifedipine
    for angina, 120
    contraindications to in non-ST-segment elevation acute coronary syndrome, 122–123
    for hypertension, 89t
Nisoldipine, 89t
Nitrates
    for angina, 120
    for diastolic dysfunction, 131
    for non-ST-segment elevation acute coronary syndrome, 122
Nitrogen mustard (mechlorethamine), 258t

Nitroglycerin
    for angina, 120
    for heart failure, 130
    for hypertensive emergency, 94
    for non-ST-segment elevation acute coronary syndrome, 122
Nitroprusside
    for heart failure, 130
    for hypertensive emergency, 94
Nitrosureas, in cancer chemotherapy, 260t
Nizoral. See Ketoconazole
NKHHC. See Nonketotic hyperglycemic-hyperosmolar coma
NMS. See Neuroleptic malignant syndrome
NNRTIs. See Non-nucleoside reverse transcriptase inhibitors
Nolvadex. See Tamoxifen
Noncompliance with therapy, behavioral/psychiatric disorders and, 277
Non-dihydropyridines, for hypertension, 89t, 93
Nonepileptic seizures, 281
Nonexperimental (observational) studies, 345
Non–insulin-dependent diabetes mellitus (NIDDM). See Diabetes mellitus, type 2
Noninvasive pressure support ventilation, 156
Nonketotic hyperglycemic-hyperosmolar coma, 216
Non-nucleoside reverse transcriptase inhibitors (NNRTIs), 41–42
Nonpeptide protease inhibitors, for HIV infection/AIDS, 42
Non–Q wave infarction, 114, 116. See also Acute coronary syndrome
    management of, 122–124
Non–Q wave, nontransmural infarction, 114, 116
Nonsteroidal anti-inflammatory drugs (NSAIDs), 196–198, 197t
    Alzheimer disease and, 288
    COX-1/COX-2 inhibition by, 196
    ocular side effects of, 197–198, 324t
    platelet function affected by, 168
    for rheumatic disorders, 196–198, 197t
    for rheumatoid arthritis, 174
Nontreponemal tests, for syphilis, 16–17, 302
Nontuberculous mycobacteria, 23
    in HIV infection/AIDS, 23
Norfloxacin, 62t, 73
Normal distribution, clinical relevance of research and, 344
Normodyne. See Labetalol
Noroxin. See Norfloxacin
North American Symptomatic Carotid Endarterectomy Trial, 108
Norvasc. See Amlodipine
Norvir. See Ritonavir
Nosocomial (hospital-acquired) infections, treatment of, 77–78
Novolog. See Aspart insulin
NPH insulin, 209, 209t
NPPIs. See Nonpeptide protease inhibitors
NPV. See Negative predictive value
NSAIDs. See Nonsteroidal anti-inflammatory drugs
NtRTIs. See Nucleotide reverse transcriptase inhibitors
Nucleic acid amplification test. See Polymerase chain reaction

Nucleoside analogues, for HIV infection/AIDS, 3, 41
    in HAART, 43
Nucleotide reverse transcriptase inhibitors (NtRTI), for
    HIV infection/AIDS, 41
Null-cell adenomas, 229
Null hypothesis, 342
Nystagmus, seizures causing, 284
Nystatin, 64t, 76

Obesity
    in diabetes mellitus type 2, 201, 202, 205
        weight reduction and, 201, 207, 208–209
    hypertension and, 85, 95
Observational studies, 345
Obstructive pulmonary disease, 143–144
    ocular surgery in patients with, 329
Obstructive shock, 317. See also Shock
Ocufen. See Flurbiprofen
Ocular adnexa
    radiation affecting, 255–256
    in systemic malignancies, 262
Ocular pharmacology, age/aging and, 235–236
Ocular (intraocular) surgery
    in elderly patients, 237–238
    perioperative management for, 327–338
        intraoperative complications and, 334t, 335–337
        medication management and, 332t
        postoperative care and, 337–338
        preoperative assessment/management and,
            327–335, 328t, 332t. See also Preoperative
            assessment/preparation for ocular surgery
Odds ratio, 361
"Off pump bypass surgery," 122
Ofloxacin, 62t, 73
OGTT. See Oral glucose tolerance test
Olanzapine, 271, 272
Older patients. See Age/aging; Geriatrics
Oligemic shock, 317. See also Shock
Oligosaccharide antibiotics, 75
Olmesartan, 88t
Omnicef. See Cefdinir
Omniflox. See Temafloxacin
Oncogenes/oncogenesis, 252
Oncovin. See Vincristine
Ondansetron, perioperative, 332t, 338
Online search, 340
Ophthalmopathy, thyroid (Graves/dysthyroid). See
    Thyroid ophthalmopathy
Opiates, abuse of, 268t, 269
Opportunistic infections, in HIV infection/AIDS,
    37–38. See also specific type
    treatment of, 45–51
Optic neuropathy
    in giant cell arteritis, 190
    radiation-induced, 256
    toxic, 271
OPV (Sabin vaccine), 304t, 307
Oral contraceptives
    hypercoagulability associated with, 171
    hypertension and, 96
    ocular effects of, 325t
Oral glucose tolerance test, 206, 207
Oral hypoglycemic agents, 211–214, 212t. See also
    specific type
    surgery in diabetic patient and, 220, 332

Oral ulcers
    in Behçet syndrome, 193
    in systemic lupus erythematosus, 179, 181t
Orbital pseudotumor, in Wegener granulomatosis, 192
Organic mental syndromes. See Mental disorders due to
    general medical condition
Orinase. See Tolbutamide
Orthostatic hypertension, 96
Orudis. See Ketoprofen
Oruvail. See Ketoprofen
Oseltamivir, 65t, 77, 291, 305
Osler-Weber-Rendu disease (hereditary hemorrhagic
    telangiectasia), 166
Osteoblasts, 241
Osteoclasts, 241
Osteocytes, 241
Osteogenesis imperfecta, bleeding disorders in, 166
Osteoid, 241
Osteopenia, definition of, 243
Osteoporosis, 240–247
    bone density levels in, 242–243
    bone physiology and, 241
    clinical features of, 242
    corticosteroid use and, 195
    definition of, 243
    diagnosis of, 242–244, 243t
    in men, 246–247
    risk factors for, 241, 242t
    testing for, 243–244
    treatment of, 244–246, 245t
Ototoxicity, of aminoglycosides, 70
Outcome/outcome measures, 362
    baseline probability of, 361
    in clinical research, 342
        case series and, 346–347
Outpatient visits, geriatric patient and, 236
Overlap syndromes (mixed connective tissue disease),
    185
Oxacarbazepine, 283t
Oxacillin, 67
Oxaprozin, 197t
Oxazolidinones, 63t, 74–75
Oxitropium, 157–158, 157t
Oxivent. See Oxitropium
Oxygen, reduction of myocardial requirements for
    for acute coronary syndrome, 122
    for angina, 121
Oxygen therapy
    for anaphylaxis, 319
    for pulmonary diseases, 156
    for shock, 318

p21, in carcinogenesis, 253
p24 antigen testing, in HIV infection/AIDS, 39
p53, in carcinogenesis, 253
P value, 344
p7 nucleocapsid zinc finger inhibitors, for HIV
    infection/AIDS, 42
Pacemakers, for heart failure, 132
Pacerone. See Amiodarone
Paclitaxel, 257, 259t
PACs. See Premature atrial complexes
Pain
    postoperative, management of, 338
    somatoform, 266

"Painless" (subacute lymphocytic) thyroiditis, 226
Pallidotomy, for Parkinson disease, 280
PAN. See Polyarteritis nodosa
Pancreas
  beta (β) cells in, in diabetes mellitus, 202
    genetic defects and, 204t
  cancer of, 297
  exocrine, disorders of in diabetes mellitus, 204t
  transplantation of, for diabetes, 214
Panic disorder, 267
Panipenem, 69
Papanicolaou test (Pap smear), for cancer screening, 294, 295t
  in HIV infection/AIDS, 41
Papillary carcinoma, of thyroid gland, 227
Papillomaviruses. See Human papillomaviruses
Parafollicular (C) cells, 221
Paranoia, in elderly, 239–240
Pareto chart, 368, 370i
Parkinson disease/parkinsonism, 278–280
  recent developments in, 263
Parlodel. See Bromocriptine
Paroxysmal atrial tachycardia, 136–137
Paroxysmal nocturnal hemoglobinuria, 162
  hypercoagulability and, 171
  screening test for, 159, 162
Partial seizures, 281, 320
Partial thromboplastin time (PTT), 165
Passive immunization, 303
PAT. See Paroxysmal atrial tachycardia
Pathergy, in Behçet syndrome, 193
Patient database, monitoring systems and, 364–365
Pauciarticular (oligoarticular) onset juvenile idiopathic arthritis, 178
PCI. See Percutaneous coronary intervention
PCP. See Pneumocystis carinii (Pneumocystis jiroveci) infections, pneumonia
PCR. See Polymerase chain reaction
PCV (pneumococcal vaccine), 291, 304t, 308
Peginterferon alfa-2a/peginterferon alfa-2b. See also Interferons
  for hepatitis C, 31
Pelvic examination, for cancer screening, 295t
Pen-Vee K. See Penicillin V
Penbutolol, 88t
Penetrex. See Enoxacin
Penicillin G, 55t, 67
Penicillin V (phenoxymethyl penicillin), 55t, 67
Penicillinase-resistant penicillins, 67
Penicillins, 54, 55–57t, 67–68. See also specific agent
  allergic reaction to, 67–68
  penicillinase-resistant, 67
  semisynthetic, 55–57t
  for syphilis, 17–18, 18t
Pentam 300. See Pentamidine
Pentamidine, 63t
  for Pneumocystis carinii (Pneumocystis jiroveci) pneumonia, 45
Pentavac. See DTacP-IPV-Hib vaccine
Penumbra, 102
Peptide fusion inhibitors, for HIV infection/AIDS, 42
Percutaneous coronary intervention (PCI), 111, 115
Percutaneous transluminal coronary angioplasty (PTCA/balloon angioplasty)
  for angina, 121
  for ST-segment elevation acute coronary syndrome, 125
  troponin levels in determining need for, 117
Perfusion-weighted magnetic resonance imaging, in cerebral ischemia/stroke, 104
Pergolide, for Parkinson disease, 279
Pericarditis, after myocardial infarction, 115
Perindopril, 88t
Peripheral airway disease, 154
Peripheral keratitis, in Wegener granulomatosis, 192
Peripheral vascular disease
  in diabetes, 216–217
  hypertension and, 96
Peripheral vascular resistance, reduction of in heart failure management, 130
Permax. See Pergolide
Pernicious anemia, 162
Personality disorders, 267
Petechiae, 166
Petit mal seizures, 282
Pharmacokinetics, age-related changes in, 235–236
Pharmacology, ocular, age/aging and, 235–236
Phenobarbital, for seizures, 283t
Phenoxymethyl penicillin. See Penicillin V
Phentolamine, for hypertension, 94
Phenylbutazone, 197t
Phenytoin, 283t, 284
Pheochromocytoma
  hypertension in, 83, 84t
  in multiple endocrine neoplasia, 230
Phosphodiesterase inhibitors, for heart failure, 130
Phospholipid antibody syndrome (antiphospholipid antibody syndrome), 171, 182–184
Photosensitivity, in systemic lupus erythematosus, 179, 181t
Physical drug dependence, 267
Physical examination, preoperative assessment and, 327, 328t
Pindolol, 88t
Pink puffers, 154
Pioglitazone, 212t, 213–214
Piperacillin, 56t, 67
  with tazobactam, 57t, 70
Pipracil. See Piperacillin
Pirbuterol, 157t
Piroxicam, 197t
  ocular effects of, 324t
Pituitary adenoma, 228–229
  MR imaging of, 229
Pituitary apoplexy, 229–230
Pituitary hormones, hypothalamic hormones and, 227–230, 229t
PJCs. See Premature junctional complexes
Plant alkaloids, in cancer chemotherapy, 257, 259t
Plaquenil. See Hydroxychloroquine
Plasma, 159
Plasmid resistance, 66
Plasminogen activator, tissue. See Tissue plasminogen activator
Platelet count, 165

Platelet glycoprotein IIb/IIIa receptor antagonists. *See* Glycoprotein IIb/IIIa receptor antagonists
Platelets, 159
 disorders of, 166–168
  drugs causing, 167–168, 331–332
  of function, 167–168
  of number, 167
 in hemostasis, 164
Platinol. *See* Cisplatin
Plavix. *See* Clopidogrel
Plendil. *See* Felodipine
Plurihormonal adenomas, 229
Pluripotential stem cells, 160
PMPA. *See* Tenofovir
Pneumocandins, 76
 for *Pneumocystis carinii (Pneumocystis jiroveci)* pneumonia, 47
Pneumococcal vaccine, 291, 304t, 308
Pneumococcus. *See* Streptococcus, pneumoniae
Pneumocystis carinii (Pneumocystis jiroveci) infections, 45
 in HIV infection/AIDS, 45–47
 pneumonia, 45–47
Pneumonia
 in HIV infection/AIDS, 45–47
 pneumococcal, 6–7, 308
  immunization against, 291, 304t, 308
Podophyllin/podophyllotoxins, in cancer chemotherapy, 257, 259t
Poker spine, in ankylosing spondylitis, 176
Polio, immunization against, 307
Polyangiitis, microscopic, 189t, 192
Polyarteritis nodosa, 189t, 191–192
Polyarthritis
 in Behçet syndrome, 193
 in systemic lupus erythematosus, 179, 181t
Polyarticular onset juvenile idiopathic arthritis, 178–179
Polychondritis, relapsing, 187–188
Polycillin. *See* Ampicillin
Polycystic kidney disease, hypertension in, 83, 84t
Polymerase chain reaction (PCR)
 in *Chlamydia trachomatis* infection, 22
 in *Haemophilus influenzae* infection, 11
 in herpes simplex infection, 27
 for HIV RNA, 43
 in infection diagnosis, 3
 in Lyme disease, 20
 in toxoplasmosis, 26
 in tuberculosis, 23, 302
Polymyalgia rheumatica, 190
Polymyositis, 186–187
Polymyxin, 54
Polyps, colorectal cancer and, 297–298
Polysaccharide encapsulation, as microbial virulence factor, 4
Polythiazide, 88t
Ponstel. *See* Mefenamic acid
Population, measurement systems and, 364
Posaconazole, 76
Positive predictive value (PPV), of screening/diagnostic test, 354
Positron emission tomography (PET), in ischemic heart disease, 119
Post-traumatic stress disorder (PTSD), 267

Postexposure prophylaxis
 hepatitis B, 305
 HIV, 45, 46–47t
 measles, 306
Postherpetic neuralgia, 28
Postictal paralysis (Todd's paralysis), 282
Postictal period, 282
Post-MI syndrome, 115
Postoperative care of ophthalmic surgery patient, 337–338
Postoperative chest physiotherapy, 156
Postoperative state, hypercoagulability and, 171
Postpartum thyroiditis, 227
Poststroke dementia, 285
Posttest probability, 358
Posttransfusion hepatitis, transfusion-transmitted virus (TTV) causing, 32
Posttransfusion isoantibody production, 167
Postural hypertension, 96
Potassium-sparing diuretics, 87, 88t
PPD test. *See* Purified protein derivative (PPD) test
PPV. *See* Positive predictive value
Pramipexole, for Parkinson disease, 279
Pramlintide, for diabetes, 214
Prandin. *See* Repaglinide
Pravachol. *See* Pravastatin
Pravastatin, for hypercholesterolemia, 149t, 150t
Prazosin
 for heart failure, 130
 for hypertension, 89t
Precose. *See* Acarbose
Prediabetic states, 206
Prednisone
 for giant cell arteritis, 190
 for rheumatoid arthritis, 174–175
Preeclampsia, 96
Pregnancy
 alcohol use during, 270
 antiphospholipid antibody syndrome and, 171, 182, 183, 184
 cocaine abuse during, 271
 cytomegalovirus infection during, 29
 diabetes during (gestational diabetes mellitus), 203t, 205t, 206
 herpes simplex virus infection during, 27
 HIV during, chemoprophylaxis and, 45
 hypertension/hypertension management and, 96–97
 immunization during, 303, 305, 307
 phenytoin use during, 284
 radiation exposure during, 255
 syphilis during, 15
 thyroiditis after, 227
 toxoplasmosis during, 26
Prehypertension, 81, 82, 82t, 292
 in children and adolescents, 97
Preload, 129
 manipulation of in heart failure, 130, 131
Premature atrial complexes, 135
Premature contractions, 135–136
Premature junctional complexes, 135
Premature ventricular complexes, 135–136
Preoperative assessment/preparation for ocular surgery, 327–335, 328t, 332t
 in adults, 327–328, 328t
 in elderly patients, 237

fasting and, 331
  medication management and, 331–334, 332t
  in pediatric patients, 328–329
  sedation and, 335
  specific concerns and, 329–331
  testing recommendations and, 327–328
Pretest probability, 357–359, 358t
Pretibial myxedema. *See* Infiltrative dermopathy
Preventive medicine, 291–311
  immunization in, 302–311
  recent developments in, 291
  screening procedures in, 291–302. *See also* Screening/diagnostic tests
Preveon. *See* Adefovir
Prevnar. *See* Pneumococcal vaccine
Primacor. *See* Milrinone
Primaquine, for *Pneumocystis carinii (Pneumocystis jiroveci)* pneumonia, 45
Primary antiphospholipid antibody syndrome, 182
Primary HIV infection (retroviral syndrome), 38
Primaxin. *See* Imipenem-cilastin
Prinivil. *See* Lisinopril
Prinzide. *See* Lisinopril
Prinzmetal (variant) angina, 113
Probability of outcome, baseline, 361
Procaine penicillin, 55t
Procardia. *See* Nifedipine
Process (content of care), 362
Progressive systemic sclerosis (scleroderma), 185–186
Prolactinomas (lactotroph adenomas), 228
Prolixin. *See* Fluphenazine
Propofol, perioperative, 332t, 335
Propranolol, 88t, 90t
Propulsid. *See* Cisapride
Propylthiouracil, for Graves hyperthyroidism, 225
Prosom. *See* Estazolam
Prostate cancer, 296
  screening for, 296
Prostate-specific antigen, in cancer screening, 296
Protease inhibitors, 3, 42
  antituberculous drug interactions and, 49
  in HAART, 43
Protease-sparing regimen, in HAART, 43
Protein C (activated protein C), 164, 165
  deficiency of/resistance to, 170
Protein kinase C, diabetes complications and, 217
Protein kinase C inhibitors, in diabetes management, 201, 217
Protein S, 164, 165
  deficiency of, 170
Proteinase-3, scleritis/retinal vasculitis in Wegener granulomatosis and, 192
Prothrombin, mutation in gene for, 170
Prothrombin time (PT), 165
  international normalized ratio and, 165
Protozoal infection, gastrointestinal, in HIV infection/AIDS, 48–49
Proventil. *See* Albuterol
Prozac. *See* Fluoxetine
PSA. *See* Prostate-specific antigen
Pseudodementia, in elderly, 240
Pseudomembranous enterocolitis, *Clostridium difficile* causing, 8
Pseudomonas aeruginosa, 14–15
Pseudotumor, orbital, in Wegener granulomatosis, 192

Pseudoxanthoma elasticum, 166
Psoriasis/psoriatic arthritis, 178
Psychiatric disorders. *See* Behavioral/psychiatric disorders
Psychic drug dependence, 267
Psychomotor seizures, 281
Psychotic disorder. *See also* Schizophrenia
  brief, 265
PT. *See* Prothrombin time
PTCA. *See* Percutaneous transluminal coronary angioplasty
PTSD. *See* Post-traumatic stress disorder
PTT. *See* Partial thromboplastin time
Pulmicort. *See* Budesonide
Pulmonary diseases, 153–158
  evaluation of, 155
  obstructive, 153–154
    ocular surgery in patients with, 329
  preoperative and postoperative considerations in patient with, 158
  recent developments in, 153
  restrictive, 154
  treatment of, 155–158, 157t
Pulmonary function tests, 155
Pulse pressure, in shock, 318
Pulseless disease (Takayasu arteritis), 189t, 191
Purified protein derivative (PPD) test, 23–24. *See also* Tuberculin skin test
Purine antagonists, in cancer chemotherapy, 258t
Purpura, 166
  Henoch-Schönlein, 189t
  idiopathic thrombocytopenic, 167
  thrombotic thrombocytopenic, 167
PVCs. *See* Premature ventricular complexes
Pyrimidine antagonists
  in cancer chemotherapy, 258t
  for rheumatic disorders, 199

Q/D. *See* Quinupristin/dalfopristin
Q wave infarction, 114, 116. *See also* Acute coronary syndrome
  management of, 124–125
Q waves, in myocardial infarction, 114, 116
QCT. *See* Dual-energy quantitative computed tomography
Quality improvement, continuous, 370, 371i
Quetiapine, 272
Quibron. *See* Theophylline
Quinapril, 88t, 90t
Quinolones, 54, 62t, 72–73. *See also* specific agent
Quinupristin/dalfopristin, 63t, 74

RA. *See* Rheumatoid arthritis
Rabies vaccination, 310
Race
  cancer and, 252, 253, 254
  hypertension and, 97
rad (R/roentgen), radiation dose measurement, 255
Radiation
  in cancer therapy, 255–256
  carcinogenic effects of, 253
  eye and adnexa affected by, 255–256
  fetal exposure and, 255
Radiation optic neuropathy, 256
Radiation retinopathy, 256

Radiation therapy, 255–256
Radioactive iodine
    for thyroid (Graves) ophthalmopathy, 225
    for thyroid scanning, 223
Radioactive iodine uptake, 223
Radiofrequency catheter ablation, for atrial fibrillation/flutter, 138
Radiography, chest, in pulmonary diseases, 155
Radionuclide scintigraphy/scans, in ischemic heart disease, 119
RAIU. *See* Radioactive iodine uptake
Raloxifene, for osteoporosis, 245t, 246
Ramipril
    for heart failure, 130
    for hypertension, 88t
    for non-ST-segment elevation acute coronary syndrome, 123
Ranbezolid, 75
Randomization, in clinical trials, 351, 351i
Ranitidine, preoperative, 331
Rapid plasma reagin (RPR) test, 16–17, 302
Ravuconazole, 76
Raynaud phenomenon
    in scleroderma, 185
    in systemic lupus erythematosus, 179, 180i
RBBB. *See* Right bundle branch block
RBCs. *See* Red blood cells
Reactive arthritis (Reiter syndrome), 176–177
Rebound hypertension, 97–98
Recall bias, 349
Receiver operating characteristics (ROC) curve, 355, 356i, 357, 357i
Recombinant tissue plasminogen activator. *See* Tissue plasminogen activator
Recombivax HB. *See* Hepatitis B vaccine
Rectal examination, in cancer screening, 295t
Red blood cells, 159
    development of, 160
Regional enteritis (Crohn disease), 177
Reglan. *See* Metoclopramide
Regular insulin, 209, 209t
Reiter syndrome (reactive arthritis), 176–177
Relafen. *See* Nabumetone
Relapsing polychondritis, 187–188
Relative risk/risk ratio (RR), 292, 360–361
Relenza. *See* Zanamivir
Reliability, 363
Remicade. *See* Infliximab
Reminyl. *See* Galantamine
Renal disease
    hypertension management and, 91t, 95
    in scleroderma, 185
    in systemic lupus erythematosus, 179, 181t
Renese. *See* Polythiazide
Renin-angiotensin-aldosterone system, in hypertension, 83, 83i
Renovascular hypertension, 83, 84t
ReoPro. *See* Abciximab
Repaglinide, 212t, 213
Reperfusion
    for angina, 121–122
    for ST-segment elevation acute coronary syndrome, 124–125
Reproducibility, 363
Requip. *See* Ropinirole
Rescriptor. *See* Delavirdine

Rescue breathing, 314
Research studies. *See* Clinical research/studies
Reserpine, 89t, 90t
Resistance (drug). *See also specific agent and specific organism*
    antibiotic, 3, 66
        new drug classes and, 74–75
    antiretroviral, 41, 43, 44
Respbid. *See* Theophylline
Respimat. *See* Fenoterol, with ipratropium
Respiratory disorders. *See* Pulmonary diseases
Restoril. *See* Temazepam
Restrictive pulmonary diseases, 154
Resuscitation (cardiopulmonary), 313–317
    medications used in, 316t
    for ventricular fibrillation, 140
Retavase. *See* Reteplase
Reteplase, for ST-segment elevation acute coronary syndrome, 124
Retina
    arteriovenous anastomoses in, in Takayasu arteritis, 191
    in systemic lupus erythematosus, 182
Retinal disease, vascular
    antiphospholipid antibody syndrome and, 184
    systemic hypertension and, 98–99, 98t
Retinal toxicity, hydroxychloroquine, 198
Retinal vasculitis, in Behçet syndrome, 194
Retinitis, cytomegalovirus, 3, 29
    cidofovir for, 29, 48
    fomivirsen for, 48
    foscarnet for, 29, 48
    ganciclovir for, 29
    in HIV infection/AIDS, 3, 29, 47–48
Retinopathy
    in antiphospholipid antibody syndrome, 184
    hydroxychloroquine causing, 198
    hypertensive, 98–99, 98t
    radiation, 256
    in scleroderma, 186
Retrobulbar anesthesia, adverse reactions to, 322, 323, 335–336
Retrovir. *See* Zidovudine
Retroviral syndrome (primary HIV infection), 38. *See also* HIV infection/AIDS
Retroviruses
    cancer association of, 254
    HIV as, 37
Revascularization procedures. *See also* Coronary artery bypass graft; Percutaneous transluminal coronary angioplasty
    for angina, 121–122
    for ST-segment elevation acute coronary syndrome, 125
Reverse transcriptase, 37
    viral carcinogenesis and, 254
Reverse transcriptase inhibitors, 41
    in HAART, 43
Reyataz. *See* Atazanavir
Rezulin. *See* Troglitazone
Rheumatic disorders, 173–200. *See also specific type*
    medical therapy for, 194–200, 197t
    recent developments in, 173
Rheumatoid arthritis, 173–175
Rheumatoid factor, 174
Rheumatoid nodules, 174

Ribavirin, 65t
　for hepatitis C, 31
Rifabutin, 49
　protease inhibitor interactions and, 49
Rifadin. See Rifampin
Rifampicin, protease inhibitor interactions and, 49
Rifampin, 24, 49, 54, 63t, 73
　ocular effects of, 324t
Right bundle branch block, 135
Rimantadine, 65t, 77
Risedronate, for osteoporosis, 245t
Risk, relative, 292, 360–361
Risk difference, 360–361
Risk factor, 361. *See also specific disorder*
　in cross-sectional studies, 349–350
　pretest probability of disease and, 357–359, 358i
Risperdal. See Risperidone
Risperidone, 271
Ritipenem, 69
Ritonavir, 42
　for postexposure HIV prophylaxis, 45, 46–47t
Rivastigmine, for Alzheimer disease, 288
RNA viruses, cancer association of, 254
ROC (receiver operating characteristics) curve, 355, 356i, 357, 357i
Rocephin. See Ceftriaxone
Rofecoxib, removal of from market, 173, 196
Roferon-A. See Interferons (IFNs), α
Rohypnol. See Flunitrazepam
Rokitamycin, 75
Ropinirole, for Parkinson disease, 279
Rosiglitazone, 212t, 213–214
　with metformin, 213
Rosuvastatin, for hypercholesterolemia, 149t, 150t
Roxithromycin, 60t, 71
RPR (rapid plasma reagin) test, 16–17, 302
Rubella, immunization against, 306–307
Rufen. See Ibuprofen
Run diagrams, 368, 371i

S-3578, 68
SA node. See Sinoatrial (SA) node
SAARDs. See Slow-acting (disease-modifying) antirheumatic drugs
Sabin vaccine (OPV), 304t, 307
Sabril. See Vigabatrin
Saccades/saccadic system, dysfunction of, in Alzheimer disease, 288
Saccular (berry) aneurysm, 105–106
Salicylates, 197t. *See also Nonsteroidal anti-inflammatory drugs*
Salk vaccine (IPV), 304t, 307
　in combination vaccines, 309
Salmeterol, 157, 157t
Salsalate, 197t
Sample size/sampling, 342, 365, 366
Sandimmune. See Cyclosporine
Saquinavir, 42
　for postexposure HIV prophylaxis, 46–47t
SARS. See Severe acute respiratory syndrome
SBE (subacute bacterial endocarditis). See Endocarditis
Scatter diagram, 368, 369i
SCD. See Sudden cardiac death
Schizoaffective disorder, 265
Schizophrenia, 264–265
　drugs for (antipsychotic drugs), 271–273, 272t

Schizophreniform disorder, 265
Scientific studies. See Clinical research/studies
Scleritis, in Wegener granulomatosis, 192
Scleroderma, 185–186
Scleroderma renal crisis (scleroderma kidney), 185
Screening/diagnostic tests, 291–302. *See also specific test or disorder*
　interpretation of, 353–360, 353i, 354i
　　clinical acceptance and, 359
　　combination strategies and, 359
　　continuous outcome and, 355, 356i
　　criteria for diagnosis and, 355–357, 357i
　　generalizability and, 359
　　pretest probability and, 357–359, 358t
Scurvy (vitamin C deficiency), 166
Sectral. See Acebutolol
Sedative-hypnotics/sedation, 273–277, 274t
　abuse and, 269
　preoperative, 335
Seizures, 280–284, 320–321
　local anesthetics causing, 336
　nonepileptic, 281
Selection bias, 341
　in case-control studies, 349
　in case series, 346
Selective estrogen receptor modulators, for osteoporosis, 246
Selective serotonin reuptake inhibitors, 275–276, 275t
Selegiline, for Parkinson disease, 279
Self–blood-glucose monitoring, 215–216
Self-examination, breast, for cancer screening, 295t
Sensitivity, of screening/diagnostic test, 292, 354
　continuous outcome and, 355, 356i
　likelihood ratio calculation and, 358
Septra. See Trimethoprim-sulfamethoxazole
Ser-Ap-Es. See Reserpine
Serevent. See Salmeterol
Seroepidemiology, of HIV infection/AIDS, 39
Seronegative spondyloarthropathies, 175–179. *See also specific type*
Seroquel. See Quetiapine
Serositis, in systemic lupus erythematosus, 181t
Serotonin, antipsychotic mechanism of action and, 271
Serotonin reuptake inhibitors, selective, 274–276, 275t
Serpasil. See Reserpine
Sertaconazole, 76
Serum, 159
Serzone. See Nefazodone
Severe acute respiratory syndrome (SARS), 33–35
Shingles. See Herpes zoster
Shock, 317–320. *See also specific type*
　assessment of, 318
　classification of, 317–318
　treatment of, 318–319
Sickle cell disease (sickle cell anemia), 163
　genetic testing for, 159, 163
Sideroblastic anemia, 162
Sigmoidoscopy, in cancer screening, 295t, 298
Significance, statistical, 366–367
Sildenafil, visual changes caused by, 324, 325t
Simultanagnosia, in Alzheimer disease, 288
Simvastatin, for hypercholesterolemia, 149t, 150t
Sinemet. See Levodopa/carbidopa
Single-photon emission computed tomography (SPECT), in ischemic heart disease, 119, 294
Singulair. See Montelukast

Sinoatrial (SA) node, 133
Sinus arrest (sinus block/SA block), 133
Sinus bradycardia, 133
Sinus tachycardia, 136
Sitagliptin, 212t, 214
Sjögren syndrome, 186, 187t
Skin disorders
   in Behçet syndrome, 193
   in dermatomyositis, 186, 187, 188i
   in scleroderma, 185
   in systemic lupus erythematosus, 179, 181t, 182
Skin tests, tuberculin, 23–25, 301–302
SLE. *See* Systemic lupus erythematosus
Sleep disorders, hypertension and, 95
Slo-Phyllin. *See* Theophylline
Slow-acting (disease-modifying) antirheumatic drugs, 174
Slow-channel calcium-blocking agents, for angina, 120–121
Smoking
   cancer and, 252, 296, 297
   cessation of, 155–156
   heart disease and, 111
   hypertension and, 85
   thyroid disease and, 201, 225
Sodium, dietary
   congestive heart failure and, 127
   hypertension and, 85, 87t
Sodium bicarbonate. *See* Bicarbonate
Sodium ferric gluconate, 159, 161
Solu-Cortef. *See* Hydrocortisone sodium succinate
Somatization disorder, 266
Somatoform disorders, 266
Somatoform pain disorder, 266
Somatotroph adenomas, 228
Somogyi phenomenon, 210
Sonata. *See* Zaleplon
Sordarins, for *Pneumocystis carinii (Pneumocystis jiroveci)* pneumonia, 47
Sparfloxacin, 62t, 73
Specificity, of screening/diagnostic test, 292, 354
   continuous outcome and, 355, 356i
   likelihood ratio calculation and, 358
SPECT. *See* Single-photon emission computed tomography
Spectracef. *See* Cefditoren
Spherocytosis, hereditary, 162
Spiramycin, 60t, 71
Spironolactone, 88t, 90t
Spondylitis, ankylosing, 175–176
   juvenile, 178
Spondyloarthropathies, 175–179. *See also specific type*
   juvenile, 178
   undifferentiated, 175
Sporadic Alzheimer disease, 286
Sporanox. *See* Itraconazole
Spore-forming intestinal protozoa, gastrointestinal infection in HIV/AIDS and, 48–49
Sputum cytology, in cancer screening, 295t, 296
SSA antigen, antibodies to (anti-Ro antibodies), in Sjögren syndrome, 186, 187t
SSB antigen, antibodies to (anti-La antibodies), in Sjögren syndrome, 186, 187t
SSRIs. *See* Selective serotonin reuptake inhibitors
ST-segment changes, in ischemic heart disease, 113, 114, 116
   management of acute coronary syndrome and, 122–125

Stable angina pectoris, 113
   management of, 120–122
   risk stratification for, 121t
Staphylococcus, 5–6
   aureus, 5
   endocarditis prophylaxis and, 7, 8–11t
   epidermidis, 5–6
   resistant strains of, 5, 71
Starlix. *See* Nateglinide
Statins
   age-related macular degeneration and, 143, 150–151, 349
   Alzheimer disease prevention and, 288
   cataracts and, 151
   heart disease prevention and, 111, 143, 148
   for hypercholesterolemia, 146, 149t, 150t
   stroke prevention and, 101
Statistics, 339–372
   clinical practice applications and, 362–370
      data presentation and, 368–370, 369i, 370i, 371i
      measurement system design and, 363–364
      monitoring system implementation and, 364–366
      quality improvement and, 370, 371i
      results analysis and, 366–368
   evaluation of research studies and, 339–344
      clinical relevance and, 344
      intervention issues and, 342
      outcome issues and, 342–343
      participants and setting and, 341
      sample size and, 342
      validity and, 343, 363
   interpreting results of studies for patients and, 360–362
   study designs and, 345–360, 345i
Status epilepticus, 320–321
Stavudine (d4T), 41
   for postexposure HIV prophylaxis, 46–47t
Stem cells, blood cell formation and, 160
Stent placement, with PTCA
   for angina, 121
   in myocardial infarction management, 111, 115, 125
Steroids. *See* Corticosteroids
Still disease (systemic onset juvenile idiopathic arthritis), 178–179
Stokes-Adams syndrome, 134
Stomach cancer, 252
Stool guaiac slide test, in cancer screening, 295t, 298
Strabismus, screening tests in diagnosis of, 353–354, 353i, 354i
Streptococcus, 6–7
   α-hemolytic, endocarditis prophylaxis and, 7, 8–11t
   pneumoniae (pneumococcus), 6–7, 308
      immunization against, 291, 304t, 308
   pyogenes (group A β-hemolytic), 6
Streptogramins, 63t, 74
Streptokinase, 172
   for ST-segment elevation acute coronary syndrome, 124
   for stroke, 104
Streptomycin, 49, 61t, 70
Stress (exercise) tests, in ischemic heart disease, 119
   echocardiography, 118
Stroke
   carotid artery disease and, 107–109
   completed, 102
   dementia after, 285

in diabetes, 218
diagnosis of, 103–104
evolving, 102
hemorrhagic, 105–106
hypertension management in prevention of, 91t, 95, 104
incidence of, 101
ischemic, 101–105
risk factors for, 103
treatment of, 104–105
  emergency transport and, 313
  recent developments in, 101
Stroke scale, 103
Structure, care system, 362
Student t test, 344
Subacute bacterial endocarditis. See Endocarditis
Subacute granulomatous thyroiditis, 226
Subacute lymphocytic ("painless") thyroiditis, 226
Subarachnoid hemorrhage, 105, 106
Subcutaneous nodules, in rheumatoid arthritis, 174
Subendocardial (non–Q wave, nontransmural) infarction, 114, 116
Sublimaze. See Fentanyl
Substance abuse disorders, 267–271, 268t. See also specific substance
  ocular trauma and, 271
Substantia nigra, in Parkinson disease, 278
Sudden cardiac death, 115–116
  ventricular fibrillation and, 140
Sufenta. See Sufentanil
Sufentanil, perioperative, 332t, 338
Suicide, SSRI use and, 276
Sular. See Nisoldipine
Sulbactam, 69–70. See also specific antibiotic combination
Sulfasalazine, 174, 199
Sulfisoxazole, 55t
Sulfonamides, 54, 55t. See also specific agent
Sulfonylureas, 211–213
Sulindac, 197t
Supraventricular tachycardias, 136–138
Suprax. See Cefixime
Surface dyslexia, in Alzheimer disease, 288
Surgery. See also specific procedure
  in diabetic patients, 220–221, 332–333
  in elderly patients, 237–238
  ocular. See Ocular surgery
  in patients with pulmonary disease, 329
Susceptibility testing, antimicrobial, 66–67
Sustiva. See Efavirenz
Symadine. See Amantadine
Symlin. See Pramlintide
Symmetrel. See Amantadine
Sympatholytics, for hypertension, 94
Sympathomimetic activity, intrinsic, beta-blocker, 92
Synercid. See Quinupristin/dalfopristin
Synergistins, 74. See also Streptogramins
Syphilis, 15–18
  congenital/intrauterine, 15, 302
  in HIV infection/AIDS, 18
  screening/testing for, 16–17, 17t, 302
Systemic lupus erythematosus, 179–182, 180i, 181t
Systemic sclerosis, progressive (scleroderma), 185–186
Systole (systolic phase), 128

Systolic dysfunction, 129
  causes of, 128
  management of, 130–131

T_3. See Triiodothyronine
T_4. See Thyroxine
T4/T8 ratio, in HIV infection/AIDS, 37
T-20. See Enfuvirtide
T-1249, 42
T cells (T lymphocytes), 4
  in HIV infection/AIDS, 37, 40
TPA. See Tissue plasminogen activator
T pallidum hemagglutination assay (TPHA), 17
T score, in osteoporosis, 243
t tests, 344
T waves, in myocardial infarction, 116
Tachyarrhythmias, 136–140
  heart failure and, 131–132
  supraventricular, 136–138
  ventricular, 138–140
Tachycardia
  junctional, 137
  narrow-complex, 136
  sinus, 136
  supraventricular, 136–138
  ventricular, 138–139
  wide-complex, 138
Tadalafil, ocular effects of, 325t
Takayasu arteritis (aortic arch arteritis/aortitis syndrome/pulseless disease), 189t, 191
Tambocor. See Flecainide
Tamiflu. See Oseltamivir
Tamoxifen, 260t
  ocular effects of, 325t
Tapazole. See Methimazole
Targocid. See Teicoplanin
Tarka. See Verapamil
Tasmar. See Tolcapone
Tau proteins, in Alzheimer disease, 286
Taxol. See Paclitaxel
Tazicef. See Ceftazidime
Tazidime. See Ceftazidime
Tazobactam, 69–70. See also specific antibiotic combination
TBG. See Thyroxine-binding globulin
3TC. See Lamivudine
Tc-99. See under Technetium-99
Td vaccine, 304t, 307
Technetium-99 pyrophosphate scintigraphy, in ischemic heart disease, 119
Technetium-99m Sestamibi scintigraphy, in ischemic heart disease, 119
Teczem. See Diltiazem
Tegopen. See Cloxacillin
Tegretol. See Carbamazepine
Teicoplanin, 61t, 72
Telangiectasias
  capillary, 106
  hereditary hemorrhagic (Osler-Weber-Rendu disease), 166
  in scleroderma, 185
Telithromycin, 60t, 71, 75
Telmisartan, 88t, 90t
Telzir. See Fosamprenavir

Temafloxacin, 62t, 73
Temazepam, 273
Temporal (giant cell) arteritis. See Arteritis, giant cell
Temporal lobe resection, for seizures, 283
Temporal lobe seizures, 281
Temporin A/temporin B, 75
Tenex. See Guanfacine
Teniposide, 257, 259t
Tenofovir (PMPA), 41
Tenoretic. See Atenolol
Tenormin. See Atenolol
Tensilon. See Edrophonium
Tequin. See Gatifloxacin
Terazosin, 89t
Terbinafine, 64t, 76
Terbutaline, 157, 157t
Test–retest reliability, 363
Testicular cancer, screening for, 296
Tetanus, immunization against, 307–308
Tetanus and diphtheria toxoid vaccine (Td vaccine), 304t, 307
Tetanus immune globulin, 308
Tetracaine, maximum safe dose of, 322t
Tetracyclines, 61t, 72. See also specific agent
 ocular effects of, 324t
Tetravac. See DTacP-IPV vaccine
Teveten. See Eprosartan
Thalassemia, 161
 β, bone marrow transplantation for, 159, 161
Thalidomide, for HIV infection/AIDS, 44
Thallium-201 myocardial scintigraphy, 119
Theo-Dur. See Theophylline
Theophylline, 156–157, 157t
Therapeutic lifestyle changes (TLCs). See Lifestyle modification
Thiamine deficiency, Wernicke-Korsakoff syndrome and, 285
Thiazide diuretics
 for diastolic dysfunction, 131
 for hypertension, 81, 86, 87, 88t, 89
 ocular effects of, 325t
Thiazolidinediones, 212t, 213–214
Thorazine. See Chlorpromazine
Thrombocytopenia, 167
Thrombocytopenic purpura
 idiopathic, 167
 thrombotic, 167
Thrombolytic therapy, 172
 for acute ischemic stroke, 104–105
  emergency transport and, 313
 for ST-segment elevation acute coronary syndrome, 124–125
Thrombophilia (thrombotic disorders), 170–172. See also Hypercoagulable states
 antiphospholipid antibody syndrome and, 171, 182–184
 fetal loss/preeclampsia and, 159
 risk factors for, 159
Thromboplastin time, partial (PTT), 165
Thrombosis. See also Hypercoagulable states; Thrombophilia
 after PTCA with stenting, 121
 stroke and, 102

Thrombotic thrombocytopenic purpura, 167
Thyroid biopsy, 223
Thyroid disease, 221–227
 in elderly, 249
 hyperthyroidism, 223–225
 hypothyroidism, 225–226
 physiology of, 221
 screening/testing for, 222–223, 301
 smoking and, 201, 225
 thyroiditis, 226–227
 tumors, 227
Thyroid follicles, 221
Thyroid hormones, 221
 adenomas producing, 228
 measurement of, 222
Thyroid medications, in perioperative setting, 334
Thyroid microsomal antibody, testing for, 223
Thyroid nodules, 227
Thyroid ophthalmopathy (Graves ophthalmopathy, dysthyroidism, thyroid orbitopathy), 224–225
 antithyroid antibodies and, 223
 in elderly, 249
 euthyroid, 224–225
 smoking and, 201, 225
Thyroid scanning, 223
 in identification of thyroid tumors, 227
Thyroid-stimulating hormone. See Thyrotropin
Thyroid storm, 224
Thyroid tumors, 227
Thyroid ultrasound, 223
Thyroiditis, 226–227. See also specific type
Thyrotoxicosis. See Hyperthyroidism
Thyrotropin (thyroid-stimulating hormone/TSH), 221
 pituitary adenoma producing, 228
 serum levels of, 222–223
Thyrotropin-releasing hormone, 221
Thyroxine-binding globulin (TBG), serum levels of, 222, 223
 screening, 301
Thyroxine (T_4), 221
 serum levels of, 222
Tiagabine, 283t
TIAs. See Transient ischemic attacks
Tiazac. See Diltiazem
Ticar. See Ticarcillin
Ticarcillin, 56t, 67
 with clavulanic acid, 56t, 69
Ticks, Lyme disease transmitted by, 18–19
Ticlid. See Ticlopidine
Ticlopidine
 for carotid disease, 107
 for cerebral ischemia/stroke, 104
Tigecycline, 75
Tilade. See Nedocromil
Timentin. See Ticarcillin, with clavulanic acid
Timolide. See Timolol
Timolol
 cholesterol levels affected by, 150
 for hypertension, 88t, 90t
Tiotropiuim, 158
Tiprinavir, 42
Tirofiban, for non-ST-segment elevation acute coronary syndrome, 123

Tissue factor pathway inhibitor, 164, 165
Tissue plasminogen activator, 101, 172
    for acute ischemic stroke, 101, 104
    for ST-segment elevation acute coronary syndrome, 124–125
TLCs (therapeutic lifestyle changes). See Lifestyle modification
TMAb. See Thyroid microsomal antibody
TMC 125, 42
TMP-SMX. See Trimethoprim-sulfamethoxazole
TNF. See Tumor necrosis factor
Tobramycin, 61t, 70
Todd's paralysis, 282
Tofranil. See Imipramine
Tolbutamide, 212t
Tolcapone, for Parkinson disease, 279
Tolectin. See Tolmetin
Tolerance (drug), 267
Tolmetin, 197t
Tomography
    computed. See Computed tomography
    myocardial perfusion, 119
Tonic-clonic seizures, 282, 320
Topamax. See Topiramate
Topiramate, 283t, 284
    ophthalmic side effects of, 263, 284, 324t
Toprol-XL. See Metoprolol
Toradol. See Ketorolac
Tornalate. See Bitolterol
Torsades de pointes, 140
Torsemide, 88t
Total T_4, 222
Toxic dementia, 285
Toxic goiter
    diffuse, 224. See also Graves hyperthyroidism
    nodular, 225
Toxic optic neuropathy, 271
Toxoplasma (toxoplasmosis), 26–27
    in HIV infection/AIDS, 50
TPA. See Tissue plasminogen activator
TPHA (*T pallidum* hemagglutination assay), 17
Trabecular bone, 241
Tracheotomy, for anaphylaxis, 319
Trandate. See Labetalol
Trandolapril, 88t, 90t
Transbronchial biopsy, 155
Transcranial Doppler, in cerebral ischemia/stroke, 103
Transesophageal Doppler echocardiography
    in amaurosis fugax, 107
    in cerebral ischemia/stroke, 103
Transfusion-transmitted virus (TTV), 32
Transient ischemic attacks, 102
    carotid disease causing, 107
    diagnosis/management of, 103
Transient visual loss, carotid artery disease and, 107
Transthyretin (prealbumin), serum levels of, 223
Trauma, hypercoagulability associated with, 171
Travel immunizations, 309–310
Trazodone, 276
Tremor, in Parkinson disease, 279
Treponema pallidum, 15–18. See also Syphilis
Treponemal antibody tests, for syphilis, 17, 302
TRH. See Thyrotropin-releasing hormone
Trial contact lens fitting, disinfection and, 51
Triamcinolone, for pulmonary diseases, 157t
Triamterene, 88t, 90t
Triazolam, 273
Tricyclic antidepressants, 275t
Triglyceride levels
    lowering, 143, 146–147. See also Lipid-lowering therapy
    risk assessment and, 144, 144t
Trihexyphenidyl, for Parkinson disease, 279
Triiodothyronine (T_3), 221
    serum levels of, 222
Triiodothyronine (T_3) resin uptake test, 222
Trileptal. See Oxacarbazepine
Trilisate. See Choline magnesium trisalicylate
Trimethoprim, 54
Trimethoprim/sulfamethoxazole, 55t, 73–74
    for *Pneumocystis carinii* (*Pneumocystis jiroveci*) pneumonia, 45, 74
    for Wegener granulomatosis, 192
Trizivir, 41
Troglitazone, withdrawal of from market, 213–214
Troponins, cardiac-specific (troponins T and I), in myocardial infarction, 117, 118i
Trovafloxacin, 62t, 73
Trovan. See Trovafloxacin
Truvada, 41
TSH (thyroid-stimulating hormone). See Thyrotropin
TTP. See Thrombotic thrombocytopenic purpura
TTV. See Transfusion-transmitted virus
Tuberculin skin test, 23–25, 301–302
Tuberculosis, 23–25, 301–302
    in HIV infection/AIDS, 24, 49–50, 301, 302
    multidrug-resistant, 24, 49
    screening for, 23–24, 301–302
    treatment of, in HIV infection/AIDS, 49–50
Tumor necrosis factor, α, drugs affecting, 199
Tumor-suppressor genes, 252
Tumors. See Cancer
Twinrix, 305
2 × 2 table, 353–354, 353t, 354t
Typhoid immunization, 309–310

UKPDS (United Kingdom Prospective Diabetes Study), 215
Ulcerative colitis, 177
Ulcers, genital and oral, in Behçet syndrome, 193
Ultrafast computed tomography, in ischemic heart disease, 119
Ultralente insulin, 209–210, 209t
Ultrasonography/ultrasound (echography)
    in amaurosis fugax, 107
    in cerebral ischemia/stroke, 103
    in ischemic heart disease, 119
    thyroid, 223
Unasyn. See Ampicillin, with sulbactam
Unipen. See Nafcillin
Uniphyl. See Theophylline
Uniretic. See Moexipril
United Kingdom Prospective Diabetes Study (UKPDS), 215
Univasc. See Moexipril
Unstable angina, 114
Urokinase, 172
    for cerebral artery occlusion, 104

Urologic cancer, screening for, 296
Uveitis
　in Behçet syndrome, 193
　HLA association in, 175, 176, 178
　in reactive arthritis, 177
　in spondyloarthropathies, 175, 178
　in toxoplasmosis, 26

V-neck sign, in dermatomyositis, 186
Vaccine-associated paralytic poliomyelitis, 307
Vaccine development, 291, 310. *See also* Immunization
　for cancer, 262
　for HIV, 44–45
Vagal nerve stimulator, for seizures, 283
Valacyclovir, 65t, 77
　for herpes simplex virus infections, 28, 77
　for herpes zoster, 28, 77
Valdecoxib, removal of from market, 173, 196
Valganciclovir, 65t, 77
　for cytomegalovirus retinitis, 29, 48
Validity, 343, 363
Valium. *See* Diazepam
Valproate/valproic acid
　as mood stabilizer, 277
　for seizures, 283t
Valsartan, 88t, 90t
Valtrex. *See* Valacyclovir
Vanceril. *See* Beclomethasone
Vancocin. *See* Vancomycin
Vancomycin, 60t, 71–72
　for endocarditis prophylaxis, 11t
　resistance and, 3, 5
Vancomycin-intermediate *S aureus* (VISA), 5
Vancomycin-resistant enterococci (VRE), 3, 5, 71
Vancomycin-resistant *S aureus* (VRSA), 3, 5, 71
Vantin. *See* Cefpodoxime
Variance (statistical), 368
Variant (Prinzmetal) angina, 113
Varicella (chickenpox), 28
Varicella vaccine (Varivax), 28, 291, 304t, 306
Varicella-zoster virus, 28–29. *See also* Herpes zoster
　vaccine against, 28, 291, 304t, 306
Varivax. *See* Varicella vaccine
Vascular dementia, 285
Vascular endothelial growth factor (VEGF)
　antibodies against, in cancer therapy, 257
　in diabetic retinopathy, 217
Vascular malformations, intracranial hemorrhage caused by, 105, 106
Vascular resistance, reduction of in heart failure management, 130
Vascular stroke. *See* Stroke
Vascular system, disorders of, 166. *See also* Vasculitis
Vasculitis, 188–192, 189t. *See also specific type*
　in Behçet syndrome, 193
　essential cryoglobulinemic, 189t
　giant cell (temporal) arteritis, 188–190, 189t
　large vessel, 188–191, 189t
　medium-sized vessel, 189t, 191–192
　small vessel, 189t, 192–193
　Takayasu arteritis, 189t, 191
　Wegener granulomatosis, 189t, 192
Vaseretic. *See* Captopril; Enalapril
Vasodilators, for hypertension, 89t, 94

Vasopressors, for shock, 318
Vasotec. *See* Enalapril
VDRL (Venereal Disease Research Laboratory) test, 16–17, 17t, 302
VEGF. *See* Vascular endothelial growth factor
Velban. *See* Vinblastine
Velosef. *See* Cephradine
Venereal Disease Research Laboratory (VDRL) test, 16–17, 17t, 302
Venlafaxine, 276
Venous thrombosis, 170–172
Ventilatory failure, in shock, 317, 318
Ventilatory support
　noninvasive, 156
　for shock, 318
Ventolin. *See* Albuterol
Ventricular complexes, premature (PVCs), 135–136
Ventricular fibrillation, 140
Ventricular tachyarrhythmias, 138–140
　tachycardia, 138–139
　　heart failure and, 131–132
Ventriculography, 119–120
VePesid. *See* Etoposide
Verapamil
　for angina, 120
　for hypertension, 89t, 90t
　for non-ST-segment elevation acute coronary syndrome, 122
Verelan. *See* Verapamil
Versed. *See* Midazolam
VF. *See* Ventricular fibrillation
Vfend. *See* Voriconazole
Viagra. *See* Sildenafil
Vibramycin. *See* Doxycycline
Vidarabine, for herpes simplex virus infections, 28
Videx. *See* Didanosine
Vigabatrin, ophthalmic side effects of, 263, 284
Vinblastine, 257, 259t
Vinca alkaloids, in cancer chemotherapy, 257, 259t
Vincristine, 257, 259t
Vioxx. *See* Rofecoxib
Viracept. *See* Nelfinavir
Viral load, testing, in HIV infection/AIDS, 40
Viramune. *See* Nevirapine
Virazole. *See* Ribavirin
Viread. *See* Tenofovir
Virtual colonoscopy, in cancer screening, 291, 299
Virulence (microbial), mechanisms of, 3–4
Viruses
　cancer and, 254
　treatment of infection caused by. *See* Antiviral agents
VISA. *See* Vancomycin-intermediate *S aureus*
Visken. *See* Pindolol
Vistide. *See* Cidofovir
Visual loss/impairment
　in Alzheimer disease, 288
　in elderly, 235
　functional, 266
Vitamin B_{12} deficiency, 162
　in elderly, 247
Vitamin C (ascorbic acid) deficiency (scurvy), 166
Vitamin D, for osteoporosis, 244
Vitamin K deficiency, coagulation disorders and, 168–169

Vitrasert. *See* Ganciclovir
Vitravene. *See* Fomivirsen
VM-26. *See* Teniposide
Voltaren. *See* Diclofenac
Volume expansion
 for anaphylaxis, 319
 for shock, 318
Volume overload, 129
von Willebrand disease, 168
von Willebrand factor, 168
Voriconazole, 64*t*, 76
VP-16. *See* Etoposide
VRE. *See* Vancomycin-resistant enterococci
VRSA. *See* Vancomycin-resistant *S aureus*
VT. *See* Ventricular tachyarrhythmias
VZV. *See* Varicella-zoster virus

Warfarin/warfarin derivatives, 171
 for antiphospholipid antibody syndrome, 184
 for heart failure, 132
 ocular effects of, 325*t*
 in perioperative setting, 332
Water-jets, for coronary revascularization, 122
Wegener granulomatosis, 189*t*, 192
Weight reduction
 diabetes management/prevention and, 201, 207, 208–209
 hypertension management and, 87*t*
Wellbutrin. *See* Bupropion
Wenckebach type atrioventricular block, 134
Wernicke-Korsakoff syndrome, 285
West Nile virus, 35
Western blot analysis
 in HIV infection/AIDS, 39
 in Lyme disease, 20
Wheezing, 153
White blood cells, 159
White coat hypertension, 82
Wide-complex tachycardias, 138
Wilcoxon rank sum test, 344
Withdrawal (abstinence) syndromes, 267. *See also specific drug*
 hypertension and, 97–98
Wolff-Parkinson-White syndrome, 137
WPW syndrome. *See* Wolff-Parkinson-White syndrome

Xanax. *See* Alprazolam
Xanthelasma, in dyslipoproteinemia/hyperlipoproteinemia, 293
Xanthine derivatives, for pulmonary diseases, 157*t*
Xibrom. *See* Bromfenac

Yeasts, *Candida albicans*, 25
Yellow fever vaccination, 309

Z score, in osteoporosis, 243
Zafirlukast, 157*t*
Zagam. *See* Sparfloxacin
Zalcitabine, 41
Zaleplon, 273
Zanamivir, 65*t*, 77, 305
Zarontin. *See* Ethosuximide
Zaroxolyn. *See* Metolazone
Zebeta. *See* Bisoprolol
Zefazone. *See* Cefmetazole
Zerit. *See* Stavudine
Zestoretic. *See* Lisinopril
Zestril. *See* Lisinopril
Ziac. *See* Bisoprolol
Ziagen. *See* Abacavir
Zidovudine, 41
 for HIV prophylaxis
  postexposure, 45, 46–47*t*
  during pregnancy, 45
 with lamivudine, 41
Zileuton, 157*t*
Zinacef. *See* Cefuroxime
Ziracin. *See* Evernimicin
Zithromax. *See* Azithromycin
Zocor. *See* Simvastatin
Zofran. *See* Ondansetron
Zolpidem, 273
Zonegran. *See* Zonisamide
Zonisamide, 283*t*
Zoster. *See* Herpes zoster
Zosyn. *See* Piperacillin, with tazobactam
Zovirax. *See* Acyclovir
Zyflo. *See* Zileuton
Zyprexa. *See* Olanzapine
Zyvox. *See* Linezolid